Mechanisms, Diagnosis and Treatment of Respiratory Diseases

Mechanisms, Diagnosis and Treatment of Respiratory Diseases

Editor: Joseph Dixon

AMERICAN
MEDICAL PUBLISHERS
www.americanmedicalpublishers.com

AMERICAN
MEDICAL PUBLISHERS
www.americanmedicalpublishers.com

Cataloging-in-Publication Data

Mechanisms, diagnosis and treatment of respiratory diseases / edited by Joseph Dixon.
p. cm.
Includes bibliographical references and index.
ISBN 979-8-88740-574-2
1. Respiratory organs--Diseases. 2. Respiratory organs--Diseases--Diagnosis.
3. Respiratory organs--Diseases--Treatment. 4. Respiratory infections. I. Dixon, Joseph.
RC731 .R47 2023
616.2--dc23

American Medical Publishers,
41 Flatbush Avenue,
1st Floor, New York,
NY 11217, USA

ISBN 979-8-88740-574-2 (Hardback)

Contents

Preface

Respiratory diseases are a group of pathological conditions that affect the lungs and other parts of the respiratory system. Some of its common types are common cold, influenza, chronic obstructive pulmonary disorder, pneumonia, acute asthma, lung cancer, tuberculosis, and severe acute respiratory syndrome. Respiratory diseases can be caused by tobacco smoking, infection, breathing second hand smoke, asbestos, radon and air pollution. Patients are examined by performing diagnostic tests, including, chest X-ray, ultrasound, blood test, lung biopsy, bronchoscopy, pulmonary function test, and CT scan. Treatments for respiratory diseases include medications, such as oral drugs, combination of inhalers, and intravenous treatment. Advanced procedures like interventional bronchoscopy, lung transplant, and stem cell therapy can also be used to treat respiratory diseases. Interventional bronchoscopy is a minimally invasive procedure used for the treatment of lung tumors, while lung transplant is appropriate for patients with severe or progressive respiratory conditions. This book outlines the mechanisms, diagnosis and treatment of respiratory diseases in detail. It will prove immensely beneficial to professionals and students involved in the study and treatment of these medical conditions at various levels.

This book is the end result of constructive efforts and intensive research done by experts in this field. The aim of this book is to enlighten the readers with recent information in this area of research. The information provided in this profound book would serve as a valuable reference to students and researchers in this field.

At the end, I would like to thank all the authors for devoting their precious time and providing their valuable contribution to this book. I would also like to express my gratitude to my fellow colleagues who encouraged me throughout the process.

Editor

1

Emerging Cell-Based Therapies in Chronic Lung Diseases: What about Asthma?

Andressa Daronco Cereta[1], *Vinícius Rosa Oliveira*[2,3], *Ivan Peres Costa*[4], *João Pedro Ribeiro Afonso*[5], *Adriano Luís Fonseca*[5], *Alan Robson Trigueiro de Souza*[5], *Guilherme Augusto Moreira Silva*[5], *Diego A. C. P. G. Mello*[5], *Luis Vicente Franco de Oliveira*[5] and *Renata Kelly da Palma*[1,2,6*]

[1]Department of Surgery, School of Veterinary Medicine and Animal Sciences, University of São Paulo, São Paulo, Brazil, [2]Department of Physical Therapy, EUSES University School, University of Barcelona/University of Girona (UB-UdG), Barcelona, Spain, [3]Research Group on Methodology, Methods, Models, and Outcomes of Health and Social Sciences (M_3O), University of Vic - Central University of Catalonia, Vic, Spain, [4]Department of Master's and and Doctoral Programs in Rehabilitation Sciences, Nove de Julho University, São Paulo, Brazil, [5]Department of Experimental Cardiorrespiratory Physiology, Postgraduate Program in Human Movement and Rehabilitation, School of Medicine, University Center of Anápolis (UniEVANGELICA), Anápolis, Brazil, [6]Institute for Bioengineering of Catalonia, Barcelona, Spain

***Correspondence:**
Renata Kelly da Palma
rekellyp@hotmail.com

Asthma is a widespread disease characterized by chronic airway inflammation. It causes substantial disability, impaired quality of life, and avoidable deaths around the world. The main treatment for asthmatic patients is the administration of corticosteroids, which improves the quality of life; however, prolonged use of corticosteroids interferes with extracellular matrix elements. Therefore, cell-based therapies are emerging as a novel therapeutic contribution to tissue regeneration for lung diseases. This study aimed to summarize the advancements in cell therapy involving mesenchymal stromal cells, extracellular vesicles, and immune cells such as T-cells in asthma. Our findings provide evidence that the use of mesenchymal stem cells, their derivatives, and immune cells such as T-cells are an initial milestone to understand how emergent cell-based therapies are effective to face the challenges in the development, progression, and management of asthma, thus improving the quality of life.

Keywords: chronic lung diseases, asthma treatments, cell-based therapies, mesenchymal stromal cells, extracellular vesicles, immune cells

INTRODUCTION

Chronic inflammation can affect the respiratory system in many ways, causing damage to the lungs and airways. Asthma is the most common condition that affects the airways, contributing to high absenteeism at work and school. It is the major respiratory disease affecting children (Guibas et al., 2015). Without a known cause, asthma has a multifactorial background and many risk factors associated with its development. Most of the risk factors are related to early life events, such as genetics, several pathogens, and environmental exposures like tobacco smoke and air pollution (Toskala and Kennedy, 2015; World Health Organisation, 2018; Tiotiu et al., 2020). Asthma is an inflammatory and heterogeneous chronic disease. It causes hyperresponsiveness of the airways and exacerbated mucous secretion. It is characterized by recurrent events of cough, wheezing, shortness of breath, and chest tightness, which persistently lead to airflow limitation. (Toskala and Kennedy, 2015; Papi et al., 2018; Mattiuzi and Lippi, 2020). Asthma prevalence has been increasing over the

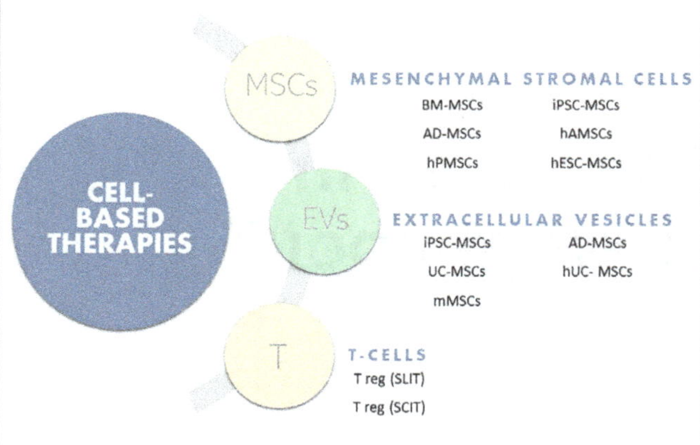

FIGURE 1 | Summary of cell-based therapies for Asthma.

past 50 years affecting around 340 million people worldwide, both adults and children (Mattiuzi and Lippi, 2020). In low and lower-middle-income countries, it accounts for most asthma-related deaths (World Health Organisation, 2018). The mortality rates of this disease have declined recently. However, there are still some associated comorbidities, such as systemic arterial hypertension and pulmonary hypertension, both of which are related to the number of asthma deaths (Kaplan et al., 2020; Miethe et al., 2020; Branco et al., 2020).

There are many recognized phenotypes designating asthma. However, they can be summarized into i) allergic, in early onset, mild, or moderate-to-severe remodeled asthma or ii) non-allergic with late-onset eosinophilic asthma or non-eosinophilic asthma (Kaur, Chupp, 2019). Moreover, asthma can be categorized by endotypes related to the biomarkers involved in the disease mechanisms (Chung, 2018). The traditional asthma treatment is corticosteroid drugs, which have been used since the middle of the last century (Baldwin et al., 1961). For many patients, inhaled corticosteroids, in combination or not with long-acting β2 agonists, are an effective treatment, suppressing airway inflammation and constriction, although it is not curative. However, 5–10% of asthmatic patients do not respond to steroid-based therapies (Wang et al., 2010). This leads to severe steroid-resistant asthma (SSR), which is associated with non-eosinophilic endotypes of the disease, including neutrophilic asthma (Kim et al., 2017) As demonstrated in **Figure 1**, some alternatives to the classical treatment of choice for asthma have arisen and most research has focused on cell-based therapies. The most common is the use of mesenchymal stem cells. However, studies on extracellular vesicles and immune modulation by using T-cells are recently increasing. Although these options are mainly in the pre-clinical step, they may be a promising approach, especially in cases of refractory asthma, in which the use of corticosteroids is no longer a viable option.

Cell-Based Therapies in Asthma

Initial studies of cell-based approaches to repair a damaged lung started two decades ago, using hematopoietic stem cells. Since then, other types of cells have been explored, such as mesenchymal stem cells, endothelial progenitor cells, or even embryonic stem cells (Kim et al., 2017). In this review, we summarized the advancements in cell therapy involving mesenchymal stem cells, extracellular vesicles, and immune cells (T-cells) in pre-clinical and clinical trial studies (**Table 1**).

Mesenchymal Stromal Cells

Because of reparative and immunological properties, such as the potential to attenuate allergic immune diseases safely, mesenchymal stem cells (MSCs) are being considered as a good approach to treat asthma (Weiss, 2018). MSCs are multipotent, nonhematopoietic, and found in both adult and neonatal tissues. They have different sources, such as bone marrow, adipose tissue, placenta, umbilical cord, and organs such as the lungs (Sueblinvong et al., 2008). However, each source of MSCs can present different anti-inflammatory or regenerative effects (Abreu et al., 2017). This results in various potential mechanisms of the action of MSCs from different sources in asthma. Even with a limited number, the bone marrow-derived mesenchymal stem cells (BM-MSCs) have been commonly used and are well characterized in experimental asthma models (Lathrop et al., 2014; Cruz et al., 2015). Habibian and colleagues (2018) demonstrated that injection of BM-MSCs into the vein reduced eosinophilia and inhibited expressions of Th2 and Th17 cytokines. In addition, it elevated levels of regulatory T cells (Tregs) cytokines in an experimental model of allergic asthma induced by ovalbumin (OVA). On the other hand, the intratracheal (IT) route delivers cells directly to affected airways. The BM-MSCs IT injection in OVA-induced asthma decreased eosinophilia, lymphocyte, total protein, IL-13, and IL-17A levels and significantly decreased airway remodeling, which persisted for 14 days after the injection (Boldrini-Leite et al., 2020).

OVA-induced asthma is widely used as an asthma model. However, it is not clinically relevant to humans compared with allergen and grass pollen. Therefore, allergens such as house dust mite (HDM) have been considered more clinically relevant, exhibiting inflammatory and ultrastructural changes in lung parenchyma and the airways, similar to human disease (Kitoko et al., 2018). However, the IT injection of BM-MSCs cannot reduce lung parenchyma inflammation, airway hyperresponsiveness, or mucus hypersecretion in HDM-induced asthma (Kitoko et al., 2018). Considering this limitation, a recent study demonstrated that a pre-treatment with eicosapentaenoic acid (EPA) could potentiate the BM-MSC-based therapy in HDM-induced asthma. This leads to the modulation of macrophages toward an anti-inflammatory phenotype, increased secretion of pro-resolution and anti-inflammatory mediators, consequently reducing the remodeling process (Abreu et al., 2018). The cockroach extract (CE) is another allergen that can lead to asthma and increase asthma morbidity in children (Pomés et al., 2019). In a murine cockroach allergen (CRE)-induced asthma model, the injection of BM-MSC modulate macrophage differentiation from a pro-inflammatory phenotype (M1) to an anti-inflammatory phenotype (M2), apparently by aryl hydrocarbon receptor (AhR) signaling activation. The AhR is a ligand-activated receptor that mediates the toxicity of environmental pollutants and can induce molecular cascade mediated by BM-MSC immunosuppression. Future studies should be addressed to understand the link between MSC and

TABLE 1 | Cell-based therapies in Asthma.

Author	Study type	Route	Therapy	Results
Kitoko et al. (2018)	PC- HDM	IT	BM-MSCs	Did not reduce lung parenchyma inflammation, airway hyperresponsiveness or mucus hypersecretion in asthma model
Habibian, et al. (2018)	PC- OVA	IV	BM-MSCs	Reduced eosinophilia, inhibited expressions of Th2 and Th17 cytokines and elevated levels of regulatory T cells (tregs) cytokines
Abreu et al. (2018)	PC- HDM	IT	BM-MSCs	Modulated macrophages toward an anti-inflammatory phenotype, increased secretion of pro-resolution and anti-inflammatory mediator, consequently reducing the remodeling process in asthma model
Boldrini-Leite et al. (2020)	PC-OVA	IT	BM-MSCs	Decreased eosinophilia, lymphocyte, total protein, IL-13, IL-17 A levels and decreased airway remodeling, which persisted 14 days after injection in asthma model
Cui et al. (2020)	PC- CE	IT	BM-MSCs and macrophages	Polarized macrophages to an anti-inflammatory phenotype (M2), apparently by aryl hydrocarbon receptor (AhR) signaling activation in asthma model
Dai et al. (2017)	PC-OVA	IV	AD-MSCs	Decreased airway responsiveness, infiltrations of inflammatory cells with are associated impaired regulation of Foxp3, IL17, IL10 and RORγ expression and restored the percentage of $CD4^{+}CD25$ + Foxp3+ tregs in the spleen in asthma model
Dai et al. (2018)	PC-OVA	IT	AD-MSCs	The restoration of Th1/Th2 cell balance in asthma model
Halim et al. (2019)	PC-OVA	Aerosol	AD-MSC-pANGPT1	Reduced the expression of pro-inflammatory cytokine genes (IL- 4, TNF, TGF-β, and MMP-9) in asthma model
Hur et al. (2020)	PC-OVA	IV	AD-MSCs or BM-MSCs	Increased Th2 levels and inflammation cell infiltration in asthma model
Li et al. (2017)	PC-OVA	IV	hPMSC	Showed a Th17/Treg rebalance mediated by increased IL-10 levels in asthma model
Li et al. (2018)	PC-OVA	IV	hPMSC	Decreased of notch pathway in asthma model
Dalouchi et al. (2021)	PC-OVA	IV	hAMSC	Decreased in oxidative stress, serum levels of immunoglobulin E (IgE), interleukin 4 (IL-4), transforming growth factor (TGF-β) and increased interferon gamma (IFN-γ) and IL-10 in asthma model
Yao et al. (2018)	PC-OVA	IT	iPSC-MSCs	Connexin 43 regulate TNTs formation by mediating the mitochondria transfer from iPSC-MSCs to epithelial cells. The mitochondria prevented epithelial cells apoptosis reducing the allergic airway inflammation in an asthma model
Zhong et al. (2019)	PC-OVA	IV	iPSC-MSCs	Reduced collagen deposition and airway thickening via regulating the expression of signaling molecules of the TGF-β1/Smad pathway in asthma model
Lin et al. (2018)	PC-OVA	IV	hESC-MSCs	Decreased Th2 and treg cells by 47 protein-coding mRNAs in asthma model
Du et al. (2018)	PC-PBMCs	*In vitro*	Exosomes secreted by BM-MSCs	Tregs modulation in IL-10 and TGF-β1 increase, probably due to antigen presenting cells (APCs) modulation and not $CD4^{+}$ T cells in asthma *in vitro* model
Lin et al. (2019)	PC-PBMCs	*In vitro*	hPMSCs	Reduced the $CD4^{+}$ and CD8+T activation and proliferation and significantly decreased IL-5 levels in asthma *in vitro* model
Aguiar et al. (2020)	CT	IV	BMMCs	No serious adverse events. Lung function remained stable throughout. A slight increase in ventilation of the right lung
Zhuansun et al. (2019)	PC-PBMCs	*In Vitro*	Exosomes secreted by BM-MSCs	miR-1470 which promote the differentiation of $CD4^{+}CD25$ + FOXP3+ tregs in PBMCs of asthmatic patients by inducing the expression of P27KIP1
Cruz et al. (2015)	PC- AHE	IV	EVs by hBM-MSC and mMSCs	EVs from hMSCs demonstrated be more potent than those from mMSCs in asthma model
de Castro et al. (2017)	PC-OVA	IV	EVs by AD-MSC	EVs acting different from MSCs regarding to lung mechanic, pro-inflammatory mediators, and regulatory T cells in asthma model
Fang et al. (2020b)	PC- OVA	IV	sEV by iPSC-MSCs	Reduced M2 macrophages in an asthma model and suggested that EVs presents 312 proteins that can be involved in the therapeutic effects
Dong et al. (2021)	PC-OVA	IV	EVs by hUC- MSC	Increased of miR-146a-5p acting on inflammation and airway remodeling by decrease pro-inflammatory mediators (IL-13and IL-4) and the expression of pro fibrogenic markers (α-SMA, collagen-1, and TGF-β1-*p*-smad2/3 signaling pathway in asthma model
Hoshino et al. (2019)	CT	SLIT	HDM tablet	Reduced FeNO (fractional exhaled nitric oxide), eosinophilic airway inflammation and improved the airflow limitation in asthmatic patients
Xian et al. (2020)	CT	SLIT and SCIT	Der-p and der-f	SLIT and SCIT upregulated $CD4^{+}CD25$ + FoxP3+ tregs, however only SLIT showed clinical improvement related to tregs in asthmatic patients
Skuljec et al. (2017)	PC- OVA	IV	CAR tregs	CAR tregs reduced airway hyper-reactivity, eosinophilic airway inflammation and cell infiltrates in the lung. Moreover, prevented excessive mucus production and increased allergen-specific IgE and Th2 cytokine levels

BM-MSC, bone marrow-derived mesenchymal stromal cells; AD-MSCs, adipose-derived mesenchymal stem cells; hAMSC, human amniotic membrane; IT, intratracheal; IV, intravenous; hPMSCs, placental-derived mesenchymal stromal cells; iPSC-MSCs human induced pluripotent stem cell; hESC-MSCs, human embryonic stem cells; PBMCs, peripheral blood mononuclear cells; EVs, Extracellular vesicles; sEV, small extracellular vesicles; UC-MSC, umbilical cord mesenchymal stromal cells; PC, Pre-clinical; CT, Clinical trial; HDM, house dust mite; OVA, ovalbumine; CE, cockroach extract; AHE, Aspergillus fumigatus hyphal extract; SLIT, sublingual immunotherapy; SCIT subcutaneous immunotherapy; Der-p, Dermatophagoides pteronyssinus; Der-f, Dermatophagoides farina.

AhR during immunomodulation activity in asthma (Cui et al., 2020).

Due to the high immunomodulatory capacity in BM-MSC, adipose-derived mesenchymal stem cells (ADMSCs) could have therapeutic potential in asthma. ADMSCs injected into the vein of a mouse with OVA-induced asthma decreased airway responsiveness, infiltrations of inflammatory cells that are associated with impaired regulation of Foxp3, interleukin (IL)

17, IL10, and RORγ expression and restored the percentage of $CD4^{+}CD25 + Foxp3+$ Tregs in the spleen (Dai et al., 2017). The restoration of Th1/Th2 cell balance mediated by ADMSCs may be the mechanism associated with airway responsiveness and inflammation decrease in OVA-induced asthma (Dai et al., 2018). However, ADMSCs can be enhanced by gene transfection. The MSC-pANGPT1 (angiopoietin 1 gene) were aerosolized in a rabbit OVA-induced asthma and reduced the expression of pro-inflammatory cytokine genes (IL-4, TNF, TGF-β, and MMP-9), which can be an additional beneficial effect in asthma treatment (Halim et al., 2019). Apart from cell source, the cell dose, cell injection frequency, and injection site are crucial in MSC therapy. Hur and colleagues (2020) showed that double injection of ADMSCs and BM-MSCs in OVA-induced asthma increased Th2 levels and inflammatory cell infiltration. Therefore, both ADMSCs and BM-MSCs can be used for asthma treatment. However, the frequency of injection should be used carefully.

MSCs derived from adult tissues can present limited therapeutic benefits due to their cell variability quality from different donors and their limitation in proliferative capacities (Crisostomo et al., 2006). Hence, human placenta MSCs (hPMSCs) could be an alternative source of stem cells for therapeutic use. The hPMSCs have few ethical issues, are easily obtained, and demonstrate prominent inhibitory effects on T cells compared with BM-MSCs (Li et al., 2014). The hPMSC, from the placental tissue of a healthy pregnant mother, was injected into a rat OVA-induced asthma for the first time in 2017. It showed a Th17/Treg rebalance mediated by increased IL-10 levels (Li et al., 2017). A further study suggested that the Notch pathway, associated with the induction of Th2 in asthma, decreased its expression after treatment with hPMSC (Li et al., 2018). Moreover, a recent study demonstrated that the human amniotic membrane (hAM) could be an ideal mesenchymal source. This is because it can decrease oxidative stress, serum levels of immunoglobulin E (IgE), IL4, transforming growth factor (TGF-β), and increase interferon-gamma (IFN-γ) and IL-10 in the OVA-induced asthma model (Dalouchi et al., 2021).

It is well known that human-induced pluripotent stem cells (iPSC-MSCs) have emerged as another valuable mesenchymal source compared with MSCs derived from adult tissue due to their higher proliferative and differentiation capacity, longer life span, and more substantial immune privilege (Gao et al., 2017). A study using an OVA-induced asthma model showed that connexin 43 regulates TNTs formation by mediating the mitochondria transfer from iPSC-MSCs to epithelial cells. The mitochondria prevent epithelial cell apoptosis, reducing the allergic airway inflammation in an asthma model (Yao et al., 2018). Furthermore, iPSC-MSC administered in a chronic asthma model can reduce collagen deposition and airway thickening via regulating the expression of signaling molecules of the TGF-β1/Smad pathway (Zhong et al., 2019). This shows a potential therapeutic effect in the treatment of acute or chronic asthma. However, iPSCs present genetic instability and tumorigenicity after reprogramming *in vivo* (Tan et al., 2014). Nonetheless, this requires further studies before their use in clinical applications. On the other hand, MSCs derived from human embryonic stem cells (hESC-MSCs) present the same advantages as iPSC-MSC with less risk of genetic instability. This may decrease Th2 and Treg cells by 47 protein-coding mRNAs, which are potential targets for asthma treatment in a future clinical study (Lin et al., 2018).

According to previous demonstrations, the use of MSCs to treat asthma has been successful in different animal models. However, there are still some issues that must be addressed before translating this therapy to humans. To the best of our knowledge, there is only one study (Aguiar et al., 2020) that demonstrated the potential efficacy of MSCs in patients with asthma and one ongoing clinical trial (NCT03137199). However, these studies (Aguiar et al., 2020) have limitations, such as a small sample size with no placebo-control and inflammatory biomarkers. Procedures for cell culture need to be appropriately standardized to produce a satisfactory number of cells and should be proliferative and maintain their regeneration properties. Also, the source of the MSCs and their effects must be accurately known as they may vary according to different types of MSCs (Yu et al., 2020). Therefore, the major challenge is to define efficient protocols to harvest, culture, and deliver the MSCs to obtain a proper therapy. Likewise, effort must be applied in future studies to finally address MSCs in human asthma treatment.

Extracellular Vesicles

Extracellular vesicles (EVs) are secreted by many types of cells, including MSCs. They circulate in the extracellular space and include exosomes, microvesicles, and apoptotic bodies. These vesicles are implicated in cell-cell communication and are considered essential for homeostasis. EVs usually contain intracellular proteins, lipids, and nucleic acids, as well as miRNAs, cytokines or chemokines, tissue factors, or caspases (Bartel et al., 2020; Nagano et al., 2019; Andres et al., 2020; Cañas et al., 2019; van den Berge and Tasena, 2019). Therefore, the biological factors secreted by MSCs can be the key mechanism in asthma treatment. Furthermore, MSC-EVs are better defined, less complicated, and easier to store compared with MSCs (Konala et al., 2016). The first experiments with EVs in asthma models demonstrated that EVs acted differently from MSCs regarding lung mechanics, pro-inflammatory mediators, and regulatory T-cells (de Castro et al., 2017). Moreover, EVs from hMSCs were more potent than those from mMSCs (Cruz et al., 2015). Therefore, their use must be encouraged with further investigation.

Recent data have shown that intravenous treatment in an experimental model of asthma with EVs derived from iPSC-MSCs can prevent the increase of group 2 innate lymphoid cells (ILC2s), which is responsible for the initiation and maintenance of type 2 allergic airway inflammation, probably through miR-146a-5p. In addition, a protocol of anion-exchange chromatography for isolation of MSC-EVs was standardized in this study. This study demonstrated some advantages when compared with the ultracentrifugation protocol due to the scalable approach and feasibility of application in industrial production (Fang et al., 2020a). Based on this protocol for isolation of MSC-EVs, the same group showed for the first time that this approach reduced M2 macrophages in an asthma model and suggested that EVs present 312 proteins that can be involved in therapeutic effects (Fang et al., 2020b). Conversely, considering that miR-146a-5p is abundant in human umbilical cord MSCs (hUCMSC-EVs) (Song et al., 2017), these EVs could be a potential choice for asthma treatment. Dong and colleagues (2021) demonstrated for the first time that a hypoxia environment for EVs extraction from hUCMSCs can increase the miR-146a-5p level even more in mice with OVA-induced asthma. The increase of miR-146a-5p acts on inflammation and airway remodeling by decreasing pro-inflammatory mediators (IL-13and IL-4) and the expression of profibrogenic markers (α-SMA, collagen-1, and TGF-β1-p-smad2/3 signaling pathway) in OVA mice. Therefore, oxygen depletion can play an important role during the EV secretion. It should, therefore, be considered during asthma treatment with EVs.

On the other hand, Exosomes derived from MSCs presents similar immunomodulatory effect as MSCs. The peripheral blood mononuclear cells (PBMCs) of patients with asthma have mainly been used associated with exosomes in *in vitro* studies. One study where exosomes secreted by BM-MSCs were isolated and cultured with PBMCs from patients with asthma demonstrated Tregs modulation in IL-10 and TGF-β1 increase. This was probably due to antigen-presenting cell (APC) modulation and not $CD4^+$ T cells. Thus, BM-MSC exosomes may prevent the disadvantages of BM-MSCs and be a potential therapeutic agent for asthma (Du et al., 2018). Moreover, BM-MSC exosomes presents high level miR-1470 which promote the differentiation of $CD4^+$CD25 + FOXP3+ Tregs in PBMCs of asthmatic patients by inducing the expression of P27KIP1(Zhuansun et al., 2019) In another recent study, hPMSCs were cultured with PBMCs from children with asthma, reducing $CD4^+$ and CD8+T activation and proliferation and significantly decreasing IL-5 levels (Lin et al., 2019). Therefore, considering the inadequate response to conventional treatment, administration of hPMSCs could be a good option.

After all, it seems that EVs secreted by MSCs are a promising cell therapy for asthma. However, these results should be interpreted with caution because of the limited number of studies. Thus, more evidence is needed.

Immune Cell Treatment: T-Cells

In response to an asthma attack, there is an elevation in the number of inflammatory cells, activated eosinophils, and T cells. The T cells are responsible for the recognition and reaction against specific antigens, which stimulate the differentiation of naive $CD4^+$ T cells into Th2 cells and Tregs. These Tregs suppress an excessive immunological response of Th2. However, when the Tregs are dysfunctional and cannot control Th2, asthma can develop (Kawayama et al., 2018). In this sense, treatment based on Tregs by increasing their number and enhancing their suppression function could be a good alternative for asthmatic patients.

Antigen-specific immunotherapy (ASIT) is the most used method for Tregs induction, and it can be administrated by sublingual immunotherapy (SLIT) (Hoshino et al., 2019) and subcutaneous immunotherapy (SCIT) (Lozano et al., 2014). There are promising clinical trials regarding the use of SCIT in asthmatic patients and HDM (house dust mite), where SLIT tablets are often used. Hoshino et al., 2019 showed that HDM SLIT tablet reduced fractional exhaled nitric oxide (FeNO), eosinophilic airway inflammation, and improved the airflow limitation in patients with asthma. On the other hand, the administration SLIT and SCIT for Dermatophagoides pteronyssinus (Der-p) and Dermatophagoides farinae (Der-f), the most common allergens in patients with asthma in China, demonstrated similar efficacy in an asthmatic patient, mediated from different mechanisms. SLIT and SCIT upregulated $CD4^+$CD25 + FoxP3+ Tregs. However, only SLIT showed clinical improvement related to Tregs (Xian et al., 2020). Despite these results, SCIT is just recommended as an adjunct to pharmacotherapy in individuals with asthma, and SLIT is not recommended (Cloutier et al., 2020).

On the other hand, Tregs can be engineered *ex vivo* with a chimeric antigen receptor (CAR) (Hombach et al., 2009) and provide more specificity regarding to diversity of asthma antigens. Skuljec and colleagues (2017) showed that injection of CAR Tregs in a mouse OVA-induced asthma was effective in reduced Th2, mucus hypersecretion, airway hyper-reactivity and allergen-specific IgE.Further studies should be addressed to identify asthma triggers and improve treatments based on Treg.

CONCLUSION

Animal models and clinical trials suggest that cell-based therapies are a potential strategy for asthma treatment, although these therapies are still on preliminary studies or the pre-clinical testing phase. The use of mesenchymal stem cells to treat asthma is still a major discussion because it lacks translation to humans. To date, most of the evidence relies on animal studies and only a few on human subjects, including an ongoing clinical trial.

Another possibility is the use of extracellular vesicles or T-cell. However, current studies still lack profound knowledge on the effects of EVs. In conclusion, the effects of these cells and derivatives can be addressed to reduce responsiveness and inflammation according to preliminary studies. This can contribute to improving lung function, immunity response, and tissue regeneration/repair at the bronchial level. Although research on these topics is still at the initial stage, more evidence and research efforts are warranted.

The use of mesenchymal stem cells, their derivatives, and immune cells such as T-cells are just the initial milestones to understand how emergent cell-based therapies are effective to face the challenges of the development, progression, and management of asthma, thus improving the quality of life.

AUTHOR CONTRIBUTIONS

JA, AF, Ad, GS, DM, and LO conceived the design and concepts. RD, AC, VO and IC wrote the manuscript. All authors contributed to the editing and revision of the manuscript and approved the submission.

REFERENCES

Abreu, S. C., Antunes, M. A., Xisto, D. G., Cruz, F. F., Branco, V. C., Bandeira, E., et al. (2017). Bone Marrow, Adipose, and Lung Tissue-Derived Murine Mesenchymal Stromal Cells Release Different Mediators and Differentially Affect Airway and Lung Parenchyma in Experimental Asthma. *Stem Cell Transl. Med.* 6 (6), 1557–1567. doi:10.1002/sctm.16-0398

Abreu, S. C., Lopes-Pacheco, M., da Silva, A. L., Xisto, D. G., de Oliveira, T. B., Kitoko, J. Z., et al. (2018). Eicosapentaenoic Acid Enhances the Effects of Mesenchymal Stromal Cell Therapy in Experimental Allergic Asthma. *Front. Immunol.* 9, 1147. doi:10.3389/fimmu.2018.01147

Aguiar, F. S., Melo, A. S., Araújo, A. M. S., Cardoso, A. P., de Souza, S. A. L., Lopes-Pacheco, M., et al. (2020). Autologous Bone Marrow-Derived Mononuclear Cell Therapy in Three Patients with Severe Asthma. *Stem Cel. Res. Ther.* 11 (1), 167. doi:10.1186/s13287-020-01675-x

Andres, J., Smith, L. C., Murray, A., Jin, Y., Businaro, R., Laskin, J. D., et al. (2020). Role of Extracellular Vesicles in Cell-Cell Communication and Inflammation Following Exposure to Pulmonary Toxicants. *Cytokine Growth Factor. Rev.* 51, 12–18. doi:10.1016/j.cytogfr.2019.12.001

Baldwin, H. S., Dworetzky, M., and Isaacs, N. J. (1961). Evaluation of the Steroid Treatment of Asthma since 1950. *J. Allergy* 32, 109–118. doi:10.1016/0021-8707(61)90063-6

Bartel, S., Deshane, J., Wilkinson, T., and Gabrielsson, S. (2020). Extracellular Vesicles as Mediators of Cellular Cross Talk in the Lung Microenvironment. *Front. Med.* 7, 326. doi:10.3389/fmed.2020.00326

Boldrini-Leite, L. M., Michelotto, P. V., Jr, de Moura, S. A. B., Capriglione, L. G. A., Barussi, F. C. M., Fragoso, F. Y. I., et al. (2020). Lung Tissue Damage Associated with Allergic Asthma in BALB/c Mice Could Be Controlled with a Single Injection of Mesenchymal Stem Cells from Human Bone Marrow up to 14 d After Transplantation. *Cel. Transpl.* 29, 096368972091325. doi:10.1177/0963689720913254

Branco, A. C. C. C., Sato, M. N., and Alberca, R. W. (2020). The Possible Dual Role of the ACE2 Receptor in Asthma and Coronavirus (SARS-CoV2) Infection. *Front. Cel. Infect. Microbiol.* 10, 550571. doi:10.3389/fcimb.2020.550571

Cañas, J. A., Sastre, B., Rodrigo-Muñoz, J. M., and Del Pozo, V. (2019). Exosomes: A New Approach to Asthma Pathology. *Clinica Chim. Acta.* 495, 139–147. doi:10.1016/j.cca.2019.04.055

Chung, K. F. (2018). Precision Medicine in Asthma. *Curr. Opin. Pulm. Med.* 24 (1), 4–10. doi:10.1097/MCP.0000000000000434

Cloutier, M. M., Dixon, A. E., Krishnan, J. A., Lemanske, R. F., Jr, Pace, W., and Schatz, M. (2020). Managing Asthma in Adolescents and Adults. *JAMA* 324 (22), 2301–2317. doi:10.1001/jama.2020.21974

Crisostomo, P. R., Wang, M., Wairiuko, G. M., Morrell, E. D., Terrell, A. M., Seshadri, P., et al. (2006). High Passage Number of Stem Cells Adversely Affects Stem Cell Activation and Myocardial Protection. *Shock* 26 (6), 575–580. doi:10.1097/01.shk.0000235087.45798.93

Cruz, F. F., Borg, Z. D., Goodwin, M., Sokocevic, D., Wagner, D. E., Coffey, A., et al. (2015). Systemic Administration of Human Bone Marrow-Derived Mesenchymal Stromal Cell Extracellular Vesicles AmelioratesAspergillusHyphal Extract-Induced Allergic Airway Inflammation in Immunocompetent Mice. *Stem Cell Transl. Med.* 4 (11), 1302–1316. doi:10.5966/sctm.2014-0280

Cui, Z., Feng, Y., Li, D., Li, T., Gao, P., and Xu, T. (2020). Activation of Aryl Hydrocarbon Receptor (AhR) in Mesenchymal Stem Cells Modulates Macrophage Polarization in Asthma. *J. immunotoxicol.* 17 (1), 21–30. doi:10.1080/1547691X.2019.1706671

Dai, R., Liu, J., Cai, S., Zheng, C., and Zhou, X. (2017). Delivery of Adipose-Derived Mesenchymal Stem Cells Attenuates Airway Responsiveness and Inflammation in a Mouse Model of Ovalbumin-Induced Asthma. *Am. J. Transl. Res.* 9 (5), 2421–2428.

Dai, R., Yu, Y., Yan, G., Hou, X., Ni, Y., and Shi, G. (2018). Intratracheal Administration of Adipose Derived Mesenchymal Stem Cells Alleviates Chronic Asthma in a Mouse Model. *BMC Pulm. Med.* 18 (1), 131. doi:10.1186/s12890-018-0701-x

Dalouchi, F., Falak, R., Bakhshesh, M., Sharifiaghdam, Z., Azizi, Y., and Aboutaleb, N. (2021). Human Amniotic Membrane Mesenchymal Stem Cell-conditioned Medium Reduces Inflammatory Factors and Fibrosis in Ovalbumin-induced Asthma in Mice. *Exp. Physiol.* 106 (2), 544–554. doi:10.1113/EP088911

de Castro, L. L., Xisto, D. G., Kitoko, J. Z., Cruz, F. F., Olsen, P. C., Redondo, P. A. G., et al. (2017). Human Adipose Tissue Mesenchymal Stromal Cells and Their Extracellular Vesicles Act Differentially on Lung Mechanics and Inflammation in Experimental Allergic Asthma. *Stem Cel. Res. Ther.* 8 (1), 151. doi:10.1186/s13287-017-0600-8

Dong, L., Wang, Y., Zheng, T., Pu, Y., Ma, Y., Qi, X., et al. (2021). Hypoxic hUCMSC-Derived Extracellular Vesicles Attenuate Allergic Airway Inflammation and Airway Remodeling in Chronic Asthma Mice. *Stem Cel. Res. Ther.* 12 (1), 4. doi:10.1186/s13287-020-02072-0

Du, Y.-M., Zhuansun, Y.-X., Chen, R., Lin, L., Lin, Y., and Li, J.-G. (2018). Mesenchymal Stem Cell Exosomes Promote Immunosuppression of Regulatory T Cells in Asthma. *Exp. Cel. Res.* 363 (1), 114–120. doi:10.1016/j.yexcr.2017.12.021

Fang, S.-B., Zhang, H.-Y., Meng, X.-C., Wang, C., He, B.-X., Peng, Y.-Q., et al. (2020b). Small Extracellular Vesicles Derived from Human MSCs Prevent Allergic Airway Inflammation via Immunomodulation on Pulmonary Macrophages. *Cell Death Dis.* 11 (6), 409. doi:10.1038/s41419-020-2606-x

Fang, S. B., Zhang, H. Y., Wang, C., He, B. X., Liu, X. Q., Meng, X. C., et al. (2020a). Small Extracellular Vesicles Derived from Human Mesenchymal Stromal Cells Prevent Group 2 Innate Lymphoid Cell-dominant Allergic Airway Inflammation through Delivery of miR-146a-5p. *J. Extracell. Vesicles* 9 (1), 1723260. doi:10.1080/20013078.2020.1723260

Gao, W.-X., Sun, Y.-Q., Shi, J., Li, C.-L., Fang, S.-B., Wang, D., et al. (2017). Effects of Mesenchymal Stem Cells from Human Induced Pluripotent Stem Cells on Differentiation, Maturation, and Function of Dendritic Cells. *Stem Cel. Res Ther.* 8 (1), 48. doi:10.1186/s13287-017-0499-0

Guibas, G. V., Megremis, S., West, P., and Papadopoulos, N. G. (2015). Contributing Factors to the Development of Childhood Asthma: Working toward Risk Minimization. *Expert Rev. Clin. Immunol.* 11 (6), 721–735. doi:10.1586/1744666X.2015.1035649

Habibian, R., Delirezh, N., and Farshid, A. A. (2018). The Effects of Bone Marrow-Derived Mesenchymal Stem Cells on Ovalbumin-Induced Allergic Asthma and Cytokine Responses in Mice. *Iran J. Basic Med. Sci.* 21 (5), 483–488. doi:10.22038/IJBMS.2018.26898.6575

Halim, N. S. S., Ch'ng, E. S., Kardia, E., Ali, S. A., Radzi, R., and Yahaya, B. H. (2019). Aerosolised Mesenchymal Stem Cells Expressing Angiopoietin-1 Enhances Airway Repair. *Stem Cel. Rev. Rep.* 15 (1), 112–125. doi:10.1007/s12015-018-9844-7

Hombach, A. A., Kofler, D., Rappl, G., and Abken, H. (2009). Redirecting Human CD4+CD25+ Regulatory T Cells from the Peripheral Blood with Pre-defined Target Specificity. *Gene. Ther.* 16 (9), 1088–1096. doi:10.1038/gt.2009.75

Hoshino, M., Akitsu, K., and Kubota, K. (2019). Effect of Sublingual Immunotherapy on Airway Inflammation and Airway Wall Thickness in Allergic Asthma. *J. Allergy Clin. Immunol. Pract.* 7 (8), 2804–2811. doi:10.1016/j.jaip.2019.06.003

Hur, J., Kang, J. Y., Kim, Y. K., Lee, S. Y., Jeon, S., Kim, Y., et al. (2020). Evaluation of Human MSCs Treatment Frequency on Airway Inflammation in a Mouse Model of Acute Asthma. *J. Korean Med. Sci.* 35 (23), e188. doi:10.3346/jkms.2020.35.e188

Kaplan, A., Szefler, S. J., and Halpin, D. M. G. (2020). Impact of Comorbid Conditions on Asthmatic Adults and Children. *NPJ Prim. Care Respir. Med.* 30 (1), 36. doi:10.1038/s41533-020-00194-9

Kaur, R., and Chupp, G. (2019). Phenotypes and Endotypes of Adult Asthma: Moving toward Precision Medicine. *J. Allergy Clin. Immunol.* 144 (1), 1–12. doi:10.1016/j.jaci.2019.05.031

Kawayama, T., Kinoshita, T., Matsunaga, K., Naito, Y., Sasaki, J., Tominaga, Y., et al. (2017). Role of Regulatory T Cells in Airway Inflammation in Asthma. *Kurume Med. J.* 64 (3), 45–55. doi:10.2739/kurumemedj.MS6430001

Kim, R. Y., Pinkerton, J. W., Essilfie, A. T., Robertson, A. A. B., Baines, K. J., Brown, A. C., et al. (2017). Role for NLRP3 Inflammasome-Mediated, IL-1β-Dependent Responses in Severe, Steroid-Resistant Asthma. *Am. J. Respir. Crit. Care Med.* 196 (3), 283–297. doi:10.1164/rccm.201609-1830OC

Kitoko, J. Z., de Castro, L. L., Nascimento, A. P., Abreu, S. C., Cruz, F. F., Arantes, A. C., et al. (2018). Therapeutic Administration of Bone Marrow-Derived Mesenchymal Stromal Cells Reduces Airway Inflammation Without Up-Regulating Tregs in Experimental Asthma. *Clin. Exp. Allergy* 48 (2), 205–216. doi:10.1111/cea.13048

Konala, V. B. R., Mamidi, M. K., Bhonde, R., Das, A. K., Pochampally, R., and Pal, R. (2016). The Current Landscape of the Mesenchymal Stromal Cell Secretome:

A New Paradigm for Cell-Free Regeneration. *Cytotherapy* 18 (1), 13–24. doi:10.1016/j.jcyt.2015.10.008

Lathrop, M. J., Brooks, E. M., Bonenfant, N. R., Sokocevic, D., Borg, Z. D., Goodwin, M., et al. (2014). Mesenchymal Stromal Cells Mediate Aspergillus Hyphal Extract-Induced Allergic Airway Inflammation by Inhibition of the Th17 Signaling Pathway. *Stem Cell Transl. Med.* 3 (2), 194–205. doi:10.5966/sctm.2013-0061

Li, X., Bai, J., Ji, X., Li, R., Xuan, Y., and Wang, Y. (2014). Comprehensive Characterization of Four Different Populations of Human Mesenchymal Stem Cells as Regards Their Immune Properties, Proliferation and Differentiation. *Int. J. Mol. Med.* 34 (3), 695–704. doi:10.3892/ijmm.2014.1821

Li, Y., Li, H., Cao, Y., Wu, F., Ma, W., Wang, Y., et al. (2017). Placenta-Derived Mesenchymal Stem Cells Improve Airway Hyperresponsiveness and Inflammation in Asthmatic Rats by Modulating the Th17/Treg Balance. *Mol. Med. Rep.* 16 (6), 8137–8145. doi:10.3892/mmr.2017.7605

Li, Y., Qu, T., Tian, L., Han, T., Jin, Y., and Wang, Y. (2018). Human Placenta Mesenchymal Stem Cells Suppress Airway Inflammation in Asthmatic Rats by Modulating Notch Signaling. *Mol. Med. Rep.* 17 (4), 5336–5343. doi:10.3892/mmr.2018.8462

Lin, S.-C., Liou, Y.-M., Ling, T.-Y., Chuang, Y.-H., and Chiang, B.-L. (2019). Placenta-Derived Mesenchymal Stem Cells Reduce the Interleukin-5 Level Experimentally in Children With Asthma. *Int. J. Med. Sci.* 16 (11), 1430–1438. doi:10.7150/ijms.33590

Lin, Y.-D., Fan, X.-L., Zhang, H., Fang, S.-B., Li, C.-L., Deng, M.-X., et al. (2018). The Genes Involved in Asthma with the Treatment of Human Embryonic Stem Cell-Derived Mesenchymal Stem Cells. *Mol. Immunol.* 95, 47–55. doi:10.1016/j.molimm.2018.01.013

Lozano, J., Cruz, M.-J., Piquer, M., Giner, M.-T., and Plaza, A. M. (2014). Assessing the Efficacy of Immunotherapy with a Glutaraldehyde-Modified House Dust Mite Extract in Children by Monitoring Changes in Clinical Parameters and Inflammatory Markers in Exhaled Breath. *Int. Arch. Allergy Immunol.* 165 (2), 140–147. doi:10.1159/000368832

Mattiuzzi, C., and Lippi, G. (2020). Worldwide Asthma Epidemiology: Insights from the Global Health Data Exchange Database. *Int. Forum Allergy Rhinol.* 10 (1), 75–80. doi:10.1002/alr.22464

Miethe, S., Karsonova, A., Karaulov, A., and Renz, H. (2020). Obesity and Asthma. *J. Allergy Clin. Immunol.* 146 (4), 685–693. doi:10.1016/j.jaci.2020.08.011

Nagano, T., Katsurada, M., Dokuni, R., Hazama, D., Kiriu, T., Umezawa, K., et al. (2019). Crucial Role of Extracellular Vesicles in Bronchial Asthma. *Int. J. Mol. Sci.* 20 (10), 2589. doi:10.3390/ijms20102589

Papi, A., Brightling, C., Pedersen, S. E., and Reddel, H. K. (2018). Asthma. *Lancet* 391 (10122), 783–800. doi:10.1016/S0140-6736(17)33311-1

Pomés, A., Glesner, J., Calatroni, A., Visness, C. M., Wood, R. A., O'Connor, G. T., et al. (2019). Cockroach Allergen Component Analysis of Children with or without Asthma and Rhinitis in an Inner-City Birth Cohort. *J. Allergy Clin. Immunol.* 144 (4), 935–944. doi:10.1016/j.jaci.2019.05.036

Skuljec, J., Chmielewski, M., Happle, C., Habener, A., Busse, M., Abken, H., et al. (2017). Chimeric Antigen Receptor-Redirected Regulatory T Cells Suppress Experimental Allergic Airway Inflammation, a Model of Asthma. *Front. Immunol.* 8 (8), 1125. doi:10.3389/fimmu.2017.01125

Song, Y., Dou, H., Li, X., Zhao, X., Li, Y., Liu, D., et al. (2017). Exosomal miR-146a Contributes to the Enhanced Therapeutic Efficacy of Interleukin-1β-Primed Mesenchymal Stem Cells against Sepsis. *Stem Cells* 35 (5), 1208–1221. doi:10.1002/stem.2564

Sueblinvong, V., Loi, R., Eisenhauer, P. L., Bernstein, I. M., Suratt, B. T., Spees, J. L., et al. (2008). Derivation of Lung Epithelium from Human Cord Blood-Derived Mesenchymal Stem Cells. *Am. J. Respir. Crit. Care Med.* 177 (7), 701–711. doi:10.1164/rccm.200706-859OC

Tan, Y., Ooi, S., and Wang, L. (2013). Immunogenicity and Tumorigenicity of Pluripotent Stem Cells and Their Derivatives: Genetic and Epigenetic Perspectives. *Curr. Stem Cell Res. Ther.* 9 (1), 63–72. doi:10.2174/1574888x113086660068

Tiotiu, A. I., Novakova, P., Nedeva, D., Chong-Neto, H. J., Novakova, S., Steiropoulos, P., et al. (2020). Impact of Air Pollution on Asthma Outcomes. *Int. J. Environ. Res. Public Health* 17 (17), 6212. doi:10.3390/ijerph17176212

Toskala, E., and Kennedy, D. W. (2015). Asthma Risk Factors. *Int. Forum Allergy Rhinol.* 5 (1), S11–S16. doi:10.1002/alr.21557

van den Berge, M., and Tasena, H. (2019). Role of microRNAs and Exosomes in Asthma. *Curr. Opin. Pulm. Med.* 25 (1), 87–93. doi:10.1097/MCP.0000000000000532

Wang, W., Jing Li, J., S. Foster, P., M. Hansbro, P., and Yang, M. (2010). Potential Therapeutic Targets for Steroid-Resistant Asthma. *Curr. Drug Targets* 11 (8), 957–970. doi:10.2174/138945010791591412

Weiss, D. J. (2018). Cell-based Therapy for Chronic Obstructive Pulmonary Disease. Rebuilding the Lung. *Ann. Am. Thorac. Soc.* 15 (Suppl. 4), S253–S259. doi:10.1513/AnnalsATS.201808-534MG

World Health Organization (2018). Asthma. http://www.who.int/news-room/fact-sheets/detail/asthma (Accessed November 15, 2020).

Xian, M., Feng, M., Dong, Y., Wei, N., Su, Q., and Li, J. (2020). Changes in CD4+CD25+FoxP3+ Regulatory T Cells and Serum Cytokines in Sublingual and Subcutaneous Immunotherapy in Allergic Rhinitis with or without Asthma. *Int. Arch. Allergy Immunol.* 181 (1), 71–80. doi:10.1159/000503143

Yao, Y., Fan, X.-L., Jiang, D., Zhang, Y., Li, X., Xu, Z.-B., et al. (2018). Connexin 43-Mediated Mitochondrial Transfer of iPSC-MSCs Alleviates Asthma Inflammation. *Stem Cel. Rep.* 11 (5), 1120–1135. doi:10.1016/j.stemcr.2018.09.012

Yu, X., Yu, L., Guo, B., Chen, R., and Qiu, C. (2020). A Narrative Review of Research Advances in Mesenchymal Stem Cell Therapy for Asthma. *Ann. Transl. Med.* 8 (21), 1461. doi:10.21037/atm-20-6389

Zhong, H., Fan, X.-L., Fang, S.-B., Lin, Y.-D., Wen, W., and Fu, Q.-L. (2019). Human Pluripotent Stem Cell-Derived Mesenchymal Stem Cells Prevent Chronic Allergic Airway Inflammation via TGF-B1-Smad2/Smad3 Signaling Pathway in Mice. *Mol. Immunol.* 109, 51–57. doi:10.1016/j.molimm.2019.02.017

Zhuansun, Y., Du, Y., Huang, F., Lin, L., Chen, R., Jiang, S., et al. (2019). MSCs Exosomal miR-1470 Promotes the Differentiation of CD4+CD25+FOXP3+ Tregs in Asthmatic Patients by Inducing the Expression of P27KIP1. *Int. Immunopharmacol.* 77, 105981. doi:10.1016/j.intimp.2019.105981

2

On the Corner of Models and Cure: Gene Editing in Cystic Fibrosis

Marjolein Ensinck[1†], Angélique Mottais[2†], Claire Detry[2], Teresinha Leal[2‡] and Marianne S. Carlon[1‡]*

[1]Molecular Virology and Gene Therapy, Department of Pharmaceutical and Pharmacological Sciences, KU Leuven, Leuven, Belgium, [2]Institut de Recherche Expérimentale et Clinique, Louvain Centre for Toxicology and Applied Pharmacology, Université Catholique de Louvain, Brussels, Belgium

***Correspondence:**
Marianne S. Carlon
marianne.carlon@kuleuven.be

†These authors share first authorship
‡These authors share last authorship

Cystic fibrosis (CF) is a severe genetic disease for which curative treatment is still lacking. Next generation biotechnologies and more efficient cell-based and *in vivo* disease models are accelerating the development of novel therapies for CF. Gene editing tools, like CRISPR-based systems, can be used to make targeted modifications in the genome, allowing to correct mutations directly in the Cystic Fibrosis Transmembrane conductance Regulator (*CFTR*) gene. Alternatively, with these tools more relevant disease models can be generated, which in turn will be invaluable to evaluate novel gene editing-based therapies for CF. This critical review offers a comprehensive description of currently available tools for genome editing, and the cell and animal models which are available to evaluate them. Next, we will give an extensive overview of proof-of-concept applications of gene editing in the field of CF. Finally, we will touch upon the challenges that need to be addressed before these proof-of-concept studies can be translated towards a therapy for people with CF.

Keywords: cystic fibrosis, CFTR, gene therapy, gene editing, CF cell models, CF animal models, humanized CF animals

INTRODUCTION

Cystic fibrosis (CF) is a rare genetic disease affecting approximately 80,000 people worldwide (Jackson and Goss, 2018). More than 2,100 mutations have been identified in the *CFTR* (Cystic Fibrosis Transmembrane conductance Regulator) gene (www.genet.sickkids.on.ca), of which currently 360 reported as disease-causing (www.CFTR2.org). The gene encodes a chloride/bicarbonate channel that plays an essential role in the fluid and electrolyte balance across secretory epithelia. Mutations in *CFTR* can disrupt the function of the protein through a variety of mechanisms, ranging from reduced or absent protein synthesis to normal apical expression of proteins with defective chloride and bicarbonate gating or conductance (De Boeck and Amaral, 2016; Veit et al., 2016). The protein loss-of-function results in dehydration of the surface liquid lining the epithelia of various organs, such as the airways, the gastrointestinal and reproductive tracts and the sweat glands. The respiratory phenotype is characterized by recurrent cycles of mucostasis, inflammation and infection that progressively destroys the lung architecture leading to respiratory failure and death (Boon et al., 2016). As CFTR is expressed in a variety of exocrine epithelia, with some of the disease symptoms already starting just after birth, or even *in utero*, this multisystemic disease requires an early, multidisciplinary management (reviewed in (Carlon et al., 2017)). Despite better symptomatic care, the median age at death remains in the early forties (Wanyama and Thomas, 2018). The development of effective CFTR modulator drugs which either improve CFTR processing (correctors) or channel gating (potentiators), brings the prospect of further increasing life quality and expectancy (Ramsey et al., 2011; Wainwright et al., 2015; Taylor-Cousar et al., 2017; Keating et al., 2018; Heijerman et al., 2019; Middleton et al., 2019). Currently, four modulator regimens are approved, consisting of Kalydeco™, a potentiator monotherapy, and three combination therapies consisting of one potentiator with one or two correctors with distinct mode of action (Orkambi™, Symdeko™, and Trikafta™). Together, they can functionally correct approximately 184 different CF-causing mutations, accounting for 90% of individuals with CF. Clinical benefits range from significant increases in lung function, to modest or even absent clinical improvements. Indeed, even the highly effective Trikafta™ showed variable clinical responses in patients with at least one F508del (c.1521–1523delCTT) allele (Heijerman et al., 2019; Middleton et al., 2019), likely influenced by the individual genetic and environmental background. Besides that, adverse events have been reported, such as chest tightness, diarrhea and drug-drug interactions, which in the context of a life-long intake is not desirable (Wainwright et al., 2015; Talamo Guevara and McColley, 2017; Guimbellot et al., 2018; Burgel et al., 2020). For Kalydeco™, the clinical benefits have been monitored over many years already, showing that after a significant increase in lung function at treatment onset, CF lung disease continues to worsen, although at a slower pace (Volkova et al., 2020). Finally, therapeutic options that tackle the CFTR defect are still missing for approximately 91% of *CFTR* mutations covering 10% of people with CF (PwCF). These carry two minimal function mutations, comprising frameshifts, large insertions and deletions (indels), nonsense and drug-refractory missense mutations. While pharmacological advances have greatly improved life quality of PwCF, and very likely will increase life expectancy as well, none of these treatments provide a cure.

Since the discovery of the *CFTR* gene 30 years ago (Kerem et al., 1989; Riordan et al., 1989; Rommens et al., 1989), scientists have been trying to bring gene therapy to PwCF. In contrast to CFTR modulators, gene therapy aims to restore the defect at the DNA level, thus providing a long-term correction. Traditionally, gene therapy efforts were focused on delivering a copy of the *CFTR* cDNA, providing cells with mutation agnostic means to produce wild type (WT) CFTR protein (Vidovic et al., 2016; Alton et al., 2017). Clinical trials investigating different gene addition strategies have not resulted in meaningful clinical benefit (reviewed in (Sondhi et al., 2017)). However, successes in other genetic diseases leading to the market approval of gene therapeutic agents, such as for retinal dystrophy (Russell et al., 2017), spinal muscular atrophy type 1 (Mendell et al., 2017), and β-thalassemia (Harrison, 2019), have in part revived the interest for CF gene therapy research. Indeed, the current priority of the CF community is to develop a causal therapy and preferably even a cure for all individuals with CF, as underscored by the Cystic Fibrosis Foundation's "Path to a Cure" mission statement (CFF, 2019).

In this review, we will discuss the most recent advances in gene editing with respect to both the development of human-relevant disease models of CF as well as proof of concept studies that have shown the feasibility and safety of correcting a variety of *CFTR* mutations. Furthermore, we discuss some of the hurdles and open questions which need to be solved, to allow further progress of these promising but early gene editing studies. Finally, we discuss possible strategies that would facilitate the further development of an *in vivo* or *ex vivo* gene therapeutic approach toward its future clinical application.

HOW TO EDIT THE GENOME: GENE EDITING TOOLS

Advances in gene editing tools have made targeted genome modifications widely available. Zinc finger nucleases (ZFN), transcription activator-like effector nucleases (TALEN) and in particular CRISPR (clustered regularly interspaced short palindromic repeats) systems have opened up a seemingly endless variety of possible alterations to be introduced into the genome. Correcting mutations at their endogenous loci heralds a new era of personalized medicine and treatment of monogenetic diseases, by correcting the underlying cause of the disease. Alternatively, mutations can be introduced in a targeted manner, allowing elucidation of disease mechanisms and testing of potential therapies. Especially when a monogenic disorder is caused by many, exceedingly rare mutations, as is the case for CF, introducing mutations into relevant cell and animal models provides a unique opportunity to study these mutations when primary material is not easily obtained. Besides, samples are usually not available in a homozygous manner, due to the low prevalence of each individual mutation, and analysis of compound heterozygous samples is complicated by the presence of another mutation on the other allele. Different editing strategies however, will be required to cover all base conversions and indels that cause CF, both for the development of gene editing-based therapies as well as new CF model systems. In the following part, we will briefly discuss the different tools available for gene-editing. Proof-of-concept applications of these tools will be discussed in the section *Gene Editing to Correct Mutations in CFTR*.

ZFN, TALEN, and Cas Nucleases

Programable nucleases like ZFN, TALEN, and CRISPR associated (Cas) nucleases, are all used to generate targeted double strand breaks (DSBs) in the genome. Editing at these sites relies on repair of the DSB by cellular DNA damage repair mechanisms. Most commonly, DSBs are repaired by a process called non-homologous end joining (NHEJ) where the two ends are re-ligated (Guirouilh-Barbat et al., 2004). As this process is imperfect, some bases can get deleted or inserted, creating indels. This can result in frameshifts disrupting the coding sequence, effectively knocking out proteins, which has been useful to study the function of genes. In the era of personalized medicine however, models harboring specific mutations are often preferred as they allow to study the disease-causing mutations in detail as well as test potential rescue strategies for these mutations. The therapeutic potential of NHEJ is rather limited since it can only be used to correct defects in certain cases e.g., gain-of-function mutations and mutations resulting in cryptic splice sites in introns where indels are tolerated. Many genetic diseases, however, including CF, are caused by loss-of-function mutations which cannot be repaired by NHEJ, with the exception of a couple of intronic splicing mutations. Introduction of specific edits relies on the alternative DNA damage repair mechanism: homology directed repair (HDR). A template, a DNA molecule containing the desired edit and homology arms on both sides, is used by the HDR machinery to repair the DSB and introduce the edit to the genome (reviewed in (Hsu et al., 2014)). HDR however is less efficient compared to NHEJ and is only active in dividing cells, as it normally protects cells against DNA damage during DNA replication. Therefore, its use in many adult cell types is limited. For a schematic overview of the two repair pathways and their possible applications, we refer to (Pranke et al., 2019; Maule et al., 2020).

The different nuclease-based gene editing tools differ mainly in their nuclease and the way specific DNA sequences are recognized. ZFNs were the first available "molecular scissors" and were built using multiple zinc finger domains (that each recognize a three bp DNA motif) fused to the FokI nuclease (reviewed in (Urnov et al., 2010)). The DNA is cleaved when two ZFNs are recruited to a target sequence, resulting in the dimerization of the FokI nuclease domains. Similarly, TALENs use transcription activator-like effectors (TALEs) rather than zinc fingers to recognize specific DNA sequences, also fused to the FokI nuclease (reviewed in (Joung and Sander, 2013)). Both ZFNs and TALENs require custom protein design for each target, in contrast to CRISPR-Cas based systems. Cas nucleases were first described as a gene editing tool in 2012 (Gasiunas et al., 2012; Jinek et al., 2012) and CRISPR-Cas gene editing rapidly became one of the cornerstones of modern biomedical research. It was hardly surprising that Jennifer Doudna and Emmanuelle Charpentier were awarded the 2020 Nobel prize in Chemistry for their pioneering work in the development of this highly versatile editing tool (Ledford and Callaway, 2020). The most used and best studied Cas protein is derived from *Streptococcus pyogenes* (SpCas9) and finds its DNA target using a short RNA, the single guide RNA (sgRNA), which consists of a 20 nucleotide spacer and a scaffold which it uses to interact with the Cas9 protein. Once the Cas9-sgRNA complex is formed, it will scan the DNA for sequences (the protospacer) that match the sgRNA-spacer motif at sites where protospacer adjacent motifs (PAM, NGG for SpCas9) are present, and if a match is found, the nuclease activity of Cas9 is activated. Cas9 however has some leniency toward mismatches between spacer and protospacer, which might result in unwanted off-targets, requiring further investigation, in particular with regard to therapeutic applications. A combination of *in silico* off-target prediction tools as well as experimental set-ups e.g., GUIDE-seq (Tsai et al., 2015), allow to identify (potential) off-target sites, which can then be evaluated by deep sequencing. For an overview of different Cas proteins and optimizations, for example to increase the number of targetable sites or improve efficacy or specificity, we refer to (Anzalone et al., 2020; Makarova et al., 2020; Maule et al., 2021).

Base Editing

Although CRISPR-Cas editing itself was still relatively new, CRISPR-Cas derived techniques rapidly emerged, one of which is base editing. One of the largest assets of base editors is the ability to perform targeted base modifications without introducing DSBs into the genome. Besides, base editing does not rely on HDR and can therefore also be performed in cells that are not actively dividing. Base editors employ a Cas9n (nickase) in which one of the nuclease sites has been knocked out (D10A) fused to a deaminase. For cytosine base editors (CBE), this is a rAPOBEC deaminase which will deaminate cytosines after the Cas9n-sgRNA complex has guided the deaminase to the target (Komor et al., 2016). Deamination results in uracil which is repaired to thymine while the Cas9n will nick the non-edited strand, pushing DNA damage repair toward incorporating the edit. Inhibition of the base excision repair (BER) pathway by adding an uracil glycosylase inhibitor (UGI) to the CBE, further increased C-to-T editing efficiencies. Alternatively, instead of inhibiting the uracil DNA glycosylase (UNG) which initiates BER, promoting it often results in uracil to guanine repair, effectively creating C-to-G base editors (CGBE) (Kurt et al., 2020; Zhao et al., 2020). Adenine base editors (ABE) on the other hand, use the adenine deaminase TadA to install A-to-G edits (Gaudelli et al., 2017). Combined, these editors can restore many disease-causing mutations, in particular ABE which can repair naturally occurring C-to-T edits. Base editing takes place in a specific window, the editing window, which is usually around four nucleotides. This somewhat limits the use of base editors, since the gRNA should place the target nucleotide within this window. Besides, if multiple cytosines or adenines, for CBE/CGBE and ABE, respectively, are present in this window, all of them can theoretically be edited, resulting in bystander edits that might alter the amino acid sequence of the protein. Prediction tools have been designed, such as BE-Hive (Arbab et al., 2020), to determine which bases will be edited most efficiently. As with Cas9 nucleases, new base editors are constantly being developed with altered PAM recognition or adjusted editing windows, to increase the number of mutations that can be corrected, or improve their specificity and efficacy as well as reduce off-targets. For an overview, we refer to (Huang et al., 2021).

Prime Editing

In 2019, another CRISPR-based tool was introduced: the prime editor (PE). Here, rather than a deaminase, a reverse transcriptase (RT) is fused to Cas9n (H840A) (Anzalone et al., 2019). In combination with a prime editing gRNA (pegRNA) that contains not just a spacer and scaffold but also a primer binding site (PBS) and an RT template, it allows to re-write all base conversions and also small insertions or deletions. Following a nick at the targeted region, the PBS anneals and the RT template is reverse transcribed. This results in an intermediate, with a 3′ and a 5′ ssDNA flap, where the former contains the edit. If this edited flap is ligated, it will create a heterodimer that can subsequently be repaired to allow incorporation of the edit. Optimizing the PE (PE2) and adding a gRNA to nick the non-edited strand (PE3) improved the

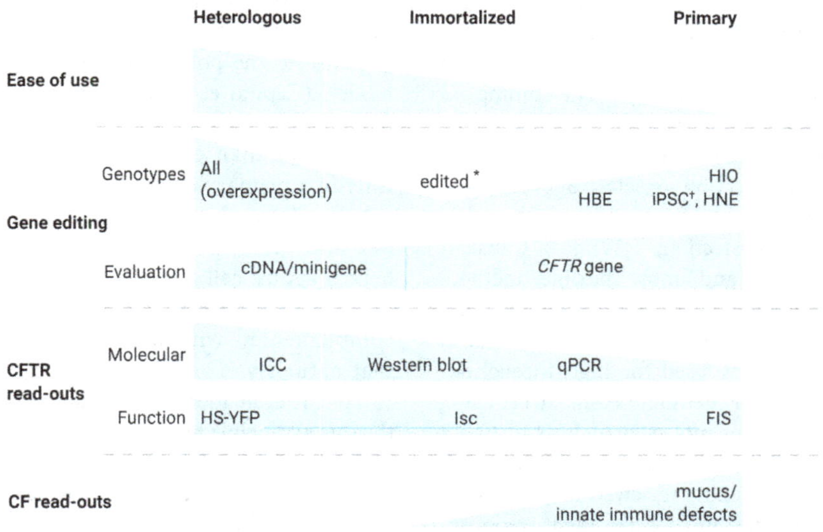

FIGURE 1 | Cystic fibrosis cell models for the evaluation of gene editing strategies. Different cell-based models are available to evaluate gene editing for CF. While heterologous, CFTR overexpressing models allow the study of any CFTR variant, and are easiest to work with, their read-outs are limited to molecular and functional analysis of CFTR and genetic correction at the cDNA or minigene level. Immortalized cells, expressing the endogenous CFTR, allow correction of the *CFTR* gene, but are only available for a limited number of the more common *CFTR* genotypes. Gene editing however, has allowed to generate immortalized lines for additional genotypes (*) (Valley et al., 2019). Primary cell models are the most relevant, since they can be used for CF specific read-outs that are important in the CF phenotype, including mucus and immune defects. Traditional molecular CFTR endpoints remain challenging for primary cells. Depending on the origin of the primary cells, genotypes might be exceedingly hard to acquire i.e., human bronchial epithelial (HBE) cells from explant lungs. On the other hand, human intestinal organoids (HIO) and human nasal epithelial (HNE) cells are more readily obtained via minimally invasive procedures. Alternatively, iPSCs were edited (†) to generate isogenic lines with different genotypes (Ruan et al., 2019). A combination of different models allows the most complete cell-based evaluation of novel gene editing strategies. Abbreviations: FIS, forskolin induced swelling; HBE, human bronchial epithelial; HIO, human intestinal organoids; HNE, human nasal epithelial; ICC, immunocytochemistry; iPSCs, induced pluripotent stem cells; Isc, short circuit currents; HS-YFP, halide sensitive yellow fluorescent protein.

efficiency of PE (Anzalone et al., 2019). In general, pegRNA design is more complicated than gRNA design for Cas9 nucleases and base editors, since there is no consensus yet on the optimal lengths of both PBS and RT. Tools have been developed to assist in the design of pegRNAs (Kim et al., 2020) but currently, multiple guides should still be empirically tested for each target.

CELL AND ANIMAL MODELS OF DISEASE

Before we discuss in detail the published proof-of-concept studies showing the feasibility to correct a variety of CFTR mutations, we first will discuss the available cell and animal models of CF, in which gene editing and a phenotypic rescue can be assessed. Cell and animal models have been invaluable for unraveling disease mechanisms in CF. They have allowed to gain insights into CF pathophysiology both at the cellular and the organ level, and have aided in the development of novel therapies to alleviate symptoms or treat the mutational defect on the DNA, RNA or protein level. For an overview of the use of different models for tailoring CFTR modulators to specific mutations, we refer to (Clancy et al., 2019). In the next section, we will discuss the different types of CF models and focus on the potential of both cell and animal models to assess a genetic correction by CRISPR-Cas or other DNA-directed editing therapies.

Cell Models

Different sorts of cell models have been used extensively to study CF(TR). Each cell model has its own advantages and limitations, balancing the ease of use with the possibility to employ specific read-outs and the translatability of the data gained (**Figure 1**). Usually, combining different complementary models allows gathering in the most complete manner all information needed to reliably confirm identified disease mechanisms and new therapeutic strategies.

CFTR Overexpressing Cell Models

In heterologous cell models a *CFTR* cDNA or minigene is overexpressed under an exogenous promoter. For this purpose, immortalized laboratory cell lines of human e.g., Human Embryonic Kidney (HEK)293T cells, or non-human e.g., Fischer Rat Thyroid (FRT) cells, origin are often used. The endogenous CFTR is usually not expressed in these models and thus allows functionally studying CFTR mutants, in the absence of endogenously expressed WT-CFTR. Some cell lines, such as FRT cells, can be grown into a polarized epithelium which allows electrophysiological read-outs like short-circuit current (I_{sc}) measurements (Sheppard et al., 1994). Non-polarized cell lines can still be used to study CFTR function, albeit indirectly, by halide-sensitive yellow fluorescent protein (HS-YFP) quenching among others (Galietta et al., 2001). Protein maturation and subcellular localization can be evaluated using biochemical assays such as Western blotting and other antibody-based methods (e.g.,

ELISA, immunocytochemistry, flow cytometry) (Okiyoneda et al., 2013; Botelho et al., 2015; Ensinck et al., 2020).

The parental cell line however, is not the only consideration when choosing a heterologous cell model. The timing of expression and form in which CFTR is expressed (cDNA or minigene) are equally important. Overexpression can be either transient e.g., by plasmid transfection or electroporation, or stable, via integration into the genome after retroviral transduction or stable transfection. While transient overexpression is the quickest and most flexible method, obtained expression levels are often variable. Stable cell lines on the other hand allow to study CFTR in a more standardized manner, and have been extensively used for high throughput screening (Van Goor et al., 2006; Pedemonte et al., 2011; Liang et al., 2017) and characterization of molecular defects of *CFTR* mutations and responses to compounds (Sosnay et al., 2013; Van Goor et al., 2014; Ensinck et al., 2020) (reviewed in (Veit et al., 2016)). Results in cell lines are indicative of treatment responses in PwCF, and have been used by the FDA to evaluate repurposing of existing CFTR modulators to rare mutations. Label extensions were approved for Kalydeco™ (2017/2020), as well as Symdeko™ (2020) and Trikafta™ (2020) based on a functional rescue, measured by I_{sc}, to at least 10% of WT current in FRT cell models (FDA, 2017; Vertex, 2020). These FRT cells express different *CFTR* mutations integrated at the same site using the Flp recombinase system to allow targeted cassette exchange at Flp recombination target sites (Flp-In™, Invitrogen) (Van Goor et al., 2014). In this way, isogenic CFTR-variant cell lines of choice can be rapidly generated, all with an identical genetic background. While recombinases are commonly used to generate heterologous cell models, Cas9 in principle also supports cassette exchange although with slightly altered characteristics, such as a higher risk of knock-out alleles, or insertion of extra pieces of DNA alongside the integrated transgene (Phan et al., 2017).

The *CFTR* cDNA is mostly chosen for overexpression since the *CFTR* gene spans at least 180 kb, although the exact size of *CFTR's* regulatory elements is not strictly defined. In any case, it is too large to be introduced efficiently into cells, unless using artificial chromosome delivery strategies (Auriche et al., 2002). The *CFTR* cDNA (4.4 kb) contains the entire *CFTR* coding sequence but is still small enough to easily transfer into most cell types, even when an external promoter and possibly a protein tag or antibiotic selection marker are added to the construct. Protein tags like small epitopes e.g., FLAG or hemagglutinin (HA), and fluorescent proteins, *e.g.* green fluorescent protein (GFP), facilitate the detection of CFTR (Ensinck et al., 2020), as CFTR antibodies often have low sensitivity or specificity (Mendes et al., 2004). While *CFTR* cDNA allows to study the biogenesis and function of the CFTR protein, there are aspects, like splicing and nonsense-mediated mRNA decay (NMD) for nonsense mutations (also see the section *Nonsense Mutations*), which are not recapitulated in these models. Minigenes are (partial) *CFTR* cDNAs in which at least one intron is included, and used to investigate splicing mutations as well as nonsense mutations sensitive to NMD (Sharma et al., 2014; Sharma et al., 2018). It can however be difficult to identify all mutations with splicing defects based on the DNA sequence alone. For example, the *CFTR* mutation G970R (c.2908G>C) was considered a stereotypical class III gating mutant based on its normal CFTR biogenesis and response to the potentiator Ivacaftor in cDNA overexpression models (Caputo et al., 2009; Yu et al., 2012). After treatment responses to Kalydeco™ in people with this G970R mutation were lower than expected, G970R was re-investigated, this time in a primary cell model, which revealed a predominant splicing defect that resulted in exon skipping or the retention of an intron (Fidler et al., 2020). This underscores that while heterologous cell models allow to elucidate many of the molecular aspects of CFTR mutants, they should still be complemented with other, preferably primary cell models that naturally express the *CFTR* gene.

For the evaluation of gene editing in heterologous cell models, the same principle holds true. These models can be used as a first proof-of-concept, to validate guide design for example or test multiple guides or editing strategies in an easy-to-use model. Read-outs will mainly include detection of editing on the cDNA or minigene level, when allele-specific (i.e., mutation is part of the target recognition sequence, such as the protospacer) or footprint-free (i.e., *CFTR* gene is already WT and thus 'correction' cannot be evaluated) editing strategies are used. Targeted integration of super-exons (also see the section *Correcting Multiple Mutations at Once*) for example could be investigated on the genomic level, although the lack of endogenous CFTR expression in these models precludes any further analysis on the RNA or protein level. If a protospacer spans an exon-boundary, gRNAs should be tested on a minigene rather than on the cDNA so that gRNA design resembles the genomic sequence. Also, when splicing mutations are edited, minigene systems are particularly interesting as they allow to not only evaluate editing of the minigene, but importantly also restoration of mRNA splicing (Sanz et al., 2017; Maule et al., 2019). Alternatively, the use of cDNA models allows to characterize the CFTR biogenesis and function of edited cells in heterologous cell models not naturally expressing CFTR.

Immortalized Models Expressing CFTR

Cells that endogenously express CFTR provide a good complement to heterologous cell models. They are more relevant as the *CFTR* gene is expressed at its normal level and with its usual regulation. Besides, these cells usually retain more epithelial features, such as their ability to form polarized epithelia that can be grown as ALI cultures, and are of human origin (in contrast to, for example, FRT cells). The endogenous CFTR expression, for example in the cystic fibrosis bronchial epithelium cell line CFBE41o- (F508del/F508del), allows to correlate genomic *CFTR* correction with functional rescue at the protein level. One major disadvantage however is the lack of models for most of the >2100 *CFTR* mutations. To overcome this issue, several of the more common *CFTR* mutations have been introduced in the non-CF 16HBE14o-parental cell line (see the section *Introducing Mutations into CFTR*) (Valley et al., 2019). Eight genotypes are currently available, all within the same isogenic background through the CFF (CFF, 2020). To date, one of them i.e., the W1282X (c.3846G>A) human bronchial epithelium cell line 16HBE14o-, has been used to study a therapeutic rescue using ABE (also see the sections *Nonsense Mutations* and *Introducing Mutations into CFTR*) (Jiang et al., 2020).

Primary Cell Models of CF

Cell models directly derived from CF patients remain the golden standard for pre-clinical testing of new therapies for CF. Since CF is a multi-organ disorder which does not exclusively affect epithelia but also for example innate immune and endothelial cells (reviewed in (Declercq et al., 2019; Lara-Reyna et al., 2020), respectively), cells from many different organs can be used to understand the diverse CFTR-associated phenotypes and study a correction by rescue strategies. Human intestinal organoids, for example, are three-dimensional stem-cell based structures derived from the crypts of rectal biopsies (Sato et al., 2009). While this is an intestinal rather than an airway-based model, it is frequently used in the study of CF therapeutics, since the stimulation of these organoids with cAMP-agonist forskolin results in CFTR-dependent organoid swelling (Dekkers et al., 2013). This correlates well with improvements in PwCF in clinical trials (Ramalho et al., 2020), and this model is therefore often used for the evaluation of new small molecules and proof-of-concept gene-editing (Dekkers et al., 2016; Maule et al., 2019; Geurts et al., 2020a; Geurts et al., 2020b). HBE cultures are a logical and frequently used primary cell model in CF as lung disease is associated with most morbidity and mortality in CF patients. HBE cells are usually isolated from explant lungs, thus limiting the availability of genotypes with many of the rare mutations. When fully differentiated, these HBE cells form pseudostratified epithelia resembling the *in vivo* epithelium. Importantly they also contain the recently identified rare but high CFTR expressing ionocyte (Montoro et al., 2018; Plasschaert et al., 2018), a cell type therefore suggested important for gene targeting. While I_{sc} measurements are classically used to assess CFTR's function as an anion channel by measuring Cl^- transport, investigating $HCO3^-$ transport is becoming increasingly important, due to the demonstrated linear relationship between CFTR levels, $HCO3^-$ transport and host defense properties (Shah et al., 2016a). Indeed, while a plateau of Cl^- transport is reached when 10–50% of cells express CFTR (Dannhoffer et al., 2009), explained by a limitation in Cl^- entry into cells at the basolateral membrane, a 50:50 mix of CF and non-CF porcine epithelial cells transported $HCO3^-$ at half the rate of non-CF epithelia (Shah et al., 2016a). These findings suggest that indeed, overexpression in a smaller fraction of cells, might still result in a clinical benefit due to the strong link between $HCO3^-$ transport and the host's ability to fight bacterial infections. Host innate defense mechanisms of the airway epithelium can be measured *in vivo* or *ex vivo*, using a variety of assays, ranging from ASL pH and height, to mucociliary clearance, mucus release from the submucosal glands (SMG) and bacterial killing (for an overview, we refer to (Carlon et al., 2017)).

While the airway epithelium is the first line of defense against invading pathogens and other inhaled particulates, these cells orchestrate the further regulation of both innate and adaptive immune responses to these challenges (reviewed in (Cohen and Prince, 2012)). CF airway epithelial cells (AEC) show intrinsic immune defects, such as aberrant Toll-like Receptor trafficking, increased nuclear factor-κB (NF-κB) signaling and increased pro-inflammatory cytokine transcription (Bruscia et al., 2011; Lara-Reyna et al., 2020). A longstanding question has been whether impaired innate immune responses of immune and endothelial cells similarly, are directly linked to CFTR impairment, or rather secondary induced. On the one hand neutrophils are recruited to inflamed CF airways, even in the absence of infection, due to continuous NF-κB signaling and pro-inflammatory cytokine secretion, however, neutrophils also show a primary defect linked to CFTR dysfunction. Indeed, CFTR plays an important role in their phagocytic capacity by moving Cl^- ions into the phagolysosome to produce the bactericidal substance, hypochlorous acid (HOCl), a process which is impaired in CF (Zhou et al., 2013). Also, for monocytes and activated macrophages, exaggerated inflammatory responses (Meyer et al., 2009) and decreased phagocytic capacity have been reported in CF, although whether these dysfunctions are intrinsic or extrinsic, requires further investigation. In that context, CFTR modulator treatment has been reported to improve the ability of macrophages to sequester iron, which is critical to prevent both oxidative tissue damage and bacterial growth (Hazlett et al., 2020). Likewise, their ability to phagocytose and kill pathogens like *Pseudomonas eruginosa* was enhanced by modulator therapy (Barnaby et al., 2018). Both studies thus provide further support for an intrinsic CFTR defect in CF macrophages. In line with these findings, a similar pro-inflammatory phenotype was identified in CFTR-deficient endothelial cells using a transcriptomic approach, which was partially reversed by CFTR modulators (Declercq et al., 2020). Altogether, it is clear that multiple cell types contribute to the hyper-inflammatory phenotype observed throughout multiple organs in CF, requiring a broad therapeutic approach that allows correcting the multiple innate immune defects associated with dysfunctional CFTR.

Besides the eminent progressive lung disease PwCF suffer from, pancreatic insufficiency (PI) affects about 85% of the CF population. Most of them are PI soon after birth, with evidence for even structural abnormalities *in utero* (reviewed in (Singh and Schwarzenberg, 2017)). PI is caused by damage and obstruction of the pancreatic ducts. Normally, CFTR is highly expressed in pancreatic ductal epithelial cells (PDECs) and allows anions and fluid to enter the ductal lumen. This ensures that the digestive enzymes produced by the acinar cells remain in a soluble state, which is not the case in severe forms of CF (reviewed in (Wilschanski and Novak, 2013)). Besides exocrine PI, also the endocrine pancreas is frequently affected, leading to CF-related diabetes (CFRD). Whether a lack of CFTR function in PwCF is directly linked with CFRD remains unclear. In that context, Mun and colleagues have developed a patient-derived pancreas-on-a-chip to allow studying in a co-culture set-up if impaired cell-cell signaling between PDECs and islet cells leads to CFRD (Shik Mun et al., 2019). Their study indeed showed that insulin secretion was strongly decreased by inhibition of CFTR function in PDECs. This organ-on-chip system will thus allow broadening the concept of personalized medicine for CF from the well-established primary lung and intestinal cultures to a pancreatic model for studying epithelial and/or endocrine dysfunctions. Even more organ-specific cell models are emerging, such as extrahepatic and intrahepatic cholangiocyte organoids (Verstegen et al., 2020), which collectively will allow to better understand the pathological mechanisms and study a therapeutic rescue in the many organs affected in CF.

In conclusion, proof-of-concept gene editing studies have mainly focused on correcting the ion channel defect of CFTR in primary cell cultures to date (see the section *Gene Editing to Correct Mutations in CFTR*). This section however points out the importance of evaluating a therapeutic rescue beyond electrophysiological end-points as ideally all pleiotropic defects caused by CFTR dysfunction should be corrected, in order to substantially improve the multi-organ nature of CF.

CF Animal Models: Possibilities for Evaluating Genetic Rescue Strategies

Even though cell models are increasing in complexity to better mimic the *in vivo* organ structure and function, none of them provide the same level of complexity as present in animal models of disease. Therefore, despite limitations in the translatability to humans, animal models still are of great value to study genotype-phenotype relationships and determine bioavailability, pharmacokinetics and drug efficacy in the different organs affected. In the next section, we will review the different animal models generated, from Cftr knock-out (KO) to knock-in (KI) of human CFTR mutations to humanized animal models of CF. For each of them, we will discuss their value and limitations in the context of studying a genetic correction of the gene defect in CF by gene editing technology.

Cftr Knock-Out Animal Models of CF

Since the identification of the *CFTR* gene, numerous animal models have been developed and widely reviewed (Grubb and Boucher, 1999; Wilke et al., 2011; Lavelle et al., 2016; Rosen et al., 2018; Semaniakou et al., 2018; McCarron et al., 2021). The conservation of this gene in mammals has made it possible to generate KO models from many different species, including mouse (Snouwaert et al., 1992; Colledge et al., 1995; Hasty et al., 1995; Rozmahel et al., 1996; van Heeckeren et al., 2004), rat (Tuggle et al., 2014; Dreano et al., 2019), rabbit (Xu et al., 2021), ferret (Sun et al., 2008; Sun et al., 2010), sheep (Fan et al., 2018) and pig (Meyerholz et al., 2010). These different models show large species-specific, and in the case of rodents, even strain-specific, phenotypic variability. For example, the KO pig and ferret present with very severe digestive and respiratory symptoms, requiring intensive postnatal symptomatic treatment such as ileostomy and antibiotics and therefore do not fully recapitulate disease progression in humans (reviewed in (Rogers et al., 2008; Sun et al., 2010)). However, these models have been extremely valuable to unravel the origin of CF lung disease (Stoltz et al., 2010; Sun et al., 2014; Keiser et al., 2015; Stoltz et al., 2015). Impaired bicarbonate secretion and reduced airway surface liquid (ASL) pH were shown to lie at the basis of viscous mucus secretions, mucostasis, impaired innate immune responses and thus the inability to efficiently clear pathogens (Stoltz et al., 2010; Hoegger et al., 2014). Mice and rats on the other hand mainly suffer from severe gastrointestinal obstruction, which requires an early and continued treatment with laxatives (Clarke et al., 1996). They show little or no respiratory phenotype, although the impairment of CFTR channel activity, measured by nasal potential difference (NPD) (Grubb and Boucher, 1999; Lubamba et al., 2008; Saussereau et al., 2013), confirms the loss of *Cftr* function. NPD is a non-invasive, translational read-out also applied in humans (Leal et al., 2008; Vermeulen et al., 2015), which allows assessing a functional rescue by gene therapy. This read-out has been used to assess the efficacy of many different gene addition rescue strategies, tested both in CF animal models (McNeer et al., 2015; Vidovic et al., 2016) and in clinical trials (Hay et al., 1995; Alton et al., 1999). For a complete overview of all *Cftr* KO animal models and their multi-organ phenotypes, we refer to the following reviews (Wilke et al., 2011; McCarron et al., 2018; Rosen et al., 2018; Semaniakou et al., 2018).

Species-Specific Differences Influence CF Lung Disease Phenotype

Several reasons have been put forward to explain the difference in lung disease severity between rodents and the larger CF animal models, such as the ferret and pig. A first reason relates to anatomical differences in SMG distribution throughout the proximal airways, which in rodents is restricted to the nose and the most proximal part of the trachea. CF airway pathology however has been shown to be largely attributed to defects in the SMGs as CFTR dysfunction is associated with abnormal mucus secretion and defective innate immunity (Stoltz et al., 2010; Hoegger et al., 2014; Keiser et al., 2015). It is also in that light that SMGs are proposed as one of the targets for gene therapy. Second, compensatory ion channels have been shown to alleviate the CFTR defect in CF mice. Besides Ca^{2+}-activated chloride channels which provide another source of Cl^- secretion, ATP12A, the non-gastric form of the H^+/K^+-ATPase, is hardly expressed in mice, explaining the absence of ASL acidification (Shah et al., 2016b). By contrast, in CF humans and CF pigs, ATP12A leads to unchecked acidification of the ASL (Shah et al., 2016b; Scudieri et al., 2018), which is not neutralized by CFTR-mediated bicarbonate transport in the case of CF, leading to prominent lung disease. A third concept relates to differences in CFTR homology and the effect of revertant or suppressive mutations contributing to a milder lung phenotype in CF mice. For example, mouse and rat CFTR show only 78 and 76% amino acid sequence homology, respectively, compared to humans (Semaniakou et al., 2018). This difference is postulated to explain why the murine CFTR channel exhibits some alterations in pharmacological and gating properties to human CFTR (Bose et al., 2019). Among these sequence differences, suppressive or reverting variants have been identified that attenuate or reverse the severity of a pre-existing disease-causing *CFTR* mutation (Hoelen et al., 2010; Dong et al., 2012; Xu et al., 2014). In the nucleotide binding domain 1 (NBD1) sequence, the amino acid at position 539

TABLE 1 | Knock-in CF animal models.

Species	Mutation	Editing technology	Insertion	CF phenotype	References
Mouse	F508del	Plasmid	HR	Peritonitis, intestinal obstruction Electrophysiological abnormalities in trachea and colon epithelium Distention and mucus hyper-accumulation in intestinal glands and colon mRNA expression lower than WT	Colledge et al. (1995)
Mouse	F508del	Plasmid	HR	Growth retardation Hypertrophy of goblet cells in intestine Residual CFTR function in nasal, intestinal and gallbladder epithelium	van Doorninck et al. (1995)
Mouse	F508del	Plasmid	HR	Growth retardation Peritonitis, intestinal obstruction Electrophysiological abnormalities in nasal, intestinal and pancreatic epithelium Inflammatory cells in broncho-alveolar lavage	Zeiher et al. (1995)
Mouse	G551D	Plasmid	HR	Intestinal obstruction, peritonitis Electrophysiological abnormalities in nasal, tracheal and intestinal epithelium	Delaney et al. (1996)
Mouse	G480C	Plasmid	HR	Hypertrophy of goblet cells in intestine Electrophysiological abnormalities in nasal epithelium	Dickinson et al. (2002)
Mouse	R117H	NR	HR	Growth retardation Electrophysiological abnormalities in nasal epithelium	van Heeckeren et al. (2004)
Pig	F508del	rAAV	HR	Intestinal obstruction Liver steatosis Pancreatic abnormalities CF lung disease: Airway obstruction, host-defense defect Residual CFTR function in nasal and pancreatic epithelium	Rogers et al. (2008), Ostedgaard et al. (2011)
Mouse	G542X	CRISPR/Cas9	HR	Growth retardation Intestinal obstruction No CFTR activity in airway and intestinal epithelium	McHugh et al. (2018)
Rat	F508del	CRISPR/Cas9	HR	Growth retardation Abnormal dentition Intestinal obstruction Residual CFTR function in airway and colon epithelium	Dreano et al. (2019)
Ferret	G551D	rAAV	HR	Intestinal obstruction mRNA expression reduced in lung and intestine Protein expression reduced in lung Electrophysiological abnormalities in intestinal organoids, jejunum and pancreatic ductal epithelium Airway obstruction Reproductive tract malformations	Sun et al. (2019)
Rat	F508del	CRISPR/Cas9	HR	Growth retardation Abnormal dentition Intestinal obstruction Residual CFTR function in nasal epithelium Reproductive tract malformations	McCarron et al. (2020)
Rat	G542X	CRISPR/Cas9	HR	Growth retardation Abnormal dentition Intestinal obstruction No CFTR activity in airway and intestinal epithelium mRNA degradation (NMD)	Sharma et al. (2020)

Abbreviations: CRISPR/Cas, Clustered Regularly Interspaced Short Palindromic Repeats/CRISPR associated protein; HR, Homologous recombination based on the presence of flanking homology arms; KO, Knock-out; NMD, Nonsense-mediated decay; NPD, Nasal potential difference; WT, Wild-type.

differs between species with an isoleucine in humans, ferrets and pigs vs. a threonine in mice. The molecular consequence of this amino acid substitution was investigated in heterologous cell models expressing a chimeric hCFTR-F508del in which the human NBD1 was substituted by murine NBD1 (Dong et al., 2012), showing that the F508del protein maturation defect was attenuated in the chimeric construct. This observation supports the hypothesis that co-expression of isoleucine at position 539 and the F508del mutation presents a possible strategy to develop novel 'humanized' CF mouse models with more prominent lung disease, a topic that will be discussed in the section *Humanized CFTR Animal Models of CF.*

Value of Cftr *KO Animal Models to Validate Gene Therapy Efficacy*

Besides the possibility to correct molecular and functional end-points related to CFTR activity, these KO models and in particular those with a prominent lung phenotype, allow studying a possible improvement of human-relevant lung disease. Two different gene addition rescue strategies conducted in the newborn gut-corrected *Cftr* KO pig, reported on the reversal of impaired bacterial killing and reduced ASL pH, two important hallmarks of CF lung disease (Cooney et al., 2016; Steines et al., 2016). These studies provide the first and exciting evidence that gene therapy holds promise to improve lung disease in a large animal model of CF, with human-relevant lung disease. Extending the use of *Cftr* KO animal models to correct the endogenous *CFTR* locus by gene editing is rather limited in that sense that most gene editing strategies are designed to correct a human disease-causing mutation. The KO models thus can only be of value for gene editing strategies aiming to integrate a super-exon (Bednarski et al., 2016; Suzuki et al., 2020) in the *Cftr* locus (also see the section *Correcting Multiple Mutations at Once*), that in case of a therapeutic super-exon encompasses all the necessary exons to correct the specific *Cftr* KO present in the animal model (Wilke et al., 2011; McCarron et al., 2018; Rosen et al., 2018; Semaniakou et al., 2018).

Human Relevant *CFTR* Mutations in the Animal Orthologue: Knock-in CF Animal Models

The development of genetic engineering tools has made it possible to generate different models expressing a human relevant *CFTR* mutation. Several frequent disease-causing *CFTR* mutations have been inserted into the animal *Cftr* gene to generate knock-in models (**Table 1**). Of the currently 2100 *CFTR* mutations reported, only five have been used to date to develop CF animal models, including R117H (c.350G>A), G480C (c.1438G>T), F508del, G542X (c.1624G>T), and G551D (c.1652G>A). Overall, these models have a generally less severe phenotype than that observed in humans, likely due to the above discussed reasons, and also less severe than their respective KO counterparts per species. As with the KO models, a difference in phenotype is observed according to species (**Table 1**).

Regarding the F508del mutation, rodent models show little airway pathology, but rather a predominant intestinal obstruction, which can be improved by a laxative diet, in contrast to the F508del pig. Although the F508del pig shows very severe digestive and lung pathology, the poor survival of this model makes longitudinal studies challenging (Rogers et al., 2008). Similarly to F508del, the G480C mutation shows impaired processing and trafficking (Smit et al., 1995; Ferec and Cutting, 2012) and likewise is coupled to a severe phenotype in patients (Kristidis et al., 1992). Contrary to human disease, the G480C mouse model only showed hypertrophy of goblet cells in the intestine and an organ-specific electrophysiological defect (defective Cl^- transport in the nose but not in the cecum) (Dickinson et al., 2002). These species-specific phenotypic differences can likely be attributed to the differences in anatomy, ion channel composition and CFTR protein sequence, as discussed above. A complete overview of all knock-in animal models of CF and their organ-specific phenotypes is given in **Table 1**. Despite these species-specific variations, these models remain of interest for the preclinical evaluation of new therapies, as well as for unraveling the mechanisms of disease initiation and progression, while considering the limitations and differences with respect to their translation to humans (Shah et al., 2016b; Scudieri et al., 2018). First, a major asset of these different animal models is that they recapitulate the complex multi-organ disease seen in PwCF and thus allow to evaluate treatment efficacy in different organs (Sun et al., 2019). Second, the complex pulmonary environment of PwCF represents a major extracellular barrier to drug and gene therapy delivery which cannot be fully recapitulated in *in vitro* models, underscoring the need to study drug penetration through the multiple barriers in relevant animals with severe lung disease (Stoltz et al., 2010; Hoegger et al., 2014; Sun et al., 2014; Keiser et al., 2015). Finally, they allow to address long-standing questions which remained unanswered even in primary cell models, such as the presumed irreversibility of exocrine pancreas insufficiency and the obliteration of the vas deferens, both already present prenatally. The first *in utero* administration of potentiator Ivacaftor (VX-770) in the G551D ferret allowed to improve pancreatic exocrine function, as well as rescue vas deferens and epididymis development, suggesting an important role for CFTR early in life in establishing organ function (Sun et al., 2019).

Value of Animal Models with Knock-in of Human CFTR *Mutations to Validate Gene Therapy Efficacy*

The availability of human relevant *CFTR* mutations in animal models is advantageous for evaluating mutation-specific treatments such as gene editing aiming at an *in vivo* delivery approach, at least for those mutations currently modeled in animals (**Table 1**). In that regard, successful *in vivo* gene editing of the F508del mutation in mice has been demonstrated using triplex-forming peptide nucleic acids (PNA) (also see the section *F508del*) (McNeer et al., 2015). By NPD, a partial but significant recovery in CFTR function was demonstrated in the nose. In the lung, a reduction in the number of inflammatory cells in broncho-alveolar lavage fluid (BALF) was indicative of a rescue by F508del-specific PNA treatment. This study hence presents promising work on the first steps toward an *in vivo* gene editing therapy, here tailored to the most common F508del mutation, further showing which read-outs can be used in a knock-in mouse model without prominent lung pathology.

In general, the severe morbidity and mortality associated with CF lung disease, have guided gene therapy efforts toward a lung-directed approach since decades (reviewed in (Carlon et al., 2017; Sondhi et al., 2017)). In that regard, animal models that recapitulate more prominent lung disease and the thereby associated extracellular barriers hampering efficient gene transfer, such as viscous mucus, chronic inflammation and infection, underscore the importance of including these models in the therapeutic development pipeline (Cooney et al., 2016; Steines et al., 2016) (and reviewed in (Mottais et al., 2017). A limitation of current knock-in models, is that despite the *CFTR* gene being phylogenetically conserved between mammals, sequence variations require a species-dependent gRNA, ZFN or TALEN design. Indeed, McNeer and colleagues had to construct two distinct PNA and donor templates to correct either the human F508del in primary HBEs or the murine

TABLE 2 | Introduction of human *CFTR* to generate humanized CFTR animal models.

Species	Background	Mutation	Construction	Insertion	CF phenotype	References
Mouse	*Cftr*^{tmUnc} null mice	h*CFTR* cDNA under control of FABP promoter	Plasmid	Random insertion	Gastro-intestinal pathology rescued by gut-specific expression of *hCFTR* under the FABP promoter	Zhou et al. (1994)
Mouse	*Cftr*^{tm1Cam} null mice	h*CFTR* full gene + regulatory elements (70 kb of flanking sequence)	YAC	Random insertion	Different function according to the founder CFTR function rescued in colon, jejunum and cecum with h*CFTR* expression under endogenous promoter	Manson et al. (1997)
Mouse	*Cftr*^{tm1Cam} null mice	*hG542X-CFTR* cDNA under control of FAPB promoter	Plasmid	Random insertion	Growth retardation Intestinal obstruction Occasional weak cAMP-stimulated current in intestinal epithelium	Du et al. (2002)
Mouse	*Cftr*^{tmUnc} null mice	*hCFTR* full gene + regulatory elements (40.1 kb At 5′; 25 kb at 3′ end of *hCFTR* gene)	BAC	Random insertion	Abnormal dentition Morphological and functional (nasal and intestinal mucosa) rescue with hCFTR expression under endogenous promoter	Gawenis et al. (2019)
Rat	WT sprague-dawley rat	*h*G551D-*CFTR* cDNA (2–27 exons) under control of endogenous promoter	ZFN and super-exon	HR	Growth retardation Abnormal dentition Intestinal obstruction ASL depletion, PCL decrease, mucus transport decrease and presence of viscous mucus	Birket et al. (2020)

Abbreviations: ASL, airway surface liquid; BAC, Bacterial artificial chromosome; FABP, Fatty acid binding protein; hCFTR, human CFTR; HR, Homologous recombination; KO, Knock-out; PCL, periciliary liquid; YAC, yeast artificial chromosome; WT, wild-type; ZFN, Zinc finger nuclease.

F508del in the CF mouse model used (McNeer et al., 2015). While at first sight, this species-specific testing might limit the direct translation of editing tools to humans, other factors likely are of more importance, such as the delivery vehicle which determines tropism and targeting efficiency. Nevertheless, one of the strategies to overcome cross-species genotype and phenotype variations, is to develop humanized animal models of CF.

Humanized *CFTR* Animal Models of CF

Humanized *CFTR* animal models of CF can be divided in two main classes (**Table 2**). The first class includes transgenic models with a random insertion of the human *CFTR* cDNA or full gene into the genome of *Cftr* KO mice. The second class corresponds to humanized models in which the *Cftr* mouse gene is replaced by the human *CFTR* cDNA via homologous recombination strategies. A first transgenic mouse model was developed in 1994, the so-called 'gut rescued' KO mouse, where the human *CFTR* cDNA under control of the intestinal fatty acid binding protein (FABP) promoter was randomly inserted into a *Cftr* KO model (Zhou et al., 1994). The local expression of this transgene made it possible to rescue CF intestinal pathology and thus increase the survival of these transgenic mice, thereby increasing the overall applicability to study therapeutic interventions among others. In a similar manner, a gut-rescued KO ferret and pig were made, though with the animal orthologue (Sun et al., 2010; Stoltz et al., 2013). Also, human relevant *CFTR* mutations have been introduced into humanized CF animal models, a first one being the most prevalent nonsense mutation, G542X. Similar to the gut corrected models, this transgenic mouse was constructed from a *Cftr* KO model in which the *G542X-CFTR* cDNA under the control of the FABP promoter ensured local expression of G542X-CFTR in the gastro-intestinal tract. So far, this model has been used to test translational read-through inducing drugs in their ability to pharmacologically correct premature termination codons (PTCs) in CFTR (Du et al., 2002; Du et al., 2006). These corrections were measured by analysis of survival rate, CFTR function (I_{sc}) and hCFTR expression in the intestine.

Two other transgenic models have been generated using yeast artificial chromosomes (YAC) (Manson et al. (1997)) and recently also bacterial artificial chromosomes (BAC) (Gawenis et al., 2019). They have as most prominent advantage the possibility to incorporate the entire h*CFTR* gene, including all necessary regulatory elements that control its expression, which is impossible using plasmid or viral vector technology. The BAC transgenic mouse with functional hCFTR was generated with the specific purpose to enable the subsequent generation of mouse models with *hCFTR* mutations, to support future *in vivo* testing of new CF therapies, pharmacologic or gene therapeutic (Gawenis et al., 2019). Phenotypically, all CF-specific organ pathologies were rescued to WT levels, with the exception of the abnormal dentition. Follow-up studies will likely follow, reporting on the introduction of human *CFTR* mutations in this BAC transgenic mouse model, which will allow studying mutations and rescue strategies in a congenic background.

Recently, a humanized transgenic G551D rat model was generated (Birket et al., 2020), the rationale being that pharmacological responses are often species-specific, such as the differential Ivacaftor response of mouse vs. human F508del-CFTR (Bose et al., 2019). A *hCFTR* cDNA super-exon, spanning exon 2–27 was inserted using ZFNs with a 5′ insertion site into the rat *Cftr* gene just beyond intron 1. This targeted insertion allows G551D-CFTR expression from the endogenous rat promoter. The G551D rat model developed a

CF phenotype similar to the KO rat and responded, as hypothesized, to potentiator Ivacaftor with a restoration of nasal and tracheal potential difference. Besides a functional recovery of CFTR, also lung disease relevant parameters were normalized, such as airway mucus viscosity, mucociliary clearance and ASL height, the latter implying a restored hydration of the airways.

Value of Humanized CF Animal Models to Validate Gene Therapy Efficacy

Generating humanized animal models of disease is an interesting approach that is gaining ground in biomedical research because of several advantages. First, disease phenotypes might more closely resemble human disease, compared to knock-in models where mutations are introduced into the animal orthologue, as interspecies sequence variations and reverting mutations are abolished. However, other confounding factors remain, such as differences in anatomy and ion channel composition. Second, expressing the human protein in an *in vivo* model is advantageous for studying drug responses, both small molecules and gene therapies, as pharmacodynamics and -kinetics ultimately determine the net uptake and tissue-specific responses to the drug. Third, the delivery of very large inserts by artificial chromosomes (YAC, BAC) opens up possibilities to not only insert cDNA, mini-genes or super-exons, but even complete genes with their regulatory elements that contribute to the tissue-specific and dynamic expression of hCFTR. This level of transcriptional control allows a more faithful and human-relevant evaluation of specific therapies for which the non-coding elements contribute to the rescue efficacy, such as PTC modulating agents and therapies aiming to correct splicing mutations (reviewed in (Clancy et al., 2019)).

On the other hand, humanized animal models hold possible limitations which should be considered. A potential risk is that the humanized protein e.g., CFTR, might interact differently with the animal-specific cellular environment, for example based on altered protein-protein interactions. In that light, the humanized G551D rat did not show a difference in the amiloride-sensitive transepithelial potential difference compared to WT-CFTR (Birket et al., 2020). We hypothesize that this might reflect a distinct, non-inhibiting interaction between human CFTR and the murine epithelial Na^+ channel. Another potential limitation of humanized models is that the animal transcription factor orthologues might not bind the inserted human regulatory regions with the same specificity, potentially resulting in altered hCFTR expression. Further, other cellular mechanisms, such as RNA splicing or chaperone-assisted CFTR folding could potentially differ between species and hinder the utility of reliable humanized animal models (Zhu et al., 2019). These theoretical limitations should be kept in mind and experimentally verified during the development process of the humanized animal model to ensure their value in the therapeutic discovery pipeline.

Possible future perspectives include the development of even closer animal mimics of human CF disease such as compound heterozygous genotypes (i.e., two different mutant *CFTR* alleles), which is frequently the case in CF patients. This would allow a better understanding of the complex genotype-phenotype relations leading to organ-specific CF pathophysiology, as well as more reliable functional responses in the development of new therapeutics.

GENE EDITING TO CORRECT MUTATIONS IN *CFTR*: WHAT HAS BEEN DONE?

Gene editing to correct mutations at the endogenous *CFTR* locus remains a rather recent field, compared to other therapeutic strategies for CF, like gene addition and CFTR modulators. Nevertheless, many proof-of-concept studies in CF cell models, including primary intestinal organoids, airway cultures and induced pluripotent stem cells (iPSCs), have already shown that correction of *CFTR* mutations is feasible. A comprehensive overview of all these studies is given in the next section.

Currently, the use of nucleases combined with HDR has been most widely investigated. Gene editing usually is highly mutation specific, and since CF is caused by at least 360 different mutations, covering base conversions as well as small and large insertions and deletions, multiple strategies will be needed to model all mutations or develop a treatment for all PwCF. For an overview of how many mutations can theoretically be covered by each gene editing strategy, we refer to (Maule et al., 2021). The *CFTR* gene spans a >180 kb region and some parts will be more suited for editing compared to others e.g., when it comes to the availability of PAM sites or GC content. Therefore, most likely different strategies will need to be tested and tailored to each specific mutation.

Before these proof-of-concept studies can be translated toward a therapy, further optimizations are needed and additional questions remain to be addressed. For example, many strategies to date used antibiotic selection to enrich edited cells, which is not compatible with *in vivo* therapies. Will genetic treatment be most effective when editing tools are delivered *in vivo,* or rather as an *ex vivo* cell therapeutic approach, requiring successful engraftment in the target organ? For some disorders this is easily decided, such as the *ex vivo* route for hematological disorders (Corbacioglu et al., 2020) and the *in vivo* strategy for inherited blindness (Editas, 2020), but for CF this question remains unanswered. Delivery of the editing machinery will have to be optimized since plasmid, mRNA or ribonucleoprotein (RNP) transfection or electroporation, while efficient in cell culture, does not translate to direct *in vivo* delivery to patients. Unlike the highly specific gene editors themselves, translation from proof-of-concept editing in cells toward a patient-directed therapy will likely be more generic, as one or a few optimized delivery vehicles can incorporate any given gene editing tool set.

Despite the current lack of immediate translational potential, these proof-of-concepts report on the efficiency and safety of editing specific *CFTR* mutations in relevant cell and animal models of CF. These preliminary but encouraging studies have set the stage to further invest in the translation of gene editing toward its future in patient use. Importantly, gene editing technology has leveraged the generation of CF cell and animal models, which allows gaining better insights into CF disease mechanisms which might be mutation specific, and hence require a tailored therapeutic intervention. In the next section we will first discuss different proof-of-concept gene editing examples for CF, correcting F508del, intronic splicing mutations, nonsense mutations, and the possibility to correct multiple mutations at once with super-exons, as well as introducing these mutations to generate CF models. Next, we will also discuss how these could be translated into therapies.

Proof-of-Concept Gene Editing for CF

F508del

So far, most CF gene editing efforts have focused on restoring F508del, as this is the most common *CFTR* mutation, accounting for ~70% of all CF alleles. Early studies used ZFNs to target the F508del region in heterologous cell lines, to validate this region could be targeted by ZFNs but did not yet correct the mutation (Maeder et al., 2008). Several years later, F508del was corrected using ZFNs and a donor DNA template containing the wild type (WT) sequence in CF tracheal epithelial cells, albeit with efficiencies below 1% (Lee et al., 2012). This could be improved to 1.9% with the use of Cas9 and an optimized repair template (Hollywood et al., 2016). Since the latter contained the complete exon 11 (containing the F508del mutation) this same strategy could potentially also be applied to any of the other twenty CF-causing mutations in this exon. Correction of F508del and I507del was also obtained using HDR following ZFN-induced DSBs in iPSCs from PwCF who were compound heterozygous for both mutations (Crane et al., 2015). Corrected cells were enriched by including a puromycin-thymidine kinase cassette in the HDR template, which allowed positive puromycin selection and subsequent negative selection with ganciclovir after excision of the selection cassette by Cre recombinase. When corrected clones were subsequently differentiated into epithelial cells, they expressed CFTR which matured correctly and functionally responded in I_{sc} measurements like WT samples. A similar selection cassette was used to correct F508del/F508del iPSCs using a Cas9 nuclease, but excision was mediated via a piggyBac transposase rather than Cre, thereby providing footprint-free editing with ~15% efficacy (Firth et al., 2015). When differentiated into proximal airway epithelial cells these clones showed corrected CFTR maturation and function, by Western blot and I_{sc} analysis, respectively.

Alternatively, F508del-containing iPSCs were corrected using TALENs and an SDF (small/short DNA fragment) donor of around 500 nt (Sargent et al., 2014; Suzuki et al., 2016). After several rounds of selection-marker-free selection, corrected clones were differentiated into airway cells, demonstrating functional CFTR. F508del homozygous iPSCs were also corrected using Cas9 and F508del-specific sgRNAs with ~2.4% efficacy (Smirnikhina et al., 2020). Recently, puromycin selection of TALEN-corrected iPSCs resulted in ~10% F508del correction efficiency (Fleischer et al., 2020). Clones were differentiated into intestinal organoids and their functional rescue was shown by CFTR-dependent organoid swelling upon stimulation with the cAMP agonist forskolin. Primary intestinal organoids homozygous for the F508del mutation had previously also directly been edited using Cas9 and an HDR template with a puromycin selection cassette (Schwank et al., 2013).

All of these examples have in common however, that either F508del was gene edited at low efficiency or that one or multiple rounds of selection were required in order to enrich the edited cells. Moreover, analysis of CFTR function took place on sequencing-verified, corrected clones. Neither selection nor screening of clones is translatable into an *in vivo* gene therapy approach, so for this strategy, editing efficiencies should be further improved. By optimizing electroporation of CRISPR-Cas9 components as RNPs combined with a single strand oligodeoxynucleotide (ssODN) repair template, F508del correction efficiencies of ~22% could be achieved without selection in iPSCs (Ruan et al., 2019). When repaired clones were differentiated into proximal lung organoids, forskolin-induced organoid swelling confirmed the genetic correction of F508del to WT or carrier (the latter phenotypically similar to WT). Also, nuclease-independent HDR-mediated editing of F508del by means of triplex-forming peptide nucleic acids (PNAs) has been described (McNeer et al., 2015). Formation of a PNA/DNA/PNA triplex will initiate DNA repair mechanisms to allow recombination. For an overview of the use of PNAs in gene editing we refer to (Ricciardi et al., 2018). CFBE41o-cells, a frequently used human F508del/F508del cell line, were corrected with an efficiency of 9.2%, while mouse *F508del-Cftr* was corrected *in vivo* at efficiencies of 5.7 and 1.2% in nasal and pulmonary epithelium, respectively, after intranasal delivery of nanoparticles (McNeer et al., 2015). The *in vivo* editing partially rescued CFTR function in the nasal epithelium, as measured by NPD.

Recently, studies have focused on correcting *F508del-CFTR* in airway progenitor cells, *i.e.* basal cells, a potentially interesting cell type for *ex vivo* stem cell therapy (Suzuki et al., 2020; Vaidyanathan et al., 2020). RNP electroporation and delivery of a donor template by adeno-associated viral vector serotype 6 (AAV6) transduction resulted in F508del correction in 28% of alleles in F508del/F508del samples and 42% in compound heterozygous samples (Vaidyanathan et al., 2020). ALI cultures derived from these upper airway basal cells (UABCs) showed rescued CFTR maturation and function. Alternatively, ZFN mRNA electroporation in combination with AAV6 donor template transduction resulted in 31% allele correction and restoration of CFTR expression and function in ALI cultures (Suzuki et al., 2020).

Due to the fact that F508del results from a three-nucleotide deletion, it cannot be corrected by base editing. However, it is an interesting target for prime editing, as this editor allows installing small insertions, like the CTT insertion needed to correct F508del. Very recently, the first prime editing attempts for the F508del mutation were reported in primary intestinal organoids, currently still a pre-print (Geurts et al., 2020b). Although efficiencies were very low compared to HDR gene editing, electroporation of PE3 (optimized prime editor, pegRNA and additional ngRNA) plasmids resulted in a genetic correction and recovery of CFTR channel function in a few corrected organoid clones.

Intronic Splicing Mutations

As CF is caused by loss-of-function mutations throughout the *CFTR* gene, the use of nucleases to correct disease-causing mutations without subsequent repair by HDR is restricted to a small group of specific mutations. Intronic mutations can create cryptic donor or acceptor splice sites which result in the incorporation of extra nucleotides into the *CFTR* mRNA. Often, this causes frameshifts, completely disrupting the remainder of the protein sequence. However, as low levels of transcripts get normally spliced, these intronic or cryptic splicing mutations are generally associated with relatively mild CF (as determined by pancreatic sufficiency) (CFTR2, 2021). Since intronic regions are less conserved compared to exons and do not code for proteins, removal of the cryptic splice site can be achieved by NHEJ which is more efficient than HDR and abolishes the need to deliver a donor template. Excising or disrupting the cryptic splice site by inducing indels is hence sufficient to restore the WT *CFTR* mRNA. In that regard, the feasibility of correcting the intronic splicing mutations 1811 + 1.6kbA > G (c.1680-886A > G), 3272-26A > G (c.3140-26A > G) and 3849 + 10kbC > T (c.3718–2477C > T) has been shown by excising these mutations using SpCas9 and two flanking sgRNAs in cell lines overexpressing the respective *CFTR* minigenes. This resulted in up to 90% of corrected minigene splicing depending on the mutation targeted (Sanz et al., 2017). In patient-derived airway cells and intestinal organoids 3272-26A > G and 3849 + 10kbC > T were corrected making use of a single mutation-specific sgRNA in combination with Cas12a (Maule et al., 2019). Specifically, 85% of mutant alleles were successfully edited in compound heterozygous organoids, while less than 1% of the other *CFTR* allele was targeted. CFTR activity of gene edited organoids reached similar levels as those transduced with a lentiviral vector encoding *WT-CFTR* cDNA without the need for prior enrichment, underscoring the efficiency and safety of this gene editing approach. While for CF this strategy to treat intronic splicing mutations has only been studied as a proof-of-concept so far, a similar strategy to cure Leber congenital amaurosis is currently already being investigated in a clinical setting (EDIT-101, NCT03872479 (Maeder et al., 2019)).

Nonsense Mutations

Nonsense mutations account for ~5% of disease-causing alleles in CF and are associated with severe CF (CFTR2, 2021). They introduce PTCs which give rise to truncated proteins. Due to the presence of the PTC there are exon boundaries on the pre-mRNA after the stop codon, which often subjects it to NMD (reviewed in (Kurosaki and Maquat, 2016)). NMD leads to very low expression levels of mutant transcripts, further complicating rescue by small molecules. To date, no causal therapies have been approved for nonsense mutations in CF. However, drug discovery efforts are ongoing to identify more effective translational read-through inducing drugs than the most advanced drug tested so far in clinical trials i.e., Ataluren, which due to lack of efficacy in patients was discontinued (Kerem et al., 2014). In parallel, also gene editing strategies are being pursued as an alternative with the potential of even providing a cure. In that light, ABE was evaluated to correct a number of nonsense mutations (R553X (c.1657C > T), R785X (c.2353C > T), R1162X (c.3484C > T) and W1282X) in primary intestinal organoids (Geurts et al., 2020a). ABE plasmids were electroporated and treated cells were enriched via selection. This resulted in editing efficiencies between 1.43 and 8.8%, depending on the mutation. Individual corrected organoids showed CFTR dependent swelling upon forskolin stimulation, confirming their functional correction and allowing to phenotypically select corrected organoids. Interestingly in a pre-print, for the R785X mutation, correction efficiencies were compared between HDR, ABE and prime editing in primary intestinal organoids. ABE resulted in approximately 6 times more forskolin-responsive organoids than HDR and prime editing, the latter both showing similar efficiencies (Geurts et al., 2020b).

W1282X, the second most common CF-causing nonsense mutation, has also been corrected by mRNA electroporation of ABE in a W1282X-encoding cell line, resulting in ~26% base conversion which rescued 10% of CFTR protein expression (Jiang et al., 2020). Of note, the editing window contained a second adenine, which was edited more efficiently than the target adenine (~45%) and introduced a missense mutation (Q1281R). This bystander edit, however, did not preclude a functional rescue of CFTR activity when both edits were present on the same allele. Nevertheless, it shows the importance of functionally evaluating the effect of possible bystander edits when applying base editing. An alternative approach for W1282X that focused on rescuing its expression by preventing NMD has also been described. The simultaneous use of two gRNAs, the first targeting exon 23 in an W1282X-specific manner, and the second exon 27, induced a 24 kb deletion which removed the exon boundaries downstream from the W1282X mutation, thereby preventing NMD (Erwood et al., 2020). Indeed, this deletion resulted in a 2.4-fold increase in the expression of the truncated mRNA and protein in human bronchial epithelial cells. The truncated protein could functionally be rescued by existing CFTR correctors and potentiators, providing a novel combination treatment potentially applicable to patients harboring this C-terminal nonsense mutation. While this approach thus allows to functionally rescue W1282X, it will likely not be translatable to other, more N-terminally located nonsense mutations, such as the most common nonsense mutation G542X, because this strategy is based on downstream deletion of the remainder of the *CFTR* gene.

Correcting Multiple Mutations at Once: Super-Exons

Most examples that have been discussed so far have focused on highly mutation-specific strategies using nucleases, base and prime editors. There is however another strategy that uses HDR to potentially correct not one but many mutations at the same time: targeted integration of a super-exon (reviewed in (Mention et al., 2019)). Super-exons code for the part of the *CFTR* cDNA downstream of the integration site, which get integrated into the endogenous *CFTR* locus. In this way, regulation of protein expression remains unaltered which is potentially advantageous over classical gene addition where an entire *CFTR* cDNA under control of an external promoter is randomly integrated into the host genome. Super-exons allow to correct all mutations included into this partial cDNA, so ultimately the integration site will determine which mutations are rescued by a super-exon strategy. In order to rescue F508del (and all other mutations located in exons 11–27 of *CFTR*) a super-exon was integrated into exon 11 in CFBE41o-cells using ZFNs followed by HDR (Bednarski et al., 2016). The super-exon also contained a puromycin cassette which allowed selection of edited clones and resulted in ~10% integration efficiency. In a corrected clone, CFTR activity was comparable to a non-CF sample. Recently, a similar approach was investigated by integrating a cDNA containing exons 9–27 into intron 8 or exons 8–27 into intron 7 of *CFTR*, using ZFN electroporation combined with AAV6 transduction to deliver the repair template in patient derived airway basal cells (Suzuki et al., 2020). Integration efficiencies ranged from ~36 (in intron 7) to ~56% (in intron 8), restoring CFTR activity to ~30 and ~40% of non-CF levels, respectively, in ALI.

Introducing Mutations into *CFTR*

Gene editing can also be applied to create new CF models by introducing disease-causing mutations into the *CFTR* gene. One such application is to generate isogenic cell lines i.e., CF and non-CF lines with the same genetic background, to allow studying the molecular defects of *CFTR* mutations in the absence of variable donor backgrounds. This is of particular interest in CF as responses to CFTR modulators have been highly variable between patients with the same *CFTR* genotype in clinical trials (Heijerman et al., 2019; Middleton et al., 2019), as well as in patient-derived samples (Dekkers et al., 2016), likely due to modifier genes and differences in the cellular environment. Isogenic cell lines have been generated starting from the often-used 16HBE14o-cell line, using CRISPR-Cas RNPs and a ssODN donor template to install the F508del, G542X, and W1282X mutations into the *CFTR* gene (Valley et al., 2019). Subsequently, the polymorphism V470M was introduced into the gene edited F508del cells, as F508del is exclusively associated with M470 which might influence disease characteristics. G542X and W1282X edited cells showed NMD levels in line with primary cell material, and responded well to NMD inhibition or PTC readthrough agents, underscoring the translational potential of these gene edited isogenic cell lines. Of note, while homozygous editing was obtained, deep sequencing of the *CFTR* gene revealed an intronic insertion from the immortalization process of the parental 16HBE14o-cells on one of the two alleles, which was consequently knocked out. Alternatively, the F508del, G551D and G542X mutations have been introduced into non-CF iPSCs, using a similar strategy, as well as the compound heterozygous F508del/G551D genotype (Ruan et al., 2019). While so far, the focus has been on generating models for the more common *CFTR* mutations, gene editing opens up opportunities to also model rare *CFTR* mutations. As homozygous samples are often not available and the presence of the other mutant *CFTR* allele (most commonly F508del) confounds the interpretation of the functional response measured, isogenic cell lines will allow to unbiasedly determine the molecular defect and treatment responses of each of these mutations.

From Proof-of-Concept to Therapy

As proof-of-concept studies have shown the feasibility to correct CF at the genomic level, enthusiasm and expectations are booming to rapidly translate these studies into therapies. However, before gene editing can be translated toward a treatment for PwCF, several questions need to be addressed. As mentioned previously, gene editing for CF could either be *ex vivo* or *in vivo*. So far, gene editing that has made it into clinical trials mainly consists of *ex vivo* examples (reviewed in (Hampton, 2020; Hirakawa et al., 2020)). *Ex vivo* cell therapy for CF however is a recent field, and no clinical trials were performed yet, either for gene editing or classical gene addition gene therapy. After sufficiently efficient correction, it will be key to successfully engraft the edited cells into the airway epithelium. Particularly in CF, this airway is severely inflamed and covered with thick mucus, which will further complicate this process. Nevertheless, edited UABCs from an F508del/F508del donor could be grown on an FDA-approved biodegradable scaffold while maintaining their differentiation potential and CFTR expression, a first step toward translation to an *ex vivo* cell therapy (Vaidyanathan et al., 2020). For an overview of the challenges for cell-based therapies for CF, we refer to (Berical et al., 2019). For *in vivo* gene therapy on the other hand, there have been many clinical trials in the past investigating gene addition gene therapy for CF (reviewed in (Sondhi et al., 2017)), although eventually all were discontinued. From these studies however, it became evident that sufficient numbers of cells need to be targeted, preferably progenitor cells i.e., basal cells, to provide long-term *CFTR* correction rather than the transient effects that were observed in clinical trials so far. Alternatively, if long-term correction cannot be achieved, repeated administrations will be necessary to maintain a functional "cure" for CF. Immune responses, both innate and pre-existing or acquired neutralizing antibodies, against vector components (reviewed in (Shirley et al., 2020)), gene editing components (reviewed in (Mehta and Merkel, 2020)), or even the CFTR protein (Figueredo et al., 2007; Limberis et al., 2007), might hamper efficacy of gene therapies and should be taken into consideration.

Delivery of the gene editing components into target cells also needs to be considered and will likely depend on the chosen strategy i.e., *in vivo* or *ex vivo*. Nuclease, guide (and donor template) should be expressed simultaneously in order to allow editing, but expression of the nuclease should, at the same time, be restricted in time so as to reduce the chance of off-targets. Gene editing components can be delivered either as plasmids, nuclease mRNA (with sgRNA) or RNP (reviewed in (Lino et al., 2018)). Equally important is the packaging of these components, so that they can efficiently reach and enter the target cells. Packaging can be either viral or non-viral (reviewed in (Maule et al., 2021)). Viral vectors are the most efficient in delivering cargo to target cells. As such, lentiviral vectors have been used to deliver Cas12a to intestinal organoids for correcting intronic splicing mutations (Maule et al., 2019). Depending on the viral vector, tropisms and immune responses vary, but transgene expression is usually medium to long-term, which is not preferred for nucleases. As an alternative, virus-like particles (VLPs) are developed to combine efficient delivery with transient transgene expression. VLPs mimic the protein structures of viruses but lack a viral

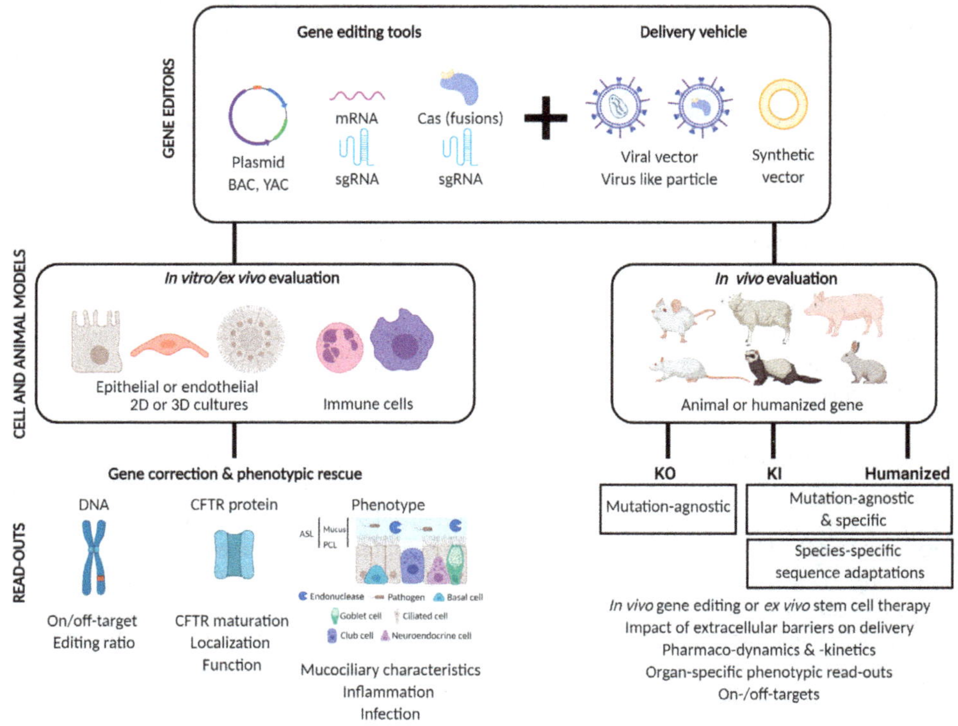

FIGURE 2 | Gene editing strategies for CF from proof-of-concept to their translation into a therapy. Gene editing for CF consists of correcting mutations in *CFTR* either by an *ex vivo* stem cell therapy approach or by directly editing target cells *in vivo*. To transfer gene editors as nucleic acids or proteins into cells, it is likely necessary, particularly for the *in vivo* approach, to encapsulate them with a vector in order to protect them and facilitate their entry into target cells. For their clinical translation, *in vitro/ ex vivo* and *in vivo* models are essential to determine the best formulation that allows efficient and safe gene editing. *In vitro* and *ex vivo* models allow evaluating gene editing efficacy at three levels: genomic, protein and physiological. Summarized, this starts by demonstrating a genetic correction with low off-targets, followed by a normalization of CFTR expression, folding and function, to end with a rescue of pathophysiological defects induced by mutant CFTR. Patient derived cell models furthermore allow developing personalized formulations for each patient. Animal models mimicking CF pathophysiology are a major asset to study the efficacy of the gene editing delivery vehicle in a clinically relevant environment. This, as extracellular barriers must be overcome such as thick and viscous mucus, pathogens or endonucleases to allow efficient gene transfer. Knock-out, knock-in and humanized models each have their specific advantages and limitations that should be considered for an *in vivo* evaluation. Abbreviations: ASL, airway surface liquid; BAC, bacterial artificial chromosome; Cas, CRISPR associated protein; KI, Knock-in models; KO, Knock-out models; PCL, periciliary liquid; sgRNA, single guide RNA; YAC, yeast artificial chromosome.

genome, and can be filled with an RNA or protein cargo (reviewed in (Roldão et al., 2017)). Finally, non-viral vectors provide an alternative to deliver gene editing components to cells. They contain lipid, polymeric or inorganic particles which are less immunogenic than viral vectors and unlike viral vectors are not restricted in their packaging capacity, allowing to incorporate large cargos (reviewed in (Wilbie et al., 2019)). Non-viral nanoparticle-based delivery of PNA/DNA was used to correct mouse F508del in CF mice (McNeer et al., 2015). Independent of the gene therapy and delivery method, it is of the utmost importance that these are evaluated well preclinically in available cell and animal models. A summary of how the different cell and animal models of CF can be included in the preclinical evaluation of gene editing strategies is given in **Figure 2**.

DISCUSSION

The advent of highly effective CFTR modulator therapies for approximately 90% of CF patients has been a major game changer for PwCF. Besides that, it has transformed therapeutic development efforts to redirect their focus to the last 10% of patients carrying two minimal function mutations, not responsive to the market approved CFTR modulators developed by Vertex Pharmaceuticals. As many of these minimal function mutations are not rescuable by current small molecules, requiring minimal amounts of CFTR protein to further enhance their folding, function, or stability, other therapies need to be developed. Gene therapy, in the form of gene addition of a healthy copy of the human *CFTR* cDNA, has been investigated in more than 25 clinical trials since the early nineties. The most recent of these trials was based on the delivery of monthly doses of a liposome *CFTR* cDNA formulation, and led to a stabilization in lung function, providing hope that further improvements in gene therapy tools will increase the efficacy of such a therapy.

Correcting mutations at the endogenous *CFTR* locus heralds a new era of personalized medicine, which has increased hopes and expectations even more as this technology holds promise to cure the disease, if sufficient numbers of progenitor cells can be targeted in a safe manner. While many promising proof-of-concept studies have shown the feasibility to efficiently and safely repair human *CFTR* mutations in primary cell models, only limited studies have progressed toward an *in vivo* or *ex vivo* stem cell therapy approach. Indeed, there lie the biggest hurdles which require further investigation in order to progress from proof-of-concept to a real therapy. How to deliver in the presence of prominent extracellular barriers in the most affected organ in CF, the lung, remains one of the major hurdles to be tackled. Solutions being pursued in that direction are to treat earlier, before established chronic inflammation, infection and remodeling, or alternatively, to pretreat the lungs with mucolytic or hydrating solutions such as hypertonic saline or mannitol. While the holy grail would be to achieve a life-long correction, repeated doses will likely be necessary, which is only possible if immune responses to vector and gene editors can be controlled. The continuous developments in delivery vehicles, ranging from viral vectors to virus like particles and synthetic vectors provides a broad portfolio for balancing the targeting efficiency with a limited expression of the editing machinery to ensure transient and thus safer gene editing. It is clear that while primary cell models will allow to elucidate which mutations are correctable by the broad portfolio of gene editing tools, animal models will play a crucial role in answering the open questions on delivery, longevity of CFTR correction and how to deal with induced immune responses.

Finally, while single cell transcriptomic approaches have identified rare but high CFTR expressers in the lung, the ionocyte, it is not yet clear how important it will be to target specific cells within the lung, as each cell type plays an important role in protecting the airways from infection. Nevertheless, the prospect of gene editing is exciting and likely in the coming years, many of the open questions and currently identified hurdles will have obtained answers that further guide the development of a gene therapy for all PwCF.

AUTHOR CONTRIBUTIONS

All authors helped conceptualize the review. ME, AM, and MC provided the draft of the manuscript. Gene editing tools and proof-of-concept gene editing in CF were discussed by ME. CF cell models were discussed by ME and MC. CF animal models were discussed by AM, CD, TL, and MC. Tables were provided by AM, figures by ME and AM. Introduction and discussion by AM and MC. All authors critically read and reviewed the final text.

ACKNOWLEDGMENTS

The figures were created using Biorender.

REFERENCES

Alton, E., Stern, M., Farley, R., Jaffe, A., Chadwick, S., Phillips, J., et al. (1999). Cationic lipid-mediated CFTR gene transfer to the lungs and nose of patients with cystic fibrosis: a double-blind placebo-controlled trial. *The Lancet* 353 (9157), 947–954. doi:10.1016/s0140-6736(98)06532-5

Alton, E. W. F. W., Beekman, J. M., Boyd, A. C., Brand, J., Carlon, M. S., Connolly, M. M., et al. (2017). Preparation for a first-in-man lentivirus trial in patients with cystic fibrosis. *Thorax* 72 (2), 137–147. doi:10.1136/thoraxjnl-2016-208406

Anzalone, A. V., Koblan, L. W., and Liu, D. R. (2020). Genome editing with CRISPR-Cas nucleases, base editors, transposases and prime editors. *Nat. Biotechnol.* 38 (7), 824–844. doi:10.1038/s41587-020-0561-9

Anzalone, A. V., Randolph, P. B., Davis, J. R., Sousa, A. A., Koblan, L. W., Levy, J. M., et al. (2019). Search-and-replace genome editing without double-strand breaks or donor DNA. *Nature* 576 (7785), 149–157. doi:10.1038/s41586-019-1711-4

Arbab, M., Shen, M. W., Mok, B., Wilson, C., Matuszek, Ż., Cassa, C. A., et al. (2020). Determinants of base editing outcomes from target library analysis and machine learning. *Cell* 182 (2), 463–480. doi:10.1016/j.cell.2020.05.037

Auriche, C., Carpani, D., Conese, M., Caci, E., Zegarra-Moran, O., Donini, P., et al. (2002). Functional human CFTR produced by a stable minichromosome. *EMBO Rep.* 3 (9), 862–868. doi:10.1093/embo-reports/kvf174

Barnaby, R., Koeppen, K., Nymon, A., Hampton, T. H., Berwin, B., Ashare, A., et al. (2018). Lumacaftor (VX-809) restores the ability of CF macrophages to phagocytose and kill *Pseudomonas aeruginosa*. *Am. J. Physiol.-Lung Cell Mol. Physiol.* 314 (3), L432–L438. doi:10.1152/ajplung.00461.2017

Bednarski, C., Tomczak, K., vom Hövel, B., Weber, W.-M., and Cathomen, T. (2016). Targeted integration of a super-exon into the CFTR locus leads to functional correction of a cystic fibrosis cell line model. *PLoS One* 11 (8), e0161072, doi:10.1371/journal.pone.0161072

Berical, A., Lee, R. E., Randell, S. H., and Hawkins, F. (2019). Challenges facing airway epithelial cell-based therapy for cystic fibrosis. *Front. Pharmacol.* 10, 74. doi:10.3389/fphar.2019.00074

Birket, S. E., Davis, J. M., Fernandez-Petty, C. M., Henderson, A. G., Oden, A. M., Tang, L., et al. (2020). Ivacaftor reverses airway mucus abnormalities in a rat model harboring a humanized g551d-CFTR. *Am. J. Respir. Crit. Care Med.* 202 (9), 1271–1282. doi:10.1164/rccm.202002-0369OC

Boon, M., Verleden, S. E., Bosch, B., Lammertyn, E. J., McDonough, J. E., Mai, C., et al. (2016). Morphometric analysis of explant lungs in cystic fibrosis. *Am. J. Respir. Crit. Care Med.* 193 (5), 516–526. doi:10.1164/rccm.201507-1281OC

Bose, S. J., Bijvelds, M. J. C., Wang, Y., Liu, J., Cai, Z., Bot, A. G. M., et al. (2019). Differential thermostability and response to cystic fibrosis transmembrane conductance regulator potentiators of human and mouse F508del-CFTR. *Am. J. Physiol.-Lung Cell Mol. Physiol.* 317 (1), L71–L86. doi:10.1152/ajplung.00034.2019

Botelho, H. M., Uliyakina, I., Awatade, N. T., Proença, M. C., Tischer, C., Sirianant, L., et al. (2015). Protein traffic disorders: an effective high-throughput fluorescence microscopy pipeline for drug discovery. *Sci. Rep.* 5 (1), 9038. doi:10.1038/srep09038

Bruscia, E. M., Zhang, P.-X., Satoh, A., Caputo, C., Medzhitov, R., Shenoy, A., et al. (2011). Abnormal trafficking and degradation of TLR4 underlie the elevated inflammatory response in cystic fibrosis. *J. Immunol.* 186 (12), 6990–6998. doi:10.4049/jimmunol.1100396

Burgel, P. R., Munck, A., Durieu, I., Chiron, R., Mely, L., Prevotat, A., et al. (2020). Real-life safety and effectiveness of lumacaftor-ivacaftor in patients with cystic fibrosis. *Am. J. Respir. Crit. Care Med.* 201 (2), 188–197. doi:10.1164/rccm.201906-1227OC

Caputo, A., Hinzpeter, A., Caci, E., Pedemonte, N., Arous, N., Di Duca, M., et al. (2009). Mutation-specific potency and efficacy of cystic fibrosis transmembrane conductance regulator chloride channel potentiators. *J. Pharmacol. Exp. Ther.* 330 (3), 783–791. doi:10.1124/jpet.109.154146

Carlon, M. S., Vidović, D., and Birket, S. (2017). Roadmap for an early gene therapy for cystic fibrosis airway disease. *Prenatal Diagn.* 37 (12), 1181–1190. doi:10.1002/pd.5164

CFF (2020). Available at: https://www.cff.org/Research/Researcher-Resources/Tools-and-Resources/CFFT-Biorepository/CFF-16HBEge-Cell-Lines.pdf (Accessed January 20, 2021)

CFF (2019). Path to a cure: Many routes One Mission | CF Foundation [Online]. Available at: https://www.cff.org/Research/About-Our-Research/Path-to-a-Cure-Many-Routes-One-Mission (Accessed October 17, 2020).

CFTR2 (2021). Clinical and functional Translation of CFTR (CFTR2) [Online]. Available at: www.CFTR2.org (Accessed January 17, 2021).

Clancy, J. P., Cotton, C. U., Donaldson, S. H., Solomon, G. M., Vandevanter, D. R., Boyle, M. P., et al. (2019). CFTR modulator theratyping: current status, gaps and future directions. *J. Cystic Fibrosis* 18 (1), 22–34. doi:10.1016/j.jcf.2018.05.004

Clarke, L. L., Gawenis, L. R., Franklin, C. L., and Harline, M. C. (1996). Increased survival of CFTR knockout mice with an oral osmotic laxative. *Lab. Anim. Sci.* 46 (6), 612–618.

Cohen, T. S., and Prince, A. (2012). Cystic fibrosis: a mucosal immunodeficiency syndrome. *Nat. Med.* 18 (4), 509–519. doi:10.1038/nm.2715

Colledge, W. H., Abella, B. S., Southern, K. W., Ratcliff, R., Jiang, C., Cheng, S. H., et al. (1995). Generation and characterization of a ΔF508 cystic fibrosis mouse model. *Nat. Genet.* 10 (4), 445–452. doi:10.1038/ng0895-445

Cooney, A. L., Abou Alaiwa, M. H., Shah, V. S., Bouzek, D. C., Stroik, M. R., Powers, L. S., et al. (2016). Lentiviral-mediated phenotypic correction of cystic fibrosis pigs. *JCI Insight* 1 (14), e88730. doi:10.1172/jci.insight.88730

Corbacioglu, S., Cappellini, M. D., Chapin, J., Chu-Osier, N., Fernandez, C. M., Foell, J., et al. (2020). "(S280) Initial safety and efficacy results with a single dose of autologous CRISPR-Cas9 modified CD34+ hematopoietic stem and progenitor cells in transfusion-dependent B-thalassemia and sickle cell disease(EHA25))," in: *European hematology association (EHA) virtual congress.*

Crane, A. M., Kramer, P., Bui, J. H., Chung, W. J., Li, X. S., Gonzalez-Garay, M. L., et al. (2015). Targeted correction and restored function of the CFTR gene in cystic fibrosis induced pluripotent stem cells. *Stem Cel Rep.* 4 (4), 569–577. doi:10.1016/j.stemcr.2015.02.005

Dannhoffer, L., Blouquit-Laye, S., Regnier, A., and Chinet, T. (2009). Functional properties of mixed cystic fibrosis and normal bronchial epithelial cell cultures. *Am. J. Respir. Cel Mol Biol* 40 (6), 717–723. doi:10.1165/rcmb.2008-0018OC

De Boeck, K., and Amaral, M. D. (2016). Progress in therapies for cystic fibrosis. *Lancet Respir. Med.* 4 (8), 662–674. doi:10.1016/S2213-2600(16)00023-0

Declercq, M., de Zeeuw, P., Vasconcelos Conchinha, N., Geldhof, V., Ramalho, A. S., García-Caballero, M., et al. (2020). Transcriptomic analysis of CFTR-impaired endothelial cells reveals a pro-inflammatory phenotype. *Eur. Respir. J.*, 2000261. doi:10.1183/13993003.00261-2020

Declercq, M., Treps, L., Carmeliet, P., and Witters, P. (2019). The role of endothelial cells in cystic fibrosis. *J. Cystic Fibrosis* 18 (6), 752–761. doi:10.1016/j.jcf.2019.07.005

Dekkers, J. F., Berkers, G., Kruisselbrink, E., Vonk, A., De Jonge, H. R., Janssens, H. M., et al. (2016). Characterizing responses to CFTR-modulating drugs using rectal organoids derived from subjects with cystic fibrosis. *Sci. Transl. Med.* 8 (344), 344ra84. doi:10.1126/scitranslmed.aad8278

Dekkers, J. F., Wiegerinck, C. L., De Jonge, H. R., Bronsveld, I., Janssens, H. M., De Winter-De Groot, K. M., et al. (2013). A functional CFTR assay using primary cystic fibrosis intestinal organoids. *Nat. Med.* 19 (7), 939–945. doi:10.1038/nm.3201

Delaney, S. J., Alton, E. W., Smith, S. N., Lunn, D. P., Farley, R., Lovelock, P. K., et al. (1996). Cystic fibrosis mice carrying the missense mutation G551D replicate human genotype-phenotype correlations. *EMBO J.* 15 (5), 955–963.

Dickinson, P., Smith, S. N., Webb, S., Kilanowski, F. M., Campbell, I. J., Taylor, M. S., et al. (2002). The severe G480C cystic fibrosis mutation, when replicated in the mouse, demonstrates mistrafficking, normal survival and organ-specific bioelectrics. *Hum. Mol. Genet.* 11 (3), 243–251. doi:10.1093/hmg/11.3.243

Dong, Q., Ostedgaard, L. S., Rogers, C., Vermeer, D. W., Zhang, Y., and Welsh, M. J. (2012). Human-mouse cystic fibrosis transmembrane conductance regulator (CFTR) chimeras identify regions that partially rescue CFTR- F508 processing and alter its gating defect. *Proc. Natl. Acad. Sci. U.S.A.* 109 (3), 917–922. doi:10.1073/pnas.1120065109

Dreano, E., Bacchetta, M., Simonin, J., Galmiche, L., Usal, C., Slimani, L., et al. (2019). Characterization of two rat models of cystic fibrosis-KO and F508del CFTR-Generated by Crispr-Cas9. *Anim. Models Exp. Med.* 2 (4), 297–311. doi:10.1002/ame2.12091

Du, M., Jones, J. R., Lanier, J., Keeling, K. M., Lindsey, R. J., Tousson, A., et al. (2002). Aminoglycoside suppression of a premature stop mutation in a Cftr−/− mouse carrying a human CFTR-G542X transgene. *J. Mol. Med.* 80 (9), 595–604. doi:10.1007/s00109-002-0363-1

Du, M., Keeling, K. M., Fan, L., Liu, X., Kovaçs, T., Sorscher, E., et al. (2006). Clinical doses of amikacin provide more effective suppression of the human CFTR-G542X stop mutation than gentamicin in a transgenic CF mouse model. *J. Mol. Med.* 84 (7), 573–582. doi:10.1007/s00109-006-0045-5

Editas (2020). Allergan and editas medicine announce dosing of first patient in landmark phase 1/2 clinical trial of CRISPR medicine. Available at: https://ir.editasmedicine.com/news-releases/news-release-details/allergan-and-editas-medicine-announce-dosing-first-patient (Accessed January 20, 2021).

Ensinck, M., De Keersmaecker, L., Heylen, L., Ramalho, A. S., Gijsbers, R., Farré, R., et al. (2020). Phenotyping of rare CFTR mutations reveals distinct trafficking and functional defects. *Cells* 9 (3), 754. doi:10.3390/cells9030754

Erwood, S., Laselva, O., Bily, T. M. I., Brewer, R. A., Rutherford, A. H., Bear, C. E., et al. (2020). Allele-specific prevention of nonsense-mediated decay in cystic fibrosis using homology-independent genome editing. *Mol. Ther. - Methods Clin. Develop.* 17, 1118–1128. doi:10.1016/j.omtm.2020.05.002

Fan, Z., Perisse, I. V., Cotton, C. U., Regouski, M., Meng, Q., Domb, C., et al. (2018). A sheep model of cystic fibrosis generated by CRISPR/Cas9 disruption of the CFTR gene. *JCI Insight* 3 (19), e123529. doi:10.1172/jci.insight.123529

FDA (2017). FDA expands approved use of Kalydeco to treat additional mutations of cystic fibrosis.

Ferec, C., and Cutting, G. R. (2012). Assessing the disease-liability of mutations in CFTR. *Cold Spring Harbor Perspect. Med.* 2 (12), a009480. doi:10.1101/cshperspect.a009480

Fidler, M. C., Buckley, A., Sullivan, J. C., Statia, M., Boj, S. F., Vries, R. G. J., et al. (2020). G970R-CFTR mutation (c.2908G>C) results predominantly in a splicing defect. *Clin. Transl Sci.* 14, 656–663. doi:10.1111/cts.12927

Figueredo, J., Limberis, M. P., and Wilson, J. M. (2007). Prediction of cellular immune responses against CFTR in patients with cystic fibrosis after gene therapy. *Am. J. Respir. Cel Mol Biol* 36 (5), 529–533. doi:10.1165/rcmb.2006-0313CB

Firth, A. L., Menon, T., Parker, G. S., Qualls, S. J., Lewis, B. M., Ke, E., et al. (2015). Functional gene correction for cystic fibrosis in lung epithelial cells generated from patient iPSCs. *Cel Rep.* 12 (9), 1385–1390. doi:10.1016/j.celrep.2015.07.062

Fleischer, A., Vallejo-Díez, S., Martín-Fernández, J. M., Sánchez-Gilabert, A., Castresana, M., Del Pozo, A., et al. (2020). iPSC-Derived Intestinal Organoids from Cystic Fibrosis Patients Acquire CFTR Activity upon TALEN-Mediated Repair of the p.F508del Mutation. *Mol. Ther. - Methods Clin. Develop.* 17, 858–870. doi:10.1016/j.omtm.2020.04.005

Galietta, L. V. J., Jayaraman, S., and Verkman, A. S. (2001). Cell-based assay for high-throughput quantitative screening of CFTR chloride transport agonists. *Am. J. Physiol.-Cell Physiol.* 281 (5), C1734–C1742. doi:10.1152/ajpcell.2001.281.5.c1734

Gasiunas, G., Barrangou, R., Horvath, P., and Siksnys, V. (2012). Cas9-crRNA ribonucleoprotein complex mediates specific DNA cleavage for adaptive immunity in bacteria. *Proc. Natl. Acad. Sci. U.S.A.* 109 (39), E2579–E2586. doi:10.1073/pnas.1208507109

Gaudelli, N. M., Komor, A. C., Rees, H. A., Packer, M. S., Badran, A. H., Bryson, D. I., et al. (2017). Programmable base editing of AT to GC in genomic DNA without DNA cleavage. *Nature* 551 (7681), 464–471. doi:10.1038/nature24644

Gawenis, L. R., Hodges, C. A., McHugh, D. R., Valerio, D. M., Miron, A., Cotton, C. U., et al. (2019). A BAC transgene expressing human CFTR under control of its regulatory elements rescues cftr knockout mice. *Sci. Rep.* 9 (1), 11828. doi:10.1038/s41598-019-48105-4

Geurts, M. H., de Poel, E., Amatngalim, G. D., Oka, R., Meijers, F. M., Kruisselbrink, E., et al. (2020a). CRISPR-based adenine editors correct nonsense mutations in a cystic fibrosis organoid biobank. *Cell Stem Cell* 26 (4), 503–510. doi:10.1016/j.stem.2020.01.019

Geurts, M. H., de Poel, E., Pleguezuelos-Manzano, C., Carrillo, L., Andersson-Rolf, A., Boretto, M., et al. (2020b). Evaluating CRISPR-based Prime Editing for cancer modeling and CFTR repair in intestinal organoids. *bioRxiv* 2010, 325837. doi:10.1101/2020.10.05.325837

Grubb, B. R., and Boucher, R. C. (1999). Pathophysiology of gene-targeted mouse models for cystic fibrosis. *Physiol. Rev.* 79 (Suppl. l), S193–S214. doi:10.1152/physrev.1999.79.1.S193

Guimbellot, J. S., Acosta, E. P., and Rowe, S. M. (2018). Sensitivity of ivacaftor to drug-drug interactions with rifampin, a cytochrome P450 3A4 inducer. *Pediatr. Pulmonol.* 53 (5), E6–E8. doi:10.1002/ppul.23971

Guirouilh-Barbat, J., Huck, S., Bertrand, P., Pirzio, L., Desmaze, C., Sabatier, L., et al. (2004). Impact of the KU80 pathway on NHEJ-induced genome rearrangements in mammalian cells. *Mol. Cel* 14 (5), 611–623. doi:10.1016/j.molcel.2004.05.008

Hampton, T. (2020). With first CRISPR trials, gene editing moves toward the clinic. *JAMA* 323 (16), 1537–1539. doi:10.1001/jama.2020.3438

Harrison, C. (2019). First gene therapy for β-thalassemia approved. *Nat. Biotechnol.* 37 (10), 1102–1103. doi:10.1038/d41587-019-00026-3

Hasty, P., O'Neal, W. K., Liu, K.-Q., Morris, A. P., Bebok, Z., Shumyatsky, G. B., et al. (1995). Severe phenotype in mice with termination mutation in exon 2 of cystic fibrosis gene. *Somat. Cel. Mol. Genet.* 21 (3), 177–187. doi:10.1007/bf02254769

Hay, J. G., McElvaney, N. G., Herena, J., and Crystal, R. G. (1995). Modification of nasal epithelial potential differences of individuals with cystic fibrosis consequent to local administration of a normal CFTR cDNA adenovirus gene transfer vector. *Hum. Gene Ther.* 6 (11), 1487–1496. doi:10.1089/hum.1995.6.11-1487

Hazlett, H. F., Hampton, T. H., Aridgides, D. S., Armstrong, D. A., Dessaint, J. A., Mellinger, D. L., et al. (2020). Altered iron metabolism in cystic fibrosis macrophages: the impact of CFTR modulators and implications for *Pseudomonas aeruginosa* survival. *Sci. Rep.* 10 (1), 10935. doi:10.1038/s41598-020-67729-5

Heijerman, H. G. M., McKone, E. F., Downey, D. G., Van Braeckel, E., Rowe, S. M., Tullis, E., et al. (2019). Efficacy and safety of the elexacaftor plus tezacaftor plus ivacaftor combination regimen in people with cystic fibrosis homozygous for the F508del mutation: a double-blind, randomised, phase 3 trial. *Lancet* 394 (10212), 1940–1948. doi:10.1016/S0140-6736(19)32597-8

Hirakawa, M. P., Krishnakumar, R., Timlin, J. A., Carney, J. P., and Butler, K. S. (2020). Gene editing and CRISPR in the clinic: current and future perspectives. *Biosci. Rep.* 40 (4), BSR20200127. doi:10.1042/BSR20200127

Hoegger, M. J., Fischer, A. J., McMenimen, J. D., Ostedgaard, L. S., Tucker, A. J., Awadalla, M. A., et al. (2014). Impaired mucus detachment disrupts mucociliary transport in a piglet model of cystic fibrosis. *Science* 345 (6198), 818–822. doi:10.1126/science.1255825

Hoelen, H., Kleizen, B., Schmidt, A., Richardson, J., Charitou, P., Thomas, P. J., et al. (2010). The primary folding defect and rescue of ΔF508 CFTR emerge during translation of the mutant domain. *PLoS One* 5 (11), e15458. doi:10.1371/journal.pone.0015458

Hollywood, J. A., Lee, C. M., Scallan, M. F., and Harrison, P. T. (2016). Analysis of gene repair tracts from Cas9/gRNA double-stranded breaks in the human CFTR gene. *Sci. Rep.* 6, 32230. doi:10.1038/srep32230

Hsu, P. D., Lander, E. S., and Zhang, F. (2014). Development and applications of CRISPR-Cas9 for genome engineering. *Cell* 157 (6), 1262–1278. doi:10.1016/j.cell.2014.05.010

Huang, T. P., Newby, G. A., and Liu, D. R. (2021). Precision genome editing using cytosine and adenine base editors in mammalian cells. *Nat. Protoc.* 16, 1089. doi:10.1038/s41596-020-00450-9

Jackson, A. D., and Goss, C. H. (2018). Epidemiology of CF: how registries can be used to advance our understanding of the CF population. *J. Cystic Fibrosis* 17 (3), 297–305. doi:10.1016/j.jcf.2017.11.013

Jiang, T., Henderson, J. M., Coote, K., Cheng, Y., Valley, H. C., Zhang, X.-O., et al. (2020). Chemical modifications of adenine base editor mRNA and guide RNA expand its application scope. *Nat. Commun.* 11 (1), 1979. doi:10.1038/s41467-020-15892-8

Jinek, M., Chylinski, K., Fonfara, I., Hauer, M., Doudna, J. A., and Charpentier, E. (2012). A programmable dual-RNA-guided DNA endonuclease in adaptive bacterial immunity. *Science* 337 (6096), 816–821. doi:10.1126/science.1225829

Joung, J. K., and Sander, J. D. (2013). TALENs: a widely applicable technology for targeted genome editing. *Nat. Rev. Mol. Cel. Biol.* 14 (1), 49–55. doi:10.1038/nrm3486

Keating, D., Marigowda, G., Burr, L., Daines, C., Mall, M. A., McKone, E. F., et al. (2018). VX-445-Tezacaftor-Ivacaftor in Patients with Cystic Fibrosis and One or Two Phe508del Alleles. *N. Engl. J. Med.* 379 (17), 1612–1620. doi:10.1056/NEJMoa1807120

Keiser, N. W., Birket, S. E., Evans, I. A., Tyler, S. R., Crooke, A. K., Sun, X., et al. (2015). Defective innate immunity and hyperinflammation in newborn cystic fibrosis transmembrane conductance regulator-knockout ferret lungs. *Am. J. Respir. Cel. Mol. Biol.* 52 (6), 683–694. doi:10.1165/rcmb.2014-0250OC

Kerem, B., Rommens, J., Buchanan, J., Markiewicz, D., Cox, T., Chakravarti, A., et al. (1989). Identification of the cystic fibrosis gene: genetic analysis. *Science* 245 (4922), 1073–1080. doi:10.1126/science.2570460

Kerem, E., Konstan, M. W., De Boeck, K., Accurso, F. J., Sermet-Gaudelus, I., Wilschanski, M., et al. (2014). Ataluren for the treatment of nonsense-mutation cystic fibrosis: a randomised, double-blind, placebo-controlled phase 3 trial. *Lancet Respir. Med.* 2 (7), 539–547. doi:10.1016/S2213-2600(14)70100-6

Kim, H. K., Yu, G., Park, J., Min, S., Lee, S., Yoon, S., et al. (2020). Predicting the efficiency of prime editing guide RNAs in human cells. *Nat. Biotechnol.* 39, 198. doi:10.1038/s41587-020-0677-y

Komor, A. C., Kim, Y. B., Packer, M. S., Zuris, J. A., and Liu, D. R. (2016). Programmable editing of a target base in genomic DNA without double-stranded DNA cleavage. *Nature* 533 (7603), 420–424. doi:10.1038/nature17946

Kristidis, P., Bozon, D., Corey, M., Markiewicz, D., Rommens, J., Tsui, L. C., et al. (1992). Genetic determination of exocrine pancreatic function in cystic fibrosis. *Am. J. Hum. Genet.* 50 (6), 1178–1184.

Kurosaki, T., and Maquat, L. E. (2016). Nonsense-mediated mRNA decay in humans at a glance. *J. Cel. Sci.* 129 (3), 461–467. doi:10.1242/jcs.181008

Kurt, I. C., Zhou, R., Iyer, S., Garcia, S. P., Miller, B. R., Langner, L. M., et al. (2020). CRISPR C-to-G base editors for inducing targeted DNA transversions in human cells. *Nat. Biotechnol.* 39, 41. doi:10.1038/s41587-020-0609-x

Lara-Reyna, S., Holbrook, J., Jarosz-Griffiths, H. H., Peckham, D., and McDermott, M. F. (2020). Dysregulated signalling pathways in innate immune cells with cystic fibrosis mutations. *Cell. Mol. Life Sci.* 77 (22), 4485–4503. doi:10.1007/s00018-020-03540-9

Lavelle, G. M., White, M. M., Browne, N., McElvaney, N. G., and Reeves, E. P. (2016). Animal models of cystic fibrosis pathology: phenotypic parallels and divergences. *Biomed. Res. Int.* 2016, 5258727. doi:10.1155/2016/5258727

Leal, T., Fajac, I., Wallace, H. L., Lebecque, P., Lebacq, J., Hubert, D., et al. (2008). Airway ion transport impacts on disease presentation and severity in cystic fibrosis. *Clin. Biochem.* 41 (10–11), 764–772. doi:10.1016/j.clinbiochem.2008.03.013

Ledford, H., and Callaway, E. (2020). Pioneers of revolutionary CRISPR gene editing win chemistry Nobel. *Nature* 586 (7829), 346–347. doi:10.1038/d41586-020-02765-9

Lee, C. M., Flynn, R., Hollywood, J. A., Scallan, M. F., and Harrison, P. T. (2012). Correction of the ΔF508 mutation in the cystic fibrosis transmembrane conductance regulator gene by zinc-finger nuclease homology-directed repair. *BioRes. Open Access* 1 (3), 99–108. doi:10.1089/biores.2012.0218

Liang, F., Shang, H., Jordan, N. J., Wong, E., Mercadante, D., Saltz, J., et al. (2017). High-throughput screening for readthrough modulators of CFTR PTC mutations. *SLAS Technol.* 22 (3), 315–324. doi:10.1177/2472630317692561

Limberis, M. P., Figueredo, J., Calcedo, R., and Wilson, J. M. (2007). Activation of CFTR-specific T Cells in cystic fibrosis mice following gene transfer. *Mol. Ther.* 15 (9), 1694–1700. doi:10.1038/sj.mt.6300210

Lino, C. A., Harper, J. C., Carney, J. P., and Timlin, J. A. (2018). Delivering CRISPR: a review of the challenges and approaches. *Drug Deliv.* 25 (1), 1234–1257. doi:10.1080/10717544.2018.1474964

Lubamba, B., Lecourt, H., Lebacq, J., Lebecque, P., De Jonge, H., Wallemacq, P., et al. (2008). Preclinical evidence that sildenafil and vardenafil activate chloride transport in cystic fibrosis. *Am. J. Respir. Crit. Care Med.* 177 (5), 506–515. doi:10.1164/rccm.200703-344OC

Maeder, M. L., Stefanidakis, M., Wilson, C. J., Baral, R., Barrera, L. A., Bounoutas, G. S., et al. (2019). Development of a gene-editing approach to restore vision loss in Leber congenital amaurosis type 10. *Nat. Med.* 25 (2), 229–233. doi:10.1038/s41591-018-0327-9

Maeder, M. L., Thibodeau-Beganny, S., Osiak, A., Wright, D. A., Anthony, R. M., Eichtinger, M., et al. (2008). Rapid "open-source" engineering of customized zinc-finger nucleases for highly efficient gene modification. *Mol. Cel.* 31 (2), 294–301. doi:10.1016/j.molcel.2008.06.016

Makarova, K. S., Wolf, Y. I., Iranzo, J., Shmakov, S. A., Alkhnbashi, O. S., Brouns, S. J. J., et al. (2020). Evolutionary classification of CRISPR-Cas systems: a burst of class 2 and derived variants. *Nat. Rev. Microbiol.* 18 (2), 67–83. doi:10.1038/s41579-019-0299-x

Manson, A. L., Trezise, A. E., MacVinish, L. J., Kasschau, K. D., Birchall, N., Episkopou, V., et al. (1997). Complementation of null CF mice with a human CFTR YAC transgene. *EMBO J.* 16 (4), 4238–4249. doi:10.1093/emboj/16.14.4238

Maule, G., Arosio, D., and Cereseto, A. (2020). Gene therapy for cystic fibrosis: progress and challenges of genome editing. *Ijms* 21 (11), 3903. doi:10.3390/ijms21113903

Maule, G., Casini, A., Montagna, C., Ramalho, A. S., De Boeck, K., Debyser, Z., et al. (2019). Allele specific repair of splicing mutations in cystic fibrosis through AsCas12a genome editing. *Nat. Commun.* 10 (1), 3556. doi:10.1038/s41467-019-11454-9

Maule, G., Ensinck, M., Bulcaen, M., and Carlon, M. S. (2021). Rewriting CFTR to cure cystic fibrosis Progress in molecular biology and translational science.

McCarron, A., Cmielewski, P., Reyne, N., McIntyre, C., Finnie, J., Craig, F., et al. (2020). Phenotypic characterization and comparison of cystic fibrosis rat models generated using CRISPR/Cas9 gene editing. *Am. J. Pathol.* 190, 977–993. doi:10.1016/j.ajpath.2020.01.009

McCarron, A., Donnelley, M., and Parsons, D. (2018). Airway disease phenotypes in animal models of cystic fibrosis. *Respir. Res.* 19 (1), 54. doi:10.1186/s12931-018-0750-y

McCarron, A., Parsons, D., and Donnelley, M. (2021). Animal and cell culture models for cystic fibrosis: which model is right for your application? *Am. J. Pathol.* 191, 228–242. doi:10.1016/j.ajpath.2020.10.017

McHugh, D. R., Steele, M. S., Valerio, D. M., Miron, A., Mann, R. J., LePage, D. F., et al. (2018). A G542X cystic fibrosis mouse model for examining nonsense mutation directed therapies. *PLoS One* 13 (6), e0199573. doi:10.1371/journal.pone.0199573

McNeer, N. A., Anandalingam, K., Fields, R. J., Caputo, C., Kopic, S., Gupta, A., et al. (2015). Nanoparticles that deliver triplex-forming peptide nucleic acid molecules correct F508del CFTR in airway epithelium. *Nat. Commun.* 6, 6952. doi:10.1038/ncomms7952

Mehta, A., and Merkel, O. M. (2020). Immunogenicity of Cas9 protein. *J. Pharm. Sci.* 109 (1), 62–67. doi:10.1016/j.xphs.2019.10.003

Mendell, J. R., Al-Zaidy, S., Shell, R., Arnold, W. D., Rodino-Klapac, L. R., Prior, T. W., et al. (2017). Single-Dose gene-replacement therapy for spinal muscular atrophy. *N. Engl. J. Med.* 377 (18), 1713–1722. doi:10.1056/NEJMoa1706198

Mendes, F., Farinha, C. M., Roxo-Rosa, M., Fanen, P., Edelman, A., Dormer, R., et al. (2004). Antibodies for CFTR studies. *J. Cystic Fibrosis* 3, 69–72. doi:10.1016/j.jcf.2004.05.016

Mention, K., Santos, L., and Harrison, P. T. (2019). Gene and base editing as a therapeutic option for cystic fibrosis-learning from other diseases. *Genes* 10 (5), 387. doi:10.3390/genes10050387

Meyer, M., Huaux, F., Gavilanes, X., van den Brûle, S., Lebecque, P., Lo Re, S., et al. (2009). Azithromycin reduces exaggerated cytokine production by M1 alveolar macrophages in cystic fibrosis. *Am. J. Respir. Cel. Mol. Biol.* 41 (5), 590–602. doi:10.1165/rcmb.2008-0155OC

Meyerholz, D. K., Stoltz, D. A., Pezzulo, A. A., and Welsh, M. J. (2010). Pathology of gastrointestinal organs in a porcine model of cystic fibrosis. *Am. J. Pathol.* 176 (3), 1377–1389. doi:10.2353/ajpath.2010.090849

Middleton, P. G., Mall, M. A., Dřevínek, P., Lands, L. C., McKone, E. F., Polineni, D., et al. (2019). Elexacaftor-Tezacaftor-Ivacaftor for Cystic Fibrosis with a Single Phe508del Allele. *N. Engl. J. Med.* 381 (19), 1809–1819. doi:10.1056/NEJMoa1908639

Montoro, D. T., Haber, A. L., Biton, M., Vinarsky, V., Lin, B., Birket, S. E., et al. (2018). A revised airway epithelial hierarchy includes CFTR-expressing ionocytes. *Nature* 560 (7718), 319–324. doi:10.1038/s41586-018-0393-7

Mottais, A., Le Gall, T., Sibiril, Y., Ravel, J., Laurent, V., d'Arbonneau, F., et al. (2017). Enhancement of lung gene delivery after aerosol: a new strategy using non-viral complexes with antibacterial properties. *Biosci. Rep.* 37 (6), BSR20160618. doi:10.1042/BSR20160618

Okiyoneda, T., Veit, G., Dekkers, J. F., Bagdany, M., Soya, N., Xu, H., et al. (2013). Mechanism-based corrector combination restores ΔF508-CFTR folding and function. *Nat. Chem. Biol.* 9 (7), 444–454. doi:10.1038/nchembio.1253

Ostedgaard, L. S., Meyerholz, D. K., Chen, J. H., Pezzulo, A. A., Karp, P. H., Rokhlina, T., et al. (2011). The DeltaF508 mutation causes CFTR misprocessing and cystic fibrosis-like disease in pigs. *Sci. Transl. Med.* 3 (74), 74ra24. doi:10.1126/scitranslmed.3001868

Pedemonte, N., Zegarra-Moran, O., and Galietta, L. J. V. (2011). *High-throughput screening of libraries of compounds to identify CFTR modulators*. Humana Press, 13–21.

Phan, Q. V., Contzen, J., Seemann, P., and Gossen, M. (2017). Site-specific chromosomal gene insertion: Flp recombinase versus Cas9 nuclease. *Sci. Rep.* 7 (1), 17771. doi:10.1038/s41598-017-17651-0

Plasschaert, L. W., Žilionis, R., Choo-Wing, R., Savova, V., Knehr, J., Roma, G., et al. (2018). A single-cell atlas of the airway epithelium reveals the CFTR-rich pulmonary ionocyte. *Nature* 560 (7718), 377–381. doi:10.1038/s41586-018-0394-6

Pranke, I., Golec, A., Hinzpeter, A., Edelman, A., and Sermet-Gaudelus, I. (2019). Emerging therapeutic approaches for cystic fibrosis. From gene editing to personalized medicine. *Front. Pharmacol.* 10, 121. doi:10.3389/fphar.2019.00121

Ramalho, A. S., Fürstová, E., Vonk, A. M., Ferrante, M., Verfaillie, C., Dupont, L., et al. (2020). Correction of CFTR function in intestinal organoids to guide treatment of Cystic Fibrosis. *Eur. Respir. J.* 57, 1902426. doi:10.1183/13993003.02426-2019

Ramsey, B. W., Davies, J., McElvaney, N. G., Tullis, E., Bell, S. C., Dřevínek, P., et al. (2011). A CFTR potentiator in patients with cystic fibrosis and theG551DMutation. *N. Engl. J. Med.* 365 (18), 1663–1672. doi:10.1056/NEJMoa1105185

Ricciardi, A., Quijano, E., Putman, R., Saltzman, W., and Glazer, P. (2018). Peptide nucleic acids as a tool for site-specific gene editing. *Molecules* 23 (3), 632. doi:10.3390/molecules23030632

Riordan, J. R., Rommens, J., Kerem, B., Alon, N., Rozmahel, R., Grzelczak, Z., et al. (1989). Identification of the cystic fibrosis gene: cloning and characterization of complementary DNA. *Science* 245 (4922), 1066–1073. doi:10.1126/science.2475911

Rogers, C. S., Hao, Y., Rokhlina, T., Samuel, M., Stoltz, D. A., Li, Y., et al. (2008). Production of CFTR-null and CFTR-ΔF508 heterozygous pigs by adeno-associated virus-mediated gene targeting and somatic cell nuclear transfer. *J. Clin. Invest.* 118 (4), 1571–1577. doi:10.1172/JCI34773

Roldão, A., Silva, A. C., Mellado, M. C. M., Alves, P. M., and Carrondo, M. J. T. (2017). Viruses and virus-like particles in biotechnology: fundamentals and applications ☆. *Compr. Biotechnol.* 1, 633–656. doi:10.1016/B978-0-12-809633-8.09046-4

Rommens, J., Iannuzzi, M., Kerem, B., Drumm, M., Melmer, G., Dean, M., et al. (1989). Identification of the cystic fibrosis gene: chromosome walking and jumping. *Science* 245 (4922), 1059–1065. doi:10.1126/science.2772657

Rosen, B. H., Chanson, M., Gawenis, L. R., Liu, J., Sofoluwe, A., Zoso, A., et al. (2018). Animal and model systems for studying cystic fibrosis. *J. Cystic Fibrosis* 17 (2S), S28–S34. doi:10.1016/j.jcf.2017.09.001

Rozmahel, R., Wilschanski, M., Matin, A., Plyte, S., Oliver, M., Auerbach, W., et al. (1996). Modulation of disease severity in cystic fibrosis transmembrane conductance regulator deficient mice by a secondary genetic factor. *Nat. Genet.* 12 (3), 280–287. doi:10.1038/ng0396-280

Ruan, J., Hirai, H., Yang, D., Ma, L., Hou, X., Jiang, H., et al. (2019). Efficient gene editing at major CFTR mutation loci. *Mol. Ther. - Nucleic Acids* 16, 73–81. doi:10.1016/j.omtn.2019.02.006

Russell, S., Bennett, J., Wellman, J. A., Chung, D. C., Yu, Z.-F., Tillman, A., et al. (2017). Efficacy and safety of voretigene neparvovec (AAV2-hRPE65v2) in patients with RPE65 -mediated inherited retinal dystrophy: a randomised, controlled, open-label, phase 3 trial. *Lancet* 390 (10097), 849–860. doi:10.1016/S0140-6736(17)31868-8

Sanz, D. J., Hollywood, J. A., Scallan, M. F., and Harrison, P. T. (2017). Cas9/gRNA targeted excision of cystic fibrosis-causing deep-intronic splicing mutations restores normal splicing of CFTR mRNA. *PLoS One* 12 (9), e0184009. doi:10.1371/journal.pone.0184009

Sargent, R. G., Suzuki, S., and Gruenert, D. C. (2014). Nuclease-mediated double-strand break (DSB) enhancement of small fragment homologous recombination

(SFHR) gene modification in human-induced pluripotent stem cells (hiPSCs). *Methods Mol. Biol.* 1114, 279–290. doi:10.1007/978-1-62703-761-7_18

Sato, T., Vries, R. G., Snippert, H. J., Van De Wetering, M., Barker, N., Stange, D. E., et al. (2009). Single Lgr5 stem cells build crypt-villus structures *in vitro* without a mesenchymal niche. *Nature* 459 (7244), 262–265. doi:10.1038/nature07935

Saussereau, E. L., Roussel, D., Diallo, S., Debarbieux, L., Edelman, A., and Sermet-Gaudelus, I. (2013). Characterization of nasal potential difference in cftr knockout and F508del-CFTR mice. *PLoS One* 8 (3), e57317. doi:10.1371/journal.pone.0057317

Schwank, G., Koo, B.-K., Sasselli, V., Dekkers, J. F., Heo, I., Demircan, T., et al. (2013). Functional repair of CFTR by CRISPR/Cas9 in intestinal stem cell organoids of cystic fibrosis patients. *Cell Stem Cell* 13 (6), 653–658. doi:10.1016/j.stem.2013.11.002

Scudieri, P., Musante, I., Caci, E., Venturini, A., Morelli, P., Walter, C., et al. (2018). Increased expression of ATP12A proton pump in cystic fibrosis airways. *JCI Insight* 3 (20), e123616. doi:10.1172/jci.insight.123616

Semaniakou, A., Croll, R. P., and Chappe, V. (2018). Animal models in the pathophysiology of cystic fibrosis. *Front. Pharmacol.* 9, 1475. doi:10.3389/fphar.2018.01475

Shah, V. S., Ernst, S., Tang, X. X., Karp, P. H., Parker, C. P., Ostedgaard, L. S., et al. (2016a). Relationships among CFTR expression, HCO3− secretion, and host defense may inform gene- and cell-based cystic fibrosis therapies. *Proc. Natl. Acad. Sci. U.S.A.* 113 (19), 5382–5387. doi:10.1073/pnas.1604905113

Shah, V. S., Meyerholz, D. K., Tang, X. X., Reznikov, L., Abou Alaiwa, M., Ernst, S. E., et al. (2016b). Airway acidification initiates host defense abnormalities in cystic fibrosis mice. *Science* 351 (6272), 503–507. doi:10.1126/science.aad5589

Sharma, J., Abbott, J., Klaskala, L., Zhao, G., Birket, S. E., and Rowe, S. M. (2020). A novel G542X CFTR rat model of cystic fibrosis is sensitive to nonsense mediated decay. *Front. Physiol.* 11, 611294, doi:10.3389/fphys.2020.611294

Sharma, N., Evans, T. A., Pellicore, M. J., Davis, E., Aksit, M. A., McCague, A. F., et al. (2018). Capitalizing on the heterogeneous effects of CFTR nonsense and frameshift variants to inform therapeutic strategy for cystic fibrosis. *Plos Genet.* 14 (11), e1007723, doi:10.1371/journal.pgen.1007723

Sharma, N., Sosnay, P. R., Ramalho, A. S., Douville, C., Franca, A., Gottschalk, L. B., et al. (2014). Experimental assessment of splicing variants using expression minigenes and comparison with in silico predictions. *Hum. Mutat.* 35 (10), 1249–1259. doi:10.1002/humu.22624

Sheppard, D. N., Carson, M. R., Ostedgaard, L. S., Denning, G. M., and Welsh, M. J. (1994). Expression of cystic fibrosis transmembrane conductance regulator in a model epithelium. *Am. J. Physiol.-Lung Cell Mol. Physiol.* 266 (Pt 1), L405–L413. doi:10.1152/ajplung.1994.266.4.L405

Shik Mun, K., Arora, K., Huang, Y., Yang, F., Yarlagadda, S., Ramananda, Y., et al. (2019). Patient-derived pancreas-on-a-chip to model cystic fibrosis-related disorders. *Nat. Commun.* 10 (1), 3124. doi:10.1038/s41467-019-11178-w

Shirley, J. L., De Jong, Y. P., Terhorst, C., and Herzog, R. W. (2020). Immune responses to viral gene therapy vectors. *Mol. Ther.* 28 (3), 709–722. doi:10.1016/j.ymthe.2020.01.001

Singh, V. K., and Schwarzenberg, S. J. (2017). Pancreatic insufficiency in cystic fibrosis. *J. Cystic Fibrosis* 16 (Suppl. 2), S70–S78. doi:10.1016/j.jcf.2017.06.011

Smirnikhina, S. A., Kondrateva, E. V., Adilgereeva, E. P., Anuchina, A. A., Zaynitdinova, M. I., Slesarenko, Y. S., et al. (2020). P.F508del editing in cells from cystic fibrosis patients. *PLOS One* 15 (11), e0242094, doi:10.1371/journal.pone.0242094

Smit, L. S., Strong, T. V., Wilkinson, D. J., Macek, M., Jr., Mansoura, M. K., Wood, D. L., et al. (1995). Missense mutation (G480C) in the CFTR gene associated with protein mislocalization but normal chloride channel activity. *Hum. Mol. Genet.* 4 (2), 269–273. doi:10.1093/hmg/4.2.269

Snouwaert, J. N., Brigman, K. K., Latour, A. M., Malouf, N. N., Boucher, R. C., Smithies, O., et al. (1992). An animal model for cystic fibrosis made by gene targeting. *Science* 257 (5073), 1083–1088. doi:10.1126/science.257.5073.1083

Sondhi, D., Stiles, K. M., De, B. P., and Crystal, R. G. (2017). Genetic modification of the lung directed toward treatment of human disease. *Hum. Gene Ther.* 28 (1), 3–84. doi:10.1089/hum.2016.152

Sosnay, P. R., Siklosi, K. R., Van Goor, F., Kaniecki, K., Yu, H., Sharma, N., et al. (2013). Defining the disease liability of variants in the cystic fibrosis transmembrane conductance regulator gene. *Nat. Genet.* 45 (10), 1160–1167. doi:10.1038/ng.2745

Steines, B., Dickey, D. D., Bergen, J., Excoffon, K. J. D. A., Weinstein, J. R., Li, X., et al. (2016). CFTR gene transfer with AAV improves early cystic fibrosis pig phenotypes. *JCI Insight* 1 (14), e88728. doi:10.1172/jci.insight.88728

Stoltz, D. A., Meyerholz, D. K., Pezzulo, A. A., Ramachandran, S., Rogan, M. P., Davis, G. J., et al. (2010). Cystic fibrosis pigs develop lung disease and exhibit defective bacterial eradication at birth. *Sci. Transl. Med.* 2 (29), 29ra31. doi:10.1126/scitranslmed.3000928

Stoltz, D. A., Meyerholz, D. K., and Welsh, M. J. (2015). Origins of cystic fibrosis lung disease. *N. Engl. J. Med.* 372 (4), 351–362. doi:10.1056/NEJMra1300109

Stoltz, D. A., Rokhlina, T., Ernst, S. E., Pezzulo, A. A., Ostedgaard, L. S., Karp, P. H., et al. (2013). Intestinal CFTR expression alleviates meconium ileus in cystic fibrosis pigs. *J. Clin. Invest.* 123 (6), 2685–2693. doi:10.1172/JCI68867

Sun, X., Olivier, A. K., Liang, B., Yi, Y., Sui, H., Evans, T. I. A., et al. (2014). Lung phenotype of juvenile and adult cystic fibrosis transmembrane conductance regulator-knockout ferrets. *Am. J. Respir. Cel. Mol. Biol.* 50 (3), 502–512. doi:10.1165/rcmb.2013-0261OC

Sun, X., Sui, H., Fisher, J. T., Yan, Z., Liu, X., Cho, H.-J., et al. (2010). Disease phenotype of a ferret CFTR-knockout model of cystic fibrosis. *J. Clin. Invest.* 120 (9), 3149–3160. doi:10.1172/JCI43052

Sun, X., Yan, Z., Yi, Y., Li, Z., Lei, D., Rogers, C. S., et al. (2008). Adeno-associated virus-targeted disruption of the CFTR gene in cloned ferrets. *J. Clin. Invest.* 118 (4), 1578–1583. doi:10.1172/JCI34599

Sun, X., Yi, Y., Yan, Z., Rosen, B. H., Liang, B., Winter, M. C., et al. (2019). In utero and postnatal VX-770 administration rescues multiorgan disease in a ferret model of cystic fibrosis. *Sci. Transl. Med.* 11 (485), eaau7531. doi:10.1126/scitranslmed.aau7531

Suzuki, S., Crane, A. M., Anirudhan, V., Barillà, C., Matthias, N., Randell, S. H., et al. (2020). Highly efficient gene editing of cystic fibrosis patient-derived airway basal cells results in functional CFTR correction. *Mol. Ther.* 28 (7), 1684–1695. doi:10.1016/j.ymthe.2020.04.021

Suzuki, S., Sargent, R. G., Illek, B., Fischer, H., Esmaeili-Shandiz, A., Yezzi, M. J., et al. (2016). TALENs Facilitate Single-step Seamless SDF Correction of F508del CFTR in Airway Epithelial Submucosal Gland Cell-derived CF-iPSCs. *Mol. Ther. - Nucleic Acids* 5, e273. doi:10.1038/mtna.2015.43

Talamo Guevara, M., and McColley, S. A. (2017). The safety of lumacaftor and ivacaftor for the treatment of cystic fibrosis. *Expert Opin. Drug Saf.* 16 (11), 1305–1311. doi:10.1080/14740338.2017.1372419

Taylor-Cousar, J. L., Munck, A., McKone, E. F., van der Ent, C. K., Moeller, A., Simard, C., et al. (2017). Tezacaftor-Ivacaftor in Patients with Cystic Fibrosis Homozygous for Phe508del. *N. Engl. J. Med.* 377 (21), 2013–2023. doi:10.1056/NEJMoa1709846

Tsai, S. Q., Zheng, Z., Nguyen, N. T., Liebers, M., Topkar, V. V., Thapar, V., et al. (2015). GUIDE-seq enables genome-wide profiling of off-target cleavage by CRISPR-Cas nucleases. *Nat. Biotechnol.* 33 (2), 187–197. doi:10.1038/nbt.3117

Tuggle, K. L., Birket, S. E., Cui, X., Hong, J., Warren, J., Reid, L., et al. (2014). Characterization of defects in ion transport and tissue development in cystic fibrosis transmembrane conductance regulator (CFTR)-knockout rats. *PLoS One* 9 (3), e91253, doi:10.1371/journal.pone.0091253

Urnov, F. D., Rebar, E. J., Holmes, M. C., Zhang, H. S., and Gregory, P. D. (2010). Genome editing with engineered zinc finger nucleases. *Nat. Rev. Genet.* 11 (9), 636–646. doi:10.1038/nrg2842

Vaidyanathan, S., Salahudeen, A. A., Sellers, Z. M., Bravo, D. T., Choi, S. S., Batish, A., et al. (2020). High-efficiency, selection-free gene repair in airway stem cells from cystic fibrosis patients rescues CFTR function in differentiated epithelia. *Cell Stem Cell* 26 (2), 161–171. doi:10.1016/j.stem.2019.11.002

Valley, H. C., Bukis, K. M., Bell, A., Cheng, Y., Wong, E., Jordan, N. J., et al. (2019). Isogenic cell models of cystic fibrosis-causing variants in natively expressing pulmonary epithelial cells. *J. Cystic Fibrosis* 18 (4), 476–483. doi:10.1016/j.jcf.2018.12.001

van Doorninck, J. H., French, P. J., Verbeek, E., Peters, R. H., Morreau, H., Bijman, J., et al. (1995). A mouse model for the cystic fibrosis delta F508 mutation. *EMBO J.* 14 (18), 4403–4411.

Van Goor, F., Straley, K. S., Cao, D., González, J., Hadida, S., Hazlewood, A., et al. (2006). Rescue of ΔF508-CFTR trafficking and gating in human cystic fibrosis airway primary cultures by small molecules. *Am. J. Physiol.-Lung Cell Mol. Physiol.* 290 (6), L1117–L1130. doi:10.1152/ajplung.00169.2005

Van Goor, F., Yu, H., Burton, B., and Hoffman, B. J. (2014). Effect of ivacaftor on CFTR forms with missense mutations associated with defects in protein processing or function. *J. Cystic Fibrosis* 13 (1), 29–36. doi:10.1016/j.jcf.2013.06.008

van Heeckeren, A. M., Schluchter, M. D., Drumm, M. L., and Davis, P. B. (2004). Role of Cftr genotype in the response to chronic *Pseudomonas aeruginosa* lung infection in mice. *Am. J. Physiol.-Lung Cell Mol. Physiol.* 287 (5), L944–L952. doi:10.1152/ajplung.00387.2003

Veit, G., Avramescu, R. G., Chiang, A. N., Houck, S. A., Cai, Z., Peters, K. W., et al. (2016). From CFTR biology toward combinatorial pharmacotherapy: expanded classification of cystic fibrosis mutations. *MBoC* 27 (3), 424–433. doi:10.1091/mbc.E14-04-0935

Vermeulen, F., Proesmans, M., Boon, M., and De Boeck, K. (2015). Improved repeatability of nasal potential difference with a larger surface catheter. *J. Cystic Fibrosis* 14 (3), 317–323. doi:10.1016/j.jcf.2014.08.006

Verstegen, M. M. A., Roos, F. J. M., Burka, K., Gehart, H., Jager, M., de Wolf, M., et al. (2020). Human extrahepatic and intrahepatic cholangiocyte organoids show region-specific differentiation potential and model cystic fibrosis-related bile duct disease. *Sci. Rep.* 10 (1), 21900. doi:10.1038/s41598-020-79082-8

Vertex (2020). "Vertex announces FDA approvals of TRIKAFTA® (elexacaftor/tezacaftor/ivacaftorand ivacaftor)," in *SYMDEKO® (tezacaftor/ivacaftor and ivacaftor) and KALYDECO® (ivacaftor) for Use in People WithCF with Certain Rare Mutations.*

Vidović, D., Carlon, M. S., da Cunha, M. F., Dekkers, J. F., Hollenhorst, M. I., Bijvelds, M. J., et al. (2016). rAAV-cftrδr rescues the cystic fibrosis phenotype in human intestinal organoids and cystic fibrosis mice. *Am. J. Respir. Crit. Care Med.* 193 (3), 288–298. doi:10.1164/rccm.201505-0914OC

Volkova, N., Moy, K., Evans, J., Campbell, D., Tian, S., Simard, C., et al. (2020). Disease progression in patients with cystic fibrosis treated with ivacaftor: data from national US and UK registries. *J. Cystic Fibrosis* 19 (1), 68–79. doi:10.1016/j.jcf.2019.05.015

Wainwright, C. E., Elborn, J. S., and Ramsey, B. W. (2015). Lumacaftor-Ivacaftor in Patients with Cystic Fibrosis Homozygous for Phe508del CFTR. *N. Engl. J. Med.* 373 (18), 1783–1784. doi:10.1056/NEJMc151046610.1056/nejmoa1409547

Wanyama, S. S., and Thomas, M. (2018). Annual report Belgian cystic fibrosis registry 2016 [Online]. Brussels: Scientific Institute of Public Health. Available at: https://www.muco.be/wp-content/uploads/2019/07/Report-Belgian-CF-registry-2016-EN_final.pdf (Accessed February 27, 2020).

Wilbie, D., Walther, J., and Mastrobattista, E. (2019). Delivery aspects of CRISPR/Cas for *in vivo* genome editing. *Acc. Chem. Res.* 52 (6), 1555–1564. doi:10.1021/acs.accounts.9b00106

Wilke, M., Buijs-Offerman, R. M., Aarbiou, J., Colledge, W. H., Sheppard, D. N., Touqui, L., et al. (2011). Mouse models of cystic fibrosis: phenotypic analysis and research applications. *J. Cystic Fibrosis* 10 (Suppl. 2), S152–S171. doi:10.1016/S1569-1993(11)60020-9

Wilschanski, M., and Novak, I. (2013). The cystic fibrosis of exocrine pancreas. *Cold Spring Harbor Perspect. Med.* 3 (5), a009746. doi:10.1101/cshperspect.a009746

Xu, J., Livraghi-Butrico, A., Hou, X., Rajagopalan, C., Zhang, J., Song, J., et al. (2021). Phenotypes of CF rabbits generated by CRISPR/Cas9-mediated disruption of the CFTR gene. *JCI Insight* 6 (1), e139813. doi:10.1172/jci.insight.139813

Xu, Z., Pissarra, L. S., Farinha, C. M., Liu, J., Cai, Z., Thibodeau, P. H., et al. (2014). Revertant mutants modify, but do not rescue, the gating defect of the cystic fibrosis mutant G551D-CFTR. *J. Physiol.* 592 (9), 1931–1947. doi:10.1113/jphysiol.2014.271817

Yu, H., Burton, B., Huang, C.-J., Worley, J., Cao, D., Johnson, J. P., et al. (2012). Ivacaftor potentiation of multiple CFTR channels with gating mutations. *J. Cystic Fibrosis* 11 (3), 237–245. doi:10.1016/j.jcf.2011.12.005

Zeiher, B. G., Eichwald, E., Zabner, J., Smith, J. J., Puga, A. P., McCray, P. B., Jr., et al. (1995). A mouse model for the delta F508 allele of cystic fibrosis. *J. Clin. Invest.* 96, 2051–2064. doi:10.1172/JCI118253

Zhao, D., Li, J., Li, S., Xin, X., Hu, M., Price, M. A., et al. (2020). Glycosylase base editors enable C-to-A and C-to-G base changes. *Nat. Biotechnol.* 39, 35. doi:10.1038/s41587-020-0592-2

Zhou, L., Dey, C., Wert, S., DuVall, M., Frizzell, R., and Whitsett, J. (1994). Correction of lethal intestinal defect in a mouse model of cystic fibrosis by human CFTR. *Science* 266 (5191), 1705–1708. doi:10.1126/science.7527588

Zhou, Y., Song, K., Painter, R. G., Aiken, M., Reiser, J., Stanton, B. A., et al. (2013). Cystic fibrosis transmembrane conductance regulator recruitment to phagosomes in neutrophils. *J. Innate Immun.* 5 (3), 219–230. doi:10.1159/000346568

Zhu, F., Nair, R. R., Fisher, E. M. C., and Cunningham, T. J. (2019). Humanising the mouse genome piece by piece. *Nat. Commun.* 10 (1), 1845. doi:10.1038/s41467-019-09716-7

GLOSSARY

ABE adenine base editors

ALI air-liquid interface

ASL airway surface liquid

BAC bacterial artificial chromosome

BALF broncho-alveolar lavage fluid

Cas CRISPR associated nuclease

CBE cytosine base editors

CF cystic fibrosis

CFBE cystic fibrosis bronchial epithelium

CFF cystic fibrosis foundation

CFTR cystic fibrosis transmembrane conductance regulator

CGBE C-to-G base editors

CRISPR clustered regularly interspaced short palindromic repeats

DSB double strand break

FRT Fisher rat thyroid

GFP green fluorescent protein

HA hemagglutinin

HBE human bronchial epithelium

hCFTR human CFTR

HS-YFP halide sensitive yellow fluorescent protein

HDR homology directed repair

HEK human embryonic kidney

iPSCs induced pluripotent stem cells

Isc short-circuit current

KI knock-in

KO knock-out

NBD nucleotide binding domain

NHEJ non-homologous end joining

NMD nonsense-mediated mRNA decay

NPD nasal potential difference

PAM protospacer adjacent motif

PBS primer binding site

PCL periciliary liquid

pegRNA prime editing gRNA

PNAs peptide nucleic acids

PTCs premature termination codon

PwCF people with CF

rAAV recombinant adeno-associated viral vector

RT reverse transcriptase

SDF small/short DNA fragment

sgRNA single guide RNA

SMG submucosal gland

ssODN single strand oligodeoxynucleotide

TALE(N) transcription activator-like effector (nuclease)

UGI uracil glycosylase inhibitor

UNG uracil DNA glycosylase

WT wild-type

YAC yeast artificial chromosome

ZFN Zinc finger nuclease

3

Salvage Therapy with Low-Dose Ruxolitinib Leads to a Significant Improvement in Bronchiolitis Obliterans Syndrome in Patients with cGVHD After Allogeneic Hematopoietic Stem Cell Transplantation

Yanmin Zhao[1,2], *Guifang OuYang*[3], *Jimin Shi*[1,2], *Yi Luo*[1,2], *Yamin Tan*[1,2], *Jian Yu*[1,2], *Huarui Fu*[1,2], *Xiaoyu Lai*[1,2], *Lizhen Liu*[1,2] *and He Huang*[1,2]*

[1]*Bone Marrow Transplantation Center, The First Affiliated Hospital, School of Medicine, Zhejiang University, Hangzhou, China,* [2]*Institute of Hematology, Zhejiang University, Hangzhou, China,* [3]*Department of Hematology, Ningbo Hospital of Zhejiang University, Ningbo, China*

Correspondence:
He Huang
huanghe@zju.edu.cn

Bronchiolitis obliterans syndrome (BOS) is a life-threatening pulmonary manifestation of chronic graft versus host disease (cGVHD) post-allogeneic hematopoietic stem cell transplantation (HSCT), without clear standard of care. This study included 30 patients undergoing an allogeneic HSCT for a hematological malignancy and the outcomes with post-HSCT BOS treated with ruxolitinib as a salvage treatment were reviewed. After a median duration of ruxolitinib therapy of 9.25 (1.5–27) months, the best overall response (BOR) rate was 66.7%: three patients (10.0%) achieved complete remission, and 17 (56.7%) achieved partial remission. The median time from initiation of ruxolitinib to achieve the best responses was 3 months. Since initiating ruxolitinib, forced expiratory volume in 1 s of predicted (FEV1%pred) slightly increased after 3 and 6 months compared with measurements before ruxolitinib in responders. Only FEV1%pred mild decline before ruxolitinib with a ratio ≤15% was an independent predictor to achieve a response to ruxolitinib. Eleven patients (36.7%) had severe pulmonary infection of ≥3 grade. Following a median follow-up of 318 days after ruxolitinib, the 2-years incidence of nonrelapse mortality and 2-years overall survival rate after ruxolitinib among patients with BOS was 25.1 and 62.6%, respectively. Ruxolitinib is a promising treatment option to improve the prognosis of post-HSCT BOS.

Keywords: ruxolitinib, bronchiolitis obliterans syndrome, allogeneic hematopoietic stem cell transplantation, chronic graft versus host disease, pulmonary function

INTRODUCTION

Bronchiolitis obliterans syndrome (BOS) is a pulmonary fibroproliferative disorder characterized by irreversible narrowing and obliteration of the small airways. (Barker et al., 2014). In the setting of allogeneic hematopoietic stem cell transplantation (allo-HSCT), BOS is the most common pulmonary manifestation of moderate/severe chronic graft versus host disease (cGVHD), and the overall prevalence of BOS is up to 14% among patients who develop cGVHD (Au et al., 2011). BOS remains a leading cause of late morbidity and mortality as well as impaired quality of life after allo-HSCT. (Dudek et al., 2003; Williams et al., 2009; Chien et al., 2010; Barker et al., 2014).

Historically, systemic corticosteroids have formed the backbone of therapy for BOS, but their side effect profile makes them disadvantageous for prolonged use. Combination of inhaled corticosteroids and bronchodilators, azithromycin and montelukast early in BOS therapy could reduce total corticosteroids exposure (Bergeron et al., 2015; Kim et al., 2016; Williams et al., 2016). Other regimens include calcineurin inhibitors (CNIs); extracorporeal photopheresis (ECP) (Lucid et al., 2011; Del Fante et al., 2016; Hefazi et al., 2018); rituximab; (Brownback et al., 2017); etanercept; (Yanik et al., 2012); and tyrosine kinase inhibitors, mainly for their inhibitory effect on fibrosis via the platelet-derived growth factor pathway (Watanabe et al., 2015; Bergeron et al., 2017; Watanabe et al., 2017). Young patients with refractory severe BOS despite all interventions and best supportive care, may be evaluated for lung transplantation (Vogl et al., 2013; Greer et al., 2018). However, no consensus has been reached regarding the optimal therapy for BOS because of suboptimal responses to medical therapies, and effective therapeutic strategies are therefore needed to stabilize lung function, reduce corticosteroid dosing, and improve quality of life for patients with BOS after HSCT.

Ruxolitinib, a Janus-associated kinase (JAK) 1/2 inhibitor approved for the treatment of patients with intermediate-2 or high-risk primary myelofibrosis (Harrison et al., 2012), has shown excellent response rates in steroid-refractory GVHD (Zeiser et al., 2015; Khoury et al., 2018; Zhao et al., 2020a; Escamilla Gómez et al., 2020; Wu et al., 2021). Presently, studies on ruxolitinib administration in patients with BOS are still in a preliminary stage, with only two published case series, which indicated ruxolitinib is an effective steroid sparing agent in BOS due to cGVHD (Schoettler et al., 2019; Streiler et al., 2020). However, the effect of ruxolitinib on pulmonary function, its toxicity profile, and factors affecting its response have not been fully determined. All these concerns must be addressed urgently. Thus, this retrospective study aimed to investigate whether ruxolitinib therapy would lead to stabilization or even improvement in pulmonary function in patients with steroid-refractory BOS. Additionally, it sought to observe the infectious events during ruxolitinib therapy. It also determined the effect of ruxolitinib in corticosteroid dosing in these patients and the clinical factors affecting the response to ruxolitinib.

METHOD

Patients

All patients who underwent an allogeneic HSCT for a hematological malignancy between January 2014 and June 2019 at the First Affiliated Hospital of Zhejiang University School of Medicine and Ningbo Hospital of Zhejiang University were retrospectively screened. Data was retrieved from the transplant databases and electronic medical. The inclusion criteria were as follows: 1) patients aged ≥14 years; 2) diagnosed with BOS related to cGVHD according to the criteria of the National Institute of Health (NIH) consensus; 3) treated with systemic glucocorticosteroids (GCSs) in combination with therapy using inhaled corticosteroids fluticasone, azithromycin, and montelukast (FAM) with/without CNIs, and had worsening lung function, which was defined as a decline in forced expiratory volume in 1 s of predicted (FEV1%pred) from baseline by 5% or more; and 4) treated with ruxolitinib as a salvage treatment for at least 30 days. The exclusion criteria were as follows: 1) Responsive to other salvage therapy except ruxolitinib; 2) other pulmonary or infectious diseases, such as asthma, lung cancer, chronic obstructive pulmonary disease, pneumonia, or tuberculosis; and 3) a history of using other JAK inhibitors. All procedures were in accordance with the Declaration of Helsinki and approved by the ethics review committee of Zhejiang University. The author had full access to the data and took responsibility for its authenticity.

BOS and cGVHD Diagnosis

BOS was diagnosed according to the National Institutes of Health 2014 criteria (Jagasia et al., 2015), namely 1) FEV1 <75% of that predicted or ≥10% absolute FEV1 decline over less than 2 years; 2) FEV1/forced vital capacity (FVC) < 70%; 3) absence of infection in the respiratory tract; and 4) one of the following two features of air trapping, that is, residual volume (RV) or predicted RV/total lung capacity >120% or evidence of air trapping on high-resolution computed tomography. cGVHD was defined according to the NIH Consensus Guidelines and classified as mild, moderate, or severe. (Jagasia et al., 2015).

Pulmonary Function Test

Pulmonary function test (PFT) was routinely performed before HSCT and at any time when complaining of respiratory symptoms, such as dry cough, wheezing or dyspnea. After initiation of ruxolitinib, PFT was carried over time (0, 3, and 6 months) during the period of ruxolitinib therapy, using body plethysmography (MasterScreen PFT System, Jaeger Corp, Germany). If a patient had an episode of infection at the indicated time points, PFT was postponed to allow the resolution of infection.

Ruxolitinib Therapy

Ruxolitinib was recommended at a dose of 5 mg orally, twice daily (BID), for patients weighing ≤60 kg, and 10 mg BID for patients weighing >60 kg. Adverse events were graded according to the

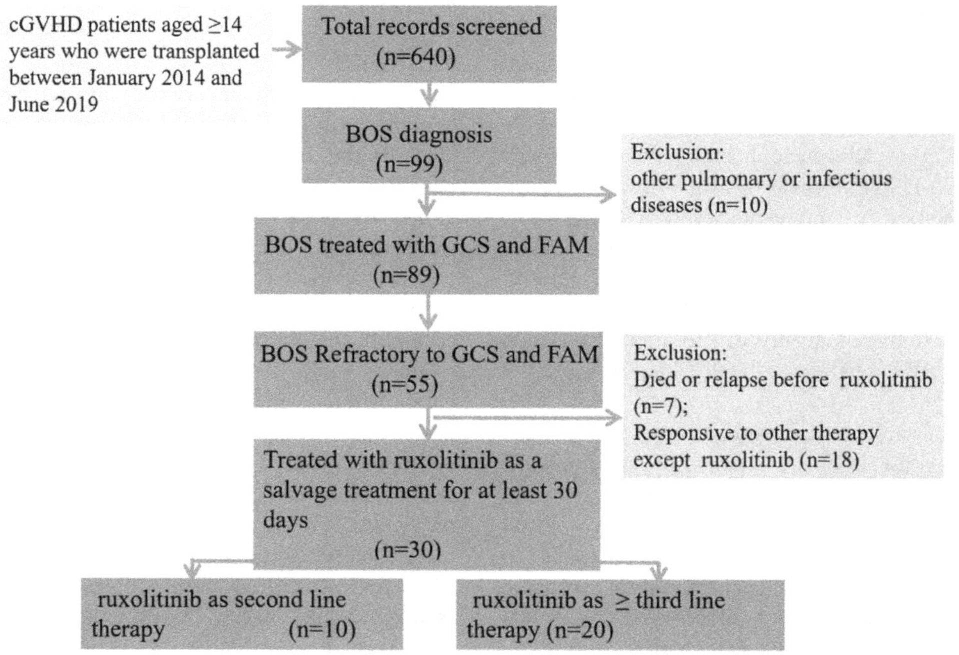

FIGURE 1 | Flow diagram of the study cohort. Eighty-nine patients were diagnosed with BOS related to cGVHD, not related to other pulmonary or infectious disease. Among these 89 patients, 30 patients who were refractory disease to first-line glucocorticosteroids plus FAM and treated with ruxolitinib as ≥ second-line therapy, were retrospectively enrolled in this analysis. cGVHD, chronic graft versus host disease; BOS, bronchiolitis obliterans syndrome.

Common Terminology Criteria for Adverse Events (CTCAE v4). If CTCAE grade 3 cytopenia occurred after ruxolitinib, the dose could be reduced according to the clinical situation. When ruxolitinib was started, the initial steroid was maintained for at least 4 weeks, after which a tapering schedule was commenced up at the discretion of the managing physician according to response.

Therapeutic Response Definitions

The response to ruxolitinib was defined as complete response (CR) when clinical symptoms decreased, and FEV1%pred increased by >75%; partial response (PR) was considered when FEV1%pred levels increased or symptoms improved with the stabilization of FEV1%pred (among partial responders, good responders were those patients reaching FEV1%pred levels above 60%); and nonresponse (NR) consisted of progression disease (PD) and stable disease (SD). PD was considered when clinical and functional findings (mainly FEV1%pred decrease from baseline by 5% or more) worsened, while SD was considered when FEV1%pred decreased to less than 5% with stable symptoms.

Statistical Analysis

Univariable analyses for treatment response risk factors were performed using the Fisher exact test and chi-square test. Logistic regression analysis was used to perform multivariable analysis for risk factors with $p < 0.1$ in univariate analysis. OS was defined as the time from stem cell infusion to death from any cause and calculated by Kaplan-Meier method. SPSS was used for the survival analysis (SPSS version 22.0.01; IBM, NY, United States). The proportional-hazards method was used to estimate the cumulative incidence of relapse and nonrelapse mortality (NRM). Relapse and nonrelapse mortality were competing risks for each other. The R statistical software (version 3.4.3; http://www.r-project.org) was used for the competing risk analysis.

RESULTS

Patient Characteristics

A total of 640 patients aged ≥14 years who were transplanted between January 2014 and June 2019 was screened. Eighty-nine patients were diagnosed with BOS related to cGVHD, not related to other pulmonary or infectious disease. Among these 89 patients, 30 patients who were refractory disease to first-line GCSs plus FAM and treated with ruxolitinib as second-line or ≥ third-line therapy, were retrospectively enrolled in this analysis (**Figure 1**). The patient characteristics are shown in **Table 1**. The median age was 27 (range 15–54) years at the time of transplantation. All the patients received a myeloablative conditioning regimen consisting of busulfan and cyclophosphamide. Antithymocyte globulin was also used in 22 (73.3%) patients, mainly for haploidentical stem cell transplantation. Fourteen (46.7%) patients received donor lymphocyte infusion as prophylaxis or preemptive intervention for relapse. Acute GVHD occurred in 21 patients, including 14 with I–II degree and 7 with III–IV degree disease. Chronic GVHD was present in all the 30 patients and graded as moderate in 6 (20%) and severe in 24 (80%) patients. For cGVHD, more than

TABLE 1 | Characteristics of the study cohort at baseline.

Characteristic	N = 30
Gender, male, n (%)	13 (43.3%)
Recipient age at SCT (yrs), median (range)	27 (15–54)
Hematologic malignancy, n (%)	
AML/AMLL	16 (53.4%)
ALL	12 (40%)
MDS	1 (3.3%)
NK/T lymphoma	1 (3.3%)
Disease status at SCT, n (%)	
CR	27 (90%)
NR	3 (10%)
Donor type, n (%)	
matched unrelated	1 (3.3%)
matched sibling	8 (26.7%)
haplo-identical related donor	21 (70%)
Stem cell source, PBMSC, n (%)	30 (100%)
Conditioning regimens, MAC, n (%)	30 (100%)
ATG in conditioning regimens, n (%)	22 (73.3%)
Prophylaxis for GVHD	
CSA, MTX plus MMF	23 (76.7%)
FK506, MTX plus MMF	7 (23.3%)
Donor lymphocyte infusion, n (%)	14 (46.7%)
Acute GVHD grade, n (%)	
0	9 (30%)
I-II	14 (46.7%)
III-IV	7 (23.3%)
Chronic GVHD sites (except lung)	
Skin	20 (66.7%)
Oral	19 (63.3%)
eyes	14 (46.7%)
Liver	6 (20%)
Joints	6 (20%)
GI	5 (16.7%)
Extrathoracic cGVHD, n (%)	
1–2	13 (43.3%)
≥3	17 (56.7%)
Chronic GVHD grade, n (%)	
Moderate	6 (20%)
Severe	24 (80%)
Time to BOS from SCT, days, median (range)	452 (106–1902)
FEV1 at the time of HSCT, mean (range)	99.6 (81.2–125.1)
FEV1 before ruxolitinib, mean (range)	43.8 (25.8–71.2)

half of patients (56.7%) had three or more organs involved apart from the lungs. The prophylaxis for fungal disease included fluconazole ($n = 11$), voriconazole ($n = 8$), or posaconazole ($n = 11$).

Before SCT, all the patients had normal PFTs, with FEV1% pred ranging from 81.2 to 125.1 (mean, 99.6). The median time from transplantation to the onset of BOS was 453 (range, 106–1902) days. At the time of BOS diagnosis, most patients presented with moderate or severe obstruction (mean FEV1% pred: 55.5%, range 39.2–76.0%). All the patients received systemic prednisone after the diagnosis of BOS, with a median dose of 0.48 (range, 0.25–0.9) mg/(kg · day), along with FAM therapy and/or CNIs, as a first-line treatment regimen. Therapies beyond front-line GCS, FAM, and CNIs included MMF ($n = 14$), imatinib ($n = 12$), MSCs infusion ($n = 5$), rituximab ($n = 2$), recombinant human α receptor antibody fusion protein of tumor necrosis factor (rhRPTN, etanercept) ($n = 1$), and pirfenidone ($n = 1$). Despite the aforementioned therapeutic intervention, these 30 patients had worsening lung function (decreased FEV1%pred from baseline by 5% or more), with or without worsening clinical symptoms; therefore, they switched to ruxolitinib.

Therapeutic Response to Ruxolitinib

Ruxolitinib was given after a median time of 125 (range 27–1,598) days from BOS diagnosis, as the second and ≥ third line of therapy in 33.3% (10/30) and 66.7% (20/30) of patients, respectively. After a median duration of ruxolitinib therapy of 9.25 (1.5–27) months, the best overall response rate (BOR) was 66.7%: three patients (10.0%) achieved a CR, and 17 (56.7%) achieved a PR. The ORR at 180 days was 56.7%. The median time from initiation of ruxolitinib to achieving the best responses was 3 (range, 1.5–8) months. Ten patients (33.3%) were nonresponders, including four with SD and six with progression. At the last follow-up, ruxolitinib was stopped in 16 patients due to continuous good response (FEV1%pred >60%, $n = 2$; FEV1% pred >75%, $n = 2$), bone marrow relapse of primary malignancy ($n = 3$), severe infectious complications ($n = 3$), and BOS progression ($n = 6$) (**Figure 2**).

Before the initiation of ruxolitinib, the mean FEV1%pred was 43.8 (range, 25.8–71.2). Since initiating ruxolitinib, PFTs improved over time in the 20 responders, whose FEV1%pred increased after 3 and 6 months compared with measurements before ruxolitinib (mean FEV1%pred in month 0 vs. month 3 vs. month 6: 49.5 vs. 53.0 vs. 60.5; month 0 vs. month 6: $p = 0.029$) (**Figure 3A**). An average reduction in prednisone dose of 44.3% after 3 months of ruxolitinib therapy and 80.9% after 6 months of ruxolitinib therapy was reported (**Figure 3B**). After a median follow-up of 318 (range, 53–730) days after ruxolitinib, nine responders (9/20, 45%) were able to stop steroids and 11 were able to wean steroids to 0.2 mg/(kg · day) with stable symptoms.

Patients with FEV1%pred >39% when receiving ruxolitinib were more likely to achieve a response compared with those with FEV1%pred ≤39%. (ORR 89.5 vs. 27.3%, $p = 0.001$). Also, the decline ratio of FEV1%pred from BOS diagnosis to ruxolitinib initiation ranged from 6.6 to 56.6%, with a median value of 15.0%. The mild-decline group with the FEV1%pred decline ratio ≤15% showed a significantly higher response rate compared with the severe-decline group whose FEV1%pred decline ratio was more than 15% (ORR 100 vs. 28.6%, $p < 0.001$). Other features related to a better response might be the use of ruxolitinib as the second line of therapy, compared with ≥third line (ORR 90.9 vs. 52.6%, $p = 0.037$). No difference in ORR was observed between early ruxolitinib group (interval from BOS diagnosis to ruxolitinib <6 months) and late ruxolitinib group (interval from BOS diagnosis to ruxolitinib ≥6 months) (61.1 vs. 75%, $p = 0.350$). Also, no significant differences related to response in age, sex, donor type, DLI history, chronic GVHD sites, BOS onset time and steroid dose at start of ruxolitinib were found. Variables with $p < 0.05$ in the univariate analysis were included in the later multivariate logistic regression analysis: FEV1%pred at ruxolitinib initiation; FEV1%pred decline ratio from BOS diagnosis to ruxolitinib initiation; ruxolitinib as different lines of salvage treatment. Only FEV1%pred mild decline before ruxolitinib was an independent predictor to achieve a response to ruxolitinib. (HR = 0.096, 95% CI 0.026–0.353, $p = 0.001$) (**Table 2**).

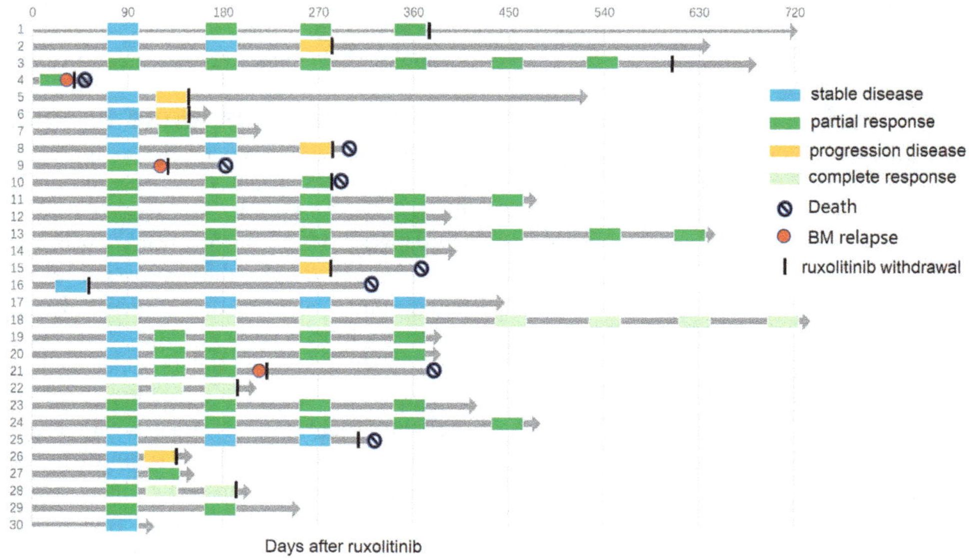

FIGURE 2 | Swimmer plot depicting response, duration of response, and patient outcome with ruxolitinib for all 30 patients.

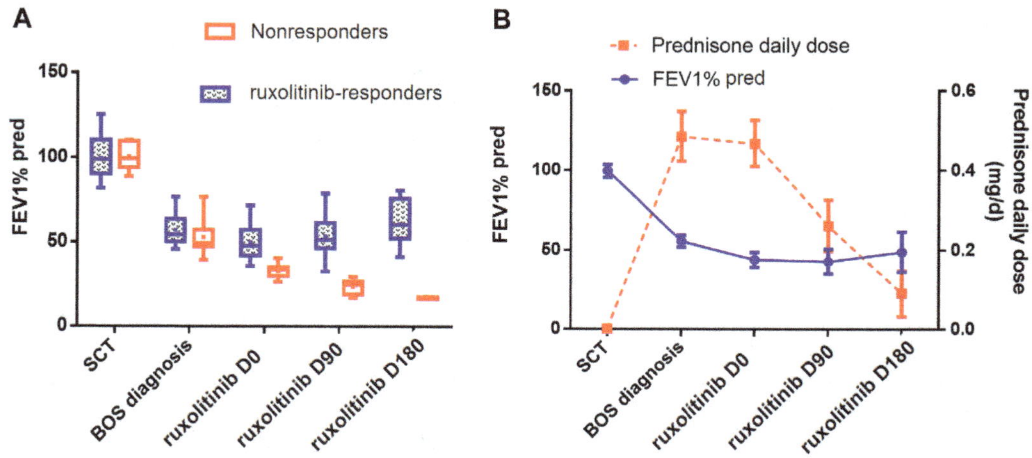

FIGURE 3 | (A) Distribution of FEV1%pred over time in ruxolitinib responders and nonresponders. **(B)** Distribution of FEV1% pred and prednisone daily dose over time in all ruxolitinib-treated patients. All the parameters were represented by the mean values and 95%CI. FEV1%pred, forced expiratory volume in 1 s of predicted; BOS, bronchiolitis obliterans syndrome; SCT, stem cell transplantation.

TABLE 2 | Clinical univariate and multivariate analysis for achieving a response to ruxolitinib.

Variable	Univariate		Multivariate	
	ORR (%)	P	Hazard ratio (CI 95%)	P
Ruxolitinib salvage therapy		0.037		
2nd line	90.9			
≥3rd line	52.6			
FEV1 at ruxolitinib initiation				
≤39%	27.3	0.001		
>39%	89.5			
FEV1 decline ratio from BOS diagnosis to ruxolitinib initiation				
≤15%	100	0.001	0.096 (95% CI 0.026–0.35)	0.001
>15%	28.6		1	

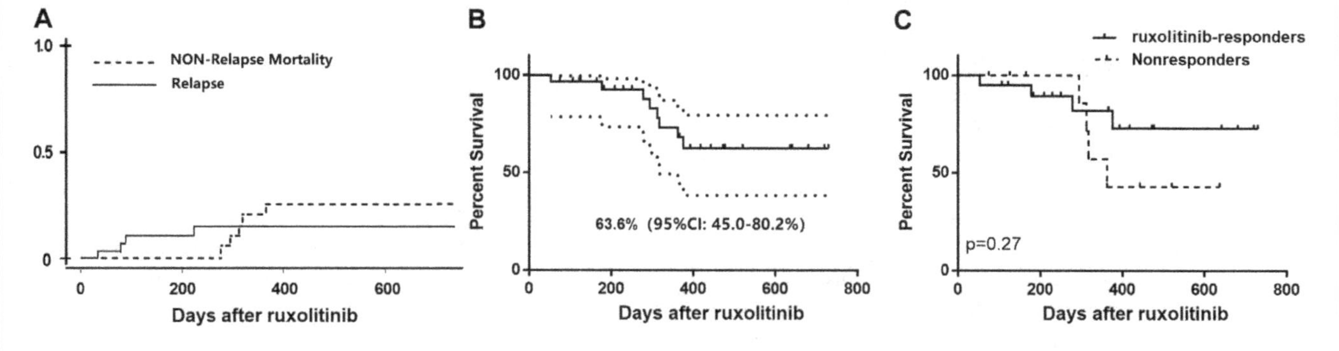

FIGURE 4 | (A) Cumulative incidence of relapse and nonrelapse mortality of all the patients with BOS receiving ruxolitinib; **(B)** Overall survival curve of all ruxolitinib-treated patients; **(C)** Overall survival of ruxolitinib-responders and nonresponders.

ADVERSE EVENTS

Any grade hematological toxicities were observed in 4 (13.3%) patients, and for grade ≥3 cytopenia, only one patient had grade ≥3 anemia. Regarding the nonhematological toxicities, two patients developed grade 3 hypertriglyceridemia. Infection-related events were frequent in the present cohort. Of the 30 patients, 100% were cytomegalovirus (CMV) IgG positive, with a CMV-seropositive donor. CMV reactivation indicated as CMV DNAemia was observed in three patients (10%). Epstein-Barr virus (EBV) reactivation was observed in 11 patients (36.7%). None of the patients developed CMV disease or EBV post-transplant lymphoproliferative disorder. Hepatitis B virus was re-activated in two patients (6.7%), both of whom were hepatitis B surface antigen-negative (HBsAg-)/hepatitis B core antibody-positive (HBcAb+)/hepatitis B surface antibody negative (HBsAb-) without any hepatitis B prophylaxis. Fourteen patients (46.7%) were complicated with pulmonary infection ≥2 grade, including invasive pulmonary fungal diseases in 10 patients, pulmonary bacterial in three patients, and mixed infection (nocardiosis/Aspergillus fumigatus/*Klebsiella pneumoniae*) in one patient. The risk for pulmonary fungal infection was 54.5% in fluconazole prophylaxis group and 26.3% in voriconazole or posaconazole group (p = 0.238). The incidence of pulmonary infection was higher in the nonresponders than in the responders (89.0 vs. 46.7%, p = 0.019). No bacteremia occurred in this cohort.

RELAPSE AND SURVIVAL AMONG PATIENTS WITH BOS TREATED WITH RUXOLITINIB

After a median follow-up of 318 (range, 53–730) days after ruxolitinib initiation, 4 out of 30 patients experienced a relapse of primary malignancy, including three bone marrow relapse and one with isolated extramedullary relapse. The cumulative 1-year incidence of relapse of the underlying malignancy was 14.7% (95%CI: 4.4–30.9%) after ruxolitinib. Eventually, eight patients died (26.7%), with causes of death predominantly resulting from infection (severe pulmonary infection/respiratory failure, n = 4; severe hepatitis B/hepatorenal syndrome, n = 1) and bone marrow relapse of original malignant disease (n = 3). The 2-years incidence of NRM and 2-years OS rate after ruxolitinib among patients with BOS were 25.1% (95%CI: 8.8–45.5%) and 62.6% (95% CI: 45.0–80.2%), respectively. There is no statistically significant difference in survival rate in ruxolitinib-responders and no responding patients (1-year OS rate: 72.9 vs. 42.9%, p = 0.27) (**Figure 4**).

DISCUSSION

Ruxolitinib, a potent anti-GVHD drug, might be a promising therapeutic option for BOS after HSCT. The present study added to a growing body of evidence for the use of ruxolitinib in SR-BOS related to cGVHD. In these heavily pretreated patients with BOS, ruxolitinib induced a relatively high response (ORR 66.7%), including FEV1 improvement and steroid sparing. The 2-years OS rate after ruxolitinib among patients with BOS was 62.6%. The present study suggests such heavily pretreated patients might benefit from salvage therapy with ruxolitinib. More importantly, relapse of the underlying malignancy in ruxolitinib-exposed patients was low (14.7%). This frequency is comparable to other currently applied immunosuppressive drugs, and other data from murine models proved that ruxolitinib does not impair the graft-vs.-leukemia (GvL) activity of alloreactive donor T cells, (Choi et al., 2014), indicating that ruxolitinib treatment is not linked to a higher relapse risk.

The pathophysiology of BOS following allo-HSCT is still not completely understood. Current evidence suggests that regulatory T (Treg) cells are effective in controlling chronic GVHD and BOS, as this cell subset can inhibit alloreactive T-cell and germinal center (GC) B-cell reactions to produce pathogenic antibodies for deposition in BOS lesion sites. (McDonald-Hyman et al., 2016). Due to the key role of JAK1/2-STAT3 pathways on T cells activation, JAK 1/2 inhibitor ruxolitinib may reduce donor alloreactive T-cell expansion and inflammatory cytokine production, and meanwhile preserve or even promote Treg recovery post-transplantation through sparing JAK3-STAT5 pathway (Spoerl et al., 2014), explaining the mechanism of action of ruxolitinib to ameliorate cGVHD related BOS. Furthermore, some components such as several chemokines, and other profibrotic factors accumulate in the airway, facilitate macrophage infiltration and collagen deposition, and hence lead to airway remodeling, and eventually, airway obstruction (Liu et al., 2001; Barker et al., 2014). In GVHD models, ruxolitinib was shown to decrease the production of chemokines and profibrotic cytokine (Spoerl et al., 2014), and in the neutrophilic asthma mouse model, it decreased the IL-17A level in bronchoalveolar lavage fluid (BALF), reduced the proportion of Th17 cells in lung tissue, and finally reduced airway inflammation. As for macrophages, ruxolitinib was shown to inhibit macrophage infiltration and prevent the upregulation of various proinflammatory cytokines in human macrophages (Maschalidi et al., 2016; Febvre-James et al., 2018). Collectively, the potent immunosuppressive and anti-inflammatory activities of ruxolitinib might be valuable for the management of BOS in the allogeneic stem cell transplantation setting.

This study demonstrated that while many patients showed an improvement in PFT with ruxolitinib, a substantial proportion of patients failed to respond to this treatment. Identifying potential responders may be more important than implementing ruxolitinib across the board in patients with BOS. Theoretically, early "inflammatory" phase might be more prone to respond to ruxolitinib than late "fibrotic" phase due to the potent anti-inflammatory effect of the drug. Actually, in our retrospective study, there is no significant difference in ORR between early ruxolitinib group and delayed ruxolitinib group. Only one element was identified to be independently related to achieving responses: FEV1% pred mild-decline before ruxolitinib with the FEV1%pred decline ratio ≤15%. It was consistent with a previous study by Kwok et al., who found that patients with BOS who manifested initial rapid lung function decline within 3 months of BOS diagnosis had significantly poorer lung function and worse OS compared with those with a gradual decline (Kwok et al., 2019). Unfortunately, despite interventions, a rapid persistent decline in FEV1 was associated with poor prognosis (Ahn et al., 2015). The ability of ruxolitinib to reverse the natural history of BOS in the FEV1 rapid decline cohort was not observed. Considering that the majority of early ruxolitinib group who moved quickly to ruxolitinib therapy belonged to the BOS progressive population, with a severe deteriorating pulmonary function, thereby the advantage of early inflammatory nature might be obscured by the more important element: rapid lung function decline. And the causes of the rapid deterioration of lung function need to be clarified and other treatment strategies need to be explored.

Ruxolitinib might increase the incidence of infections, which remained a major concern. Increasing evidence suggests that ruxolitinib may impair both innate and adaptive immunity. In detail, ruxolitinib was shown to reduced and functionally impaired dendritic cell (DC) leading to impaired T-cell activation (Heine et al., 2013a). Inhibition of JAK1 impairs cytokine production, which may result in reduced control of silent infections and increased risk of reactivation of latent infections (Heine et al., 2013b) In particular, ruxolitinib drastically reduces the quantity of natural killer (NK) cells (Schönberg et al., 2015). All these effects may result in varying degrees of immunodeficiency, leading to high risks for infectious complications. Besides, it's worth noting that the incidence of pulmonary infection (46.7%) in patients with BOS in the present study was obviously higher than that in patients with myeloproliferative neoplasms receiving ruxolitinib form Comfort II/JUMP (5.3–13.1%) and that in another cohort receiving ruxolitinib as GVHD prophylaxis (Lussana et al., 2018; Zhao et al., 2020b). indicating this high rate of coinfections was not only attributed to the effects of JAK1/2 inhibition on immunosurveillance but also associated with the innate characteristics of BOS. Like patients with bronchiectasis from other causes, patients with BOS can be colonized with Gram-negative organisms and fungus (mostly *Aspergillus*) (Hayes et al., 2013). Interestingly, in the present study, the incidence of pulmonary infection was higher in the nonresponders than in the responders. For nonresponders who relied on long-term high-dose steroids, ruxolitinib might worsen the infection status, inciting chemokines, accelerating BOS progression, and finally forming a vicious circle (Shino et al., 2013). Also, in our study, patients receiving fluconazole as antifungal prophylaxis might be even more at risk from fungal infection, indicating strong consideration should be given to voriconazole or posaconazole for prophylaxis, as mentioned by Williams, K.M (Williams, 2017). Taken together, the present study highlighted the importance of the assessment of risk factors for infectious events, along with anti-infective prophylaxis prior to initiation of ruxolitinib in patients who were already immunocompromised.

As it is considered standard of care, that every patient is required to monitor PFTs after allogeneic SCT, and in the long time, this implementation is highly recommended, thus the main limitation of the study is insufficient monitoring of PFTs in asymptomatic patients due to inadequate medical resources. The second imitation is that a small number of subjects and a retrospective nonrandomized design of this study might make a bias. However, our data still indicated ruxolitinib as a promising treatment option to improve the prognosis of post-HSCT BOS, with pulmonary function stabilization or even improvement and steroid sparing. This approach might provide a reference for the treatment of BOS in other causes including autoimmune and post lung transplantation. Also, the substantial clinical benefits and efficacy of ruxolitinib on BOS need to be balanced against infection risks. Further, hopefully prospective randomized controlled trials, are needed to definitely prove the efficacy of ruxolitinib in treatment of cGVHD-related BOS.

AUTHOR CONTRIBUTIONS

HH designed the study and supervised the analyses. YZ collected and analyzed the data, and wrote the manuscript. All authors discussed and interpreted the results. All authors approved the final version of the manuscript.

REFERENCES

Ahn, J. H., Jo, K.-W., Song, J. W., Shim, T. S., Lee, S. W., Lee, J. S., et al. (2015). Prognostic Role of FEV1for Survival in Bronchiolitis Obliterans Syndrome after Allogeneic Hematopoietic Stem Cell Transplantation. *Clin. Transpl.* 29 (12), 1133–1139. doi:10.1111/ctr.12638

Au, B. K. C., Au, M. A., and Chien, J. W. (2011). Bronchiolitis Obliterans Syndrome Epidemiology after Allogeneic Hematopoietic Cell Transplantation. *Biol. Blood Marrow Transplant.* 17 (7), 1072–1078. doi:10.1016/j.bbmt.2010.11.018

Barker, A. F., Bergeron, A., Rom, W. N., and Hertz, M. I. (2014). Obliterative Bronchiolitis. *N. Engl. J. Med.* 370 (19), 1820–1828. e-pub ahead of print 2014/05/09. doi:10.1056/NEJMra1204664

Bergeron, A., Chevret, S., Chagnon, K., Godet, C., Bergot, E., Peffault de Latour, R., et al. (2015). Budesonide/Formoterol for Bronchiolitis Obliterans after Hematopoietic Stem Cell Transplantation. *Am. J. Respir. Crit. Care Med.* 191 (11), 1242–1249. doi:10.1164/rccm.201410-1818OC

Bergeron, A., Chevret, S., Granata, A., Chevallier, P., Vincent, L., Huynh, A., et al. (2017). Effect of Azithromycin on Airflow Decline-free Survival after Allogeneic Hematopoietic Stem Cell Transplant. *JAMA* 318 (6), 557–566. doi:10.1001/jama.2017.9938

Brownback, K. R., Thomas, L. A., McGuirk, J. P., Ganguly, S., Streiler, C., and Abhyankar, S. (2017). Effect of Rituximab on Pulmonary Function in Bronchiolitis Obliterans Syndrome Due to Graft-Versus-Host-Disease. *Lung* 195 (6), 781–788. e-pub ahead of print 2017/09/13. doi:10.1007/s00408-017-0051-0

Chien, J. W., Duncan, S., Williams, K. M., and Pavletic, S. Z. (2010). Bronchiolitis Obliterans Syndrome after Allogeneic Hematopoietic Stem Cell Transplantation-An Increasingly Recognized Manifestation of Chronic Graft-Versus-Host Disease. *Biol. Blood Marrow Transplant.* 16 (1 Suppl. l), S106–S114. doi:10.1016/j.bbmt.2009.11.002

Choi, J., Cooper, M. L., Alahmari, B., Ritchey, J., Collins, L., Holt, M., et al. (2014). Pharmacologic Blockade of JAK1/JAK2 Reduces GvHD and Preserves the Graft-Versus-Leukemia Effect. *PLoS One* 9 (10), e109799. doi:10.1371/journal.pone.0109799

Del Fante, C., Galasso, T., Bernasconi, P., Scudeller, L., Ripamonti, F., Perotti, C., et al. (2016). Extracorporeal Photopheresis as a New Supportive Therapy for Bronchiolitis Obliterans Syndrome after Allogeneic Stem Cell Transplantation. *Bone Marrow Transpl.* 51 (5), 728–731. doi:10.1038/bmt.2015.324

Dudek, A. Z., Mahaseth, H., DeFor, T. E., and Weisdorf, D. J. (2003). Bronchiolitis Obliterans in Chronic Graft-Versus-Host Disease: Analysis of Risk Factors and Treatment Outcomes. *Biol. Blood Marrow Transplant.* 9 (10), 657–666. doi:10.1016/s1083-8791(03)00242-8

Escamilla Gómez, V., García-Gutiérrez, V., García-Gutiérrez, V., López Corral, L., García Cadenas, I., Pérez Martínez, A., et al. (2020). Ruxolitinib in Refractory Acute and Chronic Graft-Versus-Host Disease: a Multicenter Survey Study. *Bone Marrow Transpl.* 55 (3), 641–648. e-pub ahead of print 2019/11/09. doi:10.1038/s41409-019-0731-x

Febvre-James, M., Lecureur, V., Augagneur, Y., Mayati, A., and Fardel, O. (2018). Repression of Interferon β-regulated Cytokines by the JAK1/2 Inhibitor Ruxolitinib in Inflammatory Human Macrophages. *Int. immunopharmacol.* 54, 354–365. e-pub ahead of print 2017/12/05. doi:10.1016/j.intimp.2017.11.032

Greer, M., Berastegui, C., Jaksch, P., Benden, C., Aubert, J., Roux, A., et al. (2018). Lung Transplantation after Allogeneic Stem Cell Transplantation: a Pan-European Experience. *Eur. Respir. J.* 51 (2), 1701330, 2018 . e-pub ahead of print 2018/02/16. doi:10.1183/13993003.01330-2017

Harrison, C., Kiladjian, J.-J., Al-Ali, H. K., Gisslinger, H., Waltzman, R., Stalbovskaya, V., et al. (2012). JAK Inhibition with Ruxolitinib versus Best Available Therapy for Myelofibrosis. *N. Engl. J. Med.* 366 (9), 787–798. doi:10.1056/NEJMoa1110556

Hayes, D., Jr., Weiland, A., Kirkby, S., Galantowicz, M., McConnell, P. I., and Tobias, J. D. (2013). Gram-negative Infection and Bronchiectasis in Lung Transplant Recipients with Bronchiolitis Obliterans Syndrome. *Thorac. Cardiovasc. Surg.* 61 (3), 240–245. doi:10.1055/s-0032-1322619

Hefazi, M., Langer, K. J., Khera, N., Adamski, J., Roy, V., Winters, J. L., et al. (2018). Extracorporeal Photopheresis Improves Survival in Hematopoietic Cell Transplant Patients with Bronchiolitis Obliterans Syndrome without Significantly Impacting Measured Pulmonary Functions. *Biol. Blood Marrow Transplant.* 24 (9), 1906–1913. doi:10.1016/j.bbmt.2018.04.012

Heine, A., Held, S. A. E., Daecke, S. N., Wallner, S., Yajnanarayana, S. P., Kurts, C., et al. (2013). The JAK-Inhibitor Ruxolitinib Impairs Dendritic Cell Function *In Vitro* and *In Vivo*. *Blood* 122 (7), 1192–1202. doi:10.1182/blood-2013-03-484642

Heine, A., Brossart, P., and Wolf, D. (2013). Ruxolitinib Is a Potent Immunosuppressive Compound: Is it Time for Anti-infective Prophylaxis?. *Blood* 122 (23), 3843–3844. doi:10.1182/blood-2013-10-531103

Jagasia, M. H., Greinix, H. T., Arora, M., Williams, K. M., Wolff, D., Cowen, E. W., et al. (2015). National Institutes of Health Consensus Development Project on Criteria for Clinical Trials in Chronic Graft-Versus-Host Disease: I. The 2014 Diagnosis and Staging Working Group Report. *Biol. Blood Marrow Transplant.* 21 (3), 389–401. doi:10.1016/j.bbmt.2014.12.001

Khoury, H. J., Langston, A. A., Kota, V. K., Wilkinson, J. A., Pusic, I., Jillella, A., et al. (2018). Ruxolitinib: a Steroid Sparing Agent in Chronic Graft-Versus-Host Disease. *Bone Marrow Transpl.* 53 (7), 826–831. doi:10.1038/s41409-017-0081-5

Kim, S. W., Rhee, C. K., Kim, Y. J., Lee, S., Kim, H. J., and Lee, J. W. (2016). Therapeutic Effect of Budesonide/formoterol, Montelukast and N-Acetylcysteine for Bronchiolitis Obliterans Syndrome after Hematopoietic Stem Cell Transplantation. *Respir. Res.* 17 (1), 63. doi:10.1186/s12931-016-0380-1

Kwok, W. C., Liang, B. M., Lui, M. M. S., Tam, T. C. C., Sim, J. P. Y., Tse, E. W. C., et al. (2019). Rapid versus Gradual Lung Function Decline in Bronchiolitis Obliterans Syndrome after Haematopoietic Stem Cell Transplantation Is Associated with Survival Outcome. *Respirology* 24 (5), 459–466. doi:10.1111/resp.13472

Liu, J.-Y., Sime, P. J., Wu, T., Warshamana, G. S., Pociask, D., Tsai, S.-Y., et al. (2001). Transforming Growth Factor- β1Overexpression in Tumor Necrosis Factor- α Receptor Knockout Mice Induces Fibroproliferative Lung Disease. *Am. J. Respir. Cel Mol Biol* 25 (1), 3–7. doi:10.1165/ajrcmb.25.1.4481

Lucid, C. E., Savani, B. N., Engelhardt, B. G., Shah, P., Clifton, C., Greenhut, S. L., et al. (2011). Extracorporeal Photopheresis in Patients with Refractory Bronchiolitis Obliterans Developing after Allo-SCT. *Bone Marrow Transpl.* 46 (3), 426–429. doi:10.1038/bmt.2010.152

Lussana, F., Cattaneo, M., Rambaldi, A., and Squizzato, A. (2018). Ruxolitinib-associated Infections: A Systematic Review and Meta-Analysis. *Am. J. Hematol.* 93 (3), 339–347. e-pub ahead of print 2017/11/19. doi:10.1002/ajh.24976

Maschalidi, S., Sepulveda, F. E., Garrigue, A., Fischer, A., and de Saint Basile, G. (2016). Therapeutic Effect of JAK1/2 Blockade on the Manifestations of Hemophagocytic Lymphohistiocytosis in Mice. *Blood* 128 (1), 60–71. doi:10.1182/blood-2016-02-700013

McDonald-Hyman, C., Flynn, R., Panoskaltsis-Mortari, A., Peterson, N., MacDonald, K. P. A., Hill, G. R., et al. (2016). Therapeutic Regulatory T-Cell Adoptive Transfer Ameliorates Established Murine Chronic GVHD in a CXCR5-dependent Manner. *Blood* 128 (7), 1013–1017. doi:10.1182/blood-2016-05-715896

Schoettler, M., Duncan, C., Lehmann, L., Furutani, E., Subramaniam, M., and Margossian, S. (2019). Ruxolitinib Is an Effective Steroid Sparing Agent in Children with Steroid Refractory/dependent Bronchiolitis Obliterans Syndrome after Allogenic Hematopoietic Cell Transplantation. *Bone Marrow Transpl.* 54 (7), 1158–1160. doi:10.1038/s41409-019-0450-3

Schönberg, K., Rudolph, J., Vonnahme, M., Parampalli Yajnanarayana, S., Cornez, I., Hejazi, M., et al. (2015). JAK Inhibition Impairs NK Cell Function in Myeloproliferative Neoplasms. *Cancer Res.* 75 (11), 2187–2199. doi:10.1158/0008-5472.CAN-14-3198

Shino, M. Y., Weigt, S. S., Li, N., Palchevskiy, V., Derhovanessian, A., Saggar, R., et al. (2013). CXCR3 Ligands Are Associated with the Continuum of Diffuse Alveolar Damage to Chronic Lung Allograft Dysfunction. *Am. J. Respir. Crit. Care Med.* 188 (9), 1117–1125. doi:10.1164/rccm.201305-0861OC

Spoerl, S., Mathew, N. R., Bscheider, M., Schmitt-Graeff, A., Chen, S., Mueller, T., et al. (2014). Activity of Therapeutic JAK 1/2 Blockade in Graft-Versus-Host Disease. *Blood* 123 (24), 3832–3842. doi:10.1182/blood-2013-12-543736

Streiler, C., Shaikh, F., Davis, C., Abhyankar, S., and Brownback, K. R. (2020). Ruxolitinib Is an Effective Steroid Sparing Agent in Bronchiolitis Obliterans Due to Chronic Graft-Versus-Host-Disease. *Bone Marrow Transpl.* 55 (6), 1194–1196. e-pub ahead of print 2019/09/06. doi:10.1038/s41409-019-0662-6

Vogl, U. M., Nagayama, K., Bojic, M., Hoda, M. A. R., Klepetko, W., Jaksch, P., et al. (2013). Lung Transplantation for Bronchiolitis Obliterans after Allogeneic Hematopoietic Stem Cell Transplantation. *Transplantation* 95 (4), 623–628. doi:10.1097/TP.0b013e318277e29e

Watanabe, S., Waseda, Y., Kimura, H., Takato, H., Ohata, K., Kondo, Y., et al. (2015). Imatinib for Bronchiolitis Obliterans after Allogeneic Hematopoietic Stem Cell Transplantation. *Bone Marrow Transpl.* 50 (9), 1250–1252. doi:10.1038/bmt.2015.120

Watanabe, S., Kasahara, K., Waseda, Y., Takato, H., Nishikawa, S., Yoneda, T., et al. (2017). Imatinib Ameliorates Bronchiolitis Obliterans via Inhibition of Fibrocyte Migration and Differentiation. *J. Heart Lung Transplant.* 36 (2), 138–147. doi:10.1016/j.healun.2016.06.001

Williams, K. M., Chien, J. W., Gladwin, M. T., and Pavletic, S. Z. (2009). Bronchiolitis Obliterans after Allogeneic Hematopoietic Stem Cell Transplantation. *JAMA* 302 (3), 306–314. doi:10.1001/jama.2009.1018

Williams, K. M., Cheng, G.-S., Pusic, I., Jagasia, M., Burns, L., Ho, V. T., et al. (2016). Fluticasone, Azithromycin, and Montelukast Treatment for New-Onset Bronchiolitis Obliterans Syndrome after Hematopoietic Cell Transplantation. *Biol. Blood Marrow Transplant.* 22 (4), 710–716. e-pub ahead of print 2015/10/18. doi:10.1016/j.bbmt.2015.10.009

Williams, K. M. (2017). How I Treat Bronchiolitis Obliterans Syndrome after Hematopoietic Stem Cell Transplantation. *Blood* 129 (4), 448–455. doi:10.1182/blood-2016-08-693507

Wu, H., Shi, J., Luo, Y., Tan, Y., Zhang, M., Lai, X., et al. (2021). Evaluation of Ruxolitinib for Steroid-Refractory Chronic Graft-Vs-Host Disease after Allogeneic Hematopoietic Stem Cell Transplantation. *JAMA Netw. Open* 4 (1), e2034750. doi:10.1001/jamanetworkopen.2020.34750

Yanik, G. A., Mineishi, S., Levine, J. E., Kitko, C. L., White, E. S., Vander Lugt, M. T., et al. (2012). Soluble Tumor Necrosis Factor Receptor: Enbrel (Etanercept) for Subacute Pulmonary Dysfunction Following Allogeneic Stem Cell Transplantation. *Biol. Blood Marrow Transplant.* 18 (7), 1044–1054. doi:10.1016/j.bbmt.2011.11.031

Zeiser, R., Burchert, A., Lengerke, C., Verbeek, M., Maas-Bauer, K., Metzelder, S. K., et al. (2015). Ruxolitinib in Corticosteroid-Refractory Graft-Versus-Host Disease after Allogeneic Stem Cell Transplantation: a Multicenter Survey. *Leukemia* 29 (10), 2062–2068. e-pub ahead of print 2015/08/01. doi:10.1038/leu.2015.212

Zhao, Y., Wu, H., Shi, J., Luo, Y., Li, X., Lan, J., et al. (2020). Ruxolitinib Combined with Etanercept Induce a Rapid Response to Corticosteroid-refractory Severe Acute Graft vs Host Disease after Allogeneic Stem Cell Transplantation: Results of a Multi-center Prospective Study. *Am. J. Hematol.* 95 (9), 1075–1084. doi:10.1002/ajh.25898

Zhao, Y., Shi, J., Luo, Y., Gao, F., Tan, Y., Lai, X., et al. (2020). Calcineurin Inhibitors Replacement by Ruxolitinib as Graft-Versus-Host Disease Prophylaxis for Patients after Allogeneic Stem Cell Transplantation. *Biol. Blood Marrow Transplant.* 26 (5), e128–e133. doi:10.1016/j.bbmt.2020.01.012

4

Ferroptosis: A New Insight into Acute Lung Injury

Xiaofang Yin[1†], *Guisong Zhu*[1†], *Qian Wang*[2], *Yuan Dong Fu*[1], *Juan Wang*[1] *and Biao Xu*[1*]

[1]*Intensive Care Uint, Nanjing Hospital of Chinese Medicine Affiliated to Nanjing University of Chinese Medicine, Nanjing, China,* [2]*Department of Respiration, Jiangsu Province Hospital of Chinese Medicine, Affiliated Hospital of Nanjing University of Chinese Medicine, Nanjing, China*

***Correspondence:**
Biao Xu
20185031@njucm.edu.cn

[†]*These authors have contributed equally to this work*

Acute lung injury (ALI), a common and critical illness with high morbidity and mortality, is caused by multiple causes. It has been confirmed that oxidative stress plays an important role in the development of ALI. Ferroptosis, a newly discovered programmed cell death in 2012, is characterized by iron-dependent lipid peroxidation and involved in many diseases. To date, compelling evidence reveals the emerging role of ferroptosis in the pathophysiological process of ALI. Here, we review the role of ferroptosis in the pathogenesis of ALI and its therapeutic potential in ALI.

Keywords: ferroptosis, acute lung injury, iron metabolism, lipid peroxidation, ferrostatin-1, lipoxstatin-1, iASPP

INTRODUCTION

Acute lung injury (ALI), a common and critical illness with high morbidity and mortality, is caused by a variety of factors, including pulmonary and extrapulmonary factors (Ware et al., 2000; Mutlu et al., 2006; Matthay et al., 2019). The pathogenesis of ALI is not fully understood, and there is still no effective targeted intervention. Therefore, it is of great significance to study the pathogenesis and treatment of ALI. The pathogenesis of ALI was previously believed to involve inflammation, coagulation, oxidative stress, repair and so on (Matthay et al., 2019). In 2012, Dixon et al. proposed ferroptosis, a new concept of cell death. Studies have shown that ferroptosis is closely related to tumor, nervous system disease, infection, ischemia/reperfusion (I/R) injury, kidney injury and other diseases (Friedmann et al., 2014; Linkermann et al., 2014; Stockwell et al., 2017; Dar et al., 2018; Amaral et al., 2019; Hu et al., 2019; Mou et al., 2019; Han et al., 2020; Mao et al., 2020). In recent years, ferroptosis has also been confirmed to contribute to lipopolysaccharide (LPS)-induced ALI, intestinal I/R-induced ALI, oleic acid-induced ALI, and acute radiation-induced lung injury (RILI) (Li et al., 2019; Liu et al., 2020; Dong et al., 2020; Li et al., 2020; Zhou et al., 2019). In addition, ferroptosis inhibitors ferrostatin-1 and lipoxstatin-1, as well as inhibitor of apoptosis-stimulating protein of p53 (iASPP), can mediate protective effects against ALI by inhibiting ferroptosis (Liu et al., 2020; Li et al., 2020). This review summarizes the research progress, regulatory mechanism and therapeutic potential of ferroptosis in ALI (**Figure 1**).

Ferroptosis Is Iron-dependent Lipid Peroxidation

Ferroptosis was first discovered as a unique form of cell death by Dixon et al. when studying the mechanism of erastin killing tumor cells with RAS mutation in 2012 (Dixon et al., 2012). As a programmed cell death, ferroptosis is quite different from apoptosis and autophagy in morphology (**Table 1**). The characteristics of ferroptosis include decreased mitochondrial crista, increased mitochondrial membrane density, along with ruptured mitochondrial outer membrane as observed under electron microscopy, but the integrity of nucleus remains (Kazan et al., 2019). Besides mitochondria, other organelles such as golgi, endoplasmic reticulum and lysosome, are also

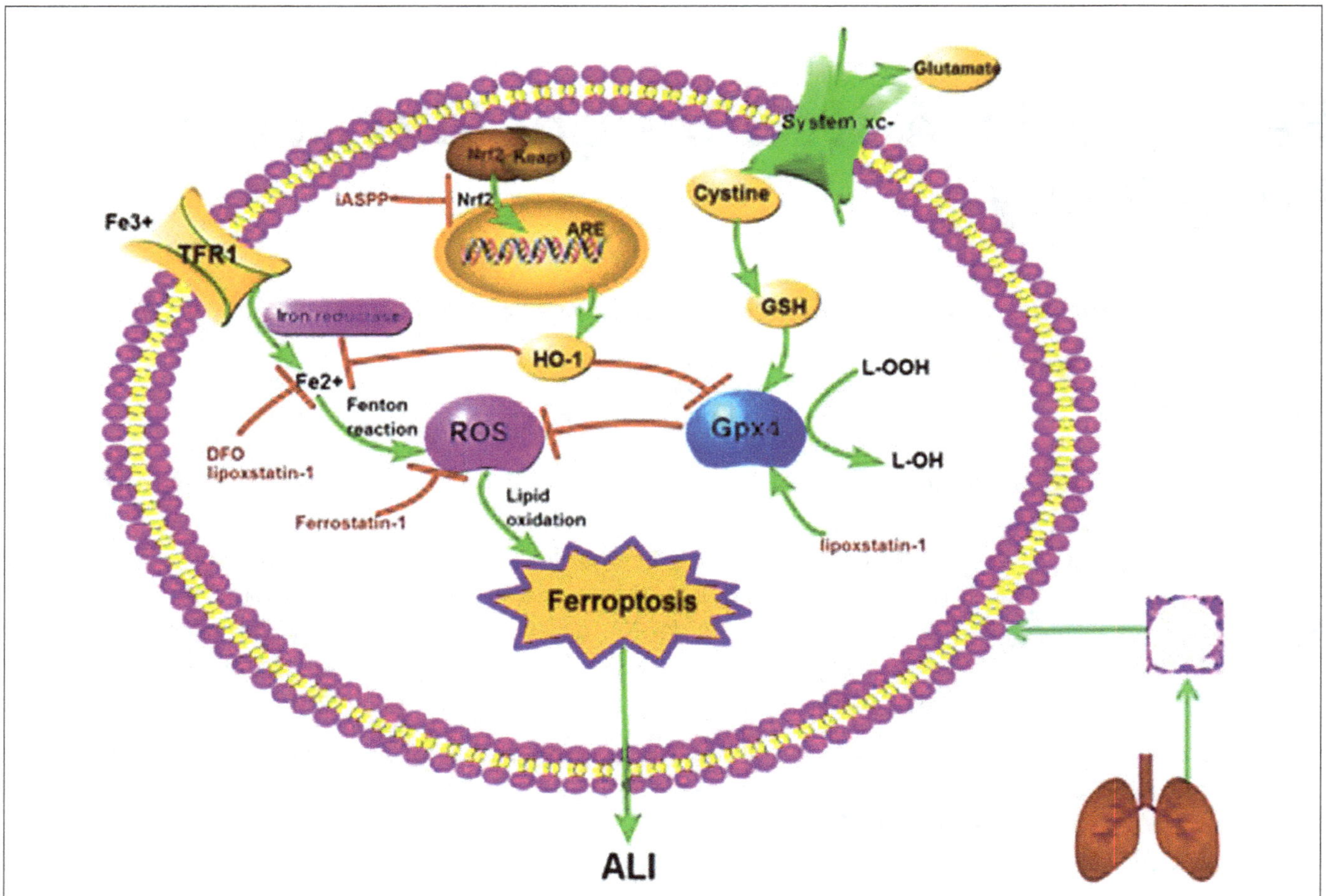

FIGURE 1 | The molecular mechanism and regulation of ferroptosis in ALI. Note: ALI: acute lung injury; GSH: glutathione peroxidase 4; ROS: reactive oxygen species; Nrf2: nuclear factor erythroid 2-related factor 2; HO-1: heme oxygenase-1; ARE: antioxidant response element; TFR1: transferrin receptor 1; DFO: deferoxamine; iASSP: inhibitor of apoptosis-stimulating protein of p53.

TABLE 1 | Morphological comparison between ferroptosis, apoptosis, necrosis, pyroptosis and autophagy (Kazan et al., 2019); (Dixon et al., 2012); (Wu et al., 2020); (Stockwell et al., 2017); (Li et al., 2020).

Cell death	Ferroptosis	Apoptosis	Necrosis	Pyroptosis	Autophagy
Morphological characteristics	Shrinkage of mitochondria, reduction of mitochondrial cristae, increase of mitochondrial density, rupture of mitochondrial outer membrane	Blebbing of plasma membrane, reduction in cellular and nuclear volume, nuclear rupture	Plasma membrane swelling, organelle swelling, moderate chromatin condensation	Karyopyknosis, cell edema, rupture of cell membrane	Formation of double-membrane autophagic lysosomes
Biochemical characteristics	Iron accumulation and lipid peroxidation, inhibition of system Xc-, depletion of GSH, and inhibition of GPX4	Caspases activation, fragmentation of oligonucleotide DNA	RIP1-RIP3 complex formation, activation of effector protein MLKL, necrotic body formation (complex IIb)	Caspase-1 mediated, assembly of inflammasome, release of inflammatory factors	The activity of lysosome increasing, digestion and degradation of many enzymes

involved in ferroptosis. Golgi stress-related lipid peroxidation, endoplasmic reticulum-related oxidative stress, and lysosome dysfunction can induce ferroptosis (Wu et al., 2020). The biological properties of ferroptosis are characterized by a large amount of iron accumulation and membrane lipid peroxidation products in the process of cell death. At present, the mechanism of ferroptosis mainly focuses on oxidative damage and iron metabolism (Stockwell et al., 2017; Li et al., 2020). Lipid

TABLE 2 | Ferroptosis in several types of ALI.

	Types of ALI	Manifestation	Signal pathway
Ferroptosis	Sepsis-induced lung injury	Down-regulation of SLC7A11 and GPx4, MDA and total iron increasing Yu et al. (2014); Yu et al. (2014); Liu et al. (2020); Liu et al. (2020)	Nrf2/ARE
	Intestinal I/R-Induced ALI	Pulmonary edema, lipid peroxidation Dong et al. (2020); Meng et al. (2016); Li et al. (2020)	Nrf2/HIF-1α/TF
	Oleic acid-induced ALI	Iron overload, decrease in glutathione, GPx4 and ferritin, increase in MDA content Lee et al. (2014); Zhou et al. (2019)	Unclear
	Radiation-induced lung injury	A large amount of ROS producing Li et al. (2019)	Unclear

peroxidation and iron metabolism signaling are recognized as the central mediators of ferroptosis (Xie et al., 2016).

Cystine/glutamate transporter (system Xc-) is an important antioxidant, composed of two subunits, SLC7A11 and SLC3A2L. It can transfer cystine into cells and excrete glutamate out of cells. Cystine and glutamate are exchanged by system Xc-in a ratio of 1: 1. Cystine is reduced to cysteine by system Xc- and participates in the synthesis of glutathione (GSH) (Chen et al., 2015). Then GSH is reduced to corresponding alcohols under the action of glutathione peroxidase 4 (Gpx4) (Bridges et al., 2012). Therefore, inhibition of system Xc- and Gpx4 can reduce Cystine uptake and GSH synthesis, leading to oxidative damage and even cell death. This process is also different from apoptosis and autophagy.

As a substrate for the synthesis of lipid signal mediators, the amount and location of polyunsaturated fatty acids (PUFA) determine the degree of lipid peroxidation in cells. The ferroptosis signal transmitted by PUFA depends on the esterification of membrane-forming phospholipids and oxidation (D'Herde et al., 2017). Acyl CoA synthase long chain family member 4 (ACSL4) and Lysophosphatidylcholine acyltransferase 3 (LPCAT3) are involved in the biosynthesis and remodeling of polyunsaturated fatty acid PE (PUFA-PE) in cell membrane. With the activation of ACSL4, the free PUFA could be esterified with the help of LPCAT3, and then bound to the membrane phospholipid to form PUFA-PE. Therefore, the up-regulation of ACSL4 is considered as a biomarker and contributor of ferroptosis. PUFA-PE can promote lipoxygenase (LOXs)-mediated enzymatic reaction to form lipid hydroperoxides. Therefore, the depletion of LOXs in cells can prevent ferroptosis induced by erastin (Yang et al., 2016).

Circulating iron exists in the form of ferric iron (Fe^{3+}) by binding to transferrin. Fe^{3+} iron is imported into the cell via the membrane protein transferrin receptor 1 (TFR1) and then locates in the endosome. Then the Fe^{3+} iron is reduced to ferrous iron (Fe^{2+}) by reductase in the endosome. The release of Fe^{2+} can be mediated by divalent metal transporter1 (DMT1) from the endosome into the cytoplasm that is a labile iron pool. Ferritin is an iron storage protein complex, where excessive iron is stored in. It includes ferritin light chain (FTL) and ferritin heavy chain1 (FTH1) (Harrison et al., 1996). FTH1 catalyzes the conversion of Fe^{2+} form into the Fe^{3+} form and then the Fe^{3+} iron is bound to the ferritin shell, thus reducing the level of free iron. Excessive iron can lead to ferroptosis by producing ROS through Fenton reaction (Wang et al., 2018).

Key Regulators of Ferroptosis

Gpx4

There are eight subtypes of glutathione peroxidase (Gpx) in mammals, among which Gpx4 is the key regulator of ferroptosis (Brigelius-Flohe et al., 2013; Conrad et al., 2015). Gpx4, a single copy gene located on chromosome 19, was isolated and purified from pig liver by Ursini and colleagues in 1982 (Forcina et al., 2019; Ursini et al., 1982; Hirschhorn et al., 2019). It is a selenoprotein that can repair oxidative damage of lipid cells. Gpx4 is unique among Gpx subtypes as it is the only enzyme capable of reducing the esterified oxidized fatty acids and cholesterol hydroperoxides (Conrad et al., 2015). Gpx4 can convert intracellular toxic lipid hydrogen peroxide (L-OOH) into nontoxic lipid alcohol (L-OH), and promote the decomposition of hydrogen peroxide (H2O2), which can protect cell membrane from oxidative damage (Forcina et al., 2019). Therefore, Gpx4 is essential for preventing cell damage and maintaining tissue homeostasis (Wortmann et al., 2013). It was found that a large number of ferroptosis occurred in renal tubular cells when Gpx4 gene was knocked out (Friedmann et al., 2014). Specific blockade of Gpx4 can lead to destruction of muscles, neurons, and other cells, suggesting that Gpx4 is essential for survival of adult cells. In conclusion, inactivation of Gpx4 can lead to accumulation of lipid peroxide and ferroptosis, and Gpx4 plays a negative regulatory role in the process of ferroptosis (Forcina et al., 2019; Kinowaki et al., 2018).

System Xc−

System Xc− is an important intracellular antioxidant system. It is an amino acid transporter expressed on mammalian cell membrane, composed of two subunits, SLC7A11 and SLC3A2L. Intracellular glutamate is exchanged with extracellular cystine via system Xc− by the ratio of 1:1. Cystine is involved in the synthesis of GSH, an important intracellular free radical scavenger. Inhibition of system Xc− can lead to a rapid decrease in intracellular GSH level and rapid ferroptosis (Bridges et al., 2012; Dixon et al., 2012). Studies have also found that tumor suppressor p53 can inhibit the uptake of cystine by inhibiting SLC7A11, thus inducing ferroptosis (Jiang et al., 2015).

Nrf2

Nuclear factor erythroid 2-related factor 2 (Nrf2) is an important transcription factor regulating cellular oxidative stress response, and antioxidant response element (ARE) is a downstream signal molecule of Nrf2(Canning et al., 2015; Xie et al., 2016; Krajka-Kuźniak et al., 2017). After activation of Nrf2/ARE signaling pathway, a classical signaling pathway, a series of cell protective genes can be induced, such as heme oxygenase−1 (HO−1), nicotinamide adenine dinucleotide phosphate quinone oxidoreductase (NQO1), glutathione peroxidase (GSH−Px) and so on (Chen et al., 2018). Nrf2 plays a very important role in ferroptosis by regulating iron homeostasis and lipid peroxidation (Sun et al., 2016; Kerins et al., 2018; Dodson et al., 2019). Studies show that Nrf2/HO-1 signaling pathway can regulate anti-inflammatory, antioxidant stress, and ferroptosis, which plays a multi-organ protective role (Zhang et al., 2019; Jiang et al., 2020). Nrf2-keap1 pathway can change tumor microenvironment and affect tumor growth by up regulating xCT (SLC7A11 or system Xc−). Nrf2 overexpression or Keap1 knockout can inhibit ferroptosis, accelerate the proliferation of glioma cells, and reduce the survival rate of tumor patients, suggesting a potential target for tumor treatment (Sartori et al., 2010).

Ferroptosis and ALI

The clinical manifestations of ALI are characterized by diffuse pulmonary infiltration, refractory hypoxemia and respiratory distress. The pathological manifestations are injury of pulmonary capillary endothelial cells and alveolar epithelial cells, and diffuse alveolar and interstitial edema. As is well known, ALI can be caused by various extrapulmonary factors (such as sepsis, surgery, burns, fluid resuscitation, severe pancreatitis,etc.) and pulmonary factors (such as pulmonary inflammation, pulmonary contusion, aspiration,etc.). However, the confirmed pathogenesis of ALI is very complex, mainly involving the uncontrolled inflammatory reaction, the regulation of aquaporin, the imbalance of coagulation/ fibrinolysis system, apoptosis, autophagy, pyrosis and so on (Sartori et al., 2010; Kovarova et al., 2012; Matthay et al., 2019).

Under normal circumstances, the lung relies on the phagocytosis of macrophages, transferrin in secretion, antioxidant molecules on the surface of respiratory tract epithelium, and respiratory ciliary expectoration system to maintain iron homeostasis. Once the protective mechanisms are destroyed by endogenous or exogenous factors, oxidative stress injury occurs in the lung (Turi et al., 2004). It was found that there was iron excess in the lower respiratory tract of ALI patients (Stites et al., 1999; Ghio et al., 2003). Iron accumulation can lead to inflammatory reaction, oxidative stress and mitochondrial dysfunction, and eventually cause lung damage through ferroptosis (Yoshida et al., 2019). Iron excess can also induce or aggravate hyperoxia-induced lung injury in patients with mechanical ventilation or diving operators, while intravenous deferoxamine can attenuate lung injury (Sha et al., 2019). Iron also plays an important role in hypoxia-induced lung injury. Iron supplementation can promote inflammatory response and oxidative stress, and aggravates lung injury induced by high altitude in rats (Salama et al., 2014). In addition, it has been found that the total GSH decreased and oxidized glutathione (GSSG) increased in alveolar epithelial lining fluid of ALI patients and animal models (Schmidt et al., 2004; Britt et al., 2014). In conclusion, in the pathological process of ALI, the release of various reactive oxygen species and the generation of free radicals can damage alveolar epithelial cells, and iron overload can further promote the conversion of hydrogen peroxide into free radicals through Fenton reaction, which increases the cytotoxicity, thus promoting the occurrence and development of ALI (Zhang et al., 2019). In conclusion, these studies suggest that iron metabolism and oxidative stress may involve in the pathogenesisof ALI. With the development of ferroptosis research, more and more studies have found that ferroptosis is involved in the pathogenesis of ALI. It has been confirmed that ferroptosis exists in some animal models or cell models of ALI.

Ferroptosis Involved in ALI

Ferroptosis in Sepsis-Induced Lung Injury

Sepsis is a systemic inflammatory response syndrome caused by severe infection, with rapid progression and poor prognosis. ALI often occurs in the early stage of sepsis, but no effective treatments are currently available for it (Rubenfeld et al., 2005). Sepsis-induced lung injury is essentially an acute pathological injury of lung tissue caused by uncontrolled inflammatory reaction. *In vitro* (Liu et al., 2020), it was found that the expression of ferroptosis markers, SLC7A11, and GPx4, were down-regulated, while the levels of malondialdehyde (MDA) and total iron were significantly increased in a dose-dependent manner after lipopolysaccharide (LPS) intervention on the human bronchial epithelial cell line, BEAS-2B. Ferrostatin-1, an inhibitor of ferroptosis, could reverse the above effects, suggesting that ferroptosis played a very important role in the pathogenesis of LPS-induced ALI. *In vivo* (Yu et al., 2014; Liu et al., 2020), similar conclusions were drawn in ALI models established by intratracheal or intravenous injection of LPS. Ferroptosis may participate in LPS-induced ALI through Nrf2/ARE signaling pathway (Yu et al., 2014; Liu et al., 2020). Another study showed that HO−1 played a protective role in the pathogenesis of sepsis-induced lung injury, and artesunate could improve sepsis-induced lung injury by activating Nrf2 and promoting HO−1 expression (Luo et al., 2014; Cao et al., 2016; see **Table 2**). In conclusion, ferroptosis may be a potential therapeutic target for sepsis-induced lung injury, thus indicating the therapeutic potential of ferroptosis inhibitors for it.

Ferroptosis in Intestinal I/R-Induced ALI

Intestinal I/R injury can be caused by severe trauma, extensive burns, severe infection, shock, intestinal obstruction, cardiac surgery, etc. Once intestinal I/R injury occurs, intestinal mucosal barrier is destroyed, intestinal bacteria and toxins are translocated, and then a large number of cytokines and inflammatory mediators are released into blood circulation, leading to systemic inflammatory response and injury of distant organs. The lung is the earliest and most vulnerable organ, known as intestinal I/R-induced ALI, which plays a vital role in the development of multiple organ dysfunction syndrome (MODS) (de Perrot et al., 2003; Marco et al., 2007;

TABLE 3 | Impact of ferroptosis inhibitors on ALI.

Reagent	Target	Impact on ALI
Ferrostatin-1	Lipid peroxidation Dong et al. (2020) GPX4, SLC7A11 Liu et al. (2020)	Alleviating sepsis-induced ALI, improving intestinal I/R-induced ALI
Panaxydol	Keap1-Nrf2/HO−1 pathway Li et al. (2021)	Alleviating LPS-induced ALI
Lipoxstatin-1	GSH and GPX4, Nrf2 pathway Li et al. (2020)	Alleviating intestinal I/R-induced ALI
IASPP	Nrf2/HIF−1α/TF Li et al. (2020)	Protecting against intestinal I/R-induced ALI
Artesunate	HO−1Cao et al. (2016); Luo et al. (2014)	Protecting against sepsis-induced lung injury
Sevoflurane	HO−1 Liu et al. (2021)	Protecting against LPS-induced ALI

Mörs et al., 2017; Li et al., 2020). So far, the pathogenesis of intestinal I/R-induced ALI has not been fully elucidated, and there is no specific medicine.

In the past, apoptosis was considered to be the main regulatory cell death mode in various ischemic injury models. However, in recent years, more and more studies have found that ferroptosis is the main driving factor of ischemic injury (Tonnus et al., 2017). Studies *in vivo* and *in vitro* have confirmed that ferroptosis occurs in type II alveolar epithelial cells of mice with intestinal I/R injury, and ferroptosis is involved in intestinal I/R-induced ALI (Dong et al., 2020; Li et al., 2020). Ferroptosis inhibitor ferrostatin-1 can improve intestinal I/R-induced ALI by alleviating pulmonary edema and inhibiting lipid peroxidation, while iron can reverse the above effects. It has been found that Nrf2 regulates ferroptosis by promoting the expression of HO−1 and SLC7A11, which plays a protective role in ferroptosis. Nrf2 may be a key regulator of intestinal I/R-induced ALI (Meng et al., 2016; Dong et al., 2020). Further research shows that iASPP can alleviate intestinal I/R-induced ALI and ferroptosis through Nrf2/HIF-1α/TF signaling pathway (Li et al., 2020; see **Table 2**). At present, the mechanism research is still in its infancy.

Ferroptosis in Oleic Acid-Induced ALI

Intravenous injection of oleic acid is one of the methods to establish ALI models (Zhou et al., 2014). Once oleic acid microbubbles enter pulmonary capillaries, it results in pulmonary vascular congestion, increased capillary permeability and pulmonary interstitial edema, which is consistent with the pathological changes of ALI (Lee et al., 2014). In mice injected with oleic acid, iron overload, decrease in glutathione levels, GPx4 (a marker of ferroptosis) and ferritin, and increase in MDA content, were observed in lung tissues, accompanied with morphological changes of ferroptosis such as mitochondrial wrinkle and mitochondrial membrane rupture (Zhou et al., 2019; see **Table 2**). However, the specific molecular signaling pathways remain unclear.

Ferroptosis in RILI

The incidence of RILI was 16.7–50.3%, which increased the mortality and disability of lung cancer patients (S N et al., 2019). Oxidative damage of lung tissue, induced by a large amount of Reactive Oxygen Species (ROS) produced by radiation, is a key factor in the pathogenesis of RILI(Li et al., 2019). It has been found that ferroptosis played an important role in RILI, and ferroptosis inhibitor significantly reduced ROS in lung tissue and inflammatory factors in serum (Li et al., 2019; see **Table 2**).

Treatment of ALI by Targeting Ferroptosis

Ferroptosis is characterized by a large amount of iron accumulation and lipid peroxidation. Accordingly, the therapeutic targets for ferroptosis should focus on inhibiting iron metabolism and lipid peroxidation. Iron metabolism inhibitors and iron chelators, such as deferoxamine (DFO), can inhibit ferroptosis by inhibiting iron uptake (Wang et al., 2020). Inhibitors of lipid metabolism inhibit polyunsaturated fatty acids (PUFA) incorporation into phospholipid membranes, such as thiazolidinediones and knockdown of long-chain acyl-CoA synthetases (ACSL4) (Dixon et al., 2015; Doll et al., 2017). Ferroptosis inhibitor ferrostatin-1 can improve intestinal I/R-induced ALI by inhibiting lipid peroxidation and alleviating pulmonary edema (Dong et al., 2020). It can also alleviate sepsis-induced ALI by promoting the expression of SLC7A11 and GPx4 and reducing the levels of MDA and iron in lung tissue (Liu et al., 2020). Another ferroptosis inhibitor, lipoxstatin-1, can promote the expression of GSH and GPx4, and reduce the content of MDA, iron and transferrin. In addition, lipoxstatin-1 can reverse the effect of erastin on promoting ferroptosis, and alleviate intestinal I/R-induced ALI, suggesting the therapeutic potential of lipoxstatin-1 (Li et al., 2020). IASPP, which is a known inhibitor of p53 transcriptional activity, mainly exists in the cytoplasm. IASPP inhibits ferroptosis through Nrf2/HIF-1α/TF signaling pathway and plays a protective role in intestinal I/R-induced ALI, as demonstrated in MLE-2 cells (Li et al., 2020). Although these ferroptosis inhibitors have been proved to have the effect of improving ALI, they are still in animal models and/or *in vitro* studies, lack of clinical evidence (see **Table 3**).

CONCLUSION AND PERSPECTIVES

As a new form of programmed cell death, ferroptosis is known to mainly involve in tumor, nervous system diseases, I/R injury and acute kidney injury. In recent years, more and more studies have found that ferroptosis is also involved in the pathogenesis of ALI. Ferroptosis has been confirmed in many ALI animal models or cell models, but its specific mechanism has not been fully elucidated. Ferroptosis may be a target for the treatment of ALI, focusing on the inhibition of iron metabolism and lipid peroxidation. Ferrostatin-1, lipoxstatin-1 and iASPP have been proved to have the effects on inhibiting ferroptosis and protecting ALI. However, they only stay in animal models and/or *in vitro* studies, lack of clinical evidence. In the future, more comprehensive and in-depth scientific researches are needed to further explore the relationship between ferroptosis and ALI, to provide more theoretical basis for clinical work.

AUTHOR CONTRIBUTIONS

All authors listed have made a substantial, direct, and intellectual contribution to the work and approved it for publication.

REFERENCES

Amaral, E. P., Costa, D. L., Namasivayam, S., Riteau, N., Kamenyeva, O., Mittereder, L., et al. (2019). A Major Role for Ferroptosis in Mycobacterium Tuberculosis-Induced Cell Death and Tissue Necrosis. *J. Exp. Med.* 216 (3), 556–570. doi:10.1084/jem.20181776

Bridges, R. J., Natale, N. R., and Patel, S. A. (2012). System Xc- Cystine/glutamate Antiporter: an Update on Molecular Pharmacology and Roles within the CNS. *Br. J. Pharmacol.* 165 (1), 20–34. doi:10.1111/j.1476-5381.2011.01480.x

Brigelius-Flohé, R., and Maiorino, M. (2013). Glutathione Peroxidases. *Biochim. Biophys. Acta (Bba) - Gen. Subjects* 1830 (5), 3289–3303. doi:10.1016/j.bbagen.2012.11.020

Britt, R. D., Velten, M., Locy, M. L., Rogers, L. K., and Tipple, T. E. (2014). The Thioredoxin Reductase-1 Inhibitor Aurothioglucose Attenuates Lung Injury and Improves Survival in a Murine Model of Acute Respiratory Distress Syndrome. *Antioxid. Redox Signaling* 20 (17), 2681–2691. doi:10.1089/ars.2013.5332

Canning, P., Sorrell, F. J., and Bullock, A. N. (2015). Structural Basis of Keap1 Interactions with Nrf2. *Free Radic. Biol. Med.* 88 (Pt B), 101–107. doi:10.1016/j.freeradbiomed.2015.05.034

Cao, T.-h., Jin, S.-g., Fei, D.-s., Kang, K., Jiang, L., Lian, Z.-y., et al. (2016). Artesunate Protects against Sepsis-Induced Lung Injury via Heme Oxygenase-1 Modulation. *Inflammation* 39 (2), 651–662. doi:10.1007/s10753-015-0290-2

Chen, L., Li, X., Liu, L., Yu, B., Xue, Y., and Liu, Y. (2015). Erastin Sensitizes Glioblastoma Cells to Temozolomide by Restraining xCT and Cystathionine-γ-Lyase Function. *Oncol. Rep.* 33 (3), 1465–1474. doi:10.3892/or.2015.3712

Chen, Q. M., and Maltagliati, A. J. (2018). Nrf2 at the Heart of Oxidative Stress and Cardiac protection. *Physiol. Genomics* 50 (2), 77–97. doi:10.1152/physiolgenomics.00041.2017

Conrad, M., and Friedmann Angeli, J. P. (2015). Glutathione Peroxidase 4 (Gpx4) and Ferroptosis: What's So Special about it? *Mol. Cell Oncol.* 2 (3), e995047. doi:10.4161/23723556.2014.995047

D'Herde, K., and Krysko, D. V. (2017). Oxidized PEs Trigger Death. *Nat. Chem. Biol.* 13 (1), 4–5. doi:10.1038/nchembio.2261

Dar, H. H., Tyurina, Y. Y., Mikulska-Ruminska, K., Shrivastava, I., Ting, H.-C., Tyurin, V. A., et al. (2018). *Pseudomonas aeruginosa* Utilizes Host Polyunsaturated Phosphatidylethanolamines to Trigger Theft-Ferroptosis in Bronchial Epithelium. *J. Clin. Invest.* 128 (10), 4639–4653. doi:10.1172/JCI99490

de Perrot, M., Liu, M., Waddell, T. K., and Keshavjee, S. (2003). Ischemia-reperfusion-induced Lung Injury. *Am. J. Respir. Crit. Care Med.* 167 (4), 490–511. doi:10.1164/rccm.200207-670so

Dixon, S. J., Lemberg, K. M., Lamprecht, M. R., Skouta, R., Zaitsev, E. M., Gleason, C. E., et al. (2012). Ferroptosis: an Iron-dependent Form of Nonapoptotic Cell Death. *Cell* 149 (5), 1060–1072. doi:10.1016/j.cell.2012.03.042

Dixon, S. J., Winter, G. E., Musavi, L. S., Lee, E. D., Snijder, B., Rebsamen, M., et al. (2015). Human Haploid Cell Genetics Reveals Roles for Lipid Metabolism Genes in Nonapoptotic Cell Death. *ACS Chem. Biol.* 10 (7), 1604–1609. doi:10.1021/acschembio.5b00245

Dodson, M., Castro-Portuguez, R., and Zhang, D. D. (2019). NRF2 Plays a Critical Role in Mitigating Lipid Peroxidation and Ferroptosis. *Redox Biol.* 23, 101107. doi:10.1016/j.redox.2019.101107

Doll, S., Proneth, B., Tyurina, Y. Y., Panzilius, E., Kobayashi, S., Ingold, I., et al. (2017). ACSL4 Dictates Ferroptosis Sensitivity by Shaping Cellular Lipid Composition. *Nat. Chem. Biol.* 13 (1), 91–98. doi:10.1038/nchembio.2239

Dong, H., Qiang, Z., Chai, D., Peng, J., Xia, Y., Hu, R., et al. (2020). Nrf2 Inhibits Ferroptosis and Protects against Acute Lung Injury Due to Intestinal Ischemia Reperfusion via Regulating SLC7A11 and HO-1. *Aging* 12 (13), 12943–12959. doi:10.18632/aging.103378

Fan, Z., Wirth, A.-K., Chen, D., Wruck, C. J., Rauh, M., Buchfelder, M., et al. (2017). Nrf2-Keap1 Pathway Promotes Cell Proliferation and Diminishes Ferroptosis. *Oncogenesis* 6 (8), e371. doi:10.1038/oncsis.2017.65

Forcina, G. C., and Dixon, S. J. (2019). GPX4 at the Crossroads of Lipid Homeostasis and Ferroptosis. *Proteomics* 19 (18), 1800311. doi:10.1002/pmic.201800311

Friedmann Angeli, J. P., Schneider, M., Proneth, B., Tyurina, Y. Y., Tyurin, V. A., Hammond, V. J., et al. (2014). Inactivation of the Ferroptosis Regulator Gpx4 Triggers Acute Renal Failure in Mice. *Nat. Cel Biol* 16 (12), 1180–1191. doi:10.1038/ncb3064

Ghio, A. J., Carter, J. D., Richards, J. H., Richer, L. D., Grissom, C. K., and Elstad, M. R. (2003). Iron and Iron-Related Proteins in the Lower Respiratory Tract of Patients with Acute Respiratory Distress Syndrome. *Crit. Care Med.* 31 (2), 395–400. doi:10.1097/01.ccm.0000050284.35609.97

Han, C., Liu, Y., Dai, R., Ismail, N., Su, W., and Li, B. (2020). Ferroptosis and its Potential Role in Human Diseases. *Front. Pharmacol.* 11, 239. doi:10.3389/fphar.2020.00239

Harrison, P. M., and Arosio, P. (1996). The Ferritins: Molecular Properties, Iron Storage Function and Cellular Regulation. *Biochim. Biophys. Acta (Bba) - Bioenerg.* 1275 (3), 161–203. doi:10.1016/0005-2728(96)00022-9

Hirschhorn, T., and Stockwell, B. R. (2019). The Development of the Concept of Ferroptosis. *Free Radic. Biol. Med.* 133, 130–143. doi:10.1016/j.freeradbiomed.2018.09.043

Hu, Z., Zhang, H., Yang, S.-k., Wu, X., He, D., Cao, K., et al. (2019). Emerging Role of Ferroptosis in Acute Kidney Injury. *Oxidative Med. Cell Longevity* 2019, 1–8. doi:10.1155/2019/8010614

Jiang, L., Kon, N., Li, T., Wang, S.-J., Su, T., Hibshoosh, H., et al. (2015). Ferroptosis as a P53-Mediated Activity during Tumour Suppression. *Nature* 520 (7545), 57–62. doi:10.1038/nature14344

Jiang, T., Cheng, H., Su, J., Wang, X., Wang, Q., Chu, J., et al. (2020). Gastrodin Protects against Glutamate-Induced Ferroptosis in HT-22 Cells through Nrf2/HO-1 Signaling Pathway. *Toxicol. Vitro* 62, 104715. doi:10.1016/j.tiv.2019.104715

Kazan, K., and Kalaipandian, S. (2019). Ferroptosis: Yet Another Way to Die. *Trends Plant Sci.* 24 (6), 479–481. doi:10.1016/j.tplants.2019.03.005

Kerins, M. J., and Ooi, A. (2018). The Roles of NRF2 in Modulating Cellular Iron Homeostasis. *Antioxid. Redox Signaling* 29 (17), 1756–1773. doi:10.1089/ars.2017.7176

Kinowaki, Y., Kurata, M., Ishibashi, S., Ikeda, M., Tatsuzawa, A., Yamamoto, M., et al. (2018). Glutathione Peroxidase 4 Overexpression Inhibits ROS-Induced Cell Death in Diffuse Large B-Cell Lymphoma. *Lab. Invest.* 98 (5), 609–619. doi:10.1038/s41374-017-0008-1

Kovarova, M., Hesker, P. R., Jania, L., Nguyen, M., Snouwaert, J. N., Xiang, Z., et al. (2012). NLRP1-dependent Pyroptosis Leads to Acute Lung Injury and Morbidity in Mice. *J.I.* 189 (4), 2006–2016. doi:10.4049/jimmunol.1201065

Krajka-Kuźniak, V., Paluszczak, J., and Baer-Dubowska, W. (2017). The Nrf2-ARE Signaling Pathway: an Update on its Regulation and Possible Role in Cancer Prevention and Treatment. *Pharmacol. Rep.* 69 (3), 393–402. doi:10.1016/j.pharep.2016.12.011

Lee, S. M., Choi, H., Yang, G., Park, K. C., Jeong, S., and Hong, S. (2014). MicroRNAs Mediate Oleic Acid-Induced Acute Lung Injury in Rats Using an Alternative Injury Mechanism. *Mol. Med. Rep.* 10 (1), 292–300. doi:10.3892/mmr.2014.2155

Li, J., Cao, F., Yin, H.-l., Huang, Z.-j., Lin, Z.-t., Mao, N., et al. (2020). Ferroptosis: Past, Present and Future. *Cell Death Dis* 11 (2), 88. doi:10.1038/s41419-020-2298-2

Li, J., Lu, K., Sun, F., Tan, S., Zhang, X., Sheng, W., et al. (2021). Panaxydol Attenuates Ferroptosis against LPS-Induced Acute Lung Injury in Mice by Keap1-Nrf2/HO-1 Pathway. *J. Transl Med.* 19 (1), 96. doi:10.1186/s12967-021-02745-1

Li, X., Zhuang, X., and Qiao, T. (2019). Role of Ferroptosis in the Process of Acute Radiation-Induced Lung Injury in Mice. *Biochem. Biophysical Res. Commun.* 519 (2), 240–245. doi:10.1016/j.bbrc.2019.08.165

Li, Y., Cao, Y., Xiao, J., Shang, J., Tan, Q., Ping, F., et al. (2020). Inhibitor of Apoptosis-Stimulating Protein of P53 Inhibits Ferroptosis and Alleviates Intestinal Ischemia/reperfusion-Induced Acute Lung Injury. *Cell Death Differ* 27 (9), 2635–2650. doi:10.1038/s41418-020-0528-x

Linkermann, A., Skouta, R., Himmerkus, N., Mulay, S. R., Dewitz, C., De Zen, F., et al. (2014). Synchronized Renal Tubular Cell Death Involves Ferroptosis. *Proc. Natl. Acad. Sci. USA* 111 (47), 16836–16841. doi:10.1073/pnas.1415518111

Liu, P., Feng, Y., Li, H., Chen, X., Wang, G., Xu, S., et al. (2020). Ferrostatin-1 Alleviates Lipopolysaccharide-Induced Acute Lung Injury via Inhibiting Ferroptosis. *Cell Mol Biol Lett* 25, 10. doi:10.1186/s11658-020-00205-0

Liu, X., Wang, L., Xing, Q., Li, K., SiMa, J. X., Ma, X., et al. (2021). Sevoflurane Inhibits Ferroptosis: A New Mechanism to Explain its Protective Role against Lipopolysaccharide-Induced Acute Lung Injury. *Life Sci.* 275, 119391. doi:10.1016/j.lfs.2021.119391

Luo, Y.-p., Jiang, L., Kang, K., Fei, D.-s., Meng, X.-l., Nan, C.-c., et al. (2014). Hemin Inhibits NLRP3 Inflammasome Activation in Sepsis-Induced Acute Lung Injury, Involving Heme Oxygenase-1. *Int. Immunopharmacology* 20 (1), 24–32. doi:10.1016/j.intimp.2014.02.017

Mao, H., Zhao, Y., Li, H., and Lei, L. (2020). Ferroptosis as an Emerging Target in Inflammatory Diseases. *Prog. Biophys. Mol. Biol.* 155, 20–28. doi:10.1016/j.pbiomolbio.2020.04.001

Matthay, M. A., Zemans, R. L., Zimmerman, G. A., Arabi, Y. M., Beitler, J. R., Mercat, A., et al. (2019). Acute Respiratory Distress Syndrome. *Nat. Rev. Dis. Primers* 5 (1), 18. doi:10.1038/s41572-019-0069-0

Meng, Q.-T., Cao, C., Wu, Y., Liu, H.-M., Li, W., Sun, Q., et al. (2016). Ischemic post-conditioning Attenuates Acute Lung Injury Induced by Intestinal Ischemia-Reperfusion in Mice: Role of Nrf2. *Lab. Invest.* 96 (10), 1087–1104. doi:10.1038/labinvest.2016.87

Mörs, K., Hörauf, J.-A., Kany, S., Wagner, N., Sturm, R., Woschek, M., et al. (2017). Ethanol Decreases Inflammatory Response in Human Lung Epithelial Cells by Inhibiting the Canonical NF-kB-Pathway. *Cell Physiol Biochem* 43 (1), 17–30. doi:10.1159/000480313

Mou, Y., Wang, J., Wu, J., He, D., Zhang, C., Duan, C., et al. (2019). Ferroptosis, a New Form of Cell Death: Opportunities and Challenges in Cancer. *J. Hematol. Oncol.* 12 (1), 34. doi:10.1186/s13045-019-0720-y

Marco, M., Andrade, C. F., Han, B., Seth, R., Zhang, Y., Bai, X. H., et al. (2007). Intestinal Ischemia-Reperfusion-Induced Acute Lung Injury and Oncotic Cell Death in Multiple Organs. *Shock* 28 (2), 227–238. doi:10.1097/01.shk.0000278497.47041.e3

Mutlu, G. M., and Budinger, G. R. (2006). Incidence and Outcomes of Acute Lung Injury. *N. Engl. J. Med.* 354 (4), 416–417. doi:10.1056/NEJMc053159

Rubenfeld, G. D., Caldwell, E., Peabody, E., Weaver, J., Martin, D. P., Neff, M., et al. (2005). Incidence and Outcomes of Acute Lung Injury. *N. Engl. J. Med.* 353 (16), 1685–1693. doi:10.1056/NEJMoa050333

Salama, S. A., Omar, H. A., Maghrabi, I. A., AlSaeed, M. S., and El-Tarras, A. E. (2014). Iron Supplementation at High Altitudes Induces Inflammation and Oxidative Injury to Lung Tissues in Rats. *Toxicol. Appl. Pharmacol.* 274 (1), 1–6. doi:10.1016/j.taap.2013.10.034

Sartori, C., Rimoldi, S. F., and Scherrer, U. (2010). Lung Fluid Movements in Hypoxia. *Prog. Cardiovasc. Dis.* 52 (6), 493–499. doi:10.1016/j.pcad.2010.02.005

Schmidt, R., Luboeinski, T., Markart, P., Ruppert, C., Daum, C., Grimminger, F., et al. (2004). Alveolar Antioxidant Status in Patients with Acute Respiratory Distress Syndrome. *Eur. Respir. J.* 24 (6), 994–999. doi:10.1183/09031936.04.00120703

Sha, X. L., Li, Y., Wang, X., Wang, J., and Chen, S. (2019). Effect of Deferoxamine on Pulmonary Surfactant Protein D and Antioxidant Enzymes in Rats Exposed to Hyperoxia Ventilation. *J. Clin. Anesthesiol* 35 (10), 1002–1005. doi:10.12089/jca.2019.10.016

S. N., S. G., Raviraj, R., Nagarajan, D., Zhao, W., and Zhao, W. (2019). Radiation-induced Lung Injury: Impact on Macrophage Dysregulation and Lipid Alteration - a Review. *Immunopharmacology and Immunotoxicology* 41 (3), 370–379. doi:10.1080/08923973.2018.1533025

Stites, S. W., Plautz, M. W., Bailey, K., O'Brien-Ladner, A. R., and Wesselius, L. J. (1999). Increased Concentrations of Iron and Isoferritins in the Lower Respiratory Tract of Patients with Stable Cystic Fibrosis. *Am. J. Respir. Crit. Care Med.* 160 (3), 796–801. doi:10.1164/ajrccm.160.3.9811018

Stockwell, B. R., Friedmann Angeli, J. P., Bayir, H., Bush, A. I., Conrad, M., Dixon, S. J., et al. (2017). Ferroptosis: a Regulated Cell Death Nexus Linking Metabolism, Redox Biology, and Disease. *Cell* 171 (2), 273–285. doi:10.1016/j.cell.2017.09.021

Sun, X., Ou, Z., Chen, R., Niu, X., Chen, D., Kang, R., et al. (2016). Activation of the P62-Keap1-NRF2 Pathway Protects against Ferroptosis in Hepatocellular Carcinoma Cells. *Hepatology* 63 (1), 173–184. doi:10.1002/hep.2825110.1002/hep.28251

Tonnus, W., and Linkermann, A. (2017). The *In Vivo* Evidence for Regulated Necrosis. *Immunol. Rev.* 277 (1), 128–149. doi:10.1111/imr.12551

Turi, J. L., Yang, F., Garrick, M. D., Piantadosi, C. A., and Ghio, A. J. (2004). The Iron Cycle and Oxidative Stress in the Lung. *Free Radic. Biol. Med.* 36 (7), 850–857. doi:10.1016/j.freeradbiomed.2003.12.008

Ursini, F., Maiorino, M., Valente, M., Ferri, L., and Gregolin, C. (1982). Purification from Pig Liver of a Protein Which Protects Liposomes and Biomembranes from Peroxidative Degradation and Exhibits Glutathione Peroxidase Activity on Phosphatidylcholine Hydroperoxides. *Biochim. Biophys. Acta (Bba) - Lipids Lipid Metab.* 710 (2), 197–211. doi:10.1016/0005-2760(82)90150-3

Wang, C., Yuan, W., Hu, A., Lin, J., Xia, Z., Yang, C., et al. (2020). Dexmedetomidine Alleviated Sepsis-induced M-yocardial F-erroptosis and S-eptic H-eart I-njury. *Mol. Med. Rep.* 22 (1), 175–184. doi:10.3892/mmr.2020.11114

Wang, S., Luo, J., Zhang, Z., Dong, D., Shen, Y., and Fang, Y. (2018). Iron and Magnetic: New Research Direction of the Ferroptosis-Based Cancer Therapy. *Am. J. Cancer Res.* 8 (10), 1933–1946.

Ware, L. B., and Matthay, M. A. (2000). The Acute Respiratory Distress Syndrome. *N. Engl. J. Med.* 342 (18), 1334–1349. doi:10.1056/NEJM200005043421806

Wortmann, M., Schneider, M., Pircher, J., Hellfritsch, J., Aichler, M., Vegi, N., et al. (2013). Combined Deficiency in Glutathione Peroxidase 4 and Vitamin E Causes Multiorgan Thrombus Formation and Early Death in Mice. *Circ. Res.* 113 (4), 408–417. doi:10.1161/CIRCRESAHA.113.279984

Wu, Y., Zhang, S., Gong, X., Tam, S., Xiao, D., Liu, S., et al. (2020). The Epigenetic Regulators and Metabolic Changes in Ferroptosis-Associated Cancer Progression. *Mol. Cancer* 19 (1), 39. doi:10.1186/s12943-020-01157-x

Xie, Y., Hou, W., Song, X., Yu, Y., Huang, J., Sun, X., et al. (2016). Ferroptosis: Process and Function. *Cel Death Differ* 23 (3), 369–379. doi:10.1038/cdd.2015.158

Yang, W. S., Kim, K. J., Gaschler, M. M., Patel, M., Shchepinov, M. S., and Stockwell, B. R. (2016). Peroxidation of Polyunsaturated Fatty Acids by Lipoxygenases Drives Ferroptosis. *Proc. Natl. Acad. Sci. USA* 113 (34), E4966–E4975. doi:10.1073/pnas.1603244113

Yoshida, M., Minagawa, S., Araya, J., Sakamoto, T., Hara, H., Tsubouchi, K., et al. (2019). Involvement of Cigarette Smoke-Induced Epithelial Cell Ferroptosis in COPD Pathogenesis. *Nat. Commun.* 10 (1), 3145. doi:10.1038/s41467-019-10991-7

Yu, J. B., Shi, J., Gong, L. R., Dong, S. A., Xu, Y., Zhang, Y., et al. (2014). Role of Nrf2/ARE Pathway in Protective Effect of Electroacupuncture against Endotoxic Shock-Induced Acute Lung Injury in Rabbits. *PLoS One* 9 (8), e104924. doi:10.1371/journal.pone.0104924

Zhang, V., Nemeth, E., and Kim, A. (2019). Iron in Lung Pathology. *Pharmaceuticals* 12 (1), 30. doi:10.3390/ph12010030

Zhang, X., Ding, M., Zhu, P., Huang, H., Zhuang, Q., Shen, J., et al. (2019). New Insights into the Nrf-2/HO-1 Signaling Axis and its Application in Pediatric Respiratory Diseases. *Oxidative Med. Cell Longevity* 2019, 1–9. doi:10.1155/2019/3214196

Zhou, H., Li, F., Niu, J. Y., Zhong, W. Y., Tang, M. Y., and Lin, D. (2019). Ferroptosis Was Involved in the Oleic Acid-Induced Acute Lung Injury in Mice. *Sheng Li Xue Bao.* 71 (5), 689–697.

Zhou, M., Osanai, K., Kobayashi, M., Oikawa, T., Nakagawa, K., Mizuno, S., et al. (2014). Adenovector-mediated Gene Transfer of Lysophosphatidylcholine Acyltransferase 1 Attenuates Oleic Acid-Induced Acute Lung Injury in Rats. *Crit. Care Med.* 42 (11), e716–e724. doi:10.1097/CCM.0000000000000633

5

Alpha-1 Antitrypsin for COVID-19 Treatment: Dual Role in Antiviral Infection and Anti-Inflammation

Chengliang Yang[1], *Shaf Keshavjee*[1,2] *and Mingyao Liu*[1,2]*

[1]*Latner Thoracic Surgery Research Laboratories, Toronto General Hospital Research Institute, University Health Network, Toronto, ON, Canada,* [2]*Institute of Medical Science and Department of Surgery, Faculty of Medicine, University of Toronto, Toronto, ON, Canada*

***Correspondence:**
Mingyao Liu
mingyao.liu@utoronto.ca

Many drugs have been approved for clinical trials for the treatment of COVID-19 disease, focusing on either antiviral or anti-inflammatory approaches. Combining antiviral and anti-inflammatory drugs or therapies together may be more effective. Human alpha-1 antitrypsin (A1AT) is a blood circulating glycoprotein that is best known as a protease inhibitor. It has been used to treat emphysema patients with A1AT deficiency for decades. We and others have demonstrated its role in reducing acute lung injury by inhibiting inflammation, cell death, coagulation, and neutrophil elastase activation. Recently, A1AT has been found to inhibit severe acute respiratory syndrome coronavirus 2 (SARS-CoV-2) infection by inhibiting transmembrane serine protease 2 (TMPRSS2), a protease involved in the entry of SARS-CoV-2 into host cells. This dual role of both antiviral infection and anti-inflammation makes A1AT a unique and excellent candidate for COVID-19 treatment. Three clinical trials of A1AT for COVID-19 treatment have recently been approved in several countries. It is important to determine whether A1AT can prevent the progress from moderate to severe lung injury and eventually to be used to treat COVID-19 patients with acute respiratory distress syndrome.

Keywords: alpha-1 antitrypsin (A1AT), severe acute respiratory syndrome coronavirus 2 (SAR-CoV-2), coronavirus disease 2019 (COVID- 19), acute lung injury, acute respiratory distress syndrome (ARDS), anti-inflammatory therapy, antiviral therapy

INTRODUCTION

The coronavirus disease 2019 (COVID-19) pandemic has caused a surge of critically ill patients in intensive care units across the world. It has been estimated that 1.7 billion people have at least one underlying condition that puts them at increased risk of severe COVID-19 if infected (Clark et al., 2020). The underlying mechanisms of COVID-19 are severe acute respiratory syndrome coronavirus 2 (SARS-CoV-2) viral infection-induced inflammatory response, cell death, microthrombus formation, and formation of neutrophil extracellular traps (NETs) (Middleton et al., 2020). Many clinical trials, therefore, have been focused on drugs that have either antiviral infection or anti-inflammatory function. It has been suggested that a combination of anti-inflammatory drugs with direct-acting antivirals could reduce viral infectivity, viral replication, and the aberrant host inflammatory response (Stebbing et al., 2020). Drugs with a dual role in both anti-inflammation and antiviral infection could be excellent candidates for COVID-19 treatment.

TABLE 1 | The current drugs or therapeutics in COVID-19 clinical studies.

Type of treatment	Name	FDA approval
Antiviral agent	Chloroquine	Not yet
	Hydroxychloroquine	Not yet
	Lopinavir/ritonavir	Not yet
	Ivermectin	Not yet
	Remdesivir	Yes
Bruton's tyrosine kinase inhibitors	Acalabrutinib	Not yet
	Ibrutinib	Not yet
	Zanubrutinib	Not yet
Janus kinase inhibitors	Baracitinib	Not yet
	Ruxolitinib	Not yet
	Tofacitinib	Not yet
Blood-derived products	Convalescent plasma	Not yet
	SARS-CoV-2 immunoglobulins	Not yet
Interleukin-1 inhibitor	Anakinra	Not yet
Interleukin-6 inhibitor	Sarilumab	Not yet
	Tocilizumab	Not yet
	Siltuximab	Not yet
Vaccines	Adenovirus type 5 vector	Not yet
	DNA plasmid vaccine electroporation device	Not yet
	Inactivated	Not yet
	Inactivated + alum	Not yet
	LNP- encapsulated mRNA	Not yet

CURRENT AVAILABLE TREATMENTS FOR CORONAVIRUS DISEASE 2019

In a large COVID-19 cohort study, 81% of patients had mild or moderate disease, 14% had severe disease, and 5% became critically ill with a life-threatening disease course. The mortality in critically ill patients with COVID-19 is approximately 49% (Wu and McGoogan, 2020). Therefore, it is urgent to have specific, effective, and safe treatments for COVID-19. Many clinical trials have been conducted to repurpose existing drugs, such as antiviral agents. To inhibit SARS-CoV-2 viral infection induced inflammatory responses, Bruton's tyrosine kinase inhibitors and Janus kinase inhibitors have been tested. Moreover, blood-derived products, antibodies (such as interleukin-1 inhibitor and interleukin-6 inhibitors), and vaccines (Lurie et al., 2020; National Institutes of Health, 2020; World Health Organization, 2020), have also been tested clinically (**Table 1**). Recently, remdesivir, an antiviral drug (Beigel et al., 2020), has been approved by the United States Food and Drug Administration (United States Food and Drug Administration, 2020). However, people have raised many questions about its worth (Cohen and Kupferschmidt, 2020). New drugs should be selected and tested.

HUMAN ALPHA-1 ANTITRYPSIN

Human alpha-1 antitrypsin (A1AT) is a 52-kDa glycoprotein that is synthesized in the liver, and is circulated in the blood, and is a natural inhibitor for a set of proteases. Adequate A1AT activity is critical for the prevention of proteolytic tissue damage (Bristow et al., 1998). In individuals with one of several inherited mutations in A1AT, low circulating A1AT levels increase the risk for destructive diseases, particularly emphysema (Chapman et al., 2015). Infusion of plasma purified A1AT protein has proven therapeutic benefits in patients with A1AT deficiency (Stoller and Aboussouan, 2005; Balbi et al., 2016; McElvaney et al., 2017). The pharmacokinetics and safety of A1AT have been well studied. It has been considered safe with infrequent and generally well-tolerated side effects (Petrache et al., 2009). Recent works from our group and others have demonstrated that human A1AT has both anti-inflammatory and anti-SARS-CoV-2 viral effects (Gao et al., 2014; Iskender et al., 2016; Lin et al., 2018; Azouz et al., 2020; Wettstein et al., 2020). This dual role makes it a unique and excellent candidate for COVID-19 treatment.

THE ROLE OF ALPHA-1 ANTITRYPSIN IN ACUTE LUNG INJURY

In addition to its anti-protease and tissue-protective function, A1AT also exerts anti-inflammatory effects, including improving mitochondrial membrane stability, inhibiting apoptosis, inhibiting nuclear factor kappa B (NFκB) activation, modulating pro-vs. anti-inflammatory cytokine balance, and promoting immunologic tolerance. For example, A1AT suppresses tumor necrosis factor-alpha and matrix metalloproteinase-12 production (Churg et al., 2007) and enhances anti-inflammatory cytokine interleukin 10 secretion in macrophages (Janciauskiene, et al., 2007; Ozeri et al., 2012). A1AT inhibits thrombin and plays a role in the regulation of proteases involved in fibrinolysis (Talens et al., 2013). In a graft-versus-host disease murine model, A1AT promoted tolerance in animal models by down-regulating early inflammation and favoring the induction and stabilization of regulatory T cells. A1AT administration promoted the expansion of donor-derived dendritic cells, regulatory T cells, and natural killer cells, and increased survival (Tawara et al., 2012).

A1AT protects the lung from acute injury. A1AT directly inhibited inflammatory responses and caspase three activation, prevented apoptosis in a human lung epithelial cell culture model that simulates preservation and reperfusion process in lung transplantation, and it also protected against ischemia-reperfusion induced acute lung injury in rat lung transplant models (Gao et al., 2014). Moreover, it inhibited coagulation activity, with reduced formation of thrombin-antithrombin complex in plasma, and it reduced inflammatory cytokines and apoptosis in pig lung allografts (Iskender et al., 2016). Furthermore, using a pig-lung transplant survival model, we demonstrated the beneficial effects of A1AT on animal recovery via the lung transplant procedure. We further demonstrated that A1AT protected pig donor lungs during *ex vivo* lung perfusion (EVLP), a technique used to assess marginal donor lungs prior to transplantation (Lin et al., 2018). In severely damaged human lungs declined for clinical transplantation, A1AT significantly improved lung function and reduced vascular leakage and pulmonary edema during EVLP. It showed direct therapeutic benefits to the lung by suppressing multiple cytokines, and inhibiting a potent vasoconstrictor, endothelin 1. Based on these translational research studies, a clinical trial for A1AT in human lung transplantation is in preparation.

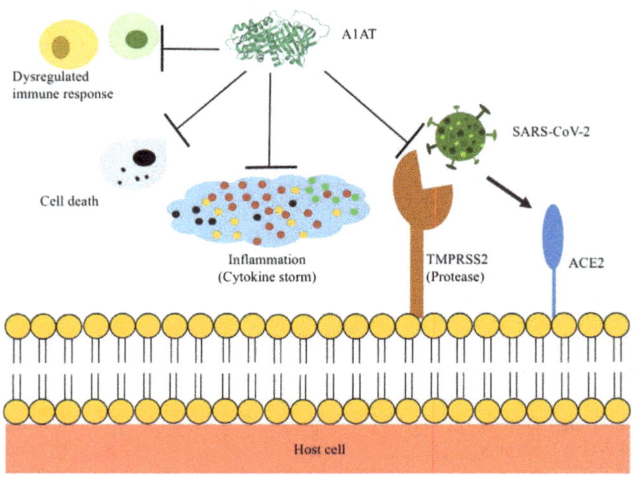

FIGURE 1 | Proposed mechanisms of alpha-1 antitrypsin (A1AT) in COVID-19 treatment. The entry of SARS-CoV2 into host cells is through the binding of viral S-protein to angiotensin converting enzyme 2 (ACE2) located on host cells, which is mediated by the transmembrane serine protease 2 (TMPRSS2). A1AT inhibits TMPRSS2, thus, reduces SARS-CoV-2 infection. In addition, A1AT can reduce acute inflammatory responses, cell death, neutrophil elastase trap formation, coagulative activity, and dysregulated immune responses.

ALPHA-1 ANTITRYPSIN AS A BIOMARKER IN CORONAVIRUS DISEASE 2019 PATIENTS

Serum interleukin 6 (IL-6) is involved in the cytokine storm seen in COVID-19 patients who developed moderate to severe symptoms (Pedersen and Ho, 2020; Vultaggio et al., 2020). The IL-6/A1AT ratio may reflect the balance between pro- and anti-inflammatory mechanisms. The ratio was markedly higher in COVID-19 patients in the intensive care unit (ICU) than in stable patients; this ratio was further increased in ICU patients with poor outcomes and decreased in cases showing clinical improvement (McElvaney et al., 2020). A1AT has been included as one of the clinical and biological predictors of COVID-19 in two clinical studies (Clinical Trial number: NCT04348396 and NCT04366089) in Italy. Interestingly, serum A1AT levels in SARS patients were significantly lower than those in healthy individuals, and truncated forms of A1AT were significantly higher in sera of SARS patients. The combination of a lower concentration and lower activity of A1AT in SARS patients is likely associated with lung failure and contributes to the development of acute respiratory distress syndrome (Ren et al., 2004). Whether A1AT is also truncated in the serum of COVID-19 patients should be determined.

ROLE OF ALPHA-1 ANTITRYPSIN IN ANTI-SEVERE ACUTE RESPIRATORY SYNDROME-CORONAVIRUS-2 INFECTION

The entry of SARS-CoV2 and other coronaviruses into host cells is through the binding of viral S-protein to angiotensin-converting enzyme 2 (ACE2) located on host cells, which is mediated by host transmembrane protease serine type 2 (TMPRSS2). TMPRSS2-deficient mice showed decreased viral spread in the airways after infection with SARS-CoV (Iwata-Yoshikawa et al., 2019). A1AT inhibits TMPRSS2 proteolytic activity in a dose-dependent manner (Azouz et al., 2020). Wettstein et al. screened a peptide/protein library derived from human bronchoalveolar lavage fluids and identified A1AT as a specific inhibitor of SARS-CoV-2 infection (Wettstein et al., 2020). Moreover, A1AT, as the major human serum protease inhibitor, potently restricts protease-mediated cellular entry of SARS-CoV-2 (Oguntuyo et al., 2020).

ALPHA-1 ANTITRYPSIN AS A DRUG FOR CORONAVIRUS DISEASE 2019

The discovery of anti-SARS-CoV-2 infection, together with the known effects of A1AT on anti-inflammation, anti-cell death, anti-protease, anti-coagulation and immunomodulation, promotes its clinical studies in COVID-19 patients (**Figure 1**).

Currently, there are three ongoing clinical trials to study A1AT therapy in patients with COVID-19 (**Table 2**). A phase I randomized placebo-controlled study has been approved on May 13, 2020, in Saudi Arabia. Hospitalized COVID-19 patients will receive A1AT through a nebulizer every 12 hours for 5 days (Clinical Trial number: NCT04385836). A phase II open labelled study has been approved on July 31, 2020, in Spain. Hospitalized patients will receive two intravenous infusion doses of A1AT at 120 mg/kg, on day 1 and day 8 (Clinical Trial number: NCT04495101). Participants in these two trials are patients with

TABLE 2 | Approved alpha-1 antitrypsin clinical trials for COVID-19 treatment.

Clinical trial	1	2	3
Trial number	NCT04385836	NCT04495101	NCT04547140
Countries	Saudi Arabia	Spain	United States
Randomized prospective	Yes	Yes	Yes
Blinded	Yes (single)	No (open label)	Yes (double)
Phase of clinical trial	I	II	II
Placebo-controlled	Yes	Yes	Yes
Number of participants	150	100	100
Clinical severity	Moderate	Moderate	Moderate
Alpha-1 antitrypsin dosage	8 ml, every 12 h for 5 days	120 mg/kg ×2 doses, day 1 and day 8	120 mg/kg ×2 doses, day 1 and day 8
Control	Usual care plus placebo	Usual care	Usual care plus placebo
Route of administration	Inhalation	Intravenous infusion	Intravenous infusion
Primary measures	Clinical improvement at day 21 according to 7-category ordinal scale	Percentage of participants dying or requiring ICU admission at day 15	Percentage of participants dying or requiring ICU admission at day 15

moderate COVID-19 only. A similar phase 2 clinical trial was posted on September 10, 2020 to be conducted in the United States of America (Clinical Trial number: NCT04547140). These trials focus on the safety and efficacy of A1AT in preventing the progression of moderate to severe manifestations. It will be important to learn whether intravenous infusion and airway inhalation have similar or different therapeutic efficacy. The success of these trials may lead to further studies using A1AT to treat COVID-19 patients with severe or critical illness. It may also shine light on whether we should give A1AT to patients with only mild symptoms and how to manage patients with A1AT deficiency when they are infected with SARS-CoV-2.

RESEARCH AGENDA

The multiple potential beneficial effects of A1AT makes it a better candidate than antiviral or anti-inflammatory drugs alone for COVID-19 treatment. However, several unanswered questions need to be addressed. First, the anti-SARS-CoV-2 viral infection of A1AT is mainly based on *in vitro* studies. This needs to be validated through *in vivo* studies, with either animal models or clinical samples. SARS-CoV-2 viral titers, TMPRSS2 activities, and levels of ACE2 in serum, bronchoalveolar lavage fluid or tissue biopsy should be examined. These can be further developed as biomarkers for A1AT or other antiviral therapy for clinical prognosis. Serum IL-6 and A1AT levels and their ratio, neutrophil elastase activity, and the formation of NETs should be measured before and during A1AT therapy. Meanwhile, basic and translational research should be conducted to elaborate on the safety, timing, and dosing of A1AT. The potential interactions of A1AT with other drugs should be determined. Moreover, the underlying mechanisms of A1AT on anti-viral, anti-inflammation, anti-cell death, anti-proteases, and anti-coagulation should be studied. Furthermore, Shapira et al. found a significant positive correlation between the combined frequencies of the A1AT deficiency alleles in 67 countries and their reported COVID-19 mortality rates (Shapira et al., 2020). Given the important role that A1AT plays in the prevention and treatment of the pathological process of SARS-CoV-2 infection, patients with A1AT deficiency may be more susceptible to SARS-CoV-2 viral infection with worse clinical outcomes. This should be confirmed through clinical epidemiology studies. These future studies will provide critical information for the clinical application of A1AT in COVID-19 patients.

AUTHOR CONTRIBUTIONS

CY, SK, and ML conceived the design and concepts. CY and ML wrote the manuscript. All authors contributed to the editing and revision of the manuscript and approved the submission.

REFERENCES

Azouz, N. P., Klingler, A. M., Callahan, V., Akhrymuk, I. V., Elez, K., Raich, L., et al. (2020). *Alpha 1 antitrypsin is an inhibitor of the SARS-CoV2–priming protease TMPRSS2.* Preprint repository name [Preprint]. Available at: bioRxiv (Accessed October 07, 2020).

Balbi, B., Ferrarotti, I., and Miravitlles, M. (2016). Efficacy of augmentation therapy for emphysema associated with α1-antitrypsin deficiency: enough is enough. *Eur. Respir. J.* 47 (1), 35–38. doi:10.1183/13993003.01145-2015

Beigel, J. H., Tomashek, K. M., Dodd, L. E., Mehta, A. K., Zingman, B. S., Kalil, A. C., et al. (2020). Remdesivir for the treatment of Covid-19–final report. *N Engl J Med.* 383, 1813–1826. doi:10.1056/NEJMoa2007764

Bristow, C. L., Di Meo, F., and Arnold, R. R. (1998). Specific activity of alpha1proteinase inhibitor and alpha2 macroglobulin in human serum: application to insulin-dependent diabetes mellitus. *Clin. Immunol. Immunopathol.* 89 (3), 247–259. doi:10.1006/clin.1998.4605

Chapman, K. R., Burdon, J. G., Piitulainen, E., Sandhaus, R. A., Seersholm, N., Stocks, J. M., et al. (2015). Intravenous augmentation treatment and lung density in severe α1 antitrypsin deficiency (RAPID): a randomised, double-blind, placebo-controlled trial. *Lancet* 386 (9991), 360–368. doi:10.1016/S0140-6736(15)60860-1

Churg, A., Wang, X., Wang, R. D., Meixner, S. C., Pryzdial, E. L., and Wright, J. L. (2007). Alpha1-antitrypsin suppresses TNF-alpha and MMP-12 production by cigarette smoke-stimulated macrophages. *Am. J. Respir. Cell Mol. Biol.* 37 (2), 144–151. doi:10.1165/rcmb.2006-0345OC

Clark, A., Jit, M., Warren-Gash, C., Guthrie, B., Wang, H. H. X., Mercer, S. W., et al. (2020). Global, regional, and national estimates of the population at increased risk of severe COVID-19 due to underlying health conditions in 2020: a modelling study. *Lancet Glob Health* 8 (8), e1003-e1017. doi:10.1016/S2214-109X(20)30264-3

Cohen, J., and Kupferschmidt, K. (2020). "A very, very bad look" for remdesivir. *Science* 370 (6517), 642–643. doi:10.1126/science.370.6517.642

Gao, W., Zhao, J., Kim, H., Xu, S., Chen, M., Bai, X., et al. (2014). α1-Antitrypsin inhibits ischemia reperfusion-induced lung injury by reducing inflammatory response and cell death. *J. Heart Lung Transplant.* 33 (3), 309–315. doi:10.1016/j.healun.2013.10.031

Iskender, I., Sakamoto, J., Nakajima, D., Lin, H., Chen, M., Kim, H., et al. (2016). Human α1-antitrypsin improves early post-transplant lung function: pre-clinical studies in a pig lung transplant model. *J. Heart Lung Transplant.* 35 (7), 913–921. doi:10.1016/j.healun.2016.03.006

Iwata-Yoshikawa, N., Okamura, T., Shimizu, Y., Hasegawa, H., Takeda, M., and Nagata, N. (2019). TMPRSS2 contributes to virus spread and immunopathology in the airways of murine models after coronavirus infection. *J. Virol.* 93 (6), e01815–e01818. doi:10.1128/JVI.01815-18

Janciauskiene, S. M., Nita, I. M., and Stevens, T. (2007). Alpha1-antitrypsin, old dog, new tricks. Alpha1-antitrypsin exerts *in vitro* anti-inflammatory activity in human monocytes by elevating cAMP. *J. Biol. Chem.* 282 (12), 8573–8582. doi:10.1074/jbc.M607976200

Lin, H., Chen, M., Tian, F., Tikkanen, J., Ding, L., Andrew Cheung, H. Y., et al. (2018). α1-Anti-trypsin improves function of porcine donor lungs during ex-vivo lung perfusion. *J. Heart Lung Transplant.* 37 (5), 656–666. doi:10.1016/j.healun.2017.09.019

Lurie, N., Saville, M., Hatchett, R., and Halton, J. (2020). Developing Covid-19 vaccines at pandemic speed. *N. Engl. J. Med.* 382 (21), 1969–1973. doi:10.1056/NEJMp2005630

McElvaney, N. G., Burdon, J., Holmes, M., Glanville, A., Wark, P. A., Thompson, P. J., et al. (2017). Long-term efficacy and safety of α1 proteinase inhibitor treatment for emphysema caused by severe α1 antitrypsin deficiency: an open-label extension trial (RAPID-OLE). *Lancet Respir. Med.* 5 (1), 51–60. doi:10.1016/S2213-2600(16)30430-1

McElvaney, O. J., McEvoy, N. L., McElvaney, O. F., Carroll, T. P., Murphy, M. P., Dunlea, D. M., et al. (2020). Characterization of the inflammatory response to severe COVID-19 illness. *Am. J. Respir. Crit. Care Med.* 202 (6), 812–821. doi:10.1164/rccm.202005-1583OC

Middleton, E. A., He, X. Y., Denorme, F., Campbell, R. A., Ng, D., Salvatore, S. P., et al. (2020). Neutrophil extracellular traps contribute to immunothrombosis in COVID-19 acute respiratory distress syndrome. *Blood* 136 (10), 1169–1179. doi:10.1182/blood.2020007008

National Institutes of Health (2020). *Coronavirus disease 2019 (COVID-19) treatment guidelines.* Available at: https://www.covid19treatmentguidelines.nih.gov (Accessed November 3, 2020).

Oguntuyo, K. Y., Stevens, C. S., Siddiquey, M. N., Schilke, R. M., Woolard, M. D., Zhang, H., et al. (2020). *In plain sight: the role of alpha-1-antitrypsin in COVID-19 pathogenesis and therapeutics.* Preprint repository name [Preprint]. Available at: bioRxiv (Accessed August 15, 2020).

Ozeri, E., Mizrahi, M., Shahaf, G., and Lewis, E. C. (2012). α-1 antitrypsin promotes semimature, IL-10-producing and readily migrating tolerogenic dendritic cells. *J. Immunol.* 189 (1), 146–153. doi:10.4049/jimmunol.1101340

Pedersen, S. F., and Ho, Y. C. (2020). SARS-CoV-2: a storm is raging. *J. Clin. Invest.* 130 (5), 2202–2205. doi:10.1172/JCI137647

Petrache, I., Hajjar, J., and Campos, M. (2009). Safety and efficacy of alpha-1-antitrypsin augmentation therapy in the treatment of patients with alpha-1-antitrypsin deficiency. *Biologics* 3, 193–204. doi:10.2147/btt.2009.3088

Ren, Y., He, Q. Y., Fan, J., Jones, B., Zhou, Y., Xie, Y., et al. (2004). The use of proteomics in the discovery of serum biomarkers from patients with severe acute respiratory syndrome. *Proteomics* 4 (11), 3477–3484. doi:10.1002/pmic.200400897

Shapira, G., Shomron, N., and Gurwitz, D. (2020). Ethnic differences in alpha-1 antitrypsin deficiency allele frequencies may partially explain national differences in COVID-19 fatality rates. *Faseb. J.* 34 (11), 14160–14165. doi:10.1096/fj.202002097

Stebbing, J., Phelan, A., Griffin, I., Tucker, C., Oechsle, O., Smith, D., et al. (2020). COVID-19: combining antiviral and anti-inflammatory treatments. *Lancet Infect. Dis.* 20 (4), 400–402. doi:10.1016/S1473-3099(20)30132-8

Stoller, J. K., and Aboussouan, L. S. (2005). Alpha1-antitrypsin deficiency. *Lancet* 365 (9478), 2225–2236. doi:10.1016/S0140-6736(05)66781-5

Talens, S., Malfliet, J. J., van Hal, P. T., Leebeek, F. W., and Rijken, D. C. (2013). Identification and characterization of α1 -antitrypsin in fibrin clots. *J. Thromb. Haemostasis.* 11 (7), 1319–1328. doi:10.1111/jth.12288

Tawara, I., Sun, Y., Lewis, E. C., Toubai, T., Evers, R., Nieves, E., et al. (2012). Alpha-1-antitrypsin monotherapy reduces graft-versus-host disease after experimental allogeneic bone marrow transplantation. *Proc. Natl. Acad. Sci. U. S. A.* 109 (2), 564–569. doi:10.1073/pnas.1117665109

United States Food and Drug Administration (2020). Frequently asked questions for veklury (remdesivir). Available at: https://www.fda.gov/media/137574/download (Accessed October 22, 2020).

Vultaggio, A., Vivarelli, E., Virgili, G., Lucenteforte, E., Bartoloni, A., and Nozzoli, C. (2020). Prompt predicting of early clinical deterioration of moderate-to-severe COVID-19 patients: usefulness of a combined score using IL-6 in a preliminary study. *J. Allergy Clin. Immunol. Pract.* 8 (8), 2575–2581. doi:10.1016/j.jaip.2020.06.013

Wettstein, L., Conzelmann, C., Müller, J. A., Weil, T., Groß, R., Hirschenberger, M., et al. (2020). *Alpha-1 antitrypsin inhibits SARS-CoV-2 infection.* Preprint repository name [Preprint]. Available at: bioRxiv (Accessed July 02, 2020).

World Health Organization (2020). *Draft landscape of Covid-19 candidate vaccines.* Available at: https://www.who.int/blueprint/priority-diseases/key-action/novel-coronavirus-landscape-ncov.pdf (Accessed April 20, 2020).

Wu, Z., and McGoogan, J. M. (2020). Characteristics of and important lessons from the coronavirus disease 2019 (COVID-19) outbreak in China: summary of a report of 72 314 cases from the chinese center for disease control and prevention. *J. Am. Med. Assoc.* 323 (13), 1239–1242. doi:10.1001/jama.2020.2648

6

Research Progress on Strategies that can Enhance the Therapeutic Benefits of Mesenchymal Stromal Cells in Respiratory Diseases with a Specific Focus on Acute Respiratory Distress Syndrome and Other Inflammatory Lung Diseases

*Sara Rolandsson Enes[1], Anna D. Krasnodembskaya[2], Karen English[3], Claudia C. Dos Santos[4] and Daniel J. Weiss[5]**

[1]Department of Experimental Medical Science, Faculty of Medicine, Lund University, Lund, Sweden, [2]Wellcome-Wolfson Institute for Experimental Medicine, School of Medicine, Dentistry, and Biomedical Sciences, Queens University, Belfast, United Kingdom, [3]Cellular Immunology Laboratory, Biology Department, Kathleen Lonsdale Institute for Human Health Research, Maynooth University, Maynooth, Ireland, [4]Interdepartmental Division of Critical Care, Department of Medicine and the Keenan Center for Biomedical Research, St. Michael's Hospital, University of Toronto, Toronto, ON, Canada, [5]Department of Medicine, 226 Health Science Research Facility, Larner College of Medicine, University of Vermont, Burlington, VT, United States

***Correspondence:**
Daniel J. Weiss
daniel.weiss@med.uvm.edu

Recent advances in cell based therapies for lung diseases and critical illnesses offer significant promise. Despite encouraging preclinical results, the translation of efficacy to the clinical settings have not been successful. One of the possible reasons for this is the lack of understanding of the complex interaction between mesenchymal stromal cells (MSCs) and the host environment. Other challenges for MSC cell therapies include cell sources, dosing, disease target, donor variability, and cell product manufacturing. Here we provide an overview on advances and current issues with a focus on MSC-based cell therapies for inflammatory acute respiratory distress syndrome varieties and other inflammatory lung diseases.

Keywords: cell therapy, mesenchymal stromal cells (MSCs), mscs, lung diseases, respiratory diseases and disorders

INTRODUCTION

Severe respiratory diseases such as the acute respiratory distress syndrome (ARDS) and other inflammatory lung diseases remain a significant cause of mortality worldwide. For many of these end-stage diseases, there is no cure and current treatments aim to treat symptoms and/or delay disease progression. New treatment strategies are therefore critically needed. Mesenchymal stromal cells (MSCs) have been widely studied in the field of regenerative medicine for applications in the treatment of lung diseases and critical illnesses. MSCs are multipotent progenitor cells with the potential to secrete a spectrum of anti-inflammatory mediators, such as cytokines and extracellular vesicles (EVs). However, due to a lack of basic understanding of the *in vivo* modes of action and of scientific consensus concerning manufacturing, disease target, and study design the translation of efficacy from preclinical studies to the clinical settings have not yet been successful. Despite fundamental discoveries regarding the potential benefits of MSCs in pre-clinical models of lung diseases and other critical illnesses, more effort needs to be made to understand the *in vivo* fate of infused MSCs, particularly in clinical settings. Importantly, in addition to the MSC cell product, conditioned media and bioactive products such as EVs isolated from MSC cultures have been used in pre-clinical settings with promising results, however, these have been reviewed extensively in other publications (Abreu et al., 2016; Abreu et al., 2021) and will not be discussed further. Understanding how the diseased environment affects MSC therapeutic potential will make it possible to design more efficient clinical trials and to include patients that are more likely to respond to this type of treatment. This is particularly relevant for ARDS in which there may be different inflammatory phenotypes (Reilly et al., 2019). Here, we identify and summarize strategies to enhance the therapeutic potential of MSCs in respiratory diseases and provide a discussion regarding challenges in the manufacturing process and the importance of patient selection.

STRATEGIES TO ENHANCE THERAPEUTIC POTENTIAL OF MESENCHYMAL STROMAL CELLS IN RESPIRATORY DISEASES

Despite the enormous interest in using MSCs in clinical settings to treat respiratory lung diseases, the knowledge regarding the exact mechanism of action is limited. Today, the generally accepted hypothesis is that MSCs modulate the immune system through different paracrine effects (such as cytokines and extracellular vesicles), a hypothesis mainly based on pre-clinical studies [reviewed in (Fernanda Ferreira Cruz, 2019)].

Inflammatory Environmental Effects on Therapeutic Behaviors

Preclinical evidence suggests that MSCs sense the environment through various damage-associated and pathogen-associated cell surface receptors and respond differentially depending on the environmental requirements (Traggiai et al., 2008; Romieu-Mourez et al., 2009; Waterman et al., 2010). For example, stimulation of Toll-like receptor 3 (TLR3) and Toll-like receptor 4 (TLR4) evoked very different MSC responses and appeared to polarize MSCs into two different immune regulatory phenotypes (Waterman et al., 2010). By exposing MSCs to LPS (a TLR4 agonist) the human MSCs differentiated toward a more pro-inflammatory phenotype with release of the cytokines IL-6 and IL-8. Poly (I:C) on the other hand (a TLR3 agonist), activated a more anti-inflammatory phenotype with release of mediators such as IDO, PGE2, and RANTES (Waterman et al., 2010). In addition, activation of MSC TLR4 signaling was demonstrated to be critical for MSC survival and therapeutic effect in a pre-clinical model of *E. coli*-induced acute lung injury, where MSCs isolated from TLR4 deficient mice had impaired survival under conditions of inflammatory stress *in vitro*, and were not therapeutically active *in vivo*. Mechanistically, it was shown that TLR4 pathway regulates signaling through PAR1 on MSCs and TLR4 stimulation leads to expression and secretion of prothrombin by MSCs (Gupta et al., 2018).

To understand the mechanisms by which MSCs act *in vivo*, Islam *et al.* induced ARDS by intratracheal installation of hydrochloric acid, mechanical ventilation, or a combination of the two methods (two-hit model). Following lung injury, MSCs were administered and the outcome was evaluated for each different lung injury model with relevant markers including Ashcroft lung injury score, pulmonary elastance, and lung collagen content (Islam et al., 2019). The authors found that the therapeutic effect of MSCs depended on the microenvironment at the time of administration. For example, MSCs administered into the mechanical ventilation induced ARDS were found to be protective. In contrast, no beneficial effect of MSC administration was noted following hydrochloric acid induced ARDS. To further investigate the microenvironment in the different models, a proteomic analysis of the BALF samples was performed. It was clearly demonstrated that the most enriched clusters of proteins upregulated in the hydrochloric acid model, in which the MSCs did not have a beneficial effect, consisted of proteins involved in inflammation, coagulation, and fibrosis. These proteomic data are somewhat surprising and contradictory since it would seem reasonable that injected MSCs would have effects on at least the inflammatory proteins.

In line with the findings by Islam *et al.*, human MSCs (hMSCs) exposed to clinical bronchoalveolar lavage fluid (BALF) samples obtained from patients with ARDS were less effective in promoting an anti-inflammatory monocyte phenotype than hMSCs exposed to BALF obtained from patients with other lung diseases including acute respiratory exacerbations of cystic fibrosis (CF) (Abreu et al., 2019a). Interestingly, neutralizing IL-6 resulted in promotion of the anti-inflammatory monocyte phenotype (Abreu et al., 2019b). This was a proof-of-concept study and the primary etiology on the ARDS patients used in these experiments were described as either pneumonia or other, and therefore it is not possible to compare these data with the results from the Islam *et al.* study. In another study, Morrison *et al.* exposed hMSCs to pooled samples from ARDS patients and found that ARDS-exposed MSCs promoted anti-inflammatory macrophage marker expression and increased the phagocytic capacity of human macrophages. The increased phagocytic capacity was partly attributed to the acquisition of the phagocytic receptor CD44 expressed in extracellular vesicles secreted by MSCs after exposure to ARDS BALF (Morrison et al., 2017). In similarity with the Abreu *et al.* study, the details of the etiology of ARDS were not well described, making it difficult to compare findings from the two studies. Moreover, the monocytes used in each study came from different species (murine RAW cells vs. human monocyte-derived macrophages), which might explain why different pathways were activated and thereby different outcomes were obtained. Another important difference is that the control group to which the results were compared to were very different, hMSCs exposed to BALF from other lung diseases vs. hMSCs exposed to healthy control BALF samples.

In parallel, hMSCs exposed *ex vivo* to BALF samples obtained from cystic fibrosis patients who had *Aspergillus* infection were

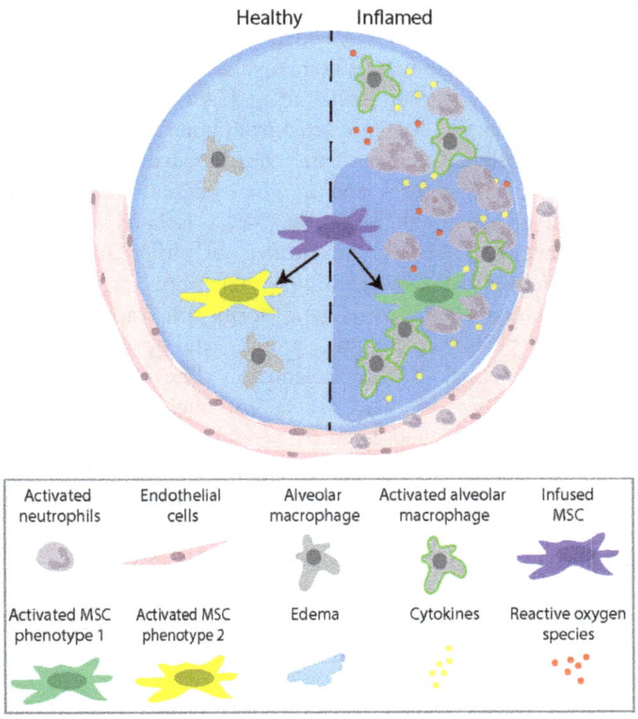

FIGURE 1 | A schematic illustration describing the role of the microenvironment (healthy vs. inflamed) in activating MSCs to induce different therapeutic Phenotypes. Abbreviations: MSC, mesenchymal stromal cell.

rapidly killed. This effect on hMSCs was at least partly related to the mycotoxin, gliotoxin, produced by the fungus (Sara Rolandsson Enes, 2020). In line with these findings, exposure to serum from asthmatic mice resulted in increased levels of MSC cell death. Interestingly, in addition to increased cell death, exposure to serum also induced increased expression of anti-inflammatory mediators including IDO-1, TSG-6, IFN-γ, and IL-10. Administration of these pre-exposed MSCs into house dust mite (HDM)-induced allergic asthma model demonstrated that serum-exposed MSCs improved lung mechanics to a greater extent that unexposed MSCs (Abreu et al., 2019a).

The notion that the ability to "react" to MSCs is associated with their potential therapeutic benefit is supported by results from patients with graft-versus-host disease (GvHD) treated with MSCs. In these patients, only those who demonstrated high cytotoxic activity against the infused MSCs responded to the treatment. Using a murine GvHD model, it was demonstrated that recipient cytotoxic cells activated MSCs to undergo apoptosis through a perforin-dependent pathway. Perforin-induced MSC apoptosis was then further demonstrated to induce immunosuppression via indoleamine 2,3-diocygenase (IDO) production in recipient phagocytes (Galleu et al., 2017). This illustrates a growing appreciation that, whatever the MSCs themselves might do, the host responses to dead or dying MSCs can play a significant role in mitigating inflammation and injury (Weiss et al., 2019). Collectively, these studies demonstrate that an inflammatory microenvironment plays an important role in activating MSCs to induce different therapeutic and/or apoptotic phenotypes, which further highlight the need to understand the complex interaction between MSCs and the host environment (**Figure 1**).

Pre-Activation of Mesenchymal Stromal Cells Prior to Administration

One way to take advantage of the current knowledge that MSCs are being activated by the inflammatory environment, is to pre-activate MSCs before administration. This could be done using different approaches; however, the most common method is to expose MSCs *ex vivo* to inflammatory cytokines such as IFN-γ and TNF-α (English et al., 2010). For example, MSCs exposed to IFN-γ had an increased immunosuppressive effect on T-lymphocytes. This suppressive effect was inhibited when an IFN-γ blocking antibody was added to the system (Krampera et al., 2006). Similarly, by using an IFN-γ knock out system it was demonstrated that endogenous IFN-γ was essential for MSC actions (Polchert et al., 2008). Functionally, pre-stimulation of hMSCs had superior protective effects in a humanized mouse model of acute GvHD (Tobin et al., 2013). In another study, MSCs stimulated with TNF-α demonstrated increased IL-6, IL-8, IL-2, and IFN-γ production compared to control MSCs. In this study, the investigators were also able to demonstrate that TNF-α was more important than IFN-γ regarding MSC secretion of IL-8 (Hemeda et al., 2010). By exposing MSCs to TNF-α in combination with IL-1β Murphey *et. al* observed that the immunomodulatory effects were enhanced compared to control cells (Murphy et al., 2019). In a recent study, it was demonstrated that TNF-α/IFN-γ/IL-1β exposed MSCs had a stronger IL-8 secretion than MSCs exposed to TNF-α/IFN-γ only. Moreover, this increased expression of IL-8 enhanced neutrophil recruitment, a recruitment that was suggested to be mediated trough activation of STAT5 and p38-MAPK signaling (Hackel et al., 2020). This is but one example of potential means of pre-activating MSCs.

Although hypoxia and high levels of oxidative stress are often seen in tissues with pathological inflammation and it is well known that oxygen levels can affect cell function (Cooper et al., 1958; Ivanovic et al., 2000; Choi et al., 2014; Choi et al., 2015), MSCs tend to be cultured at normal atmospheric oxygen levels. MSCs cultured at oxygen levels that better recapitulate the "destination" environment after administration significantly impacted their function. For example, MSCs cultured at low oxygen levels formed a greater number of colonies, had higher proliferation rates, and secreted higher levels of cytokines such as VEGF and FGF compared to MSCs cultured at 20% oxygen (Lennon et al., 2001; Choi et al., 2017; Kwon et al., 2017; Elabd et al., 2018). Moreover, MSCs co-cultured with bone marrow-derived lineage positive blood cells under hypoxic condition contributed to an increased proliferation and differentiation toward anti-inflammatory macrophages (Takizawa et al., 2017). More recently, the metabolic pathway used by MSCs has been shown to be important in determining immunomodulatory capacity (Liu et al., 2019). HIF-1α, the master hypoxia inducible transcription factor, regulated MSC immunomodulation and was associated with a metabolic switch from oxidative phosphorylation to glycolysis (Contreras-Lopez et al., 2020). These are all very interesting results, however, additional studies are needed in order to understand whether hypoxia activates an angiogenic phenotype that could be more appropriate for issue healing rather than immune modulatory. Altogether, modulating culture condition oxygen levels is an interesting approach to pre-activate MSCs, however there are still limited knowledge on this topic, particularly with respect to use of MSCs in respiratory diseases, and further studies are warranted.

Another physiological condition which frequently develops in chronic lung diseases or due to low tidal volume mechanical ventilation is hypercapnic acidosis. A study by Fergie *et al.* have demonstrated that culture of MSCs in 15% CO_2 induced significant mitochondrial dysfunction and inhibited MSCs ability to promote reparative capacity of primary human pulmonary endothelial and distal lung epithelial cells (Fergie et al., 2019).

Genetic Engineering of Mesenchymal Stromal Cells to Enhance Therapeutic Properties

Genetic engineering has been used to enhance MSC survival and therapeutic potential. Genetic engineering of MSCs has been used to induce expression of different cytokines, growth factors, transcription factors, miRNA, and enzymes (Damasceno et al., 2020). For example, overexpressing the pluripotent genes Oct4 and Sox2 in MSCs using liposomal transfection resulted in increased proliferation and differentiation capacity (Han et al., 2014). Moreover, rat bone marrow-derived MSCs transfected with the nerve growth factor receptor tropomyosin receptor kinase A (TrkA) showed increased survival and Schwann-like cell differentiation (Zheng et al., 2016), as well as improved nerve functional recovery and enhanced efficacy *in vivo* (Zheng et al., 2017). In a separate study, it was demonstrated that MSCs overexpressing insulin-like growth factor I (IGF-I) decreased collagen deposition in a liver fibrosis model compared to animals treated with GFP-MSCs or recombinant IGF-I (Fiore et al., 2015). Genetically engineered MSCs overexpressing anti-inflammatory cytokines such as IL-10 resulted in a reduction of pro-inflammatory cytokines such as IL-1β and TNF, and increased viability (Meng et al., 2018). Interestingly, MSCs overexpressing angiopoietin-1 were demonstrated to prevent LPS-induced acute lung injury and were more potent in decreasing inflammatory cells in bronchoalveolar lavage fluid (BALF) compared to untreated MSCs and saline treated groups. Also, levels of proinflammatory cytokines measured in BALF were further reduced in mice treated with angiopoietin-1 overexpressing MSCs compared to non-treated control MSCs (Mei et al., 2007).

Mesenchymal Stromal Cells functional Heterogeneity and Tissue-specificity

Another important factor that likely plays a role in the absence of success of clinical trials is the lack of consistency between different studies such as use of MSCs isolated from different tissues and organs. Increasing evidence demonstrates that MSCs are tissue-specific cells that retain many tissue- and organ-specific functions and properties [reviewed in (Sara Rolandsson Enes, 2019)]. For example, MSCs isolated from bone marrow, skeletal muscle, periosteum, and perinatal cord blood differed in their transcriptomic signatures and *in vivo* differentiation profiles (Sacchetti et al., 2016). Moreover, MSCs isolated from lung tissue have also been demonstrated to differ from bone marrow-derived MSCs regarding proliferation rate, colony-forming potential, *in vivo* bone formation capacity, gene expression profile, secretome profile, and protein profile (Rolandsson et al., 2014; Rolandsson Enes et al., 2016; Rolandsson Enes et al., 2017). Although, tissue-specific properties have been observed by several investigators (Abreu et al., 2017), further parallel studies comparing MSCs from different sources need to be performed in order to roll out if one source is better than others to treat lung diseases. In addition to the MSC tissue-specificity, MSCs are also known to be a very heterogenous population, at least after standard *in vitro* tissue culture expansion. Whether it is possible to sort out specific MSC sub-populations with increased or specific therapeutic properties remains to be further explored.

STRATEGIES TO IMPROVE THE MANUFACTURING PROCESS AND CLINICAL OUTCOME

Given the fairly high number of MSC-based clinical trials performed to date, it is surprising that there are no established consensus concerning MSC product manufacturing, dosing strategies, and which patient group or groups to target. It is well known that MSC properties change depending on the isolation process, number of passages, seeding density, culture surface, and if they have been cryopreserved or not. Regardless of this knowledge, a survey provided by the MSC committee of the International Society of Cell and Gene Therapy discovered that the current MSC manufacturing practice differs significant among different US academic centers (Phinney et al., 2019). Comparable lack of harmonization exists among MSC manufacturing facilities in Europe when a similar survey was performed (Trento et al., 2018). In this section, we will summarize and discuss some of the current strategies that could be used to improve the manufacturing process and clinical outcome.

The Impact of Donor Variance on Mesenchymal Stromal Cells Properties

In addition to the above mentioned challenges such as source, seeding density, and cryopreservation, it is important to acknowledge the impact of donor variance on MSC numbers, but more importantly, on the MSC therapeutic potential. It is well known that MSC properties are affected by factors such as donor age, gender, and harvest site (Zaim et al., 2012; Martin et al., 2016; Rolandsson Enes et al., 2016; Mehrian et al., 2020). For example, MSCs isolated from donors at different ages will have different proliferation rates and *in vitro* differentiation potentials (Zaim et al., 2012; Mehrian et al., 2020). Therefore, it is important to take this into account when manufacturing MSCs for both basic studies and clinical trials and to find strategies that facilitate easy identification of clinically potent MSCs. One such strategy could potentially be to maximize the number of batches that one can obtain from a good donor. However, it is important to remember that MSCs manufactured in large quantities can become ineffective or altered, even from that single donor. When finally obtaining expanded MSCs of desired qualities from a good donor, it is important to pay attention to how the cells are being stored and finally administered to patients. In the report from the MSC pre-conference organized by the International Society of Cell Therapy (ISCT) held in 2018, the difference in potency between cryopreserved MSCs given as a "bedside thaw" formulation and cultured MSCs was highlighted (Nolta et al., 2020). Further, it has also been demonstrated by Francois *et. al.* that cryopreserved MSCs need a recovery phase before infused to patients in order to retain their immunomodulatory activity *in vitro* (Francois et al., 2012). However, interestingly recent data by Tan *et al.* demonstrated that there was comparable immunomodulatory efficacy of fresh and thawed MSCs (Tan et al., 2019).

Predicting the Best Suited Mesenchymal Stromal Cells Cell Product Using Machine Learning

Artificial intelligence, including machine learning, is an interesting area of research which has been given a lot of attention during the last years. Machine learning algorithms and other artificial intelligence approaches may be trained to recognize underlaying relationships in a dataset and thereby perform tasks such as classification, recognition, and counting of lung nodules on chest CT to predict cancer risk and navigate clinical decision options (Khemasuwan et al., 2020). This approach has also been tested in an attempt to characterize MSCs as a step forward toward improved MSC manufacturing process and a better MSC cell product. In a recent study, machine learning was used to profile MSCs based on cell morphology. Here, images of MSCs at low and high passages from 10 different donors exposed to different doses of IFN-γ (0, 10, and 50 ng/ml) were taken and analyzed using visual stochastic neighbor embedding (viSNE) technique. Several morphological sub-populations of MSCs were found after IFN-γ exposure, and it was further suggested that this model could be used to predict immunosuppressive capacity of different MSC lots (Marklein et al., 2019). In another study, machine learning was used to predict MSC population doubling time using *ex vivo* expanded MSCs from multiple donors at different ages and passages. Data from 131 donors from all ages were used to build a predictive model for cultured MSC population doubling time in passage 1 to 4. As suggested by the authors, this model can be used as a tool during the manufacturing process in order to predict the time it takes to reach a desired number of MSCs from a specific donor (Mehrian et al., 2020). This is a new and very exciting area, which hopefully can lead to improvements, standardization, and simplifications in the MSC manufacturing process.

The Importance of Predicting Clinical Responders

In addition to optimizing MSC manufacturing and potential pre-conditioning, it is equally important to predict patients that are more likely to respond to this type of treatment. In previous clinical studies, MSCs have been administered to patients with a variety of lung diseases including both chronic and acute diseases (Tzouvelekis et al., 2013; Weiss et al., 2013; Chambers et al., 2014; Zheng et al., 2014; Wilson et al., 2015; Glassberg et al., 2017). However, based on the general hypothesis that MSCs mainly act via secreted factors in combination with the fact that MSCs have been demonstrated to be cleared from the lungs within a few days, makes it unlikely that MSC-based therapy can remodel destroyed tissue found in patients with end-stage chronic lung diseases (Armitage et al., 2018; Rolandsson Enes and Weiss, 2020). It is more likely that patients with lung diseases involving acute inflammatory response and/or infection such as sepsis/septic shock and ARDS will respond better to this type of treatment. Even if preferentially well suited for the treatment of acute lung injury, patient heterogeneity as in the case of ARDS is critical and identifying those individuals or sub-populations that are more likely to benefit from MSC treatment is critical. For example, in a multicenter phase II clinical trial using MSCs to treat graft-versus-host disease (GvHD) it was demonstrated that a sub-population of MSC-treated patients had a complete response, and those patients further had an increased survival rate compared to partial-responders and non-responders (Le Blanc et al., 2008). Similarly, in a retrospectively study of children suffering from GvHD that were treated with MSCs, it was observed that complete responders had an increased survival rate compared to partial-responders and non-responders (Ball et al., 2013). Therefore, it would be very interesting, and important, to identify biological factors that differentiate the complete responders from the other two groups. While there may be different strategies to accomplish this, Martin *et al.* makes a compelling argument on investing more resources on mechanistical studies and the design of future clinical trials based on molecular markers found in subpopulations of patients (Martin et al., 2019).

The Importance of Large-Scale Cell Manufacturing and Successful Cell Delivery

For clinical translation several challenges need to be addressed including how to generate the high number of good quality MSCs needed for large human trials, as well as how to produce and store MSCs for future clinical treatments. For example, ARDS is an acute severe disease with a very rapid onset and there is insufficient time to start cultivating MSCs when the patient is admitted to hospital thus the cell product needs to be a cryopreserved ready-to-use product. Furthermore, isolation processes, passage number, density strategies, growth media and cultivation properties (e.g., plastic vs 3D environments) each can influence the biological properties of MSCs (reviewed in (Sara Rolandsson Enes DJW and Burgess IHH, 2019)) are necessary to ensure therapeutic efficient MSCs. Another challenge is that the lung is a complex organ, and it is critical to find the most optimal delivery route where MSCs reach all compartments in the lung. In preclinical studies of lung diseases, the most common delivery route is still intravenous administration, however for lung diseases there are a number of examples in which intratracheal administration can be as or even more effective (Sally Yunsun Kim WC and Burgess IHH, 2019). For example, using a naphthalene-induced airway injury model Wong *et al.* demonstrated that a larger number of epithelial cells reached the lung when they were administered through transtracheal delivery over intravenous cell delivery (Wong et al., 2007). It is however important to remember that some lung diseases, such as COPD and ARDS, are systemic diseases and therefore different delivery routes might be good for some but not others.

Challenges Related to Conducting Clinical Trials During the COVID-19 Outbreak

The global coronavirus pandemic has increased the number of initiated MSC clinical trials dramatically, and there are a number of challenges related to the conducting trials such as having a good cell product, as discussed above, enrolling patients, assessing outcomes, and ethical issues. For example, a global pandemic aim to find a rapid and effective treatment however it is important that this occurs in a transparent manner following appropriate ethical guidelines (Khoury et al., 2020; Khoury et al., 2021). As discussed by Khoury *et al.* it is also very important to include recognized end-point such as length of ICU, ventilator-free days, and overall mortality. Another important issue to considerate, especially for treatment of COVID-19 induced ARDS, is when to enroll patients and when to initiate MSC treatment, but also which COVID-19 patient population to target (Khoury et al., 2020). The issues discussed in this section is highly relevant for the ongoing COVID-19 MSC clinical trials, however they are equally important to consider in all cell-based therapies for pulmonary diseases.

SUMMARY AND FINAL REMARKS

The enthusiasm for using MSC-based therapy to treat severe lung disorders is great and it is currently increasing due to the COVID-19 pandemic. Unfortunately, the very promising pre-clinical studies performed in animal models of lung diseases has not yet translated into improved clinical outcomes in clinical trials. The field is still struggling with the lack of knowledge regarding the fate of administered MSCs, lack of standardized protocols for manufacturing of MSCs, and how to determine which patients are more likely to respond to this type of treatment. Despite these limitations, there are several interesting studies demonstrating that MSCs can be activated and modified in order to enhance their therapeutic efficacy using either genetic modifications or environmental factors including inflammatory cytokines and hypoxia. Moreover, recent studies have used artificial intelligence as a tool to predict which MSCs are better to be used in clinical trials, a strategy that would improve the manufacturing process substantially and hopefully lead to a better and more effective MSC cell product. We can conclude that currently there is no clear path to reconcile the issues discussed in this review, however one potential solution might be that investigators begin to combine all aspects of potential benefits into a unified effort to establish a greater search for where benefit could occur.

AUTHOR CONTRIBUTIONS

SRE and DW conceived the design, concept, and wrote the manuscript. AK, KE, and CDS contributed with references, critically reviewed and provided comments on the manuscript draft. All authors read and approved the final version of this manuscript.

REFERENCES

Abreu, S. C., Weiss, D. J., and Rocco, P. R. (2016). Extracellular vesicles derived from mesenchymal stromal cells: a therapeutic option in respiratory diseases? *Stem Cel Res Ther* 7 (1), 53. doi:10.1186/s13287-016-0317-0

Abreu, S. C., Antunes, M. A., Xisto, D. G., Cruz, F. F., Branco, V. C., Bandeira, E., et al. (2017). Bone marrow, adipose, and lung tissue-derived murine mesenchymal stromal cells release different mediators and differentially affect airway and lung parenchyma in experimental asthma. *Stem Cell Transl Med* 6 (6), 1557–1567. doi:10.1002/sctm.16-0398

Abreu, S. C., Xisto, D. G., de Oliveira, T. B., Blanco, N. G., de Castro, L. L., Kitoko, J. Z., et al. (2019a). Serum from asthmatic mice potentiates the therapeutic effects of mesenchymal stromal cells in experimental allergic asthma. *STEM CELLS Translational Med.* 8 (3), 301–312. doi:10.1002/sctm.18-0056

Abreu, S. C., Enes, S. R., Dearborn, J., Goodwin, M., Coffey, A., Borg, Z. D., et al. (2019b). Lung inflammatory environments differentially alter mesenchymal stromal cell behavior. *Am J Physiol Lung Cell Mol Physiol.* 317 (6), L823-L831. doi:10.1152/ajplung.00263.2019

Abreu, S. C., Lopes-Pacheco, M., Weiss, D. J., and Rocco, P. R. M. (2021). Mesenchymal stromal cell-derived extracellular vesicles in lung diseases: current status and perspectives. *Front Cel Dev Biol* 9, 600711. doi:10.3389/fcell.2021.600711

Armitage, J., Tan, D. B. A., Troedson, R., Young, P., Lam, K. V., Shaw, K., et al. (2018). Mesenchymal stromal cell infusion modulates systemic immunological responses in stable COPD patients: a phase I pilot study. *Eur. Respir. J.* 51 (3). doi:10.1183/13993003.02369-2017

Ball, L. M., Bernardo, M. E., Roelofs, H., van Tol, M. J., Contoli, B., Zwaginga, J. J., et al. (2013). Multiple infusions of mesenchymal stromal cells induce sustained remission in children with steroid-refractory, grade III-IV acute graft-versus-host disease. *Br. J. Haematol.* 163 (4), 501–509. doi:10.1111/bjh.12545

Chambers, D. C., Enever, D., Ilic, N., Sparks, L., Whitelaw, K., Ayres, J., et al. (2014). A phase 1b study of placenta-derived mesenchymal stromal cells in patients with idiopathic pulmonary fibrosis. *Respirology.* 19 (7), 1013–1018. doi:10.1111/resp.12343

Choi, J. R., Pingguan-Murphy, B., Wan Abas, W. A. B., Noor Azmi, M. A., Omar, S. Z., Chua, K. H., et al. (2014). Impact of low oxygen tension on stemness, proliferation and differentiation potential of human adipose-derived stem cells. *Biochem. Biophysical Res. Commun.* 448 (2), 218–224. doi:10.1016/j.bbrc.2014.04.096

Choi, J. R., Pingguan-Murphy, B., Wan Abas, W. A., Yong, K. W., Poon, C. T., Noor Azmi, M. A., et al. (2015). *In situ* normoxia enhances survival and proliferation rate of human adipose tissue-derived stromal cells without increasing the risk of tumourigenesis. *PLoS One.* 10 (1), e0115034. doi:10.1371/journal.pone.0115034

Choi, J. R., Yong, K. W., and Wan Safwani, W. K. Z. (2017). Effect of hypoxia on human adipose-derived mesenchymal stem cells and its potential clinical applications. *Cell. Mol. Life Sci.* 74 (14), 2587–2600. doi:10.1007/s00018-017-2484-2

Contreras Lopez, R., Elizondo-Vega, R., Paredes, M. J., Luque-Campos, N., Torres, M. J., Tejedor, G., et al. (2020). HIF1α-dependent metabolic reprogramming governs mesenchymal stem/stromal cell immunoregulatory functions. *FASEB J.* 34 (6), 8250–8264. doi:10.1096/fj.201902232R

Cooper, P. D., Burt, A. M., and Wilson, J. N. (1958). Critical effect of oxygen tension on rate of growth of animal cells in continuous suspended culture. *Nature.* 182 (4648), 1508–1509. doi:10.1038/1821508b0

Damasceno, P. K. F., de Santana, T. A., Santos, G. C., Orge, I. D., Silva, D. N., Albuquerque, J. F., et al. (2020). Genetic engineering as a strategy to improve the therapeutic efficacy of mesenchymal stem/stromal cells in regenerative medicine. *Front. Cel Dev Biol.* 8, 737. doi:10.3389/fcell.2020.00737

Elabd, C., Ichim, T. E., Miller, K., Anneling, A., Grinstein, V., Vargas, V., et al. (2018). Comparing atmospheric and hypoxic cultured mesenchymal stem cell transcriptome: implication for stem cell therapies targeting intervertebral discs. *J. Transl Med.* 16 (1), 222. doi:10.1186/s12967-018-1601-9

English, K., French, A., and Wood, K. J. (2010). Mesenchymal stromal cells: facilitators of successful transplantation? *Cell Stem Cell.* 7 (4), 431–442. doi:10.1016/j.stem.2010.09.009

Fergie, N., Todd, N., McClements, L., McAuley, D., O'Kane, C., and Krasnodembskaya, A. (2019). Hypercapnic acidosis induces mitochondrial dysfunction and impairs the ability of mesenchymal stem cells to promote distal lung epithelial repair. *FASEB j.* 33 (4), 5585–5598. doi:10.1096/fj.201802056r

Fernanda Ferreira Cruz, P. R. M. R. (2019). in: Janette K. Burgess IHH ed. *Stem Cell-Based Therapy for Lung Disease.* Cham, Switzerland: Springer.

Fiore, E. J., Bayo, J. M., Garcia, M. G., Malvicini, M., Lloyd, R., Piccioni, F., et al. (2015). Mesenchymal stromal cells engineered to produce IGF-I by recombinant adenovirus ameliorate liver fibrosis in mice. *Stem Cell Development* 24 (6), 791–801. doi:10.1089/scd.2014.0174

Francois, M., Copland, I. B., Yuan, S., Romieu-Mourez, R., Waller, E. K., and Galipeau, J. (2012). Cryopreserved mesenchymal stromal cells display impaired immunosuppressive properties as a result of heat-shock response and impaired interferon-gamma licensing. *Cytotherapy* 14 (2), 147–152. doi:10.3109/14653249.2011.623691

Galleu, A., Riffo-Vasquez, Y., Trento, C., Lomas, C., Dolcetti, L., Cheung, T. S., et al. (2017). Apoptosis in mesenchymal stromal cells induces *in vivo* recipient-mediated immunomodulation. *Sci. Transl Med.* 9 (416). doi:10.1126/scitranslmed.aam7828

Glassberg, M. K., Minkiewicz, J., Toonkel, R. L., Simonet, E. S., Rubio, G. A., DiFede, D., et al. (2017). Allogeneic human mesenchymal stem cells in patients with idiopathic pulmonary fibrosis via intravenous delivery (aether): a phase I safety clinical trial. *Chest.* 151 (5), 971–981. doi:10.1016/j.chest.2016.10.061

Gupta, N., Sinha, R., Krasnodembskaya, A., Xu, X., Nizet, V., Matthay, M. A., et al. (2018). The TLR4-PAR1 *Axis* regulates bone marrow mesenchymal stromal cell survival and therapeutic capacity in experimental bacterial pneumonia. *Stem Cells.* 36 (5), 796–806. doi:10.1002/stem.2796

Hackel, A., Aksamit, A., Bruderek, K., Lang, S., and Brandau, S. (2020). TNF-alpha and IL-1beta sensitize human MSC for IFN-gamma signaling and enhance neutrophil recruitment. *Eur. J. Immunol.* 51 (2), 319-330. doi:10.1002/eji.201948336

Han, S.-M., Han, S.-H., Coh, Y.-R., Jang, G., Chan Ra, J., Kang, S.-K., et al. (2014). Enhanced proliferation and differentiation of Oct4- and Sox2-overexpressing human adipose tissue mesenchymal stem cells. *Exp. Mol. Med.* 46, e101. doi:10.1038/emm.2014.28

Hemeda, H., Jakob, M., Ludwig, A.-K., Giebel, B., Lang, S., and Brandau, S. (2010). Interferon-γ and tumor necrosis factor-α differentially affect cytokine expression and migration properties of mesenchymal stem cells. *Stem Cell Development* 19 (5), 693–706. doi:10.1089/scd.2009.0365

Islam, D., Huang, Y., Fanelli, V., Delsedime, L., Wu, S., Khang, J., et al. (2019). Identification and modulation of microenvironment is crucial for effective mesenchymal stromal cell therapy in acute lung injury. *Am. J. Respir. Crit. Care Med.* 199 (10), 1214–1224. doi:10.1164/rccm.201802-0356oc

Ivanovic, Z., Sbarba, P. D., Trimoreau, F., Faucher, J.-L., and Praloran, V. (2000). Primitive human HPCs are better maintained and expanded *in vitro* at 1 percent oxygen than at 20 percent. *Transfusion.* 40 (12), 1482–1488. doi:10.1046/j.1537-2995.2000.40121482.x

Khemasuwan, D., Sorensen, J. S., and Colt, H. G. (2020). Artificial intelligence in pulmonary medicine: computer vision, predictive model and COVID-19. *Eur. Respir. Rev.* 29 (157), 200181. doi:10.1183/16000617.0181-2020

Khoury, M., Cuenca, J., Cruz, F. F., Figueroa, F. E., Rocco, P. R. M., and Weiss, D. J. (2020). Current status of cell-based therapies for respiratory virus infections: applicability to COVID-19. *Eur. Respir. J.* 55 (6), 2000858. doi:10.1183/13993003.00858-2020

Khoury, M., Ikonomou, L., Dominici, M., LeBlanc, K., Levine, B. L., and Weiss, D. J. (2021). The coronavirus pandemic: a pitfall or a fast track for validating cell therapy products? *Stem Cell Dev* 30 (3), 119–127. doi:10.1089/scd.2020.0122

Krampera, M., Cosmi, L., Angeli, R., Pasini, A., Liotta, F., Andreini, A., et al. (2006). Role for interferon-γ in the immunomodulatory activity of human bone marrow mesenchymal stem cells. *Stem Cells.* 24 (2), 386–398. doi:10.1634/stemcells.2005-0008

Kwon, S. Y., Chun, S. Y., Ha, Y.-S., Kim, D. H., Kim, J., Song, P. H., et al. (2017). Hypoxia enhances cell properties of human mesenchymal stem cells. *Tissue Eng. Regen. Med.* 14 (5), 595–604. doi:10.1007/s13770-017-0068-8

Le Blanc, K., Frassoni, F., Ball, L., Locatelli, F., Roelofs, H., Lewis, I., et al. (2008). Mesenchymal stem cells for treatment of steroid-resistant, severe, acute graft-versus-host disease: a phase II study. *Lancet.* 371 (9624), 1579–1586. doi:10.1016/S0140-6736(08)60690-X

Lennon, D. P., Edmison, J. M., and Caplan, A. I. (2001). Cultivation of rat marrow-derived mesenchymal stem cells in reduced oxygen tension: effects on *in vitro* and *in vivo* osteochondrogenesis. *J. Cel. Physiol.* 187 (3), 345–355. doi:10.1002/jcp.1081

Liu, Y., Yuan, X., Muñoz, N., Logan, T. M., and Ma, T. (2019). Commitment to aerobic glycolysis sustains immunosuppression of human mesenchymal stem cells. *STEM CELLS Translational Med.* 8 (1), 93–106. doi:10.1002/sctm.18-0070

Marklein, R. A., Klinker, M. W., Drake, K. A., Polikowsky, H. G., Lessey-Morillon, E. C., and Bauer, S. R. (2019). Morphological profiling using machine learning reveals emergent subpopulations of interferon-gamma-stimulated mesenchymal stromal cells that predict immunosuppression. *Cytotherapy.* 21 (1), 17–31. doi:10.1016/j.jcyt.2018.10.008

Martin, I., De Boer, J., and Sensebe, L.Therapy MSCCotISfC (2016). A relativity concept in mesenchymal stromal cell manufacturing. *Cytotherapy.* 18 (5), 613–620. doi:10.1016/j.jcyt.2016.02.004

Martin, I., Galipeau, J., Kessler, C., Le Blanc, K., and Dazzi, F. (2019). Challenges for mesenchymal stromal cell therapies. *Sci. Transl Med.* 11 (480), eaat2189. doi:10.1126/scitranslmed.aat2189

Mehrian, M., Lambrechts, T., Marechal, M., Luyten, F. P., Papantoniou, I., and Geris, L. (2020). Predicting *in vitro* human mesenchymal stromal cell expansion based on individual donor characteristics using machine learning. *Cytotherapy.* 22 (2), 82–90. doi:10.1016/j.jcyt.2019.12.006

Mei, S. H. J., McCarter, S. D., Deng, Y., Parker, C. H., Liles, W. C., and Stewart, D. J. (2007). Prevention of LPS-induced acute lung injury in mice by mesenchymal stem cells overexpressing angiopoietin 1. *Plos Med.* 4 (9), e269. doi:10.1371/journal.pmed.0040269

Meng, X., Li, J., Yu, M., Yang, J., Zheng, M., Zhang, J., et al. (2018). Transplantation of mesenchymal stem cells overexpressing IL10 attenuates cardiac impairments in rats with myocardial infarction. *J. Cel Physiol.* 233 (1), 587–595. doi:10.1002/jcp.25919

Morrison, T. J., Jackson, M. V., Cunningham, E. K., Kissenpfennig, A., McAuley, D. F., O'Kane, C. M., et al. (2017). Mesenchymal stromal cells modulate macrophages in clinically relevant lung injury models by extracellular vesicle mitochondrial transfer. *Am. J. Respir. Crit. Care Med.* 196 (10), 1275–1286. doi:10.1164/rccm.201701-0170oc

Murphy, N., Treacy, O., Lynch, K., Morcos, M., Lohan, P., Howard, L., et al. (2019). TNF-α/IL-1β-licensed mesenchymal stromal cells promote corneal allograft survival via myeloid cell-mediated induction of Foxp3 + regulatory T cells in the lung. *FASEB j.* 33 (8), 9404–9421. doi:10.1096/fj.201900047r

Nolta, J. A., Galipeau, J., and Phinney, D. G. (2020). Improving mesenchymal stem/stromal cell potency and survival: proceedings from the International Society of Cell Therapy (ISCT) MSC preconference held in May 2018, Palais des Congres de Montreal, Organized by the ISCT MSC Scientific Committee. *Cytotherapy.* 22 (3), 123–126. doi:10.1016/j.jcyt.2020.01.004

Phinney, D. G., Galipeau, J., and Gene, T.Msc Committee Of The International Society Of C (2019). Manufacturing mesenchymal stromal cells for clinical applications: a survey of Good Manufacturing Practices at U.S. academic centers. *Cytotherapy.* 21 (7), 782–792. doi:10.1016/j.jcyt.2019.04.003

Polchert, D., Sobinsky, J., Douglas, G., Kidd, M., Moadsiri, A., Reina, E., et al. (2008). IFN-γ activation of mesenchymal stem cells for treatment and prevention of graft versus host disease. *Eur. J. Immunol.* 38 (6), 1745–1755. doi:10.1002/eji.200738129

Reilly, J., Calfee, C., and Christie, J. (2019). Acute respiratory distress syndrome phenotypes. *Semin. Respir. Crit. Care Med.* 40 (1), 019–030. doi:10.1055/s-0039-1684049

Rolandsson Enes, S., Ahrman, E., Palani, A., Hallgren, O., Bjermer, L., Malmstrom, A., et al. (2017). Quantitative proteomic characterization of lung-MSC and bone marrow-MSC using DIA-mass spectrometry. *Sci. Rep.* 7 (1), 9316. doi:10.1038/s41598-017-09127-y

Rolandsson Enes, S., Andersson Sjoland, A., Skog, I., Hansson, L., Larsson, H., Le Blanc, K., et al. (2016). MSC from fetal and adult lungs possess lung-specific properties compared to bone marrow-derived MSC. *Sci. Rep.* 6, 29160. doi:10.1038/srep29160

Rolandsson Enes, S., and Weiss, D. J. (2020). Cell therapy for lung disease: current status and future prospects. *Curr. Stem Cel Rep* 6, 30–39. doi:10.1007/s40778-020-00171-5

Rolandsson, S., Andersson Sjoland, A., Brune, J. C., Li, H., Kassem, M., Mertens, F., et al. (2014). Primary mesenchymal stem cells in human transplanted lungs are CD90/CD105 perivascularly located tissue-resident cells. *BMJ Open Respir. Res.* 1 (1), e000027. doi:10.1136/bmjresp-2014-000027

Romieu-Mourez, R., François, M., Boivin, M.-N., Bouchentouf, M., Spaner, D. E., and Galipeau, J. (2009). Cytokine modulation of TLR expression and activation in mesenchymal stromal cells leads to a proinflammatory phenotype. *J. Immunol.* 182 (12), 7963–7973. doi:10.4049/jimmunol.0803864

Sacchetti, B., Funari, A., Remoli, C., Giannicola, G., Kogler, G., Liedtke, S., et al. (2016). No identical "mesenchymal stem cells" at different times and sites: human committed progenitors of distinct origin and differentiation potential are incorporated as adventitial cells in microvessels. *Stem Cel Rep.* 6 (6), 897–913. doi:10.1016/j.stemcr.2016.05.011

Sara Rolandsson Enes GW-T (2019). In: Janette K. Burgess IHH ed. *Stem Cell-Based Therapy for Lung Disease.* Cham, Switzerland: Springer.

Soraia, C., Abreu, T. H. H., Hoffman, Evan., Jacob, Dearborn., Ashare, Alix., Singh Sidhu, Karatatiwant., et al.Sara Rolandsson Enes (2020). Differential effects of the cystic fibrosis lung inflammatory environment on mesenchymal stromal cells. *Am J Physiol Lung Cell Mol Physiol.* 319 (6), L908-L925. doi:10.1152/ajplung.00218.2020

Sara Rolandsson Enes DJW (2019). In: Janette K. Burgess IHH ed. *Stem Cell-Based Therapy for Lung Disease.* Cham, Switzerland: Springer.

Sally Yunsun Kim WC (2019). In: Janette K. Burgess IHH ed. *Stem Cell-Based Therapy for Lung Disease.* Cham, Switzerland: Springer.

Takizawa, N., Okubo, N., Kamo, M., Chosa, N., Mikami, T., Suzuki, K., et al. (2017). Bone marrow-derived mesenchymal stem cells propagate immunosuppressive/anti-inflammatory macrophages in cell-to-cell contact-independent and -dependent manners under hypoxic culture. *Exp. Cel Res.* 358 (2), 411–420. doi:10.1016/j.yexcr.2017.07.014

Tan, Y., Salkhordeh, M., Wang, J. P., McRae, A., Souza-Moreira, L., McIntyre, L., et al. (2019). Thawed mesenchymal stem cell product shows comparable immunomodulatory potency to cultured cells in vitro and in polymicrobial septic animals. *Sci. Rep.* 9 (1), 18078. doi:10.1038/s41598-019-54462-x

Tobin, L. M., Healy, M. E., English, K., and Mahon, B. P. (2013). Human mesenchymal stem cells suppress donor CD4+T cell proliferation and reduce pathology in a humanized mouse model of acute graft-versus-host disease. *Clin. Exp. Immunol.* 172 (2), 333–348. doi:10.1111/cei.12056

Traggiai, E., Volpi, S., Schena, F., Gattorno, M., Ferlito, F., Moretta, L., et al. (2008). Bone marrow-derived mesenchymal stem cells induce both polyclonal expansion and differentiation of B cells isolated from healthy donors and systemic lupus erythematosus patients. *Stem Cells.* 26 (2), 562–569. doi:10.1634/stemcells.2007-0528

Trento, C., Bernardo, M. E., Nagler, A., Kuci, S., Bornhauser, M., Kohl, U., et al. (2018). Manufacturing mesenchymal stromal cells for the treatment of graft-versus-host disease: a survey among centers affiliated with the European society for blood and marrow transplantation. *Biol. Blood Marrow Transpl.* 24 (11), 2365 2370. doi:10.1016/j.bbmt.2018.07.015

Tzouvelekis, A., Paspaliaris, V., Koliakos, G., Ntolios, P., Bouros, E., Oikonomou, A., et al. (2013). A prospective, non-randomized, no placebo-controlled, phase Ib clinical trial to study the safety of the adipose derived stromal cells-stromal vascular fraction in idiopathic pulmonary fibrosis. *J. Transl Med.* 11, 171. doi:10.1186/1479-5876-11-171

Waterman, R. S., Tomchuck, S. L., Henkle, S. L., and Betancourt, A. M. (2010). A new mesenchymal stem cell (MSC) paradigm: polarization into a pro-inflammatory MSC1 or an Immunosuppressive MSC2 phenotype. *PLoS One.* 5 (4), e10088. doi:10.1371/journal.pone.0010088

Weiss, D. J., Casaburi, R., Flannery, R., LeRoux-Williams, M., and Tashkin, D. P. (2013). A placebo-controlled, randomized trial of mesenchymal stem cells in COPD. *Chest.* 143 (6), 1590–1598. doi:10.1378/chest.12-2094

Weiss, D. J., English, K., Krasnodembskaya, A., Isaza-Correa, J. M., Hawthorne, I. J., and Mahon, B. P. (2019). The necrobiology of mesenchymal stromal cells affects therapeutic efficacy. *Front. Immunol.* 10, 1228. doi:10.3389/fimmu.2019.01228

Wilson, J. G., Liu, K. D., Zhuo, H., Caballero, L., McMillan, M., Fang, X., et al. (2015). Mesenchymal stem (stromal) cells for treatment of ARDS: a phase 1 clinical trial. *Lancet Respir. Med.* 3 (1), 24–32. doi:10.1016/S2213-2600(14)70291-7

Wong, A. P., Dutly, A. E., Sacher, A., Lee, H., Hwang, D. M., Liu, M., et al. (2007). Targeted cell replacement with bone marrow cells for airway epithelial regeneration. *Am. J. Physiol. Lung Cel Mol Physiol.* 293 (3), L740–L752. doi:10.1152/ajplung.00050.2007

Zaim, M., Karaman, S., Cetin, G., and Isik, S. (2012). Donor age and long-term culture affect differentiation and proliferation of human bone marrow mesenchymal stem cells. *Ann. Hematol.* 91 (8), 1175–1186. doi:10.1007/s00277-012-1438-x

Zheng, G., Huang, L., Tong, H., Shu, Q., Hu, Y., Ge, M., et al. (2014). Treatment of acute respiratory distress syndrome with allogeneic adipose-derived mesenchymal stem cells: a randomized, placebo-controlled pilot study. *Respir. Res.* 15, 39. doi:10.1186/1465-9921-15-39

Zheng, M., Duan, J., He, Z., Wang, Z., Mu, S., Zeng, Z., et al. (2017). Transplantation of bone marrow stromal stem cells overexpressing tropomyosin receptor kinase A for peripheral nerve repair. *Cytotherapy.* 19 (8), 916–926. doi:10.1016/j.jcyt.2017.04.007

Zheng, M., Duan, J., He, Z., Wang, Z., Mu, S., Zeng, Z., et al. (2016). Overexpression of tropomyosin receptor kinase A improves the survival and Schwann-like cell differentiation of bone marrow stromal cells in nerve grafts for bridging rat sciatic nerve defects. *Cytotherapy.* 18 (10), 1256–1269. doi:10.1016/j.jcyt.2016.06.015

7

Implications for Extracellular Matrix Interactions with Human Lung Basal Stem Cells in Lung Development, Disease and Airway Modeling

*Shana M. Busch[1], Zareeb Lorenzana[1] and Amy L. Ryan[1,2]**

[1]Hastings Center for Pulmonary Research, Division of Pulmonary, Critical Care and Sleep Medicine, Department of Medicine, University of Southern California, Los Angeles, CA, United States, [2]Department of Stem Cell Biology and Regenerative Medicine, University of Southern California, Los Angeles, CA, United States

***Correspondence:**
Amy L. Ryan
afirth@usc.edu

The extracellular matrix (ECM) is not simply a quiescent scaffold. This three-dimensional network of extracellular macromolecules provides structural, mechanical, and biochemical support for the cells of the lung. Throughout life, the ECM forms a critical component of the pulmonary stem cell niche. Basal cells (BCs), the primary stem cells of the airways capable of differentiating to all luminal cell types, reside in close proximity to the basolateral ECM. Studying BC-ECM interactions is important for the development of therapies for chronic lung diseases in which ECM alterations are accompanied by an apparent loss of the lung's regenerative capacity. The complexity and importance of the native ECM in the regulation of BCs is highlighted as we have yet to create an *in vitro* culture model that is capable of supporting the long-term expansion of multipotent BCs. The interactions between the pulmonary ECM and BCs are, therefore, a vital component for understanding the mechanisms regulating BC stemness during health and disease. If we are able to replicate these interactions in airway models, we could significantly improve our ability to maintain basal cell stemness *ex vivo* for use in *in vitro* models and with prospects for cellular therapies. Furthermore, successful, and sustained airway regeneration in an aged or diseased lung by small molecules, novel compounds or via cellular therapy will rely upon both manipulation of the airway stem cells and their immediate niche within the lung. This review will focus on the current understanding of how the pulmonary ECM regulates the basal stem cell function, how this relationship changes in chronic disease, and how replicating native conditions poses challenges for *ex vivo* cell culture.

Keywords: airway modeling, chronic lung disease, cellular niche, extracellular matrix, basal stem cells, regeneration

INTRODUCTION

The extracellular matrix (ECM) is a three-dimensional (3-D) network of extracellular macromolecules that provides structural, mechanical, and biochemical support for the cells and tissues that make up complex organisms. It is becoming increasingly apparent that the ECM plays a vital role in development and maintenance of healthy adult tissues. This review will focus on the ECM of the tracheo-bronchial airways, discussing our current knowledge of how the pulmonary ECM facilitates lung development, influences the stem cell niche, changes with chronic disease, and poses challenges for cell culture in an *ex vivo* environment. If we are to look forward to regenerative strategies for the human lung it is critical that we understand the mechanisms by which the immediate cellular environment of the basal airway stem cell regulates its long-term regenerative capacity for restoring functional mucociliary clearance.

The pulmonary ECM changes significantly throughout lung development. In addition to providing a progressive scaffold for the complex structure of the lung from the trachea to alveoli, the ECM influences stem cell specification and differentiation to the diverse cell types of the adult lung (McGowan, 1992; Burgstaller et al., 2017; Zhou et al., 2018). This is thought to occur through compartment-specific ECM composition, substrate-stiffness, and other mechanical properties, as well as biochemical signaling (Yayon et al., 1991; McGowan, 1992; Coraux et al., 2002; Izvolsky et al., 2003; Arteaga-Solis et al., 2012; Enomoto et al., 2013; Burgstaller et al., 2017; Zhou et al., 2018). Several growth factors and cytokines have been shown to influence lung development and regulate ECM deposition and basal cell (BC) phenotype. Fibroblast growth factor 10 (FGF10) and transforming growth factor beta 1 (TGF-β1) are both examples of such factors that interact with and/or influence the pulmonary ECM (Yayon et al., 1991; Sekine et al., 1999; Izvolsky et al., 2003; Alcorn et al., 2008; Arteaga-Solis et al., 2012; Li et al., 2017; Schittny, 2017; Velden et al., 2018). In the adult lung, the ECM forms a critical component of the pulmonary stem cell niche. Basal cells (BCs), the primary stem cells of the airways, reside in close proximity to the basolateral ECM and will be the primary focus of this review due to their interactions with the basement membrane and importance in regeneration of the mucociliary epithelium of the airways. While BCs are known to have the capacity to regenerate all the cells comprising the epithelium of the cartilaginous airways, the mechanisms regulating this are still poorly understood. There is increasing evidence that supports the existence of multiple sub-types of BCs *in vivo* with varying capacity for differentiation (Watson et al., 2015; Greaney et al., 2020; Travaglini et al., 2020; Carraro et al., 2020a; Carraro et al., 2020b) and distinct phenotypic changes in disease (Watson et al., 2015; Greaney et al., 2020; Travaglini et al., 2020; Carraro et al., 2020a; Carraro et al., 2020b). Despite an increase in our knowledge of both the pulmonary ECM and lung BCs there is still a paucity of information on how the ECM may influence BC stemness. As such, it is imperative that we develop a better understanding of the interactions between BCs and the ECM. Studying BC-ECM interactions is also important for the development of therapies for chronic lung diseases in which ECM alterations are accompanied by an apparent loss of the lung's regenerative capacity (Gohy et al., 2015; Jonsdottir et al., 2015; Burgstaller et al., 2017; Ghosh et al., 2017). Such disorders include asthma. chronic obstructive pulmonary disease (COPD) and idiopathic pulmonary fibrosis (IPF) (Burgess et al., 2016; Burgstaller et al., 2017).

The impact of the ECM on cell survival and phenotype becomes apparent in an *ex vivo* culture environment. While a variety of culture matrices have been developed commercially, such as Matrigel® and PureCol®, to recreate the native ECM composition and mechanical properties, numerous studies have reported significant differences in phenotype and differentiation between native BCs and those expanded *ex vivo* (Zabner et al., 2003; Cortiella et al., 2010; Greaney et al., 2020; Carraro et al., 2020a; Carraro et al., 2020b). Furthermore, these matrices are poorly defined and thus variable batch to batch. Such discrepancies pose a great challenge for both healthy and diseased airway modeling, as we are unable to determine, for instance, whether a change in BC phenotype during *ex vivo* culture reflects the same BC attrition observed with aging or injury *in vivo* or is just an artifact of inadequate culture conditions. The complexity and importance of the native ECM in the regulation of BCs is highlighted as we have yet to create an *in vitro* culture model that is capable of the long-term expansion of BCs while maintaining their phenotypic stability (Zabner et al., 2003; Cortiella et al., 2010; Liu et al., 2012; Mou et al., 2016; Gentzsch et al., 2017; Peters-Hall et al., 2018; Greaney et al., 2020; Carraro et al., 2020b). To circumnavigate the difficulties of culturing airway cells on an artificial matrix, some have turned to decellularization and recellularization of the lung or trachea (Cortiella et al., 2010; Ott et al., 2010; Price et al., 2010; Badylak et al., 2011b; Au - Bonvillain et al., 2013; Keane et al., 2015; Uriarte et al., 2018; Greaney et al., 2020). Decellularization methods attempt to remove all cellular material, leaving behind the intact ECM (Ott et al., 2010; Price et al., 2010; Badylak et al., 2011b; Uriarte et al., 2018). With present techniques, some DNA and other cytoplasmic and/or nuclear material is usually retained by the scaffold, but the composition and mechanical properties of the ECM are largely preserved (Badylak et al., 2011b; Uriarte et al., 2018). Several laboratories have attempted to repopulate the ECM with *ex vivo* expanded cells (Cortiella et al., 2010; Au - Bonvillain et al., 2013; Gilpin et al., 2014; Keane et al., 2015; Burgstaller et al., 2018; Gilpin and Wagner, 2018; Uriarte et al., 2018; Greaney et al., 2020; Ravindra et al., 2021). While this has yielded promising results, there are many aspects, particularly in the recellularization process, that must be refined before decellularization/recellularization can be widely used in clinical applications.

Determining the precise nature of the interactions between the pulmonary ECM and BCs is, therefore, a vital component of BC regulation in lung development, regeneration, and disease pathogenesis. As lungs age, or acquire disease, their capacity for functional regeneration depletes; understanding how ECM-BC interactions are altered by aging or disease should inform new therapeutic approaches for restoring long-term airway function. In addition, improving *ex vivo* cell culture will create a more physiological model of disease offering a superior platform for evaluating the mechanisms that drive chronic lung disease and providing a pathway to breakthroughs in the development of regenerative therapeutics, including cellular therapy. In this review, the role of the ECM in lung development, disease, and as a niche for basal stem cells will be reviewed and complement recent reviews focusing more on the ECM in the distal-alveolar airspace (Tschumperlin, 2015; Gu et al., 2018; Zhou et al., 2018).

Lung Development and the ECM

To understand the importance of the ECM in regulating BCs, it is essential to first discuss its role as a key component in regulating lung development and maintaining homeostasis (McGowan, 1992; Zhou et al., 2018). The composition of the pulmonary ECM changes with maturation from the fetal, to neonatal, and subsequently adult lung tissue (McGowan, 1992; Coraux et al., 2002; Burgstaller et al., 2017; Gilpin et al., 2017; Zhou et al., 2018). There are two principal concepts surrounding the role of ECM in lung development: 1) it provides a scaffold for cells and contributes to the mechanical properties of the lung, while supporting signaling between multiple cell types, and 2) its production and deposition is controlled by many cells throughout lung development (McGowan, 1992). In early lung morphogenesis, a respiratory diverticulum (or lung bud), is generated from the foregut endoderm in the human embryo approximately 5 weeks after conception (Warburton et al., 2010; Zhou et al., 2018). In humans, development then continues in four stages: pseudoglandular (5–17 weeks of gestation), canalicular (16–25 weeks), terminal saccular (24–32 weeks), and alveolar (32 or 36 weeks extending to childhood or early adolescence) (Burri, 1984; Warburton et al., 2010; Schittny, 2017; Zhou et al., 2018). Each stage is briefly discussed below, and we also refer the readers to comprehensive reviews on airway development (Burri, 1984; McGowan, 1992; Mund et al., 2008; Warburton et al., 2010; Schittny, 2017).

The Pseudoglandular Stage

The pseudoglandular stage is marked by airway branching. Branching morphogenesis is facilitated by ECM components including fibronectin, syndecan, laminin, and tenascin, along with interactions between the epithelium and mesenchyme (McGowan, 1992; Zhou et al., 2018). The cells primarily responsible for the production of such ECM proteins are pulmonary fibroblasts (Blaauboer et al., 2014; Kendall and Feghali-Bostwick, 2014; White, 2015). Epithelial branching can be induced by transplanting mesenchyme from an actively branching region into a normally unbranched region, demonstrating the importance of epithelial interactions with the mesenchyme (Shannon et al., 1998). The ECM expresses proteoglycans (PGs) decorin, lumican, and biglycan, along with collagens I, III, and VI at the epithelial-mesenchymal interface forming a sleeve around the bronchiolar ducts (Godoy-Guzman et al., 2012). Sulfated proteoglycans, heparin sulfates (HS), in the ECM may also contribute to the regulation airway branching due to their ability to regulate growth factor binding and signaling (Yayon et al., 1991; Aviezer et al., 1994; Izvolsky et al., 2003; Zhang et al., 2012). FGF-10 deficient mice do not survive post-natal due to lack of lung development, while the trachea is formed, pulmonary branching morphogenesis is disrupted (Yayon et al., 1991; Sekine et al., 1999; Izvolsky et al., 2003). HS are expressed in the lung mesenchyme at prospective bud sites in close proximity to FGF-10 expressing regions, and highly sulfated HS are also found in the basement membranes of epithelial tubule branches (Izvolsky et al., 2003; Zhang et al., 2012). This suggests that FGF-10′s ability to induce budding is significantly changed by the developmental patterns of HS sulfation (Izvolsky et al., 2003). By the conclusion of the pseudoglandular stage, all of the prospective conducting airways have been formed and the acinar outlines have appeared (Coraux et al., 2002; Warburton et al., 2010; Schittny, 2017).

The Canalicular and Saccular Stage

There are three critical events that occur during the canalicular stage: 1) the appearance of the distal alveolar air sac (acinus), 2) the development of the air-blood interface and differentiation of the pulmonary epithelium, and 3) the commencement of surfactant production (McGowan, 1992). Type 1 and 2 alveolar epithelial cells (AT1 and AT2 respectively), the latter being responsible for surfactant synthesis, arise from the differentiation of the glycogen-rich cuboidal epithelial cells of the future alveolar ducts (Schittny, 2017). AT1s, with AT2s integrated between them, form the thin lining of the alveolar ducts and sacculi (Schittny, 2017). The future air-blood barrier will form at the locations where the capillary endothelium comes into close contact with the AT1s (Schittny, 2017). By the end of the canalicular stage, the airways have been divided to form the future alveolar, also known as transitory, ducts (McGowan, 1992).

During the terminal saccular stage, air spaces continue to widen, and the air-blood interface becomes more closely related through the rearrangement of capillaries (McGowan, 1992; Warburton et al., 2010; Schittny, 2017). A significant decrease in the mass of the mesenchymal ECM accompanies this sophistication of the membrane between the capillary and alveolar wall (Burri, 1984; McGowan, 1992). This process seems to be mediated by elastin, as an organized deposition of elastin fibrils occurs beneath the transitory duct epithelium (McGowan, 1992; Schittny, 2017). Elastin, a structural ECM protein, is principally responsible for the elasticity of the alveolar walls and its deposition is maximal along the sites of future secondary crests (McGowan, 1992). To facilitate alveolar septation the precursor of elastin, tropoelastin, is produced and cross-linked by lysyl oxidase (Zhou et al., 2018). The elevation and suspension of the secondary crests that subdivide the primary saccules is a consequence of elastin deposition (Amy et al., 1977; Zhou et al., 2018). The importance of elastin for developing lung structure during the saccular stage is demonstrated when epithelial-driven inflammation is induced in murine models. Such inflammation disrupts elastin fiber organization and causes a decreased regulation in elastin assembly components such as fibulins 4/5, lysyl oxidase, and fribrillin-1 leading to impaired structural development during the saccular stage (Benjamin et al., 2016). Inflammation, as a result incomplete lung development, has also been implicated in human infants born prematurely (Kramer et al., 2009). The saccular stage appears to be an intermediate stage in which branching is concluded and the scaffold for future alveolarization is set into place.

The Alveolar Stage

In humans, alveolarization begins at approximately 20 weeks post-conception and is not completed until at least 7 years of age; in mice however, alveolarization takes place entirely postnatally (Mund et al., 2008; Warburton et al., 2010). The saccules are divided into alveoli by the formation of secondary crests that appear as narrow ridges (Amy et al., 1977; Branchfield et al., 2016). It has been demonstrated that secondary crests develop, through the deposition of elastic tissue, at the juxtaposition of a capillary, AT1 cell, and an epithelial cell (Amy et al., 1977). These observations suggest that portions of the primary saccular wall are tethered by the elastin and collagen fibers in the expanding secondary crest while the free regions of the wall enlarge outward into alveoli (Amy et al., 1977). FGF signaling is considered to be the director of elastin deposits during this stage by restricting the expression of the elastogenic machinery in the mesenchyme to allow for controlled and ordered formation of elastic ECM (Li et al., 2017). Alveolar myofibroblasts are considered to be the elastin producing cells of the lung due to their physical proximity to sites of elastin deposition (Vaccaro and Brody, 1978; Noguchi et al., 1989). In addition, platelet derived growth factor subunit A (PDGF-A) has been demonstrated to have an essential and highly specific function in lung development by promoting differentiation of fibroblasts to alveolar myofibroblasts and, as a consequence, alveolarization (Bostrom et al., 1996). PDGF-A deficient mice surviving birth show failed alveolar septation leading to lung emphysema (Bostrom et al., 1996; Lindahl et al., 1997). This appears to be the result of a lack of alveolar myofibroblasts and their associated elastin deposits (Bostrom et al., 1996). The degree of sulfation of proteoglycans (PGs) is also thought to play a role in alveolus formation. Sulfation of PGs is affected by sulfatases, activated by sulfatase-modifying factor 1 (SUMF1), through the removal of sulfate groups (Arteaga-Solis et al., 2012). Mice lacking the SUMF1 enzyme show normal lung development until the start of alveolarization when an increase in sulfated PGs is detected in the lung parenchyma along with a decrease in alveolar septa formation (Arteaga-Solis et al., 2012). These mice also showed an increase in TGF-β1 signaling (Arteaga-Solis et al., 2012). Removal of sulfatase activity seems to increase the deposition of sulfated PGs which leads to a deregulation of TGF-β1 signaling and a halt in alveolarization (Arteaga-Solis et al., 2012).

Adult Lung ECM Composition

Two major structural types compose the adult pulmonary ECM. First, basement membranes, thin glycoprotein sheets, line the basal surface of the epithelia and endothelia, and also envelop muscle, peripheral nerve cells, and fat (Sannes and Wang, 1997; Moore et al., 2005; Burgstaller et al., 2017). Second, interstitial matrices interconnect structural cells and maintain 3-D structure and biomechanical characteristics through a loose, fibril-like meshwork (Burgstaller et al., 2017). ECM proteins, glycosaminoglycans, and modifying enzymes assemble into insoluble composite materials to provide a binding interface for the hundreds of secreted proteins within the lung (Burgstaller et al., 2017; He et al., 2017; Wigen et al., 2019). This allows for the complex signaling that is thought to direct cell function and differentiation. Collagen and elastin are the two major ECM proteins of the lung. While collagens (types I, II, III, V, and XI) provide overall structure to the lung, elastic fibers are responsible for elastic recoil (Burgstaller et al., 2017; Mereness et al., 2018). Glycoproteins, fibulins, elastin microfibril interface-located proteins, and elastin-crosslinking lysyl oxidases are other proteins that are associated with elastic fibers (Ge et al., 2015; Liu et al., 2016; Burgstaller et al., 2017; Philp et al., 2018; Ito et al., 2019). PGs contribute to the viscoelasticity of the lung due to their hydrophilic nature (Burgstaller et al., 2017; Iravani et al., 2020). Post-translational modifications of ECM proteins, such as enzymatic or chemical crosslinking, glycation and glycosylation, and oxidation, allow for further structural and/or function diversity (Burgstaller et al., 2017; Merl-Pham et al., 2019; Rani et al., 2021). The remainder of this review will focus on current knowledge of how the ECM regulates lung stem cell function, and we refer readers to Burgstaller and colleagues (Burgstaller et al., 2017) for an in-depth review of the adult pulmonary ECM composition.

The ECM and Regulation of Stem Cells

Decoding the regenerative capacity of the lungs is a vital step toward identifying potential therapies for chronic lung diseases. This has proven to be difficult because the lung is relatively quiescent under normal conditions with infrequent divisions of progenitor cells to maintain the respiratory epithelium (Beers and Morrisey, 2011; Stabler and Morrisey, 2017). As such, it is challenging to study epithelial regeneration under steady-state conditions, especially in relevant human cells, and artificial injury to activate stem cells and regenerate airways is required in animal models (Zhu et al., 2007; Rock et al., 2009; Mereness et al., 2018; Yuan et al., 2019). Additionally, there are limited studies on how the ECM facilitates and regulates stem cell differentiation and maintenance, and the relationship between changes in ECM composition in diseased states and the impact on the stem cell niche has yet to be fully elucidated. As BCs are known to be the major stem cell population in the conducting airways, we will focus on their interactions with the ECM *in vivo* and in *ex vivo* models.

The Pulmonary Stem Cell Niche

BCs are multipotent stem cells that reside in close proximity to the basal lamina in the pseudostratified epithelium of the tracheobronchial tree (Rock et al., 2009; Donne et al., 2015). They are present in approximately equal proportions to ciliated and secretory cells in the conducting airways (Rock et al., 2009; Donne et al., 2015). With their ability to self-renew and differentiate into all luminal cell types (Hong et al., 2004; Rock et al., 2009), BCs are thought to be important in maintaining epithelium homeostasis. As previously mentioned, the lung has a relatively slow cell-turnover rate during homeostasis (Beers and Morrisey, 2011; Stabler and Morrisey, 2017). To date BCs have been characterized by their expression of transcription factor tumor protein 63 (TP63), cytokeratin 5 (KRT5), podoplanin (PDPN), nerve growth factor receptor (NGFR), and cytokeratin 14 (KRT14) (Rock et al., 2009; Donne et al., 2015); however, the situation is likely more complex. New transcriptomic data has emerged that suggests the presence of a number of BC subpopulations (Watson et al., 2015; Smirnova et al., 2016; Carraro et al., 2020a). Each sub-type of BC may have a different physiological and functional role in airway maintenance and regeneration. A collaborative study by Carraro *et al.* has identified 5 BC sub-types in the native human proximal epithelium (Carraro et al., 2020a). The sub-types include one highly expressing canonical markers such as TP63, KRT5, and cytokeratin 15 (KRT15), and another with proliferative characteristics including DNA topoisomerase II alpha, and the marker of proliferation antigen Ki-67 (Carraro et al., 2020a). Of the various BC sub-populations, it has been suggested that ciliated and secretory "primed" cells exist as intermediates between BCs and their differentiated progeny (Watson et al., 2015; Carraro et al., 2020a). Watson *et al.* proposes that multipotent BCs give rise to luminal precursors (BLPs) that show upregulation of cytokeratin 8 (KRT8), and that these BLPs eventually differentiate to secretory or ciliated cells (Watson et al., 2015). Furthermore, the concept of "hillock" cells, originally described by Montoro and colleagues, was reconfirmed in a study that identified two populations within this KRT13 expressing "hillock" population, one which was notably high in markers of squamous/cornified epithelium (Montoro et al., 2018; Deprez et al., 2020). Further studies will be required to determine the precise functional differences that specifically define the BC sub-populations observed and determine if they are universally expressed in humans and other species.

Due to the important role of the ECM in directing lung development, it is thought to perform an equally important role in the maintenance of the pulmonary stem cell niche and the regulation of regeneration. These mechanisms and interactions between BCs and the ECM are historically poorly studied and defined; however, in more recent years there has been a greater push to advance our understanding in this area. Age related changes in the ECM have been shown to have a significant impact on epithelial phenotype and gene expression (Godin et al., 2016; Gilpin et al., 2017). Isolated human BCs demonstrated higher proliferative markers, PCNA and Ki67, and a higher percentage of living cells when cultured on a scaffold derived from a human early post-natal lung than an adult lung (Gilpin et al., 2017). The glycoproteins Fibrillin-2 and Tenascin-C were found to be significantly enriched in the post-natal lung and labeled as potential mediators of the reported results (Gilpin et al., 2017). Lung growth that occurs most robustly during the early post-natal period may explain why proliferation-stimulating ECM components are more highly expressed during this phase. In another study, collagen VI (COLVI) was found *in vivo* in a position to interact with epithelial cells in both the airways and alveoli (Mereness et al., 2018). In an *in vitro* experiment, primary human lung epithelial cells displayed a heightened rate of "healing" in response to scratch injury when plated on COLVI as opposed to Matrigel, collagen I (COLI), or a combination of Matrigel and COLI or COLVI (Mereness et al., 2018). Studies that follow up on these initial observations to determine the precise BC-ECM interactions that occur in early post-natal lung compared to the adult lung. This knowledge could inform on the development of better *in vitro* culture systems as well as identify new regulators of BC stemness and proliferation.

One of the early studies on the airway BC transcriptome identified gene clusters postulated to be associated with the cells ability to maintain the structural integrity of the airway epithelium (Hackett et al., 2011). Over 201 genes in the focal adhesion pathway overlapped with BCs inclusive of these associated with adherens junction formation, ECM-receptor interactions, and regulation of the actin cytoskeleton. Among these genes overrepresented in BCs were 5 laminin subunits (α, β1, β3, γ1, γ3), and 6 integrin subunits (α3, α5, α6, β1, β4, β6) associated with cell-cell and cell-ECM interactions (Evans et al., 2001; Hackett et al., 2011). To date most transcriptomic studies have included minimal validation of the findings with no specific functional characterization (Hackett et al., 2011; Hackett et al., 2012; Xu et al., 2016; Carraro et al., 2020a; Carraro et al., 2020b). The BC signature highlights the array of integrins, extracellular laminins and collagen, and adaptor proteins including actinin, vinculin and filamin essential for functional interaction with other cells and the ECM and also demonstrates differences between mouse and human BCs. For example, ITGA5 and ITGB6 are expressed in human, but not mouse BCs and, in humans, ITGA5 is known to mediate fibronectin-dependent epithelial cell proliferation through activation of EGFR (Kuwada and Li, 2000). Recently we have gained significant transcriptomic insight into BC subpopulations, however the field now needs to determine the regional-specific distribution and also validate the functional properties, cell: cell, and cell: ECM interactions that are relevant to homeostasis and to disease pathogenesis. Information acquired at the transcriptomic level does not always correlate to changes at the functional and physiological level (Kuwada and Li, 2000).

Understanding how the ECM influences the regeneration of an injured airway epithelium is a pre-requisite to the development of regenerative therapeutics for patients with acute and chronic lung disease. The scratch injury, mentioned above, is one model of airway wound repair in which epithelial-ECM interactions can be evaluated. Initial migration of airway BCs involves the formation of heterodimers of integrin α and β subunits, with the ECM expressing the ligands for integrins expressed on BCs regulating ECM-cell adhesion (Coraux et al., 2008; Hamilton et al., 2020). The importance of the various integrin subunits for BC migration directly depends on the ECM and, therefore, many *ex vivo* culture systems do not accurately reflect the specific process of *in vivo* airway regeneration. Matrix proteins, especially cellular fibronectin, are key in the successful migration of BCs and blocking their function substantially impairs wound repair (Hocking and Chang, 2003). It has been long established that as lungs age there is an age dependent change in the expression of fibronectin in the alveolar regions of the lung (D'Errico et al., 1989) and recent studies have supported such changes in the ECM, however there is still a paucity of information on how such age-related changes correlate to tissue formation and degradation and how ECM signals regulate injury repair and disease progression (Meiners et al., 2015; Brandenberger and Mühlfeld, 2017; Burgess et al., 2019). Given the increasing amount of data documenting ECM changes in the aging lung it is important that we start to understand the aging-related signature and its implications in the repair and regeneration of the lung epithelium.

In addition to being regulated by the matrix, BCs are also implicated in the production of ECM. During wound repair, the

TABLE 1 | Matrices available for the culture of pulmonary basal stem cells.

Matrix (ECM)	Composition	Biological source	References
Matrigel®[a] Geltrex®[a] Cultrex®[b]	Laminin, collagen IV, enactin, heparin sulfate proteoglycans, growth factors	Murine engelbreth-holm-swarm tumor	Hughes et al. (2010); Badylak et al. (2011b)
PureCol®	97% Type I atelocollagen, 3% Type III collagen	Bovine hide	Dodmane et al. (2018)
Type I Collagen	Collagen I	Rat tail	Mereness et al. (2018)
Type IV Collagen	Collagen IV	Human cell culture	Gilpin et al. (2017)
Fibronectin	Fibronectin (Human plasma)	Human plasma	Hamilton et al. (2020)
Laminin	Laminin	Human placenta, human fibroblasts, murine engelbreth-holm-swarm tumor	Hamilton et al. (2020)

[a]*Multiple varieties available including high concentration and reduced growth factor.*
[b]*Variety optimized for stem cell culture available.*

production of matrix components by BCs is influenced by the secretion of factors, such as TGF-β, either from BCs themselves or from inflammatory cells in the airways. The functional implications of these secreted factors remain somewhat unclear. For example, treatment with TGF-β impairs airway epithelial sheet migration due to increased cellular adhesion via integrins (Neurohr et al., 2006) and, conversely, TGF-β1 has also been shown to upregulate MMP2 accelerating the rate of epithelial repair (Coraux et al., 2008). Matrix metalloproteases (MMPs) regulate ECM secreted by the wound closing migratory BCs, these include MMP-9 (also known as gelatinase B), MMP-3 and MMP-11. These reparative BC often also express vimentin suggesting that acquisition of a mesenchymal phenotype is needed for effective wound closure via cell migration. Studies of mouse tracheal BCs have also demonstrated similar upregulation of markers of an epithelial to mesenchymal transition (EMT) (Velden et al., 2018). BCs subsequently plated on matrix secreted by TGF-β1-treated BCs have increased expression of EMT markers and acquire a spindle-like, fibroblastic appearance (Alcorn et al., 2008; Gohy et al., 2015; Velden et al., 2018; Adams et al., 2020).

BC-ECM interactions, although extensively investigated in the process of would repair, have been substantially less studied in the subsequent differentiation and restoration of functional mucociliary clearance. As BCs progress toward potential cellular therapy applications a detailed understanding of such interactions will be critical. Furthermore, determining the mechanisms driving changes in cellular phenotype and stemness during the *ex vivo* expansion of BCs will rely upon this information to design methods for effective cellular expansion while maintaining BC stemness. Many *ex vivo* culture systems study epithelial function and regeneration in monocultures comprising of epithelium alone. While these models can be used to study cell-matrix interactions critical modulation by exogenous influences such as inflammatory cells and their secreted mediators, and the surrounding mesenchyme limits the physiological interpretation of the model system. In the next section we will focus on how ECM components and mechanics are critical for maintaining BC stemness in an *in vitro* culture environment.

Culture and Airway Modeling

A variety of medias, matrices, and techniques are commonly used to culture BCs and/or drive differentiation into airway epithelium via culture at an air-liquid-interface (ALI) (Jiang et al., 2018) or in 3-D organoids or spheroids (Barkauskas et al., 2017). Commercially available ECMs used for BC expansion include Matrigel® (a protein mixture including laminin, collagen IV, and enactin that is derived from mouse tumor cells) (Hughes et al., 2010; Greaney et al., 2020) and PureCol® (a combination of collagens I and III) (Dodmane et al., 2018). A more extensive inventory of ECMs suitable for BC expansion and differentiation can be found in **Table 1**. However, BCs that are isolated and expanded *ex vivo* lose stemness within a few passages, differentiation capacity is reduced, and expression of genes that are critical for function, such as the cystic fibrosis transmembrane regulator (CFTR), decline (Zabner et al., 2003; Peters-Hall et al., 2018). In ALI cultures, primary BCs show a rapid linear decrease in CFTR function and ciliated cell formation with increased passages (Zabner et al., 2003; Peters-Hall et al., 2018). Often by passage 4, a significant decrease in differentiation capacity and CFTR expression/function is observed, and by passage 10 growth tends to stop (Zabner et al., 2003; Peters-Hall et al., 2018). In addition, airway epithelium produced by differentiation at ALI shows notable deviations from native samples. In the Carraro *et al.* study, 5 BC subtypes were identified in native human bronchial epithelium; however, only four subtypes were found in their ALI generated epithelia (Carraro et al., 2020a). While three subtypes were similar between the native and ALI samples, the fourth ALI subtype was high in KRT14 and lacked a native counterpart (Carraro et al., 2020a). The presence of a unique BC subtype in the ALI generated samples suggests that this subtype developed in response to culture conditions and demonstrates that the ALI culture platform may not be completely analogous *to in vivo* airway conditions.

Advanced media formulations have also extended our capacity to effectively maintain stem cell characteristics over prolonged *in vitro* expansion. The addition of a combination of three small molecules to the media, Rho-associated protein kinase (ROCK) inhibitor, dorsomorphin homolog 1 (DMH-1) [inhibitor of bone morphogenic proteins (BMP) signaling], and A-83-01 (inhibitor of TGF-β1 signaling), allows for extended airway BC expansion in the undifferentiated state; this is thought to be the result of dual SMAD inhibition (Mou et al., 2016). Cells grown in this media were positive for TP63 and KRT5, markers of multipotent epithelial BCs, and also expressed cell proliferation marker Ki-67, expanding for 18–25 passages without a loss of replicative potential (Mou et al., 2016). BMP and TGF-β1 inhibitors produced similar results when added to commercially available stem cell culture mediums bronchial epithelial cell growth medium (BEGM) and primary human airway epithelial cell media (HTEC) (Mou et al., 2016).

Prior to the addition of dual SMAD inhibitors to the media, the gold standard for preservation of stemness across serially passaged human bronchial epithelial cells (HBECs) was the addition of Rho kinase inhibitor (Y-27632) and co-culture on a layer of fibroblast feeder cells, specifically NIH-3T3-J2 cells (Liu et al., 2012; Gentzsch et al., 2017; Peters-Hall et al., 2018). Cells reprogrammed in this way are referred to as "conditionally reprogrammed cells" (CRCs). They retain a normal karyotype and remain non-tumorigenic (Liu et al., 2012). However, ALI cultures derived from CRC cells still show morphological differences and reduced CFTR expression compared to non-CRC ALIs (Gentzsch et al., 2017). Recently, a modified CRC (Mod-CRC) method has been presented that demonstrates improved preservation of differentiation capacity and CFTR function of HBECs (Peters-Hall et al., 2018). In a modified-CRC method, BEGM is used along with 2% O_2, as opposed to a serum free expansion media and 21% O_2 used in traditional CRC expansion (Peters-Hall et al., 2018).

To overcome culture constraints and improve the viability of BCs *ex vivo*, researchers are now exploring the decellularization of lung and airway tissues to more closely recapitulate the ECM and mechanical properties seen *in vivo* (Ott et al., 2010; Price et al., 2010; Wagner et al., 2014; Gilpin and Wagner, 2018). Decellularization methods strive for total removal of the cellular material, while preserving the structure, protein and molecular composition, and mechanical properties of the ECM scaffold (Badylak et al., 2011b; Keane et al., 2015; Uriarte et al., 2018). The ultimate goal is to re-populate this scaffold with stem cells to completely regenerate a functional organ or tissue (Badylak et al., 2011b; Uriarte et al., 2018). While currently practiced methods of decellularization leave much of the ECM intact, including the structural geography of the airways, alveoli and vessels, there is a reduction in many components such as elastin, collagen, and sulfonated PGs (Price et al., 2010; Pouliot et al., 2016). Creation of a functional tissue from a decellularized scaffold has been attempted for multiple organs including heart, liver, urinary bladder, trachea, and lung (Cortiella et al., 2010; Badylak et al., 2011b). Decellularized lungs have been successfully re-populated with cells (Cortiella et al., 2010; Ott et al., 2010; Au - Bonvillain et al., 2013; Halabi and Mecham, 2018); however, keeping distinct cell populations in their proper areas and creating functional gas-exchange units has not been achieved (Uriarte et al., 2018). Ott and colleagues were successful in perfusing repopulated rat lung scaffolds with blood and performing ventilation, however transplantation of the lungs was only able to maintain gas exchange for 6 h (Ott et al., 2010). Although bio scaffolds generated from ECM of decellularized source tissues have been successfully used in the clinic (Badylak et al., 2011a; Dziki et al., 2016; Keane et al., 2017), for the trachea they have been unsuccessful due to the immediate need for a complete epithelium capable of functional mucociliary clearance. While an exciting advance to the field there is still a long way to go before the concept of a bioartificial lung will be a therapeutic reality.

Although decellularization and recellularization techniques must be significantly refined before they are capable of generating a functional lung, researchers are demonstrating that there are advantages to using a native ECM scaffold for BC culture and epithelium generation (**Figure 1A**). Recently, a study by Greaney *et al.* compared the differences in differentiation of murine BCs across four different culture platforms: organoid, ALI, decellularized trachea, and decellularized lung (Greaney et al., 2020). They concluded that the decellularized or "engineered" scaffolds produced the most mature epithelial tissues *in vitro* over the artificial culture platforms (Greaney et al., 2020). Demonstrating the regional specificity of ECM and effect on differentiation, the engineered trachea contained the most mature proximal epithelium and ciliated cells, while the engineered lung showed early surfactant production suggesting distalization (Greaney et al., 2020). In the artificial platforms, the organoid culture presented a less developed epithelium and a non-physiological EMT population was observed at ALI (Greaney et al., 2020). This study supports the results of previous work by Cortiella *et al.* which compared the attachment, differentiation, and development of complex tissue of murine embryonic stem cells (ESCs) when expanded on several artificial culture matrices, including Matrigel and COLI, and whole decellularized lung (Cortiella et al., 2010). The lung scaffold produced more differentiated ESCs of epithelial and endothelial lineages, retained a higher ratio of living cells, and showed evidence of differentiated ESCs arranging into 3-D structures similar to those seen *in vivo* (2010). Such comprehensive studies have yet to be carried out for human airways and will be essential if a functional lung derived from a repopulated ECM scaffold is to become reality.

Instead of using a decellularized lung a scaffold for repopulation, some researchers are further processing native ECM into a hydrogel for 2-D or 3-D culture. These hydrogels exhibit characteristics such as self-assembly, architecture, and mechanical properties of the native tissue (Pouliot et al., 2016; de Hilster et al., 2020; Petrou et al., 2020). Mesenchymal stem cells, for example, encapsulated in hydrogels derived from porcine lung demonstrate attachment, proliferation, and viability at a comparable or greater level than cells grown in commercially available collagen-based matrices (Pouliot et al., 2016). Hydrogels have also been generated from human lungs that retained native stiffness in the range of 15–60 Pa (Pouliot et al., 2016; de Hilster et al., 2020). Changes in ECM-derived hydrogel stiffness induce significant changes in cultured cells. Petrou *et al.* reported that on hydrogels with increased elastic moduli, similar to native fibrotic ECM, ECM producing myofibroblasts showed heightened expression of myofibroblast transgenes and fibroblasts

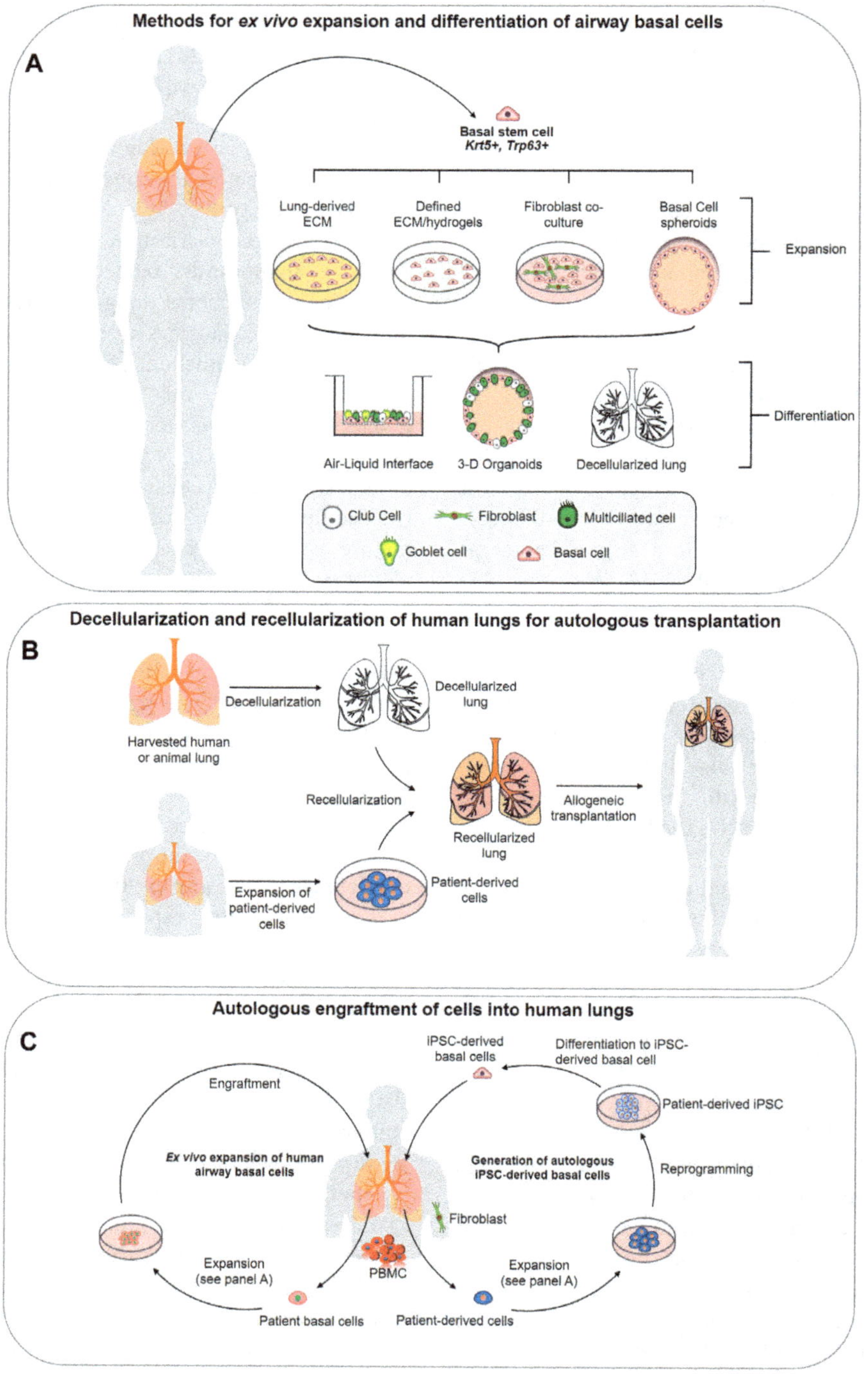

FIGURE 1 | Strategies for utilizing airway basal stem cells in regenerative medicine approaches. **(A)** *Methods for ex vivo expansion and differentiation of airway basal cells.* Basal cells (BCs) can be isolated from the human lung epithelium and expanded in 3-D culture, co-culture with 3T3 fibroblasts, or potentially on specifically designed hydrogels or extracellular matrix (ECM)-derived from decellularized lungs. Expanded basal cells are capable of complete differentiation into a pseudostratified airway epithelium at the air-liquid interface, in 3-D spheroid cultures or in decellularized lung scaffolds. **(B)** *Decellularization and recellularization of human lungs for autologous transplantation.* Decellularization of human donor lungs, followed by recellularization with patient-derived cells (generated via methods described in panels c (primary airway cell expansion) and d (iPSC-derived basal cell generation. The concept is designed to achieve functional lung tissues or indeed, entire lungs, for autologous transplantation. **(C)** *Ex vivo expansion of human airway basal cells.* BCs can be isolated from human lung biopsy or bronchoscopy and expanded on defined ECM to maintain stemness and phenotype. The goal is to engraft these stem cells into the lung to restore airway function. *Generation of autologous iPSC-derived basal cells.* Using accessible cells such as peripheral blood mononucleocytes (PBMCs) or fibroblasts from skin biopsies, iPSC can be generated via reprogramming. Protocols now exist for their precise differentiation to lung basal cells (Hawkins et al., 2020) generating a potentially unlimited source of autologous cells for engraftment.

demonstrated a 60% increase in levels of collagen 1a1 and alpha smooth muscle actin compared to soft matrices (Petrou et al., 2020). These results may have significant implications for the understanding of cellular changes in response to fibrotic lung diseases. Further development of 2-D culture matrices derived from native pulmonary ECM will have important implications for 2-D culture of BCs and airway modeling, however, to date, there have been relatively few studies investigating the culture of airway BCs on these hydrogels. One recent study by Ravindra and colleagues compared HBEC attachment and functional differentiation on tracheal and urinary bladder ECM substrates. (Ravindra et al., 2021). Both hydrogels successfully supported cell proliferation and generation of a continuous basement membrane, however, while both substrates supported epithelial differentiation, this was not quantified or functionally evaluated. Critical next steps are to understand the components of the hydrogels that specifically support functional specification of the tracheal epithelium (Ravindra et al., 2021).

Most recently, progress in the development and use of synthetic ECM materials for cell culture have emerged. Biomaterial inks have been developed from regenerated silk fibroin (SF) and 2,2,6,6-tetramethylpiperidine-1-oxyl (TEMPO)-oxidized bacterial cellulose (OBC) nanofibrils and engineered for 3D printing of lung tissue scaffolds (Huang et al., 2020). Another group has developed a tissue-specific hybrid bioinks from the naturally occurring polymer alginate along with ECM derived from decellularized tissue (De Santis et al., 2021). In both models HBECs were able to adhere and proliferate, maintaining expression of basal cell markers TP63 and KRT5. De Santis and colleagues evaluated differentiation over a month on 3D bio-printed human airways composed of regionally specified airway smooth muscle and human bronchial epithelial cells and observed basolateral localization of BCs and evidence of differentiation to mucus-producing cells ($MUC5AC^+$) and ciliated cells shown directly through scanning electron microscopy and alpha-tubulin expression (De Santis et al., 2021). The results of this study do demonstrate that a combination of exogenously and endogenously derived ECM materials supports epithelial development and offers the potential of printing customized airway scaffolds which has not yet been achieved with native ECM alone. Huang suggested that by manipulating the alignment of the OBC nanofibrils within the scaffold, ECM remodeling could be recreated and consequently manipulate cell fate (Huang et al., 2020). Unfortunately, neither study comprehensively evaluated functional differentiation, mucociliary clearance, and regenerative capacity, all core criteria in creating bio scaffolds for lung repair. (Huang et al., 2020) (Huang et al., 2020). While extensive validation is necessary before the creation of functional organs derived from decellularized ECM scaffolds is feasible, these studies do support the notion that ECMs derived from native tissues produce more physiologic BC populations and airway epithelia in an *in vitro* setting.

Disease Pathogenesis

It is becoming increasingly apparent that changes in the ECM are associated with the development of many chronic lung diseases. As such, increasing our understanding of the role ECM alterations play in disease pathogenesis offers a new potential route for the development therapies for chronic conditions. COPD, IPF, asthma, and lung cancers are several diseases in which significant changes in the pulmonary ECM have been observed (Fukuda et al., 1989; Bensadoun et al., 1996; Black et al., 2008; Merrilees et al., 2008; Löfdahl et al., 2011; Estany et al., 2014; Eurlings et al., 2014; Abdillahi et al., 2015; Burgess et al., 2016; Burgstaller et al., 2017; Elowsson Rendin et al., 2019). There are very few viable treatments available for these diseases and, in their most serious forms, complete lung transplantation is often the only option (Arcasoy and Kotloff, 1999). Unfortunately, there is a significant lack of suitable donors and, at most, a lung transplantation is a temporary cure with post-transplant survival averaging only 5 years (Arcasoy and Kotloff, 1999; Cypel et al., 2015). Regenerative therapeutic options include: 1) decellularization and repopulation of donor lung and/or animal sourced organs with patient specific stem cells (Cortiella et al., 2010; Badylak et al., 2011b; Au - Bonvillain et al., 2013) (**Figure 1B**), 2) engraftment of *ex vivo* expanded autologous BCs (Ghosh et al., 2016; Ma et al., 2018) (**Figure 1C**), 3) derivation of autologous iPSC-derived airway cells (**Figure 1C**) (Firth et al., 2014; Huang et al., 2014; Miller et al., 2018; Hawkins et al., 2020; Kanagaki et al., 2020; Yamamoto et al., 2020) or 4) activation of endogenous basal stem cells to repair the damaged tissues. We refer the readers to Ikonomou *et al.* who have thoroughly reviewed the current state of cell-based therapies for respiratory diseases (Ikonomou et al., 2019). All of these options rely upon a receptive cellular microenvironment to preserve BC stemness and the ECM is likely a critical component for this. Our current knowledge of the ECM changes linked to asthma, COPD and IPF will be reviewed primarily focusing on changes in the proximal airways.

Asthma

Asthma is a chronic inflammatory disease of the airways marked by hyperresponsiveness of the airways to triggers or irritants such as allergens, viruses, and exercise resulting in exaggerated narrowing of the airways (Mims, 2015; Quirt et al., 2018). This causes the individual to experience recurrent bouts of wheezing, breathlessness, feeling tightness in the chest, and/or coughing varying in intensity from mild to, in some cases, fatal severity (Mims, 2015; Quirt et al., 2018). These symptoms are the result of wide-spread airflow obstruction within the lungs. Despite extensive evaluation of changes in airway smooth muscle (ASM) phenotype and ECM interactions there is relatively little known about how ECM changes in asthma regulate epithelial-mesenchymal communication and subsequently BC function. We will summarize some of the key findings specific to the regulation of airway BCs and ECM in asthmatic airways.

It is clear that the profile of ECM proteins in altered in asthmatic airways with the degree of ECM remodeling correlating to the severity of the patient's symptoms. The deposition of fibronectin, tenascin, hyaluronan, versican, laminin $\alpha2/\beta2$, and collagens I, III, and V has been shown to increase, while the deposition of collagen IV and elastin is decreased (Bousquet et al., 1992; Chetta et al., 1997; Roberts and Burke, 1998; Araujo et al., 2008; Nihlberg et al., 2010; Weitoft et al., 2014). When investigating asthma, it is critical to consider complex interactions within the immediate microenvironment of the airway epithelium, a structural and immunological barrier known as the epithelial mesenchymal trophic unit (EMTU) (Vignola et al., 2000; Heijink et al., 2014). Furthermore, the change in deposition of ECM can have considerable changes on matrix stiffness which, in turn, can differentiate fibroblasts to myofibroblasts leading to further matrix production (Shi et al., 2013). *In vitro* experiments replicate this phenotype with TGF-β-stimulated fibroblasts grown on polydimethylsiloxane (PDMS) substrates having increased expression of collagen 1 and alpha-smooth muscle actin indicative of their differentiation to myofibroblasts. As myofibroblast differentiation increased, substrate stiffness also increased from 1 to 50 kPa (Shi et al., 2013). Cells involved in the inflammatory response underlying asthma can interact with, and induce, structural changes in the airway, including synthesis of ECM by fibroblasts (Chan et al., 2006; Shi et al., 2013; Osei et al., 2020). Interleukin signaling has been shown to be one of the key pathways that can stimulate changes in the secretion of ECM proteins including fibronectin and collagen (Chan et al., 2006; Osei et al., 2020). IL-1 expression is increased in asthmatic HBECs compared to those cultured from non-asthmatic lungs, this has a significant impact of pro-inflammatory responses in airway fibroblasts, production of collagen, fibronectin and periostin and leads to abnormal collagen remodeling of the asthmatic-EMTU. Further studies need to be carried out to fully evaluate IL-1 signaling as a therapeutic option for treating chronic asthma (Osei et al., 2020). Another potential target is fibulin-1 (Fbln1) which has recently been shown to both stabilize collagen and other ECM proteins and to regulate the expression of mucins including MUC5AC, and inflammatory mediators, such as CXCL1, in airway epithelial cells (Liu et al., 2017). Another example of changes in asthmatic HBEC regulating the ECM is highlighted in work studying the production of Hyaluronan (HA) a non-sulfate glycosaminoglycan synthesized at the cell membrane. Studies have shown that HA is increased in both bronchioalveolar fluid (Bousquet et al., 1991; Zhu et al., 2010; Ge et al., 2018) and in ECM produced when HBECs of asthmatics are cultured with human lung fibroblasts (Reeves et al., 2018). Its ability to suppress airway inflammation and mucus secretion, indicating that HA may be a potential therapeutic option for reducing remodeling in asthma (Ko et al., 2020).

Other mechanisms driving abnormal ECM composition include increased synthesis of new ECM proteins, decreased activity of ECM-degrading enzymes [metalloproteinases (MMPs) in particular] (Bajbouj et al., 2021), and upregulation of the tissue-specific inhibitors of metalloproteinases (TIMP) (Bajbouj et al., 2021). The role of MMPs in asthma pathogenesis is not as simple as it may seem with disagreement in the field on the destructive vs protective impact of MMPs in chronic lung diseases like asthma (Grzela et al., 2016). Discrepancies may be attributed to the severity of the disease or localization of specific MMP responses (Araujo et al., 2008), significant research still needs to be carried out in this area and likely requires the use of more complex, human tissue-level studies comprising of all the cells in an EMTU. MMP-9 and MMP-12 are increased in the airway smooth muscle of the large airways in fatal cases of asthma (Araujo et al., 2008) and it has been shown that HA may play a role in suppressing MMP9 production and be of potential therapeutic benefit (Ko et al., 2020). More recently a role for MMP2, expressed by HBECs, has been considered in ECM remodeling and data suggests that MMP2 may be key in mediating crosstalk between HBEC and their underlying myofibroblasts in the EMTU and that a net change in MMP2 activity in asthma may promote fibrosis and increased deposition of ECM, despite its role in ECM degradation (Xu et al., 2002). This contrasts data from mice where MMP2 is proposed to provide a protective role (Takahashi et al., 2019). Most recently a study of over 80 bronchial biopsies identified significant overexpression of MMP-10 and MET in biopsies with high mucosal eosinophil numbers. These genes are involved in ECM organization and their increased expression in these tissues corelated to increased submucosal thickness (Kuo et al., 2019). Mechanisms pertaining to MMP regulation and function in asthma remain to be fully validated and regulation of MMP production is likely to be a potential therapeutic option in the treatment of chronic asthma (Kuo et al., 2019).

The data in *in vitro* models of asthma are supported by changes observed in the lungs of asthmatic patients. Recently, Vieira Braga et al. completed a comprehensive scRNAseq profile of biopsies from asthmatic airways. The data revealed a significant increase in goblet cell numbers compared healthy control samples supporting prior observations in asthmatic lung tissues (Vieira Braga et al., 2019). The transcriptome of the goblet cells was deviant from goblet cells from control lungs with an up regulation of proinflammatory and remodeling genes including nitric oxide synthase 2 (NOS2), Carcinoembryonic antigen-related cell adhesion molecule 5 (CEACAM5), and Cystatin-SN (CST)1. Furthermore, asthmatic airways present a novel cell state the authors label as mucous ciliated cells which resemble ciliated cells (FOXJ1 expressing), but also co-express some mucous genes including MUC5AC and CEACAM5 (Vieira Braga et al., 2019). In addition, these mucous ciliated cells express the genes CST1 and Periostin (POSTN) that have been previously shown to play a role in the remodeling of asthmatic airways. Clinical trials to evaluate allergen exposure in asthmatic patients have also shown that exposures correlate with significant transcriptomic changes in the airway epithelium, including upregulation of markers of cell proliferation, and differentiation, as well as extracellular proteins, interleukin receptors, and transcription factors in subjects clinically diagnosed with asthma (Lilly et al., 2005). These genetic changes suggest that the epithelial response to allergens involves genes likely to change the function of airway epithelial cells. Despite detailed analysis of changes in the extracellular matrix and cellular phenotype being studied in asthma there is still a paucity of data to understand how the changes in ECM influence the changes in BC phenotype and differentiation that have been observed.

Inhaled corticosteroids and beta-2-agonists are commonly used as asthma treatments to reduce inflammation and relax the airway smooth muscle; these treatment options are effective at preventing exacerbations, but they are not able to treat airway remodeling (Castillo et al., 2017). More recently, therapy routes are being explored that seek to target the ECM and airway smooth muscle as a means to reverse asthmatic airway remodeling (ClinicalTrials.gov Identifier: NCT03388359). While still in early development, this seems to be the most promising avenue for restoring asthmatic airways and potentially eliminating completely the associated symptoms.

Chronic Obstructive Pulmonary Disease

COPD is a progressive disease that is characterized by emphysema, reduction of gas exchange within the lung, chronic bronchitis, constant irritation, inflammation, and excess mucus production in the airways. Cigarette smoking is the primary cause of COPD with around 75% of the patients being current or past smokers. COPD is currently the 4th leading cause of death in the United States, and it is predicted that it will soon be the 3rd. The ECM of COPD patients shows abnormalities in both structure and composition. Finely disrupted fibers, electron-dense deposits and vacuoles, and indications of abnormal elastogenesis are seen in the elastic fibers (Fukuda et al., 1989). Further, the overall presence of elastic fibers is reduced in the small airways, possibly contributing to the development of airflow obstruction in the alveoli (Black et al., 2008; Merrilees et al., 2008; Eurlings et al., 2014). In contrast, other ECM elements, including tenascin-C (Löfdahl et al., 2011; Annoni et al., 2012), fibronectin (Annoni et al., 2012), versican (Merrilees et al., 2008), and collagens (Eurlings et al., 2014; Abdillahi et al., 2015) have been shown to be overexpressed in COPD. It is suspected that the changes in the ECM contribute to the dysfunction of the airway epithelium observed in COPD by regulating the function of airway BCs, possibly by acting as storage for inflammatory mediators, growth factors and cytokines. Basal stem cell number, self-renewal, and multipotency are all reduced in COPD, with impaired lung function as a consequence of impaired BC differentiation (Ghosh et al., 2017). Instead of a multipotent basal stem cell a more differentiated progenitor cell progeny persists. Squamous metaplasia is a hall mark of COPD lungs in which an increase in proliferative TP63 expressing basal cells contributes to significant airway thickening (Araya et al., 2007). Upregulation of squamous cell markers including IVL and KRT6 is observed in the absence of mucociliary differentiation and correlates to the severity of COPD (Araya et al., 2007). Several studies have suggested that a partial EMT transition is part of this process and characteristic of COPD occurring through TGF-β1-dependent regulation of BCs (Gohy et al., 2015). In these instances, the EMT transition is characterized by upregulation of EMT associated markers Twist1, Twist2, Snai2 vimentin and N-cadherin and a reduction in the expression of E-cadherin (Nishioka et al., 2015). In *in vitro* assays, however, the abnormal mesenchymal phenotype only persists for two weeks in ALI models, after which mesenchymal markers progressively declined, suggesting that there are other *in vivo* microenvironmental factors necessary to maintain EMT or that EMT is specific to *in vitro* culture systems which mimic airway epithelial repair (Gohy et al., 2015). In this particular study there was a significant difference in EMT between control and COPD patient derived basal cells suggestive of an augmented EMT phenotype in COPD and this is supported by evidence of active EMT in patient tissues (Sohal et al., 2011). EMT has previously been described as an active process in the large and small airways of patients with mild to moderate COPD validating these observations (Sohal et al., 2010; Soltani et al., 2010; Soltani et al., 2012; Milara et al., 2013; Nishioka et al., 2015). Most recently, Cullin4A (CUL4A), an E3 ubiquitin ligase associated with EMT in non-small cell lung cancer, is also overexpressed in the lung epithelium of COPD patients and could be associated with the poor differentiation and function of the small airway epithelium (Ren et al., 2019) There still remains some controversy over the specific role for an active EMT transition in the pathogenesis of COPD. What can be concluded is that a significant change in the matrix associated genes and a reprogramming of airway BCs are core factors in COPD pathophysiology, however significantly more work needs to be completed to fully understand the mechanisms driving this BC dysfunction.

A role for TGF-β1 impairing mucociliary differentiation of ALI cultures, offers a potential explanation for the reduced number of ciliated cells observed in COPD patient airway samples (Gohy et al., 2019). Interestingly, HBECs grown on decellularized bronchial scaffolds from COPD patients show patterns of gene expression during early differentiation that deviate from cultures on healthy scaffolds (Hedström et al., 2018). These differences indicate altered activity of upstream mediators of regeneration and remodeling through hepatocyte growth factor (HGF) and TGF-β1 respectively (Hedström et al., 2018). HGF activity was down regulated which impairs proliferation and survival of airway epithelial cells, while several genes known to be induced by TGF-β1 were upregulated indicating increased TGF-β1 activity and consequently ECM dysregulation (Hedström et al., 2018). While the precise mechanisms have yet to be unraveled, these results indicate that the ECM changes that accompany or prelude COPD are involved in the further progression of the disease. A decrease in ciliated cell differentiation is likely congruent with squamous BC metaplasia that is also associated with COPD as a result of smoking and is thought to be induced, at least in part, through chronic inflammation (Herfs et al., 2012). Compared to healthy pseudostratified epithelium from non-smoking patients, squamous metaplasia and epithelial hyperplasia are accompanied by a significant increase in proinflammatory cytokines TNF-α, IL-1β, and IL-6 (Herfs et al., 2012). Changes in signaling mediated by extracellular vesicles from (Herfs et al., 2012; Gohy et al., 2015; Brandenberger and Mühlfeld, 2017) HBECs are able to induce fibroblast differentiation to myofibroblasts in *in vitro* experiments (Xu et al., 2018). It will be interesting to further study these effects in *in vivo* models (Fujita et al., 2015; Xu et al., 2018). Such increases in the myofibroblast population in the lungs may in part explain the elevated levels of some ECM components observed in COPD. The study by Xu and colleagues also demonstrates how changes induced in one cell type, in this case HBECs, can significantly impact other cell types (Ghosh et al., 2017). Refining our understanding of the relationship between ECM changes and abnormal BC phenotype in COPD can open new possibilities for the early identification and treatment of the disease.

Idiopathic Pulmonary Fibrosis

IPF is another chronic lung disease in which significant modifications of the ECM and changes in BC phenotype have been observed. IPF is characterized by significant deposition of ECM components throughout the alveolar parenchyma and, to a lesser extent, the terminal airways (Burgess et al., 2016). This process is facilitated by fibroblastic foci, which are clusters of myofibroblasts and fibroblasts, neighboring apoptotic or hyperplastic alveolar epithelial cells (Burgess et al., 2016; Burgstaller et al., 2017). Abnormal populations of both fibroblasts and myofibroblasts are present in the foci. Fibroblasts exhibit increased expression of hyaluronan synthase 1 (HAS1), hyaluronan synthase 2 (HAS2), fibrillin 1 (FBN1), and chemokine ligand 14 (CXCL14), and myofibroblasts fibrillar collagens and smooth muscle alpha-2 actin (ACTA2) (Adams et al., 2020). An overall decrease in the proportion of alveolar epithelial cells is reported as well (Adams et al., 2020). Repeated lung injury and repair are responsible for ongoing destruction of the elastic parenchymal lung tissue which is then replaced by scar tissue that develops into fibroblastic foci (Burgstaller et al., 2017). As the lung tissue is progressively remodeled, bronchiectasis, thicken interlobular septae, and subpleural honeycombing develop (Burgstaller et al., 2017).

Similar to the response to acute lung injury, the development of fibrosis in IPF seems to result from exudate within the airspaces, and fibroblasts increase collagen and fibronectin synthesis throughout the process (Kuhn et al., 1989; Elowsson Rendin et al., 2019). The ECM compounds versican and tenascin C have also been shown to be upregulated in the fibroblastic foci (Bensadoun et al., 1996; Estany et al., 2014). However, the basement membrane portion of the ECM is depleted of proteins such as laminin and collagen IV and shows overall disorganization (Elowsson Rendin et al., 2019). Increases in the elastic fiber proportion of the ECM associated with IPF have been correlated to worse patient survival outcomes because excess elastin alters the stiffness of the lungs which increases the effort of breathing due to higher elastic recoil (Enomoto et al., 2013). IPF lungs show a 60% increase in stiffness and three-fold increase in tissue density compared to healthy lungs (Elowsson Rendin et al., 2019).

The ECM changes originating from the fibrotic foci seem to have a significant effect on the overlying basal epithelium. The airway epithelium over the fibrotic foci contains a layer of TP63-positive BCs and lacks ciliated and goblet cells (Jonsdottir et al., 2015; Adams et al., 2020). Increased expression of KRT14, Vimentin, and N-cadherin is also observed in the epithelial cells; however, the underlying foci shows N-cadherin and E-cadherin-positive cells (Jonsdottir et al., 2015). These alterations indicate that BCs acquire mesenchymal traits due to signals originating from the foci or, alternatively, that the EMT of the epithelium directly contributes to foci formation (Jonsdottir et al., 2015). Distally, IPF lungs demonstrate a larger population of KRT5 positive cells, a subpopulation of KRT5/KRT14 positive cells, and morphological changes in these BCs (Smirnova et al., 2016). In this study, KRT5/KRT14/TP63 positive BCs were totally absent in the healthy distal lungs, while they were abundantly found in the IPF lungs (Smirnova et al., 2016). The KRT14 positive population also did not express bronchial or alveolar differentiation markers in IPF (Smirnova et al., 2016). In a recent publication, Adams *et at.* demonstrated a more precise characterization of the abnormal BC phenotypes observed in IPF lungs (Adams et al., 2020). They report a population of BCs, aberrant BCs, unique to IPF that express BC markers TP63, cytokeratin 17 (KRT17), laminin subunit beta-3 (LAMB3), and laminin subunit gamma-2 (LAMC2), but also lack other accepted BC markers such as KRT5 and KRT15 (Adams et al., 2020). These aberrant BCs also show evidence of EMT, senescence-related genes, and high expression of IPF-associated molecules including matrix metallopeptidase 7 (MMP7) (Adams et al., 2020). Aberrant BCs are found consistently in the epithelial layer covering fibroblastic foci (Adams et al., 2020). The exact mechanisms of IPF development related to abnormal ECM production and BC phenotype remain unknown, however the significant upregulation of ECM-related (such as FN1, COL1A1 and VCAN) and ECM-interacting genes (such as Integrins B8, AV and B6) in the aberrant basaloid cells suggests that changes in the ECM may influence the change in cellular phenotype. The publication of large scRNA sequencing studies comparing IPF basal cells to non-IPF basal cells may start to provide clues regarding the phenotypic switch in basal cell phenotypes; however further studies will be essential to uncover the relationship between ECM changes and BC phonotype if effective therapies are to be developed (Carraro et al., 2020b).

Conclusion and Future Implications

An absolute understanding of the pulmonary ECM and its interactions with, and effects on, the cells of the lung may be the key to developing everything from a physiological airway model to a functional recellularized lung. The ECM is part of the complex environment of the lung, with regional variations, that supports and maintains the overlying tissue. As BCs are the primary stem cells of the lung and are positioned to have the most direct contact with the ECM, deciphering their reliance on the ECM for the maintenance stemness and differentiation capacity will allow for advancements in airway modeling and understanding of disease pathogenesis. Regional variations in BC distribution, function and ECM localization to specific BC niches are still relatively poorly understood. Furthermore, we need a greater understanding of how age-related changes in ECM correlate to changes in basal cell function as we progress toward cellular therapy and regenerative therapeutics for the lung. Continued research in the areas discussed in this review will have momentous implications for the modeling of healthy and diseased airways, understanding the relationship between ECM alterations and abnormal BCs in chronic lung disease, therapy development for such diseases, and decellularization/recellularization capacity.

The current standard methods of BC culture and airway modeling fall short in producing cells and tissue that fully maintain their native phenotype. While commercial culture ECMs, medias, and differentiation platforms, such as Matrigel®, BEGM with Y-27632, and ALI inserts respectively, have improved the culture of airway cells considerably, abnormal gene expression and differentiation is still observed. If our airway models do not entirely simulate *in vivo* cells and conditions, there are caveats associated with experiments conducted on them. By improving our understanding of the *in vivo* pulmonary ECM and how it supports BCs and other cell types, we will become better equipped to create an *ex vivo* culture ECM that supports native conditions. Variables such as stiffness, stretch, and molecular composition are proving to be of particular importance. A promising direction of ECM research is the conversion of the 3-D native lung ECM scaffold into a hydrogel that can be plated on a 2-D surface. Ideally, this will allow for the preservation of the ECM components and stiffness found *in vivo*. This technique also offers the option of using ECM from diseased lungs to study disease-specific ECM alterations and the subsequent changes in cellular response. It will be interesting to follow this, and the progression in 3-D bioinks where the impact of 3-D structure and curvature of the airways can also be accounted for in the regulation of BC function. Complete understanding of BC-ECM interactions may have a significant impact on our capacity to efficiently repopulate decellularized lungs/tracheas to generate functional tissues for engraftment. While there has been substantial progress made on techniques for decellularization and recellularization there is still a paucity in the characterization of the ECM, adherence and functional quality of the recellularized tissues [reviewed in (Uriarte et al., 2018)]. Current protocols for decellularization vary considerably in reagents used and length of digestion which pose challenges in balancing the structural and chemical composition of the ECM with complete cellular removal. Evaluation of the remaining ECM including the level of residual proteins will require more quantitative proteomic approaches (Schiller et al., 2015; Gilpin et al., 2017), in addition to a more complete understanding of basal stem cell homing, niche, subtypes and differentiation will be critical as the field of lung tissue engineering moves forward.

Abnormal ECM and BC phenotype appear to be closely related in the context of chronic lung disease. As such, BCs have become a target for regenerative therapy development in conditions such as COPD and IPF where lung transplantation is currently the only curative option. Engraftment of *ex vivo* expanded autologous BCs, derivation of autologous iPSC-derived BCs, and activation of endogenous basal stem cells to repair damaged tissues are currently under investigation as patient-specific cell therapies that could provide a superior alternative to transplantation. However, these techniques rely upon a receptive cellular microenvironment for both *ex vivo* expansion and *in vivo* engraftment, further highlighting the necessity for improved knowledge of ECM mechanisms in the context of native physiology and culture platforms.

Perhaps the most impressive and challenging application of ECM-BC research is the potential to repopulate a decellularized ECM scaffold to create a functional lung. Decellularization of donor lungs and recellularization with autologous stem cells is thought to be a solution to overcome the deficiency of donor lungs suitable for direct transplantation and avoid complications such as organ rejection. While there has been some success with simpler structures such as the trachea alone, researchers still face significant challenges in the complex and diverse structural and biochemical environment of the whole lung. Such challenges include the effective removal of cellular material while preserving the structural and mechanical properties of the ECM, seeding of cells to maintain compartmentalization (i.e., airways vs. vasculature), and differentiation to produce functional gas exchange units. Advancements in our awareness of the often subtle, differences in ECM composition in different regions of the lung and how these differences produce diverse tissue types will aid in our ability to contain seeded cells to their designated area and direct them to differentiate appropriately.

While at the surface level the ECM may appear to be simple scaffold, in reality it plays a critical role in lung physiology through mechanical and biochemical factors. Further study of the pulmonary ECM and its relationship with cells will progress airway modeling, therapy development for chronic diseases, and overall understanding of lung physiology.

AUTHOR CONTRIBUTIONS

SB and AR conceived, wrote, edited, and finalized the manuscript. ZL created the figure.

REFERENCES

Abdillahi, S. M., Bober, M., Nordin, S., Hallgren, O., Baumgarten, M., Erjefält, J., et al. (2015). Collagen VI Is Upregulated in COPD and Serves Both as an Adhesive Target and a Bactericidal Barrier for ***Moraxella Catarrhalis***. *J. Innate Immun.* 7, 506–517. doi:10.1159/000381213

Adams, T. S., Schupp, J. C., Poli, S., Ayaub, E. A., Neumark, N., Ahangari, F., et al. (2020). Single-cell RNA-Seq Reveals Ectopic and Aberrant Lung-Resident Cell Populations in Idiopathic Pulmonary Fibrosis. *Sci. Adv.* 6, eaba1983. doi:10.1126/sciadv.aba1983

Alcorn, J. F., Guala, A. S., van der Velden, J., McElhinney, B., Irvin, C. G., Davis, R. J., et al. (2008). Jun N-Terminal Kinase 1 Regulates Epithelial-To-Mesenchymal Transition Induced by TGF-β1. *J. Cel Sci.* 121, 1036–1045. doi:10.1242/jcs.019455

Amy, R. W., Bowes, D., Burri, P. H., Haines, J., and Thurlbeck, W. M. (1977). Postnatal Growth of the Mouse Lung. *J. Anat.* 124, 131–151.

Annoni, R., Lanças, T., Yukimatsu Tanigawa, R., de Medeiros Matsushita, M., de Morais Fernezlian, S., Bruno, A., et al. (2012). Extracellular Matrix Composition in COPD. *Eur. Respir. J.* 40, 1362–1373. doi:10.1183/09031936.00192611

Araujo, B. B., Dolhnikoff, M., Silva, L. F. F., Elliot, J., Lindeman, J. H. N., Ferreira, D. S., et al. (2008). Extracellular Matrix Components and Regulators in the

Airway Smooth Muscle in Asthma. *Eur. Respir. J.* 32, 61–69. doi:10.1183/09031936.00147807

Araya, J., Cambier, S., Markovics, J. A., Wolters, P., Jablons, D., Hill, A., et al. (2007). Squamous Metaplasia Amplifies Pathologic Epithelial-Mesenchymal Interactions in COPD Patients. *J. Clin. Invest.* 117, 3551–3562. doi:10.1172/jci32526

Arcasoy, S. M., and Kotloff, R. M. (1999). Lung Transplantation. *N. Engl. J. Med.* 340, 1081–1091. doi:10.1056/nejm199904083401406

Arteaga-Solis, E., Settembre, C., Ballabio, A., and Karsenty, G. (2012). Sulfatases Are Determinants of Alveolar Formation. *Matrix Biol.* 31, 253–260. doi:10.1016/j.matbio.2012.02.001

Au - Bonvillain, R. W., Au - Scarritt, M. E., Au - Pashos, N. C., Au - Mayeux, J. P., Au - Meshberger, C. L., Au - Betancourt, A. M., et al. (2013). Nonhuman Primate Lung Decellularization and Recellularization Using a Specialized Large-Organ Bioreactor. *JoVE*, e50825. doi:10.3791/50825

Aviezer, D., Hecht, D., Safran, M., Eisinger, M., David, G., and Yayon, A. (1994). Perlecan, Basal Lamina Proteoglycan, Promotes Basic Fibroblast Growth Factor-Receptor Binding, Mitogenesis, and Angiogenesis. *Cell* 79, 1005–1013. doi:10.1016/0092-8674(94)90031-0

Badylak, S. F., Hoppo, T., Nieponice, A., Gilbert, T. W., Davison, J. M., and Jobe, B. A. (2011a). Esophageal Preservation in Five Male Patients after Endoscopic Inner-Layer Circumferential Resection in the Setting of Superficial Cancer: a Regenerative Medicine Approach with a Biologic Scaffold. *Tissue Eng. A.* 17, 1643–1650. doi:10.1089/ten.tea.2010.0739

Badylak, S. F., Taylor, D., and Uygun, K. (2011b). Whole-organ Tissue Engineering: Decellularization and Recellularization of Three-Dimensional Matrix Scaffolds. *Annu. Rev. Biomed. Eng.* 13, 27–53. doi:10.1146/annurev-bioeng-071910-124743

Bajbouj, K., Ramakrishnan, R. K., and Hamid, Q. (2021). Role of Matrix Metalloproteinases in Angiogenesis and its Implications in Asthma. *J. Immunol. Res.* 2021, 6645072. doi:10.1155/2021/6645072

Barkauskas, C. E., Chung, M.-I., Fioret, B., Gao, X., Katsura, H., and Hogan, B. L. M. (2017). Lung Organoids: Current Uses and Future Promise. *Development* 144, 986–997. doi:10.1242/dev.140103

Beers, M. F., and Morrisey, E. E. (2011). The Three R's of Lung Health and Disease: Repair, Remodeling, and Regeneration. *J. Clin. Invest.* 121, 2065–2073. doi:10.1172/jci45961

Benjamin, J. T., van der Meer, R., Im, A. M., Plosa, E. J., Zaynagetdinov, R., Burman, A., et al. (2016). Epithelial-Derived Inflammation Disrupts Elastin Assembly and Alters Saccular Stage Lung Development. *Am. J. Pathol.* 186, 1786–1800. doi:10.1016/j.ajpath.2016.02.016

Bensadoun, E. S., Burke, A. K., Hogg, J. C., and Roberts, C. R. (1996). Proteoglycan Deposition in Pulmonary Fibrosis. *Am. J. Respir. Crit. Care Med.* 154, 1819–1828. doi:10.1164/ajrccm.154.6.8970376

Blaauboer, M. E., Boeijen, F. R., Emson, C. L., Turner, S. M., Zandieh-Doulabi, B., Hanemaaijer, R., et al. (2014). Extracellular Matrix Proteins: A Positive Feedback Loop in Lung Fibrosis? *Matrix Biol.* 34, 170–178. doi:10.1016/j.matbio.2013.11.002

Black, P. N., Ching, P. S. T., Beaumont, B., Ranasinghe, S., Taylor, G., and Merrilees, M. J. (2008). Changes in Elastic Fibres in the Small Airways and Alveoli in COPD. *Eur. Respir. J.* 31, 998–1004. doi:10.1183/09031936.00017207

Boström, H., Willetts, K., Pekny, M., Levéen, P., Lindahl, P., Hedstrand, H., et al. (1996). PDGF-A Signaling Is a Critical Event in Lung Alveolar Myofibroblast Development and Alveogenesis. *Cell* 85, 863–873. doi:10.1016/s0092-8674(00)81270-2

Bousquet, J., Chanez, P., Lacoste, J., Enander, I., Venge, P., Peterson, C., et al. (1991). Indirect Evidence of Bronchial Inflammation Assessed by Titration of Inflammatory Mediators in BAL Fluid of Patients with Asthma. *J. Allergy Clin. Immunol.* 88, 649–660. doi:10.1016/0091-6749(91)90159-l

Bousquet, J., Chanez, P., Lacoste, J. Y., White, R., Vic, P., Godard, P., et al. (1992). Asthma: a Disease Remodeling the Airways. *Allergy* 47, 3–11. doi:10.1111/j.1398-9995.1992.tb02242.x

Branchfield, K., Li, R., Lungova, V., Verheyden, J. M., McCulley, D., and Sun, X. (2016). A Three-Dimensional Study of Alveologenesis in Mouse Lung. *Developmental Biol.* 409, 429–441. doi:10.1016/j.ydbio.2015.11.017

Brandenberger, C., and Mühlfeld, C. (2017). Mechanisms of Lung Aging. *Cell Tissue Res.* 367, 469–480. doi:10.1007/s00441-016-2511-x

Burgess, J. K., Mauad, T., Tjin, G., Karlsson, J. C., and Westergren-Thorsson, G. (2016). The Extracellular Matrix - the Under-recognized Element in Lung Disease? *J. Pathol.* 240, 397–409. doi:10.1002/path.4808

Burgess, J. K., Weckmann, M., and Karsdal, M. A. (2019). The Message from the Matrix-Should We Listen More Closely? *J. Thorac. Dis.* 11, S230–S233. doi:10.21037/jtd.2019.01.68

Burgstaller, G., Oehrle, B., Gerckens, M., White, E. S., Schiller, H. B., and Eickelberg, O. (2017). The Instructive Extracellular Matrix of the Lung: Basic Composition and Alterations in Chronic Lung Disease. *Eur. Respir. J.* 50, 1601805. doi:10.1183/13993003.01805-2016

Burgstaller, G., Sengupta, A., Vierkotten, S., Preissler, G., Lindner, M., Behr, J., et al. (2018). Distinct Niches within the Extracellular Matrix Dictate Fibroblast Function in (Cell Free) 3D Lung Tissue Cultures. *Am. J. Physiology-Lung Cell Mol. Physiol.* 314, L708–L723. doi:10.1152/ajplung.00408.2017

Burri, P. H. (1984). Fetal and Postnatal Development of the Lung. *Annu. Rev. Physiol.* 46, 617–628. doi:10.1146/annurev.ph.46.030184.003153

Carraro, G., Langerman, J., Sabri, S., Lorenzana, Z., Purkayastha, A., Konda, B., et al. (2020a). A Molecular Atlas of Proximal Airway Identifies Subsets of Known Airway Cell Types Revealing Details of the Unique Molecular Pathogenesis of Cystic Fibrosis, *bioRxiv* 2005. doi:10.1101/2020.05.01.072876

Carraro, G., Mulay, A., Yao, C., Mizuno, T., Konda, B., Petrov, M., et al. (2020b). Single-Cell Reconstruction of Human Basal Cell Diversity in Normal and Idiopathic Pulmonary Fibrosis Lungs. *Am. J. Respir. Crit. Care Med.* 202, 1540–1550. doi:10.1164/rccm.201904-0792oc

Castillo, J. R., Peters, S. P., and Busse, W. W. (2017). Asthma Exacerbations: Pathogenesis, Prevention, and Treatment. *J. Allergy Clin. Immunol. Pract.* 5, 918–927. doi:10.1016/j.jaip.2017.05.001

Chan, V., Burgess, J. K., Ratoff, J. C., O'Connor, B. J., Greenough, A., Lee, T. H., et al. (2006). Extracellular Matrix Regulates Enhanced Eotaxin Expression in Asthmatic Airway Smooth Muscle Cells. *Am. J. Respir. Crit. Care Med.* 174, 379–385. doi:10.1164/rccm.200509-1420oc

Chetta, A., Foresi, A., Del Donno, M., Bertorelli, G., Pesci, A., and Olivieri, D. (1997). Airways Remodeling Is a Distinctive Feature of Asthma and Is Related to Severity of Disease. *Chest* 111, 852–857. doi:10.1378/chest.111.4.852

Coraux, C., Meneguzzi, G., Rousselle, P., Puchelle, E., and Gaillard, D. (2002). Distribution of Laminin 5, Integrin Receptors, and Branching Morphogenesis during Human Fetal Lung Development. *Dev. Dyn.* 225, 176–185. doi:10.1002/dvdy.10147

Coraux, C., Roux, J., Jolly, T., and Birembaut, P. (2008). Epithelial Cell-Extracellular Matrix Interactions and Stem Cells in Airway Epithelial Regeneration. *Proc. Am. Thorac. Soc.* 5, 689–694. doi:10.1513/pats.200801-010aw

Cortiella, J., Niles, J., Cantu, A., Brettler, A., Pham, A., Vargas, G., et al. (2010). Influence of Acellular Natural Lung Matrix on Murine Embryonic Stem Cell Differentiation and Tissue Formation. *Tissue Eng. Part A* 16, 2565–2580. doi:10.1089/ten.tea.2009.0730

Cypel, M., Levvey, B., Van Raemdonck, D., Erasmus, M., Dark, J., Love, R., et al. (2015). International Society for Heart and Lung Transplantation Donation after Circulatory Death Registry Report. *J. Heart Lung Transplant.* 34, 1278–1282. doi:10.1016/j.healun.2015.08.015

D'Errico, A., Scarani, P., Colosimo, E., Spina, M., Grigioni, W. F., and Mancini, A. M. (1989). Changes in the Alveolar Connective Tissue of the Ageing Lung. *Vichows Archiv A. Pathol. Anat.* 415, 137–144. doi:10.1007/bf00784351

de Hilster, R. H. J., Sharma, P. K., Jonker, M. R., White, E. S., Gercama, E. A., Roobeek, M., et al. (2020). Human Lung Extracellular Matrix Hydrogels Resemble the Stiffness and Viscoelasticity of Native Lung Tissue. *Am. J. Physiology-Lung Cell Mol. Physiol.* 318, L698–L704. doi:10.1152/ajplung.00451.2019

De Santis, M. M., Alsafadi, H. N., Tas, S., Bolukbas, D. A., Prithiviraj, S., Da Silva, I. A. N., et al. (2021). Extracellular-Matrix-Reinforced Bioinks for 3D Bioprinting Human Tissue. *Adv. Mater.* 33, e2005476. doi:10.1002/adma.202005476

Deprez, M., Zaragosi, L.-E., Truchi, M., Becavin, C., Ruiz García, S., Arguel, M.-J., et al. (2020). A Single-Cell Atlas of the Human Healthy Airways. *Am. J. Respir. Crit. Care Med.* 202, 1636–1645. doi:10.1164/rccm.201911-2199oc

Dodmane, P. R., Schulte, N. A., Heires, A. J., Band, H., Romberger, D. J., and Toews, M. L. (2018). Biphasic Changes in Airway Epithelial Cell EGF Receptor

Binding and Phosphorylation Induced by Components of Hogbarn Dust. *Exp. Lung Res.* 44, 443–454. doi:10.1080/01902148.2019.1575931

Donne, M. L., Lechner, A. J., and Rock, J. R. (2015). Evidence for Lung Epithelial Stem Cell Niches. *BMC Developmental Biol.* 15, 32. doi:10.1186/s12861-015-0082-9

Dziki, J., Badylak, S., Yabroudi, M., Sicari, B., Ambrosio, F., Stearns, K., et al. (2016). An Acellular Biologic Scaffold Treatment for Volumetric Muscle Loss: Results of a 13-patient Cohort Study. *NPJ Regen. Med.* 1, 16008. doi:10.1038/npjregenmed.2016.8

Elowsson Rendin, L., Lofdahl, A., Ahrman, E., Muller, C., Notermans, T., Michalikova, B., et al. (2019). Matrisome Properties of Scaffolds Direct Fibroblasts in Idiopathic Pulmonary Fibrosis. *Int. J. Mol. Sci.* 20, 4013. doi:10.3390/ijms20164013

Enomoto, N., Suda, T., Kono, M., Kaida, Y., Hashimoto, D., Fujisawa, T., et al. (2013). Amount of Elastic Fibers Predicts Prognosis of Idiopathic Pulmonary Fibrosis. *Respir. Med.* 107, 1608–1616. doi:10.1016/j.rmed.2013.08.008

Estany, S., Vicens-Zygmunt, V., Llatjós, R., Montes, A., Penín, R., Escobar, I., et al. (2014). Lung Fibrotic Tenascin-C Upregulation Is Associated with Other Extracellular Matrix Proteins and Induced by TGFβ1. *BMC Pulm. Med.* 14, 120. doi:10.1186/1471-2466-14-120

Eurlings, I. M. J., Dentener, M. A., Cleutjens, J. P. M., Peutz, C. J., Rohde, G. G. U., Wouters, E. F. M., et al. (2014). Similar Matrix Alterations in Alveolar and Small Airway Walls of COPD Patients. *BMC Pulm. Med.* 14, 90. doi:10.1186/1471-2466-14-90

Evans, M. J., Van Winkle, L. S., Fanucchi, M. V., and Plopper, C. G. (2001). Cellular and Molecular Characteristics of Basal Cells in Airway Epithelium. *Exp. Lung Res.* 27, 401–415. doi:10.1080/019021401300317125

Firth, A. L., Dargitz, C. T., Qualls, S. J., Menon, T., Wright, R., Singer, O., et al. (2014). Generation of Multiciliated Cells in Functional Airway Epithelia from Human Induced Pluripotent Stem Cells. *Proc. Natl. Acad. Sci.* 111, E1723–E1730. doi:10.1073/pnas.1403470111

Fujita, Y., Araya, J., Ito, S., Kobayashi, K., Kosaka, N., Yoshioka, Y., et al. (2015). Suppression of Autophagy by Extracellular Vesicles Promotes Myofibroblast Differentiation in COPD Pathogenesis. *J. Extracellular Vesicles* 4, 28388. doi:10.3402/jev.v4.28388

Fukuda, Y., Masuda, Y., Ishizaki, M., Masugi, Y., and Ferrans, V. J. (1989). Morphogenesis of Abnormal Elastic Fibers in Lungs of Patients with Panacinar and Centriacinar Emphysema. *Hum. Pathol.* 20, 652–659. doi:10.1016/0046-8177(89)90152-4

Ge, Q., Chen, L., Jaffar, J., Argraves, W. S., Twal, W. O., Hansbro, P., et al. (2015). Fibulin1C Peptide Induces Cell Attachment and Extracellular Matrix Deposition in Lung Fibroblasts. *Sci. Rep.* 5, 9496. doi:10.1038/srep09496

Ge, X. N., Bastan, I., Ha, S. G., Greenberg, Y. G., Esko, J. D., Rao, S. P., et al. (2018). Regulation of Eosinophil Recruitment and Allergic Airway Inflammation by Heparan Sulfate Proteoglycan (HSPG) Modifying Enzymes. *Exp. Lung Res.* 44, 98–112. doi:10.1080/01902148.2018.1451574

Gentzsch, M., Boyles, S. E., Cheluvaraju, C., Chaudhry, I. G., Quinney, N. L., Cho, C., et al. (2017). Pharmacological Rescue of Conditionally Reprogrammed Cystic Fibrosis Bronchial Epithelial Cells. *Am. J. Respir. Cel Mol Biol.* 56, 568–574. doi:10.1165/rcmb.2016-0276ma

Ghosh, M., Ahmad, S., White, C. W., and Reynolds, S. D. (2016). Transplantation of Airway Epithelial Stem/Progenitor Cells: A Future for Cell-Based Therapy. *Am. J. Respir. Cel Mol Biol* 56, 1–10. doi:10.1165/rcmb.2016-0181MA

Ghosh, M., Miller, Y. E., Nakachi, I., Kwon, J. B., Barón, A. E., Brantley, A. E., et al. (2017). Exhaustion of Airway Basal Progenitor Cells in Early and Established Chronic Obstructive Pulmonary Disease. *Am. J. Respir. Crit. Care Med.* 197, 885–896. doi:10.1164/rccm.201704-0667OC

Gilpin, S. E., Li, Q., Evangelista-Leite, D., Ren, X., Reinhardt, D. P., Frey, B. L., et al. (2017). Fibrillin-2 and Tenascin-C Bridge the Age Gap in Lung Epithelial Regeneration. *Biomaterials* 140, 212–219. doi:10.1016/j.biomaterials.2017.06.027

Gilpin, S. E., Ren, X., Okamoto, T., Guyette, J. P., Mou, H., Rajagopal, J., et al. (2014). Enhanced Lung Epithelial Specification of Human Induced Pluripotent Stem Cells on Decellularized Lung Matrix. *Ann. Thorac. Surg.* 98, 1721–1729. doi:10.1016/j.athoracsur.2014.05.080

Gilpin, S. E., and Wagner, D. E. (2018). Acellular Human Lung Scaffolds to Model Lung Disease and Tissue Regeneration. *Eur. Respir. Rev.* 27. doi:10.1183/16000617.0021-2018

Godin, L. M., Sandri, B. J., Wagner, D. E., Meyer, C. M., Price, A. P., Akinnola, I., et al. (2016). Decreased Laminin Expression by Human Lung Epithelial Cells and Fibroblasts Cultured in Acellular Lung Scaffolds from Aged Mice. *PLoS One* 11, e0150966. doi:10.1371/journal.pone.0150966

Godoy-Guzman, C., San Martin, S., and Pereda, J. (2012). Proteoglycan and Collagen Expression during Human Air Conducting System Development. *Eur. J. Histochem.* 56, e29. doi:10.4081/ejh.2012.e29

Gohy, S., Carlier, F. M., Fregimilicka, C., Detry, B., Lecocq, M., Ladjemi, M. Z., et al. (2019). Altered Generation of Ciliated Cells in Chronic Obstructive Pulmonary Disease. *Sci. Rep.* 9, 17963. doi:10.1038/s41598-019-54292-x

Gohy, S. T., Hupin, C., Fregimilicka, C., Detry, B. R., Bouzin, C., Gaide Chevronay, H., et al. (2015). Imprinting of the COPD Airway Epithelium for Dedifferentiation and Mesenchymal Transition. *Eur. Respir. J.* 45, 1258–1272. doi:10.1183/09031936.00135814

Greaney, A. M., Adams, T. S., Brickman Raredon, M. S., Gubbins, E., Schupp, J. C., Engler, A. J., et al. (2020). Platform Effects on Regeneration by Pulmonary Basal Cells as Evaluated by Single-Cell RNA Sequencing. *Cel Rep.* 30, 4250–4265. doi:10.1016/j.celrep.2020.03.004

Grzela, K., Litwiniuk, M., Zagorska, W., and Grzela, T. (2016). Airway Remodeling in Chronic Obstructive Pulmonary Disease and Asthma: the Role of Matrix Metalloproteinase-9. *Arch. Immunol. Ther. Exp.* 64, 47–55. doi:10.1007/s00005-015-0345-y

Gu, B.-H., Madison, M. C., Corry, D., and Kheradmand, F. (2018). Matrix Remodeling in Chronic Lung Diseases. *Matrix Biol.* 73, 52–63. doi:10.1016/j.matbio.2018.03.012

Hackett, N. R., Butler, M. W., Shaykhiev, R., Salit, J., Omberg, L., Rodriguez-Flores, J. L., et al. (2012). RNA-seq Quantification of the Human Small Airway Epithelium Transcriptome. *BMC Genomics* 13, 82. doi:10.1186/1471-2164-13-82

Hackett, N. R., Shaykhiev, R., Walters, M. S., Wang, R., Zwick, R. K., Ferris, B., et al. (2011). The Human Airway Epithelial Basal Cell Transcriptome. *PLoS One* 6, e18378. doi:10.1371/journal.pone.0018378

Halabi, C. M., and Mecham, R. P. (2018). Elastin Purification and Solubilization. *Methods Cel Biol* 143, 207–222. doi:10.1016/bs.mcb.2017.08.012

Hamilton, N. J. I., Lee, D. D. H., Gowers, K. H. C., Butler, C. R., Maughan, E. F., Jevans, B., et al. (2020). Bioengineered Airway Epithelial Grafts with Mucociliary Function Based on Collagen IV- and Laminin-Containing Extracellular Matrix Scaffolds. *Eur. Respir. J.* 55. doi:10.1183/13993003.01200-2019

Hawkins, F. J., Suzuki, S., Beermann, M. L., Barilla, C., Wang, R., Villacorta-Martin, C., et al. (2020). Derivation of Airway Basal Stem Cells from Human Pluripotent Stem Cells. *Cell Stem Cell* 28, 79-95. doi:10.1016/j.stem.2020.09.017

He, H., Huang, M., Sun, S., Wu, Y., and Lin, X. (2017). Epithelial Heparan Sulfate Regulates Sonic Hedgehog Signaling in Lung Development. *Plos Genet.* 13, e1006992. doi:10.1371/journal.pgen.1006992

Hedström, U., Hallgren, O., Öberg, L., DeMicco, A., Vaarala, O., Westergren-Thorsson, G., et al. (2018). Bronchial Extracellular Matrix from COPD Patients Induces Altered Gene Expression in Repopulated Primary Human Bronchial Epithelial Cells. *Scientific Rep.* 8, 3502. doi:10.1038/s41598-018-21727-w

Heijink, I. H., Nawijn, M. C., and Hackett, T.-L. (2014). Airway Epithelial Barrier Function Regulates the Pathogenesis of Allergic Asthma. *Clin. Exp. Allergy* 44, 620–630. doi:10.1111/cea.12296

Herfs, M., Hubert, P., Poirrier, A.-L., Vandevenne, P., Renoux, V., Habraken, Y., et al. (2012). Proinflammatory Cytokines Induce Bronchial Hyperplasia and Squamous Metaplasia in Smokers. *Am. J. Respir. Cel Mol Biol.* 47, 67–79. doi:10.1165/rcmb.2011-0353oc

Hocking, D. C., and Chang, C. H. (2003). Fibronectin Matrix Polymerization Regulates Small Airway Epithelial Cell Migration. *Am. J. Physiology-Lung Cell Mol. Physiol.* 285, L169–L179. doi:10.1152/ajplung.00371.2002

Hong, K. U., Reynolds, S. D., Watkins, S., Fuchs, E., and Stripp, B. R. (2004). Basal Cells Are a Multipotent Progenitor Capable of Renewing the Bronchial Epithelium. *Am. J. Pathol.* 164, 577–588. doi:10.1016/s0002-9440(10)63147-1

Huang, L., Yuan, W., Hong, Y., Fan, S., Yao, X., Ren, T., et al. (2020). 3D Printed Hydrogels with Oxidized Cellulose Nanofibers and Silk Fibroin for the Proliferation of Lung Epithelial Stem Cells. *Cellulose (Lond)*, 1–17. doi:10.1007/s10570-020-03526-7

Huang, S. X. L., Islam, M. N., O'Neill, J., Hu, Z., Yang, Y.-G., Chen, Y.-W., et al. (2014). Efficient Generation of Lung and Airway Epithelial Cells from Human Pluripotent Stem Cells. *Nat. Biotechnol.* 32, 84–91. doi:10.1038/nbt.2754

Hughes, C. S., Postovit, L. M., and Lajoie, G. A. (2010). Matrigel: a Complex Protein Mixture Required for Optimal Growth of Cell Culture. *Proteomics* 10, 1886–1890. doi:10.1002/pmic.200900758

Ikonomou, L., Wagner, D. E., Turner, L., and Weiss, D. J. (2019). Translating Basic Research into Safe and Effective Cell-Based Treatments for Respiratory Diseases. *Ann. ATS* 16, 657–668. doi:10.1513/annalsats.201812-890cme

Iravani, A., Thambyah, A., and Burrowes, K. S. (2020). A Viscoelastic Two-Dimensional Network Model of the Lung Extracellular Matrix. *Biomech. Model. Mechanobiol* 19, 2241–2253. doi:10.1007/s10237-020-01336-1

Ito, J. T., Lourenco, J. D., Righetti, R. F., Tiberio, I., Prado, C. M., and Lopes, F. (2019). Extracellular Matrix Component Remodeling in Respiratory Diseases: What Has Been Found in Clinical and Experimental Studies? *Cells* 8, 342. doi:10.3390/cells8040342

Izvolsky, K. I., Shoykhet, D., Yang, Y., Yu, Q., Nugent, M. A., and Cardoso, W. V. (2003). Heparan Sulfate-FGF10 Interactions during Lung Morphogenesis. *Developmental Biol.* 258, 185–200. doi:10.1016/s0012-1606(03)00114-3

Jiang, D., Schaefer, N., and Chu, H. W. (2018). "Air-Liquid Interface Culture of Human and Mouse Airway Epithelial Cells," in *Lung Innate Immunity and Inflammation: Methods and Protocols*. Editors S. Alper and W. J. Janssen (New York, NY: Springer New York), 91–109. doi:10.1007/978-1-4939-8570-8_8

Jonsdottir, H. R., Arason, A. J., Palsson, R., Franzdottir, S. R., Gudbjartsson, T., Isaksson, H. J., et al. (2015). Basal Cells of the Human Airways Acquire Mesenchymal Traits in Idiopathic Pulmonary Fibrosis and in Culture. *Lab. Invest.* 95, 1418–1428. doi:10.1038/labinvest.2015.114

Kanagaki, S., Ikeo, S., Suezawa, T., Yamamoto, Y., Seki, M., Hirai, T., et al. (2020). Directed Induction of Alveolar Type I Cells Derived from Pluripotent Stem Cells via Wnt Signaling Inhibition. *Stem Cells*. doi:10.1002/stem.3302

Keane, T. J., Dziki, J., Castelton, A., Faulk, D. M., Messerschmidt, V., Londono, R., et al. (2017). Preparation and Characterization of a Biologic Scaffold and Hydrogel Derived from Colonic Mucosa. *J. Biomed. Mater. Res.* 105, 291–306. doi:10.1002/jbm.b.33556

Keane, T. J., Swinehart, I. T., and Badylak, S. F. (2015). Methods of Tissue Decellularization Used for Preparation of Biologic Scaffolds and In Vivo Relevance. *Methods* 84, 25–34. doi:10.1016/j.ymeth.2015.03.005

Kendall, R. T., and Feghali-Bostwick, C. A. (2014). Fibroblasts in Fibrosis: Novel Roles and Mediators. *Front. Pharmacol.* 5. doi:10.3389/fphar.2014.00123

Ko, J. W., Kwon, H. J., Seo, C. S., Choi, S. J., Shin, N. R., Kim, S. H., et al. (2020). 4-Hydroxycinnamic Acid Suppresses Airway Inflammation and Mucus Hypersecretion in Allergic Asthma Induced by Ovalbumin Challenge. *Phytotherapy Res.* 34, 624–633. doi:10.1002/ptr.6553

Kramer, B. W., Kallapur, S., Newnham, J., and Jobe, A. H. (2009). Prenatal Inflammation and Lung Development. *Semin. Fetal Neonatal Med.* 14, 2–7. doi:10.1016/j.siny.2008.08.011

Kuhn, C., Boldt, J., King, T. E., Crouch, E., Vartio, T., and McDonald, J. A. (1989). An Immunohistochemical Study of Architectural Remodeling and Connective Tissue Synthesis in Pulmonary Fibrosis. *Am. Rev. Respir. Dis.* 140, 1693–1703. doi:10.1164/ajrccm/140.6.1693

Kuo, C.-H. S., Pavlidis, S., Zhu, J., Loza, M., Baribaud, F., Rowe, A., et al. (2019). Contribution of Airway Eosinophils in Airway Wall Remodeling in Asthma: Role ofMMP-10andMET. *Allergy* 74, 1102–1112. doi:10.1111/all.13727

Kuwada, S. K., and Li, X. (2000). Integrin α5/β1 Mediates Fibronectin-dependent Epithelial Cell Proliferation through Epidermal Growth Factor Receptor Activation. *MBoC* 11, 2485–2496. doi:10.1091/mbc.11.7.2485

Li, R., Herriges, J. C., Chen, L., Mecham, R. P., and Sun, X. (2017). FGF Receptors Control Alveolar Elastogenesis. *Development* 144, 4563–4572. doi:10.1242/dev.149443

Lilly, C. M., Tateno, H., Oguma, T., Israel, E., and Sonna, L. A. (2005). Effects of Allergen Challenge on Airway Epithelial Cell Gene Expression. *Am. J. Respir. Crit. Care Med.* 171, 579–586. doi:10.1164/rccm.200404-532oc

Lindahl, P., Karlsson, L., Hellström, M., Gebre-Medhin, S., Willetts, K., Heath, J. K., et al. (1997). Alveogenesis Failure in PDGF-A-Deficient Mice Is Coupled to Lack of Distal Spreading of Alveolar Smooth Muscle Cell Progenitors during Lung Development. *Development* 124, 3943–3953. doi:10.1242/dev.124.20.3943

Liu, G., Cooley, M. A., Jarnicki, A. G., Hsu, A. C., Nair, P. M., Haw, T. J., et al. (2016). Fibulin-1 Regulates the Pathogenesis of Tissue Remodeling in Respiratory Diseases. *JCI Insight* 1. doi:10.1172/jci.insight.86380

Liu, G., Cooley, M. A., Nair, P. M., Donovan, C., Hsu, A. C., Jarnicki, A. G., et al. (2017). Airway Remodelling and Inflammation in Asthma Are Dependent on the Extracellular Matrix Protein Fibulin-1c. *J. Pathol.* 243, 510–523. doi:10.1002/path.4979

Liu, X., Ory, V., Chapman, S., Yuan, H., Albanese, C., Kallakury, B., et al. (2012). ROCK Inhibitor and Feeder Cells Induce the Conditional Reprogramming of Epithelial Cells. *Am. J. Pathol.* 180, 599–607. doi:10.1016/j.ajpath.2011.10.036

Löfdahl, M., Kaarteenaho, R., Lappi-Blanco, E., Tornling, G., and Sköld, M. C. (2011). Tenascin-C and Alpha-Smooth Muscle Actin Positive Cells Are Increased in the Large Airways in Patients with COPD. *Respir. Res.* 12, 48. doi:10.1186/1465-9921-12-48

Ma, Q., Ma, Y., Dai, X., Ren, T., Fu, Y., Liu, W., et al. (2018). Regeneration of Functional Alveoli by Adult Human SOX9+ Airway Basal Cell Transplantation. *Protein Cell* 9, 267–282. doi:10.1007/s13238-018-0506-y

McGowan, S. E. (1992). Extracellular Matrix and the Regulation of Lung Development and Repair 1. *FASEB j.* 6, 2895–2904. doi:10.1096/fasebj.6.11.1644255

Meiners, S., Eickelberg, O., and Königshoff, M. (2015). Hallmarks of the Ageing Lung. *Eur. Respir. J.* 45, 807–827. doi:10.1183/09031936.00186914

Mereness, J. A., Bhattacharya, S., Wang, Q., Ren, Y., Pryhuber, G. S., and Mariani, T. J. (2018). Type VI Collagen Promotes Lung Epithelial Cell Spreading and Wound-Closure. *PLoS One* 13, e0209095. doi:10.1371/journal.pone.0209095

Merl-Pham, J., Basak, T., Knüppel, L., Ramanujam, D., Athanason, M., Behr, J., et al. (2019). Quantitative Proteomic Profiling of Extracellular Matrix and Site-specific Collagen Post-translational Modifications in an In Vitro Model of Lung Fibrosis. *Matrix Biol. Plus* 1, 100005. doi:10.1016/j.mbplus.2019.04.002

Merrilees, M. J., Ching, P. S. T., Beaumont, B., Hinek, A., Wight, T. N., and Black, P. N. (2008). Changes in Elastin, Elastin Binding Protein and Versican in Alveoli in Chronic Obstructive Pulmonary Disease. *Respir. Res.* 9, 41. doi:10.1186/1465-9921-9-41

Milara, J., Peiró, T., Serrano, A., and Cortijo, J. (2013). Epithelial to Mesenchymal Transition Is Increased in Patients with COPD and Induced by Cigarette Smoke. *Thorax* 68, 410–420. doi:10.1136/thoraxjnl-2012-201761

Miller, A. J., Hill, D. R., Nagy, M. S., Aoki, Y., Dye, B. R., Chin, A. M., et al. (2018). *In Vitro* Induction and *In Vivo* Engraftment of Lung Bud Tip Progenitor Cells Derived from Human Pluripotent Stem Cells. *Stem Cel Rep.* 10, 101–119. doi:10.1016/j.stemcr.2017.11.012

Mims, J. W. (2015). Asthma: Definitions and Pathophysiology. *Int. Forum Allergy Rhinology* 5 (Suppl. 1), S2–S6. doi:10.1002/alr.21609

Montoro, D. T., Haber, A. L., Biton, M., Vinarsky, V., Lin, B., Birket, S. E., et al. (2018). A Revised Airway Epithelial Hierarchy Includes CFTR-Expressing Ionocytes. *Nature* 560, 319–324. doi:10.1038/s41586-018-0393-7

Moore, K. A., Polte, T., Huang, S., Shi, B., Alsberg, E., Sunday, M. E., et al. (2005). Control of Basement Membrane Remodeling and Epithelial Branching Morphogenesis in Embryonic Lung by Rho and Cytoskeletal Tension. *Dev. Dyn.* 232, 268–281. doi:10.1002/dvdy.20237

Mou, H., Vinarsky, V., Tata, P. R., Brazauskas, K., Choi, S. H., Crooke, A. K., et al. (2016). Dual SMAD Signaling Inhibition Enables Long-Term Expansion of Diverse Epithelial Basal Cells. *Cell Stem Cell* 19, 217–231. doi:10.1016/j.stem.2016.05.012

Mund, S. I., Stampanoni, M., and Schittny, J. C. (2008). Developmental Alveolarization of the Mouse Lung. *Dev. Dyn.* 237, 2108–2116. doi:10.1002/dvdy.21633

Neurohr, C., Nishimura, S. L., and Sheppard, D. (2006). Activation of Transforming Growth Factor-β by the Integrin αvβ8 Delays Epithelial Wound Closure. *Am. J. Respir. Cel Mol Biol.* 35, 252–259. doi:10.1165/rcmb.2006-0013oc

Nihlberg, K., Andersson-Sjöland, A., Tufvesson, E., Erjefält, J. S., Bjermer, L., and Westergren-Thorsson, G. (2010). Altered Matrix Production in the Distal Airways of Individuals with Asthma. *Thorax* 65, 670–676. doi:10.1136/thx.2009.129320

Nishioka, M., Venkatesan, N., Dessalle, K., Mogas, A., Kyoh, S., Lin, T. Y., et al. (2015). Fibroblast-epithelial Cell Interactions Drive Epithelial-Mesenchymal Transition Differently in Cells from Normal and COPD Patients. *Respir. Res.* 16, 72. doi:10.1186/s12931-015-0232-4

Noguchi, A., Reddy, R., Kursar, J. D., Parks, W. C., and Mecham, R. P. (1989). Smooth Muscle Isoactin and Elastin in Fetal Bovine Lung. *Exp. Lung Res.* 15, 537–552. doi:10.3109/01902148909069617

Osei, E. T., B Mostaço-Guidolin, L., Hsieh, A., Warner, S. M., Al-Fouadi, M., Wang, M., et al. (2020). Epithelial-interleukin-1 Inhibits Collagen Formation by Airway Fibroblasts: Implications for Asthma. *Sci. Rep.* 10, 8721. doi:10.1038/s41598-020-65567-z

Ott, H. C., Clippinger, B., Conrad, C., Schuetz, C., Pomerantseva, I., Ikonomou, L., et al. (2010). Regeneration and Orthotopic Transplantation of a Bioartificial Lung. *Nat. Med.* 16, 927–933. doi:10.1038/nm.2193

Peters-Hall, J. R., Coquelin, M. L., Torres, M. J., LaRanger, R., Alabi, B. R., Sho, S., et al. (2018). Long-term Culture and Cloning of Primary Human Bronchial Basal Cells that Maintain Multipotent Differentiation Capacity and CFTR Channel Function. *Am. J. Physiology-Lung Cell Mol. Physiol.* 315, L313–L327. doi:10.1152/ajplung.00355.2017

Petrou, C. L., D'Ovidio, T. J., Bölükbas, D. A., Tas, S., Brown, R. D., Allawzi, A., et al. (2020). Clickable Decellularized Extracellular Matrix as a New Tool for Building Hybrid-Hydrogels to Model Chronic Fibrotic Diseases In Vitro. *J. Mater. Chem. B.* 8, 6814–6826. doi:10.1039/d0tb00613k

Philp, C. J., Siebeke, I., Clements, D., Miller, S., Habgood, A., John, A. E., et al. (2018). Extracellular Matrix Cross-Linking Enhances Fibroblast Growth and Protects against Matrix Proteolysis in Lung Fibrosis. *Am. J. Respir. Cel Mol Biol.* 58, 594–603. doi:10.1165/rcmb.2016-0379oc

Pouliot, R. A., Link, P. A., Mikhaiel, N. S., Schneck, M. B., Valentine, M. S., Kamga Gninzeko, F. J., et al. (2016). Development and Characterization of a Naturally Derived Lung Extracellular Matrix Hydrogel. *J. Biomed. Mater. Res.* 104, 1922–1935. doi:10.1002/jbm.a.35726

Price, A. P., England, K. A., Matson, A. M., Blazar, B. R., and Panoskaltsis-Mortari, A. (2010). Development of a Decellularized Lung Bioreactor System for Bioengineering the Lung: the Matrix Reloaded. *Tissue Eng. Part A* 16, 2581–2591. doi:10.1089/ten.tea.2009.0659

Quirt, J., Hildebrand, K. J., Mazza, J., Noya, F., and Kim, H. (2018). Asthma. *Allergy Asthma Clin. Immunol.* 14, 50. doi:10.1186/s13223-018-0279-0

Rani, A., Chin, C., Bremner, R., Mohanakumar, T., and Angara, S. (2021). Targeting Chromatin Dysregulation in Organ Fibrosis. *Cytokine Growth Factor. Rev.* 57, 64–72. doi:10.1016/j.cytogfr.2020.08.004

Ravindra, A., D'Angelo, W., Zhang, L., Reing, J., Johnson, S., Myerburg, M., et al. (2021). Human Bronchial Epithelial Cell Growth on Homologous versus Heterologous Tissue Extracellular Matrix. *J. Surg. Res.* 263, 215–223. doi:10.1016/j.jss.2021.01.040

Reeves, S. R., Kang, I., Chan, C. K., Barrow, K. A., Kolstad, T. K., White, M. P., et al. (2018). Asthmatic Bronchial Epithelial Cells Promote the Establishment of a Hyaluronan-Enriched, Leukocyte-Adhesive Extracellular Matrix by Lung Fibroblasts. *Respir. Res.* 19, 146. doi:10.1186/s12931-018-0849-1

Ren, Y., Zhang, Y., Fan, L., Jiao, Q., Wang, Y., and Wang, Q. (2019). The cullin4A Is Up-Regulated in Chronic Obstructive Pulmonary Disease Patient and Contributes to Epithelial-Mesenchymal Transition in Small Airway Epithelium. *Respir. Res.* 20, 84. doi:10.1186/s12931-019-1048-4

Roberts, C. R., and Burke, A. K. (1998). Remodelling of the Extracellular Matrix in Asthma: Proteoglycan Synthesis and Degradation. *Can. Respir. J.* 5, 48–50.

Rock, J. R., Onaitis, M. W., Rawlins, E. L., Lu, Y., Clark, C. P., Xue, Y., et al. (2009). Basal Cells as Stem Cells of the Mouse Trachea and Human Airway Epithelium. *Proc. Natl. Acad. Sci.* 106, 12771–12775. doi:10.1073/pnas.0906850106

Sannes, P. L., and Wang, J. (1997). Basement Membranes and Pulmonary Development. *Exp. Lung Res.* 23, 101–108. doi:10.3109/01902149709074023

Schiller, H. B., Fernandez, I. E., Burgstaller, G., Schaab, C., Scheltema, R. A., Schwarzmayr, T., et al. (2015). Time- and Compartment-resolved Proteome Profiling of the Extracellular Niche in Lung Injury and Repair. *Mol. Syst. Biol.* 11, 819. doi:10.15252/msb.20156123

Schittny, J. C. (2017). Development of the Lung. *Cel Tissue Res* 367, 427–444. doi:10.1007/s00441-016-2545-0

Sekine, K., Ohuchi, H., Fujiwara, M., Yamasaki, M., Yoshizawa, T., Sato, T., et al. (1999). Fgf10 Is Essential for Limb and Lung Formation. *Nat. Genet.* 21, 138–141. doi:10.1038/5096

Shannon, J. M., Nielsen, L. D., Gebb, S. A., and Randell, S. H. (1998). Mesenchyme Specifies Epithelial Differentiation in Reciprocal Recombinants of Embryonic Lung and Trachea. *Dev. Dyn.* 212, 482–494. doi:10.1002/(sici)1097-0177(199808)212:4<482::aid-aja2>3.0.co;2-d

Shi, Y., Dong, Y., Duan, Y., Jiang, X., Chen, C., and Deng, L. (2013). Substrate Stiffness Influences TGF-β1-Induced Differentiation of Bronchial Fibroblasts into Myofibroblasts in Airway Remodeling. *Mol. Med. Rep.* 7, 419–424. doi:10.3892/mmr.2012.1213

Smirnova, N. F., Schamberger, A. C., Nayakanti, S., Hatz, R., Behr, J., and Eickelberg, O. (2016). Detection and Quantification of Epithelial Progenitor Cell Populations in Human Healthy and IPF Lungs. *Respir. Res.* 17, 83. doi:10.1186/s12931-016-0404-x

Sohal, S. S., Reid, D., Soltani, A., Ward, C., Weston, S., Muller, H. K., et al. (2011). Evaluation of Epithelial Mesenchymal Transition in Patients with Chronic Obstructive Pulmonary Disease. *Respir. Res.* 12, 130. doi:10.1186/1465-9921-12-130

Sohal, S. S., Reid, D., Soltani, A., Ward, C., Weston, S., Muller, H. K., et al. (2010). Reticular Basement Membrane Fragmentation and Potential Epithelial Mesenchymal Transition Is Exaggerated in the Airways of Smokers with Chronic Obstructive Pulmonary Disease. *Respirology* 15, 930–938. doi:10.1111/j.1440-1843.2010.01808.x

Soltani, A., Muller, H. K., Sohal, S. S., Reid, D. W., Weston, S., Wood-Baker, R., et al. (2012). Distinctive Characteristics of Bronchial Reticular Basement Membrane and Vessel Remodelling in Chronic Obstructive Pulmonary Disease (COPD) and in Asthma: They Are Not the Same Disease. *Histopathology* 60, 964–970. doi:10.1111/j.1365-2559.2011.04147.x

Soltani, A., Reid, D. W., Sohal, S. S., Wood-Baker, R., Weston, S., Muller, H. K., et al. (2010). Basement Membrane and Vascular Remodelling in Smokers and Chronic Obstructive Pulmonary Disease: a Cross-Sectional Study. *Respir. Res.* 11, 105. doi:10.1186/1465-9921-11-105

Stabler, C. T., and Morrisey, E. E. (2017). Developmental Pathways in Lung Regeneration. *Cel Tissue Res.* 367, 677–685. doi:10.1007/s00441-016-2537-0

Takahashi, Y., Kobayashi, T., D'Alessandro-Gabazza, C. N., Toda, M., Fujiwara, K., Okano, T., et al. (2019). Protective Role of Matrix Metalloproteinase-2 in Allergic Bronchial Asthma. *Front. Immunol.* 10, 1795. doi:10.3389/fimmu.2019.01795

Travaglini, K. J., Nabhan, A. N., Penland, L., Sinha, R., Gillich, A., Sit, R. V., et al. (2020). A Molecular Cell Atlas of the Human Lung from Single-Cell RNA Sequencing. *Nature* 587, 619–625. doi:10.1038/s41586-020-2922-4

Tschumperlin, D. J. (2015). Matrix, Mesenchyme, and Mechanotransduction. *Ann. ATS* 12 (Suppl. 1), S24–S29. doi:10.1513/annalsats.201407-320mg

Uriarte, J. J., Uhl, F. E., Rolandsson Enes, S. E., Pouliot, R. A., and Weiss, D. J. (2018). Lung Bioengineering: Advances and Challenges in Lung Decellularization and Recellularization. *Curr. Opin. Organ. Transpl.* 23, 673–678. doi:10.1097/mot.0000000000000584

Vaccaro, C., and Brody, J. S. (1978). Ultrastructure of Developing Alveoli. I. The Role of the Interstitial Fibroblast. *Anat. Rec.* 192, 467–479. doi:10.1002/ar.1091920402

van der Velden, J. L., Wagner, D. E., Lahue, K. G., Abdalla, S. T., Lam, Y. W., Weiss, D. J., et al. (2018). TGF-β1-induced Deposition of Provisional Extracellular Matrix by Tracheal Basal Cells Promotes Epithelial-To-Mesenchymal Transition in a C-Jun NH2-terminal Kinase-1-dependent Manner. *Am. J. Physiol. Lung Cel Mol Physiol.* 314, L984–L997. doi:10.1152/ajplung.00053.2017

Vieira Braga, F. A., Kar, G., Berg, M., Carpaij, O. A., Polanski, K., Simon, L. M., et al. (2019). A Cellular Census of Human Lungs Identifies Novel Cell States in Health and in Asthma. *Nat. Med.* 25, 1153–1163. doi:10.1038/s41591-019-0468-5

Vignola, A. M., Kips, J., and Bousquet, J. (2000). Tissue Remodeling as a Feature of Persistent Asthma. *J. Allergy Clin. Immunol.* 105, 1041–1053. doi:10.1067/mai.2000.107195

Wagner, D. E., Bonenfant, N. R., Sokocevic, D., DeSarno, M. J., Borg, Z. D., Parsons, C. S., et al. (2014). Three-dimensional Scaffolds of Acellular Human and Porcine Lungs for High Throughput Studies of Lung Disease and Regeneration. *Biomaterials* 35, 2664–2679. doi:10.1016/j.biomaterials.2013.11.078

Warburton, D., El-Hashash, A., Carraro, G., Tiozzo, C., Sala, F., Rogers, O., et al. (2010). "Lung Organogenesis," in *Current Topics in Developmental Biology.* Editor P. Koopman (Academic Press), 73–158. doi:10.1016/s0070-2153(10)90003-3

Watson, J. K., Rulands, S., Wilkinson, A. C., Wuidart, A., Ousset, M., Van Keymeulen, A., et al. (2015). Clonal Dynamics Reveal Two Distinct Populations of Basal Cells in Slow-Turnover Airway Epithelium. *Cel Rep.* 12, 90–101. doi:10.1016/j.celrep.2015.06.011

Weitoft, M., Andersson, C., Andersson-Sjöland, A., Tufvesson, E., Bjermer, L., Erjefält, J., et al. (2014). Controlled and Uncontrolled Asthma Display Distinct Alveolar Tissue Matrix Compositions. *Respir. Res.* 15, 67. doi:10.1186/1465-9921-15-67

White, E. S. (2015). Lung Extracellular Matrix and Fibroblast Function. *Ann. ATS* 12 (Suppl. 1), S30–S33. doi:10.1513/annalsats.201406-240mg

Wigén, J., Elowsson-Rendin, L., Karlsson, L., Tykesson, E., and Westergren-Thorsson, G. (2019). Glycosaminoglycans: A Link between Development and Regeneration in the Lung. *Stem Cell Development* 28, 823–832. doi:10.1089/scd.2019.0009

Xu, H., Ling, M., Xue, J., Dai, X., Sun, Q., Chen, C., et al. (2018). Exosomal microRNA-21 Derived from Bronchial Epithelial Cells Is Involved in Aberrant Epithelium-Fibroblast Cross-Talk in COPD Induced by Cigarette Smoking. *Theranostics* 8, 5419–5433. doi:10.7150/thno.27876

Xu, J., Benyon, R. C., Leir, S.-H., Zhang, S., Holgate, S. T., and Lackie, P. M. (2002). Matrix Metalloproteinase-2 from Bronchial Epithelial Cells Induces the Proliferation of Subepithelial Fibroblasts. *Clin. Exp. Allergy* 32, 881–888. doi:10.1046/j.1365-2745.2002.01386.x

Xu, Y., Mizuno, T., Sridharan, A., Du, Y., Guo, M., Tang, J., et al. (2016). Single-cell RNA Sequencing Identifies Diverse Roles of Epithelial Cells in Idiopathic Pulmonary Fibrosis. *JCI Insight* 1, e90558. doi:10.1172/jci.insight.90558

Yamamoto, Y., Korogi, Y., Hirai, T., and Gotoh, S. (2020). A Method of Generating Alveolar Organoids Using Human Pluripotent Stem Cells. *Methods Cel Biol.* 159, 115–141. doi:10.1016/bs.mcb.2020.02.004

Yayon, A., Klagsbrun, M., Esko, J. D., Leder, P., and Ornitz, D. M. (1991). Cell Surface, Heparin-like Molecules Are Required for Binding of Basic Fibroblast Growth Factor to its High Affinity Receptor. *Cell* 64, 841–848. doi:10.1016/0092-8674(91)90512-w

Yuan, T., Volckaert, T., Redente, E. F., Hopkins, S., Klinkhammer, K., Wasnick, R., et al. (2019). FGF10-FGFR2B Signaling Generates Basal Cells and Drives Alveolar Epithelial Regeneration by Bronchial Epithelial Stem Cells after Lung Injury. *Stem Cel Rep.* 12, 1041–1055. doi:10.1016/j.stemcr.2019.04.003

Zabner, J., Karp, P., Seiler, M., Phillips, S. L., Mitchell, C. J., Saavedra, M., et al. (2003). Development of Cystic Fibrosis and Noncystic Fibrosis Airway Cell Lines. *Am. J. Physiology-Lung Cell Mol. Physiol.* 284, L844–L854. doi:10.1152/ajplung.00355.2002

Zhang, H., Newman, D. R., and Sannes, P. L. (2012). HSULF-1 Inhibits ERK and AKT Signaling and Decreases Cell Viability In Vitro in Human Lung Epithelial Cells. *Respir. Res.* 13, 69. doi:10.1186/1465-9921-13-69

Zhou, Y., Horowitz, J. C., Naba, A., Ambalavanan, N., Atabai, K., Balestrini, J., et al. (2018). Extracellular Matrix in Lung Development, Homeostasis and Disease. *Matrix Biol.* 73, 77–104. doi:10.1016/j.matbio.2018.03.005

Zhu, L., Zhuo, L., Kimata, K., Yamaguchi, E., Watanabe, H., Aronica, M. A., et al. (2010). Deficiency in the Serum-Derived Hyaluronan-Associated Protein-Hyaluronan Complex Enhances Airway Hyperresponsiveness in a Murine Model of Asthma. *Int. Arch. Allergy Immunol.* 153, 223–233. doi:10.1159/000314362

Zhu, M., Tian, D., Li, J., Ma, Y., Wang, Y., and Wu, R. (2007). Glycogen Synthase Kinase 3β and β-catenin Are Involved in the Injury and Repair of Bronchial Epithelial Cells Induced by Scratching. *Exp. Mol. Pathol.* 83, 30–38. doi:10.1016/j.yexmp.2007.02.001

8

AGR3 Regulates Airway Epithelial Junctions in Patients with Frequent Exacerbations of COPD

*Rui Ye, Cuihong Wang, Pengbo Sun, Shuang Bai and Li Zhao**

Department of Pulmonary and Critical Care Medicine, Shengjing Hospital of China Medical University, Shenyang, China

***Correspondence:**
Li Zhao
lzhaoli@163.com

Background: The mechanisms underlying differences in the susceptibility to chronic obstructive pulmonary disease (COPD) exacerbations between patients are not well understood. Recent studies have shown that the patients with frequent COPD exacerbations is related to specific protein expression in lung tissue. Anterior gradient 3 (AGR3) is expressed in airway epithelial cells in the lung and proteomic analysis revealed that its expression is decreased in patients with frequent COPD exacerbations. Moreover, the loss of epithelial integrity might facilitate trans-epithelial permeability of pathogens in such patients. This study was performed to determine that AGR3 protein play a role in COPD frequency exacerbators.

Methods: Human lung tissues were collected from current-smoking patients (Control; n = 15) as well as patients with infrequent COPD exacerbations (IFCOPD; n = 18) and frequent COPD exacerbations (FCOPD; n = 8). While AGR3 protein expression was measured by immunohistochemistry and western blotting, *AGR* mRNA expression was determined by real time quantitative polymerase chain reaction (RT-qPCR). Furthermore, adherent junctions (AJs) and tight junctions (TJs) protein expression in human lung tissues were measured by immunohistochemistry. The effects of cigarette smoke extract (CSE) on AJ and TJ protein and mRNA expression in BEAS-2B cells were assessed by western blotting and RT-qPCR. In addition, the effect of AGR3 overexpression and knockdown on AJ and TJ protein expression was determined.

Results: AGR3 was mainly expressed in the airway epithelium and AGR3-positive products were localized in the cytoplasm. Western blotting and RT-qPCR results showed that AGR3 protein (p = 0.009) and mRNA (p = 0.04) expression in the FCOPD group was significantly lower than that in the IFCOPD group. Moreover, E-cadherin, occludin, and zonula occludens-1 (ZO-1) expression was lower in the FCOPD group than in the IFCOPD group. The protein and mRNA expression of E-cadherin, occludin, and ZO-1 was decreased within 24 h post-CSE exposure. AGR3 overexpression rescued CSE-induced downregulation of E-cadherin, occludin, and ZO-1.

Abbreviations: AGR, anterior gradient; AGR2, anterior gradient 2; AGR3, anterior gradient 3; AJ, adherens junction; COPD, chronic obstructive pulmonary disease; CSE, cigarette smoke extract; PDI, protein disulphide isomerase; TJ, tight junction

Conclusion: Difference in AGR3 expression in the lung tissue might be correlated with increased susceptibility to COPD exacerbation. AGR3 can prevent CSE-induced downregulation of E-cadherin, occludin, and ZO-1 in airway epithelial cells. Loss of AGR3 might promote viral and bacterial infection and induce immune inflammation to increase COPD exacerbation.

Keywords: COPD, AGR3, frequent exacerbator, human lung tissue, airway epithelial barrier

INTRODUCTION

Chronic obstructive pulmonary disease (COPD) is a worldwide public health problem that accounts for 5% of all deaths each year and is associated with increasing morbidity and mortality (Wang et al., 2018). Among various COPD phenotypes, the frequent-exacerbation phenotype has the most marked impact on accelerating the decline of lung function, reducing physical activity, decreasing quality of life, and increasing mortality (Donaldson et al., 2002). The frequent-exacerbation phenotype of COPD was first described by Hurst et al., in 2010 and its clinical importance was demonstrated (Hurst et al., 2010; From the Global Strategy for the Diagnosis, Management and Prevention of COPD, Global Initiative for Chronic Obstructive Lung Disease (GOLD), 2018). So far it is no primary outcome that reduces the frequency and severity of COPD exacerbations for almost any development of new drugs in COPD, especially for target therapies. Unfortunately, two kinds of monoclonal antibodies that bind to receptors related to eosinophil reduction were found to be ineffective in their clinical trials in COPD patients, including frequent exacerbation phenotype (Pavord et al., 2017; Criner et al., 2019). The underlying mechanisms and predisposing factors of the frequent-exacerbation COPD phenotype are still unclear. A previous study on the proteomics of lung tissues in patients with frequent COPD exacerbations identified 23 differentially expressed proteins (Sun et al., 2019), including anterior gradient 3 (AGR3).

The AGR protein family consists of three subfamilies: AG1, AGR2, and AGR3. The AGR family proteins share high sequence homology to the non-secreted protein disulphide isomerase (PDI) family proteins (Ivanova et al., 2013). The PDI family proteins harbor core thioredoxin folds (CxxC or CxxS motifs), which can promote protein folding via modulation of disulphide bond formation and calcium homeostasis in the endoplasmic reticulum (Persson et al., 2005). AGR3, also known as HAG-3, AG3, or BCMP11, was first identified in breast cancer cell membrane fractions using a proteomics screen (Adam et al., 2003). AGR3 is a highly related homologue of pro-oncogenic AGR2, and both genes are located on chromosome 7p21 (Petek et al., 2000). The effects of AGR3 on ciliary beat frequency in airway epithelial cells were demonstrated using a knockout mouse model (Bonser et al., 2015). However, limited information is available about AGR3 function in the respiratory system. AGR3 is involved in mucociliary system which plays an important role in defense to foreign pathogens. Epithelial tight junctions (TJs) and adherens junctions (AJs) also plays an important role in host defense against foreign pathogens (Nawijn et al., 2011). The disruption of these structures might increase the susceptibility of patients with COPD to viral and bacterial infection. Most patients with COPD exacerbations have viral and bacterial infection (Hiemstra et al., 2015). To our knowledge, the effect of AGR3 on airway epithelial barriers in patients with frequent COPD exacerbations has not been studied. The present study was conducted to identify potential therapeutic targets of patients with frequent COPD exacerbations. Furthermore, AGR3 expression was measured in the lung tissues of patients with frequent and infrequent COPD exacerbations and the role of AGR3 on epithelial junctions was determined both in lung tissues and vitro.

MATERIALS AND METHODS

Lung Tissue Sample Collection

The study was approved by the Ethics Review Committee for Human Studies at Shengjing Hospital of China Medical University, and informed written consent was obtained from each patient (2016PS342K). The inclusion criteria for patients with COPD were as follows: 1) 40–80 years of age; 2) history of 10 or more pack-years of smoking; 3) ratio of forced expiratory volume in 1 s (FEV1) to forced vital capacity (FVC) (FEV1/FVC ratio) of 70% or less after bronchodilator use (Wang et al., 2019); and 4) stable clinical pulmonary condition of COPD, with no acute exacerbations for at least 4 weeks prior to enrollment. The severity of airway limitation was graded based on FEV1post%, as described in the GOLD guidelines (Wang et al., 2018). Patients with COPD were assigned to two groups based on their medical history: infrequent exacerbations (IFCOPD) and frequent exacerbations (FCOPD). Patients in the FCOPD group must have experienced at least two or more exacerbations per year that required treatment with additional antibiotics or a systemic steroid, or hospitalization (Wang et al., 2018). Each exacerbation must have occurred at least 4 weeks after the end of treatment for the previous exacerbation or 6 weeks after its onset (Spencer and Jones, 2003; Soler-Cataluña and Rodriguez-Roisin, 2010). These criteria were included to distinguish a new exacerbation from a "treatment failure" (Soler-Cataluña and Rodriguez-Roisin, 2010). In addition, subjects with normal lung function and current-smoking history >10 pack-years were enrolled as the control group. Patients with other respiratory diseases such as asthma, pulmonary fibrosis, and hilar lung cancer, or other chronic diseases such as rheumatoid arthritis and chronic colitis were excluded from the study. Two professional pulmonologists assembled a detailed clinical history for each patient and conducted comprehensive lung function tests using standard spirometric techniques. Lung tissue specimens were retrieved from Biobank, Shengjing Hospital of China Medical University. All biopsy tissues were obtained from patients who underwent pulmonary lobectomy. These resected tissue samples included non-diseased regions near lung nodules and tumors, bullectomy (at least 5 cm from the tumor edge) and appeared to be normal when inspected as previously described (Bi et al., 2015). The location and amount (approximately 1 cm^3) of each sample were standardized and paired according to tumor type and grade (Kelsen et al., 2008). The resected samples were immediately frozen in liquid nitrogen and stored at −80°C until use.

Immunofluorescence and Immunohistochemistry

Lung tissue blocks were fixed in 10% neutral buffered formalin for 24 h and embedded in paraffin wax. Immunohistochemical analysis was performed on 2.5-μm-thick sections cut from formalin-fixed, paraffin-embedded archival tissue blocks. These sections were mounted on slides, deparaffinized in xylene, and rehydrated in phosphate-buffered saline (PBS) through a graded ethanol series. Endogenous peroxidase activity was quenched in 3% H_2O_2 in PBS for 15 min. Antigen retrieval was performed in citrate buffer, pH 6 at 100°C for 7.5 min. For AGR3 immunodetection, the sections were incubated overnight at 4°C with rabbit monoclonal anti-AGR3 (1:200, Proteintech, Chicago, IL, United States), anti-E-cadherin (1:1,000, Proteintech), anti-ZO-1 (1:400, Proteintech), and anti-occludin (1:500, Proteintech). A streptavidin–biotin peroxidase detection system was used according to the manufacturer's protocol (Ultrasensitive™ S-P Kit, Maxim Biotechnologies, Fuzhou, China) for immunohistochemical studies. In addition, each section was stained using the DAB color reagent kit (ZSGB-BIO, Beijing, China).

For immunofluorescence, primary antibodies were rabbit monoclonal anti-AGR3 (1:200, Proteintech), monoclonal anti-cytokeratin (1:100, Sigma-Aldrich, Darmstadt, Germany), rabbit anti-E-cadherin (1:100, Proteintech), anti-ZO-1 (1:100, Proteintech), and anti-occludin (1:100, Proteintech) and Alexa Fluor-conjugated secondary antibodies were goat anti-rabbit (488 nm) (1:100, Proteintech), goat anti-mouse (594 nm) (1: 100, Proteintech) and donkey anti-rabbit (594 nm) (1:100, Sigma-Aldrich). Immunofluorescence staining was visualized under Olympus FV1000 confocal microscope with a 60× oil-immersion objective. Images were acquired and analyzed by NIS-Elements F 3.0 and NIS- Elements Br 3.0.

Western Blot

Total protein was extracted from frozen lung tissues using RIPA and phenylmethylsulfonyl fluoride (PMSF) (99:1) (Beyotime, Shanghai, China). Protein concentrations were determined using the BCA kit (Beyotime). Protein extracts were subjected to SDS-PAGE and visualized with SuperSignal West Pico Chemiluminescent substrate (Thermo Fisher, MA, United States). The following primary antibodies were purchased from Proteintech and used for western blotting: anti-GAPDH (1:5,000), anti-AGR3 (1:500), anti-E-cadherin (1: 8,000), anti-occludin (1:5,000), and anti-ZO-1 (1:5,000).

TABLE 1 | RT-PCR primers.

Gene	Sequence	Length (nt)
GAPDH-F	5′-CCTGGTATGACAACGAATTTG-3′	131
GAPDH-R	5′-CAGTGAGGGTCTCTCTCTTCC-3′	
AGR3-F	5′-CATCACCTGGAGGATTGTCAATAC-3′	91
AGR3-R	5′-TGAACTTATTCTGAGCCATTTCTTGT-3′	
Occludin-F	5′-TGCATGTTCGACCAATGC-3′	235
Occludin-R	5′-AAGCCACTTCCTCCATAAGG-3′	
ZO-1-F	5′-AAGATGTCCGCCAGAGCTGC-3′	80
ZO-1-R	5′-AGCGTCACTGTATGTTGTTCCC-3′	
E-cadherin-F	5′-AGGGGTTAAGCACAACAGCA-3′	161
E-cadherin-R	5′-GGTATTGGGGGCATCAGCAT-3′	

TABLE 2 | Demographic characteristics of patients.

	Control	IFCOPD	FCOPD	p
	(n=15)	(n=18)	(n=8)	
Age	57.87 ± 6.97	59.00±6.94	65.00±6.41	0.061
Gender (M/F)	11/4	15/3	7/1	
Packs/year	26.67 ± 15.99	30.61 ± 15.67	37.50 ± 11.65	0.275
FEV1 (%predict)	100.49 ± 18.27	71.80 ± 14.75	57.92 ± 14.95	0.051[a]
FVC (%predict)	101.57 ± 12.68	91.91 ± 15.48	80.06 ± 15.44	0.062[a]
FEV1/FVC	80.77 ± 10.26	62.48 ± 6.65	56.86 ± 5.97	0.113[a]

All values are represented as mean ± SD.

[a]p > 0.05 in FEV1 (%predict), FVC(%predict), and FEV1/FVC between IFCOPD and FCOPD groups.

Real Time Polymerase Chain Reaction

The primers used for real time polymerase chain reaction (RT-PCR) are shown in **Table 1**. Total RNA was extracted from lung tissues using TRIzol reagent (Takara, Ohtsu, Shiga, Japan), according to the manufacturer's instructions. The transcribed cDNA concentration was adjusted to 120 ng/ml with RNase-free water before PCR analysis. PCR was performed using the SYBR Green PCR Kit (Takara) with a Roche 480 Real-Time PCR System (Roche, Basel, Switzerland). The PCR cycling parameters were as follows: pre-incubation for 2 min at 42°C and 40 cycles of denaturation at 95°C for 5 s. RT-PCR was performed in triplicate for both endogenous controls and each target gene. Relative gene expression was calculated using the $2^{-\Delta\Delta ct}$ method. Melting curve analysis and 2% agarose gel electrophoresis were performed to confirm the PCR product.

Cell Culture

BEAS-2B (CRL-9609) cell line was obtained from the Cell Bank of the Chinese Academy of Sciences (Shanghai, China) and cultured in high-glucose Dulbecco's Modified Eagle's Medium (H-DMEM) supplemented with 10% foetal bovine serum, 100 U/ml penicillin, and 100 mg/ml streptomycin (growth medium) at 37°C in a 5% CO_2, 95% air atmosphere. Unless otherwise stated, cells were grown to 70–80% confluency prior to treatment.

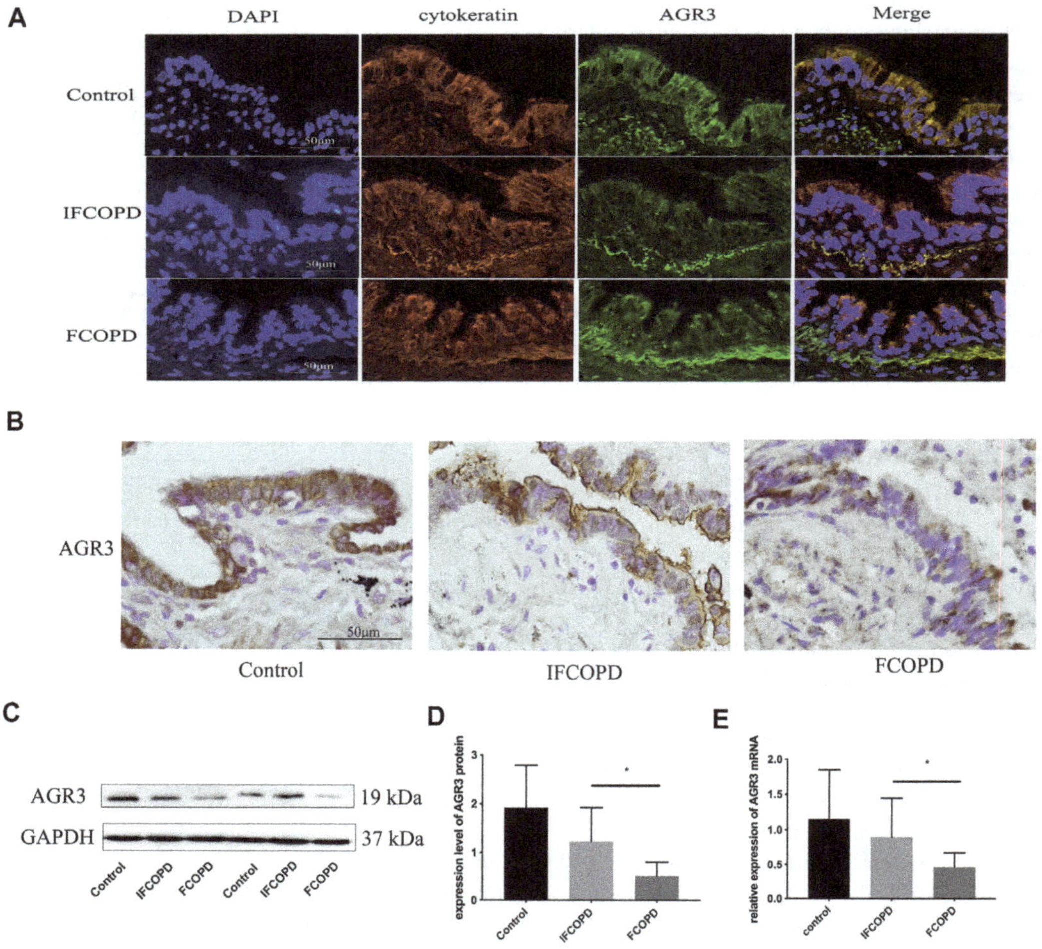

FIGURE 1 | AGR3 expression in airway epithelial cells of frequent COPD exacerbators. The control group included subjects with normal lung function and a current smoking history of >10 pack years. **(A)** Immunofluorescence staining for AGR3 (green) and cytokeratin (red) in human airway epithelial cells **(B)** Immunohistochemical staining for AGR3 in human airway epithelial cells of Control (n = 15), IFCOPD (n = 18), and FCOPD (n = 8) groups. The control group included subjects with normal lung function and a current smoking history of >10 pack years. Cells were stained with anti-AGR3 antibody. AGR3 expression in the airway epithelium of patients with COPD and control subjects was determined by IHC (400×). **(C,D)** Western blot analysis of AGR3 expression in FCOPD, IFCOPD, and control groups. $*p < 0.05$. **(E)** qPCR analysis of *AGR3* mRNA expression in lung tissues of FCOPD, IFCOPD, and control groups. $*p < 0.05$.

Plasmid Construction and Cell Transfection

For lentiviral AGR3 overexpression in BEAS-2B cells, full-length *AGR3* was cloned into the pHBLV-CMV-MCS-3FLAG-EF1-ZsGreen-T2A-PURO vector. Lentivirus packaging, cellular transfection, and selection of puromycin-resistant cells were performed according to the instruction manual provided by Hanbio Biotechnology (Shanghai, China). shAGR3 and shNC were purchased form GenePharma (Suzhou, China). Cells were transfected with Lipofectamine 3,000 (Invitrogen), following the product manual. The nucleotide sequences of all constructed plasmids were confirmed by DNA sequencing.

Cigarette Smoke Extract Preparation

Cigarette smoke extract (CSE) was prepared by bubbling smoke from two filtered cigarettes (Hongmei cigarettes, tobacco type, tar: 10 mg, nicotine content: 0.8 mg, and carbon monoxide fumes: 12 mg; Hongta Tobacco Industry LLC, Yunnan, China) in a 50-ml centrifuge tube containing 20 ml H-DMEM by vacuum extraction. The extracts were sterilized by passing through a 0.22-μm filter and considered full concentrations of CSE (Kelsen et al., 2008).

Statistical Analysis

Statistical analyses were performed using SPSS 22.0 software (Chicago, IL, United States) and GraphPad Prism 7 (La Jolla, CA, United States). Data are expressed as the mean ± SD. ANOVA was used to compare differences between groups. $p < 0.05$ was considered statistically significant.

RESULTS

Patient Information

Lung tissues from 41 patients (15 controls, 18 IFCOPD, and 8 FCOPD) were collected from September 2016 to September 2018.

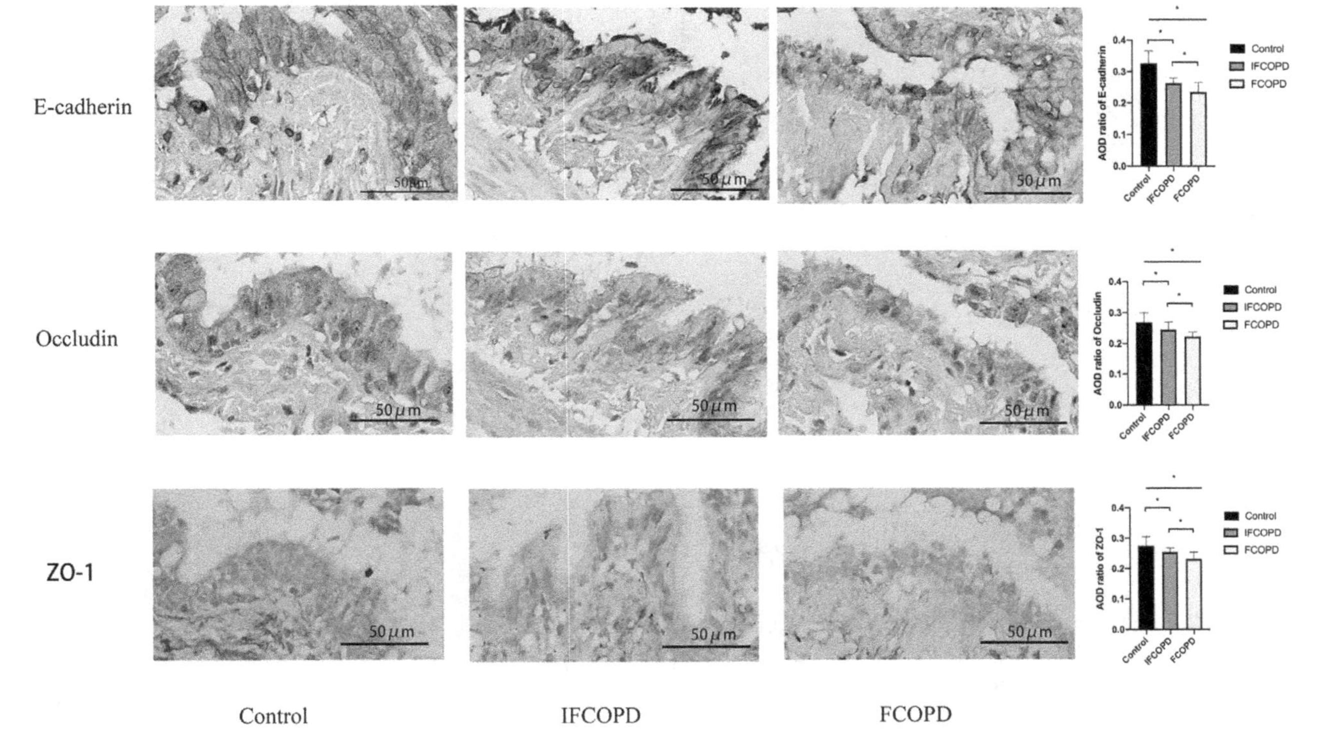

FIGURE 2 | Immunohistochemical analysis of E-cadherin, occludin, and ZO-1 expression in the airway epithelium cells of Control (n = 15), IFCOPD (n = 18), and FCOPD (n = 8) groups. The control group included subjects with normal lung function and a current smoking history of >10 pack years. Cells were stained with anti-E-cadherin, anti-occludin, and anti-ZO-1 antibody. All subjects were determined by IHC (400×). Data are displayed as mean ± SD, *$p < 0.05$ by one-way ANOVA. Results represent significant differences in the expression of E-cadherin, occludin, and ZO-1 in airway epithelium cells, compared to the Control group.

There were no significant differences in the age or gender between the three groups. In addition, there were no significant differences in FEV1 (%predict), FVC (%predict), and FEV1/FVC between the IFCOPD and FCOPD groups (**Table 2**).

AGR3 Is Downregulated in the Airway Epithelial Cells of Patients with Frequent COPD Exacerbation

Histological analysis showed that AGR3 is mainly expressed in the airway epithelial cells of the lung tissue and AGR3-positive products are localized in the cytoplasm (**Figure 1A**). AGR3 protein expression in the IFCOPD and FCOPD groups was significantly lower than that in the control group (**Figures 1A,B**, $p = 0.009$). Moreover, *AGR3* mRNA expression in the FCOPD group was lower than that in the IFCOPD group (**Figure 1C**, $p = 0.04$).

Epithelial Junction Proteins are Downregulated in Patients with Frequent COPD Exacerbation

Epithelial junction proteins in the bronchial epithelium consist of apical TJ proteins such as occludins, zonula occludins (ZO), and claudin family and junctional adhesion molecule, and AJ proteins such as E-cadherin (Heijink et al., 2014). The expression of E-cadherin, occludin, and ZO-1 was assessed by immunohistochemistry in the FCOPD and IFCOPD groups. Compared to Control group, the expression of E-cadherin in airway epithelial cells was decreased in COPD groups ($p = 0.004$) and markedly lower in IFCOPD group ($p = 0.006$). As same as the expression of E-cadherin, the expression of occludin, and ZO-1 was respectively decreased in COPD groups ($p = 0.001$and $p = 0.001$), and markedly lower in IFCOPD group ($p = 0.03$ and $p = 0.004$) (**Figure 2**).

CSE Downregulates TJ and AJ Proteins in Airway Epithelial Cells

The effects of CSE exposure on the expression of TJ proteins (occludin and ZO-1) and an AJ protein (E-cadherin) were determined. BEAS-2B cells were treated with 5 and 10% CSE for 24 h. The gene and protein expression of occludin, ZO-1, and E-cadherin were analyzed by qPCR and western blotting, respectively. The treatment of cells with 10% CSE significantly decreased gene and protein expression of occludin, ZO-1, and E-cadherin (**Figure 3**).

AGR3 Rescue CSE-Induced Downregulation of AJs and TJs in Airway Epithelial Cells

The ability of AGR3 to rescue CSE-induced downregulation of TJs and AJs in bronchial epithelial cells was assessed. At first, *AGR3* was overexpressed or silenced in BEAS-2B cells. Western

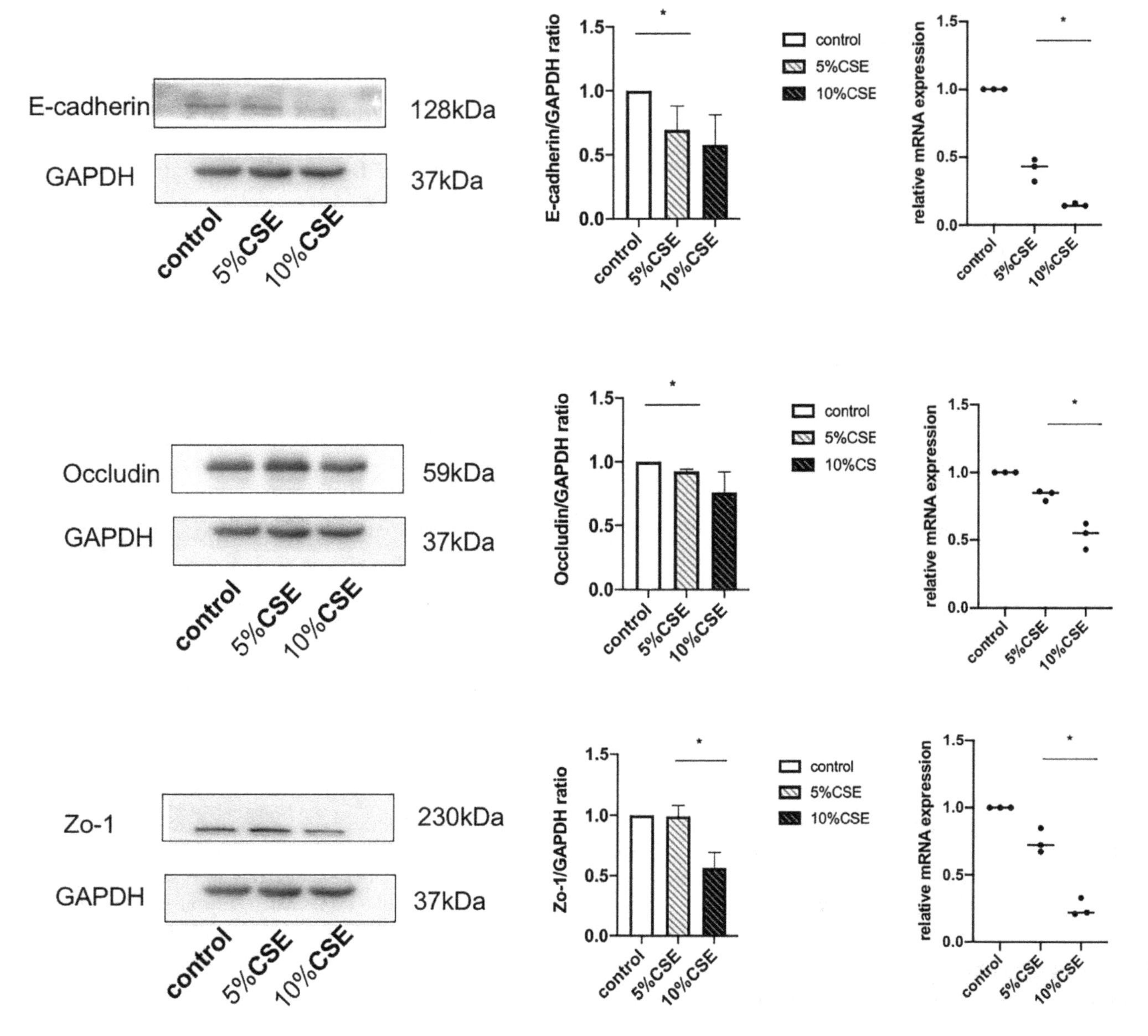

FIGURE 3 | Western blotting and real-time quantitative reverse-transcriptase PCR results showing TJ and AJ protein expression in BEAS-2B cells in the presence or absence of 5 and 10% CSE for 24 h. Band intensity was quantitated using densitometry. All results are representative of at least three independent experiments. Data are shown as the mean ± SD. $^*p < 0.05$ by one-way ANOVA.

blot analysis showed that the expression of occludin, ZO-1, and E-cadherin was significantly increased in AGR3-overexpressed BEAS-2B cells and decreased in AGR3-silenced BEAS-2B cells. Next, the ability of AGR3 to rescue CSE-induced downregulation of TJ and AJ proteins was determined. Western blot analysis showed increased expression of occludin, ZO-1, and E-cadherin in CSE-exposed AGR3-overexpressing cells (**Figure 4**).

DISCUSSION

COPD is characterized by airway inflammation with periods of symptom exacerbation that leads to irreversible airflow limitation, lung damage, and mucus hypersecretion. The treatment strategies for patients with COPD remain a challenge due the wide range of COPD phenotypes and their unpredictable clinical course (Wang et al., 2018). The frequency of COPD exacerbation can determine COPD phenotype. Patients with more than two exacerbations per year have been defined as having frequent COPD exacerbations. These individuals have high levels of inflammatory cytokines such as interleukin-6 in sputum (Bhowmik et al., 2000), and show a high risk of adverse health outcomes. In our previous study on patients with frequent COPD exacerbations, proteomics analysis showed low expression of several proteins in lung tissues (Sun et al., 2019). Moreover, AGR3 was significantly decreased and previous study (Bonser

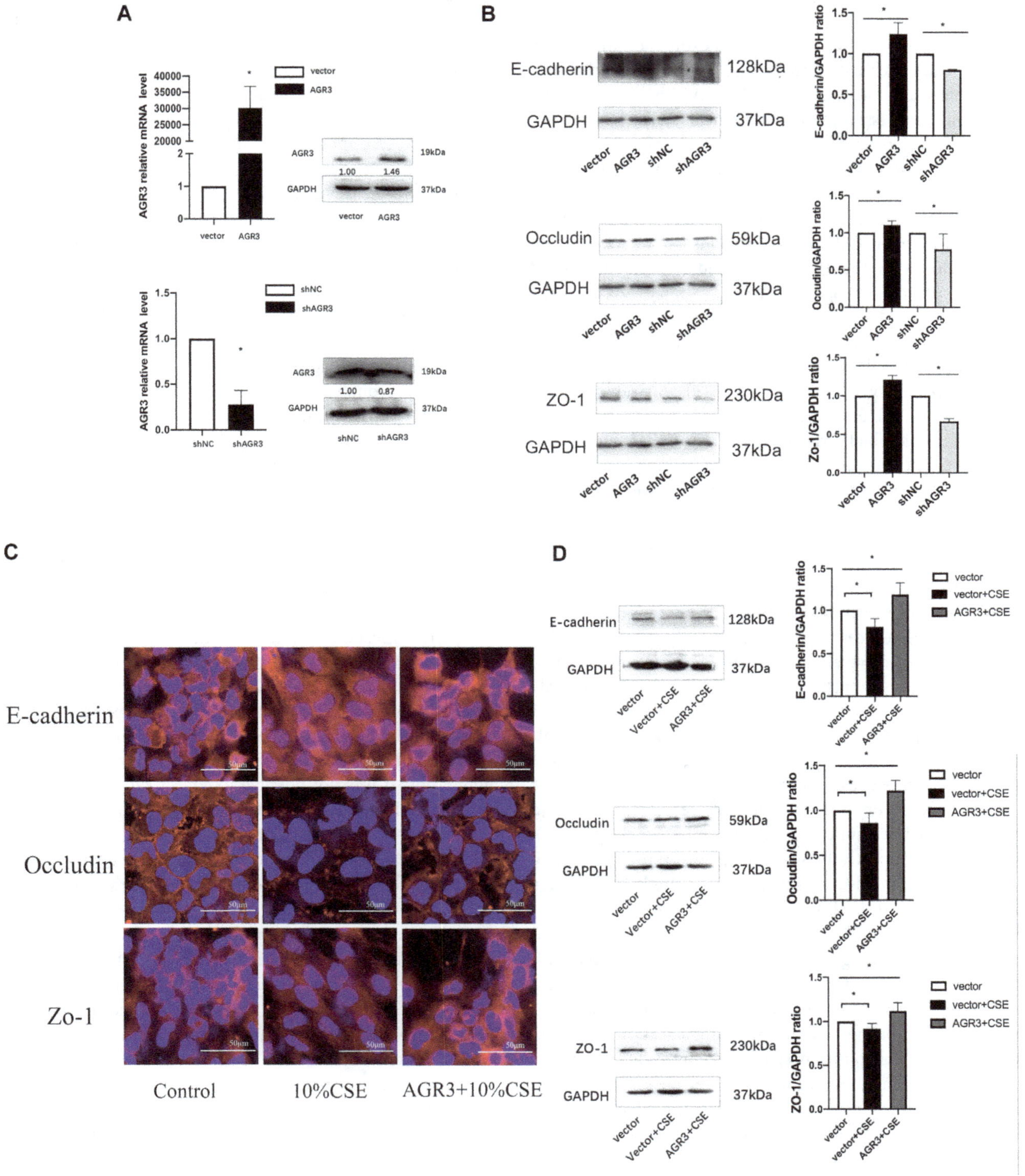

FIGURE 4 | Effects of AGR3 on E-cadherin, Occludin, and ZO-1 expression in BEAS-2B cells. **(A)** AGR3 overexpressed and silenced in BEAS-2B cells. **(B)** Protein expression of occludin, ZO-1, and E-cadherin in AGR3 overexpressed and silenced BEAS-2B cells. **(C)** Immunofluorescence staining for E-cadherin, Occludin, and ZO-1 in Control cells or AGR3 overexpressed cells with 10% CSE exposed for 24 h. **(D)** Western blot analysis for E-cadherin, Occludin, and ZO-1 in Control cells or AGR3 overexpressed cells with 10% CSE exposed for 24 h. Band intensity was quantitated using densitometry. All results are representative of at least three independent experiments. Data are shown as the mean ± SD. *$p < 0.05$ by one-way ANOVA.

et al., 2015) showed AGR3 expressed in the respiratory airway epithelium.

In this study, we first measured AGR3 expression in the lung tissue of patients with frequent COPD exacerbations. Histochemical analysis revealed that AGR3 proteins are predominantly expressed in airway epithelial cells. In addition, AGR3 protein and mRNA expression in lung tissues of patients with frequent COPD exacerbations was significantly lower than that of patients with infrequent COPD exacerbations. Thus, AGR3 protein and gene expression is downregulated in patients with frequent COPD exacerbations.

AGR3 belongs to the PDI family and is a highly related homologue of pro-oncogenic AGR2. Unlike AGR2, the functional role of AGR3 remains unclear. A previous study has shown that AGR3 is expressed in ciliated cells and is required for mucociliary clearance and calcium-modulated ciliary beat frequency (Bonser et al., 2015). Airway epithelial barriers are required for innate immunity as the first line of defense against microbial invasion in the lung. Other studies have shown that COPD at a high risk of exacerbations is associated with excessive microbiota colonization in the lower respiratory track (Miravitlles et al., 1999; Yawn et al., 2013). Thus, we speculated that the downregulation of AGR3 might predict the reduction of airway microbiota clearance or innate immune system, and then inducing lung microbiota easy to be inhaled into low respiratory track and colonized. These event increases the risk for COPD exacerbations.

However, AGR3 have also been detected in no multiciliated organs such colon, stomach, prostate, and liver (Persson et al., 2005; Brychtova et al., 2014). A recent study showed that AGR3 can promote stemness of colorectal cancer by modulating Wnt/β-catenin signaling (Chi et al., 2020). Wnt signaling functions in branching morphogenesis and airway formation in the developing lung, maintains an epithelial cell phenotype, and forms proper cell-cell junctions (Pongracz & Stockley, 2006). The junctional complexes between neighboring cells consist of TJs and AJs, which also maintain airway epithelial barriers (Nawijn et al., 2011). Previous studies have shown that occludin, ZO-1, and E-cadherin expression in bronchial epithelial cells and lung tissue sections from patients with COPD is lower than that in healthy individuals (Heijink et al., 2014; Nishida et al., 2017; Aghapour et al., 2018). The disruption of airway epithelial barriers can promote translocation of inhaled particles into the subepithelial space, thereby inducing airway inflammation and innate immune cell response (Rezaee and Georas, 2014). However, to our knowledge, the effect of AGR3 on airway epithelial junction proteins in patients with frequent COPD exacerbations has not been studied. Histochemical analysis showed that the expression of occludin, ZO-1, and E-cadherin in airway epithelial cells of the lung tissue from patients with frequent COPD exacerbations was lower than that from patients with infrequent COPD exacerbations. These results suggest that the injured junction complexes in the airway epithelium of patients with frequent COPD exacerbations damage the airway epithelial physical barrier and promote microbial invasion, leading to COPD exacerbation.

Despite evidence of the association between AGR3 and Wnt signaling (Chi et al., 2020), there have been no reports about the effects of AGR3 on airway epithelial cell junction protein expression. Our results showed that AGR3 silencing or overexpression can decrease or increase the expression of occludin, ZO-1, and E-cadherin. Furthermore, AGR3 attenuated CSE-induced downregulation of occludin, ZO-1, and E-cadherin expression. AGR family was first found from X. laevis. In X. laevis, the XAG family of genes appear to be important factors during differentiation of the cement gland (Sive et al., 1989), and human AGR genes had shown to be involved in the epithelial barrier function in inflammatory bowel disease (Zheng et al., 2006). Previous studies showed that AGR2 play a crucial role for maintaining the epithelial phenotype by preventing the expression of E-cadherin (Sommerova et al., 2017), and the E-cadherin-mediated adhesion was shown to specifically promote cell signaling toward formation of other junctions (van Roy and Berx, 2008). AGR3 is a highly related homologue of AGR2, and may be involved in the formation of epithelial junctions through maintaining the expression of E-cadherin. Moreover, AGR3 had shown to promote Wnt/β-catenin signaling (Chi et al., 2020) which play a role to form cell-cell junctions. Although the protective mechanism of AGR3 remains unknown, future studies are warranted to identify the molecular role of AGR3 in cellular junction activity and signaling.

A strict selection criterion for enrollment of eligible patients was implemented in our study. To eliminate individual differences within a group, the patients were grouped according to age, sex, lung function, and tumor type. All lung tissues were tumor free and were obtained from areas away from the tumor. Despite our promising results, our study has several limitations. It was not possible to collect sufficient sputum and BALF samples in patients with stable COPD for AGR3 analysis in future studies. Moreover, comparison between the exacerbation stage and stable stage for frequent COPD exacerbations was not performed due to inability to obtain lung tissue sample during the COPD exacerbation stage.

In our previous study, proteomic analysis showed that AGR3 expression in the lung tissues of patients with frequent COPD exacerbations were low. Herein, we showed that the expression of AGR3 and cell junction proteins (occludin, ZO-1, and E-cadherin) in the lung tissues of patients with frequent COPD exacerbations were decreased. AGR3 plays a role in regulating the expression of junction proteins and can revert CSE-induced downregulation of occludin, ZO-1, and E-cadherin. Thus, AGR3 deficiency can disrupt airway epithelial barriers and enhance translocation of inhaled particles into the subepithelial space to induce airway inflammatory responses, which might increase susceptibility to COPD exacerbation.

AUTHOR CONTRIBUTIONS

RY performed the scientific work and conceive the study design, was a major contributor in writing the manuscript. CW analyzed and interpreted the patient data. PS analyzed and interpreted the patient data and edited the figures and tables. SB prepared the manuscript and figures. LZ was a major contributor in designing the study and takes responsibility of the integrity of the work. All authors read and approved the final manuscript.

ACKNOWLEDGMENTS

The authors would like to acknowledge Lili Wang for her technical assistance.

REFERENCES

Adam, P. J., Boyd, R., Tyson, K. L., Fletcher, G. C., Stamps, A., Hudson, L., et al. (2003). Comprehensive Proteomic Analysis of Breast Cancer Cell Membranes Reveals Unique Proteins with Potential Roles in Clinical Cancer. *J. Biol. Chem.* 278 (8), 6482–6489. doi:10.1074/jbc.m210184200

Aghapour, M., Raee, P., Moghaddam, S. J., Hiemstra, P. S., and Heijink, I. H. (2018). Airway Epithelial Barrier Dysfunction in Chronic Obstructive Pulmonary Disease: Role of Cigarette Smoke Exposure. *Am. J. Respir. Cel Mol Biol* 58 (2), 157–169. doi:10.1165/rcmb.2017-0200tr

Bhowmik, A., Seemungal, T. A., Sapsford, R. J., and Wedzicha, J. A. (2000). Relation of Sputum Inflammatory Markers to Symptoms and Lung Function Changes in COPD Exacerbations. *Thorax* 55 (2), 114–120. doi:10.1136/thorax.55.2.114

Bi, H., Zhou, J., Wu, D., Gao, W., Li, L., Yu, L., et al. (2015). Microarray Analysis of Long Non-coding RNAs in COPD Lung Tissue. *Inflamm. Res.* 64 (2), 119–126. doi:10.1007/s00011-014-0790-9

Bonser, L. R., Schroeder, B. W., Ostrin, L. A., Baumlin, N., Olson, J. L., Salathe, M., et al. (2015). The Endoplasmic Reticulum Resident Protein AGR3. Required for Regulation of Ciliary Beat Frequency in the Airway. *Am. J. Respir. Cel Mol Biol* 53 (4), 536–543. doi:10.1165/rcmb.2014-0318oc

Brychtova, V., Zampachova, V., Hrstka, R., Fabian, P., Novak, J., Hermanova, M., et al. (2014). Differential Expression of Anterior Gradient Protein 3 in Intrahepatic Cholangiocarcinoma and Hepatocellular Carcinoma. *Exp. Mol. Pathol.* 96 (3), 375–381. doi:10.1016/j.yexmp.2014.04.002

Chi, J., Zhang, H., Hu, J., Song, Y., Li, J., Wang, L., et al. (2020). AGR3 Promotes the Stemness of Colorectal Cancer via Modulating Wnt/β-Catenin Signalling. *Cell Signal.* 65, 109419. doi:10.1016/j.cellsig.2019.109419

Criner, G. J., Celli, B. R., Brightling, C. E., Agusti, A., Papi, A., Singh, D., et al. (2019). Benralizumab for the Prevention of COPD Exacerbations. *N. Engl. J. Med.* 381 (11), 1023–1034. doi:10.1056/nejmoa1905248

Donaldson, G. C., Seemungal, T. A., Bhowmik, A., and Wedzicha, J. A. (2002). Relationship between Exacerbation Frequency and Lung Function Decline in Chronic Obstructive Pulmonary Disease. *Thorax* 57, 847–852. doi:10.1136/thorax.57.10.847

From the Global Strategy for the Diagnosis, Management and Prevention of COPD, Global Initiative for Chronic Obstructive Lung Disease (GOLD). 2018. Available from: http://goldcopd.org/.

Heijink, I. H., Noordhoek, J. A., Timens, W., van Oosterhout, A. J. M., and Postma, D. S. (2014). Abnormalities in Airway Epithelial junction Formation in Chronic Obstructive Pulmonary Disease. *Am. J. Respir. Crit. Care Med.* 189 (11), 1439–1442. doi:10.1164/rccm.201311-1982le

Hiemstra, P. S., McCray, P. B., Jr, and Bals, R. (2015). The Innate Immune Function of Airway Epithelial Cells in Inflammatory Lung Disease. *Eur. Respir. J.* 45 (4), 1150–1162. doi:10.1183/09031936.00141514

Hurst, J. R., Vestbo, J., Anzueto, A., Locantore, N., Müllerova, H., Tal-Singer, R., et al. (2010). Susceptibility to Exacerbation in Chronic Obstructive Pulmonary Disease. *N. Engl. J. Med.* 363, 1128–1138. doi:10.1056/nejmoa0909883

Ivanova, A. S., Tereshina, M. B., Ermakova, G. V., Belousov, V. V., and Zaraisky, A. G. (2013). Agr Genes, Missing in Amniotes, Are Involved in the Body Appendages Regeneration in Frog Tadpoles. *Sci. Rep.* 3, 1279. doi:10.1038/srep01279

Kelsen, S. G., Duan, X., Ji, R., Perez, O., Liu, C., and Merali, S. (2008). Cigarette Smoke Induces an Unfolded Protein Response in the Human Lung. *Am. J. Respir. Cel Mol Biol* 38 (5), 541–550. doi:10.1165/rcmb.2007-0221oc

Miravitlles, M., Espinosa, C., Fernández-Laso, E., Martos, J. A., Maldonado, J. A., and Gallego, M. (1999). Relationship between Bacterial Flora in Sputum and Functional Impairment in Patients with Acute Exacerbations of COPD. *Chest* 116 (1), 40–46. doi:10.1378/chest.116.1.40

Nawijn, M. C., Hackett, T. L., Postma, D. S., van Oosterhout, A. J. M., and Heijink, I. H. (2011). E-cadherin: Gatekeeper of Airway Mucosa and Allergic Sensitization. *Trends Immunol.* 32 (6), 248–255. doi:10.1016/j.it.2011.03.004

Nishida, K., Brune, K. A., Putcha, N., Mandke, P., O'Neal, W. K., Shade, D., et al. (2017). Cigarette Smoke Disrupts Monolayer Integrity by Altering Epithelial Cell-Cell Adhesion and Cortical Tension. *Am. J. Physiology-Lung Cell Mol. Physiol.* 313 (3), L581–L591. doi:10.1152/ajplung.00074.2017

Pavord, I. D., Chanez, P., Criner, G. J., Kerstjens, H. A. M., Korn, S., Lugogo, N., et al. (2017). Mepolizumab for Eosinophilic Chronic Obstructive Pulmonary Disease. *N. Engl. J. Med.* 377 (17), 1613–1629. doi:10.1056/nejmoa1708208

Persson, S., Rosenquist, M., Knoblach, B., Khosravi-Far, R., Sommarin, M., and Michalak, M. (2005). Diversity of the Protein Disulfide Isomerase Family: Identification of Breast Tumor Induced Hag2 and Hag3 as Novel Members of the Protein Family. *Mol. Phylogenet. Evol.* 36 (3), 734–740. doi:10.1016/j.ympev.2005.04.002

Petek, E., Windpassinger, C., Egger, H., Kroisel, P. M., and Wagner, K. (2000). Localization of the Human Anterior Gradient-2 Gene (AGR2) to Chromosome Band 7p21.3 by Radiation Hybrid Mapping and Fluorescence *In Situ* Hybridisation. *Cytogenet. Cel Genet* 89 (3-4), 141–142. doi:10.1159/000015594

Pongracz, J. E., and Stockley, R. A. (2006). Wnt Signalling in Lung Development and Diseases. *Respir. Res.* 7 (1), 15. doi:10.1186/1465-9921-7-15

Rezaee, F., and Georas, S. N. (2014). Breaking Barriers. New Insights into Airway Epithelial Barrier Function in Health and Disease. *Am. J. Respir. Cel Mol Biol* 50 (5), 857–869. doi:10.1165/rcmb.2013-0541rt

Sive, H. L., Hattori, K., and Weintraub, H. (1989). Progressive Determination during Formation of the Anteroposterior axis in *Xenopus laevis*. *Cell* 58, 171–180. doi:10.1016/0092-8674(89)90413-3

Soler-Cataluña, J. J., and Rodriguez-Roisin, R. (2010). Frequent Chronic Obstructive Pulmonary Disease Exacerbators: How Much Real, How Much Fictitious?. *COPD: J. Chronic Obstructive Pulm. Dis.* 7 (4), 276–284. doi:10.3109/15412555.2010.496817

Sommerova, L., Ondrouskova, E., Vojtesek, B., and Hrstka, R. (2017). Suppression of AGR2 in TGF-β-Induced Smad Regulatory Pathway Mediates Epithelial-Mesenchymal Transition. *BMC cancer* 17 (1), 546. doi:10.1186/s12885-017-3537-5

Spencer, S., and Jones, P. W. GLOBE Study Group (2003). Time Course of Recovery of Health Status Following an Infective Exacerbation of Chronic Bronchitis. *Thorax* 58 (7), 589–593. doi:10.1136/thorax.58.7.589

Sun, P., Ye, R., Wang, C., Bai, S., and Zhao, L. (2019). Identification of Proteomic Signatures Associated with COPD Frequent Exacerbators. *Life Sci.* 230, 1–9. doi:10.1016/j.lfs.2019.05.047

van Roy, F., and Berx, G. (2008). The Cell-Cell Adhesion Molecule E-Cadherin. *Cell. Mol. Life Sci.* 65 (23), 3756–3788. doi:10.1007/s00018-008-8281-1

Wang, C., Xu, J., Yang, L., Xu, Y., Zhang, X., Bai, C., et al. (2018). Prevalence and Risk Factors of Chronic Obstructive Pulmonary Disease in China (The China Pulmonary Health [CPH] Study): a National Cross-Sectional Study. *The Lancet* 391 (10131), 1706–1717. doi:10.1016/s0140-6736(18)30841-9

Wang, Z., Zhao, J., Wang, T., Du, X., and Xie, J. (2019). Fine-particulate Matter Aggravates Cigarette Smoke Extract-Induced Airway Inflammation via Wnt5a-ERK Pathway in COPD. *Copd* Vol. 14 (14), 979–994. doi:10.2147/copd.s195794

Yawn, B., Li, Y., Tian, H., Zhang, J., Arcona, S., and Kahler, K. H. (2013). Inhaled Corticosteroid Use in Patients with Chronic Obstructive Pulmonary Disease and the Risk of Pneumonia: a Retrospective Claims Data Analysis. *Copd* 8, 295–304. doi:10.2147/copd.s42366

Zheng, W., Rosenstiel, P., Huse, K., Sina, C., Valentonyte, R., Mah, N., et al. (2006). Evaluation of AGR2 and AGR3 as Candidate Genes for Inflammatory Bowel Disease. *Genes Immun.* 7 (1), 11–18. doi:10.1038/sj.gene.6364263

9

Assessment of Lentiviral Vector Mediated CFTR Correction in Mice using an Improved Rapid *in vivo* Nasal Potential Difference Measurement Protocol

P. Cmielewski[1,2,3], J. Delhove[1,2,3], M. Donnelley[1,2,3] and D. Parsons[1,2,3]*

[1]Respiratory and Sleep Medicine, Women's and Children's Hospital, Adelaide, SA, Australia, [2]Robinson Research Institute, University of Adelaide, Adelaide, SA, Australia, [3]Adelaide Medical School, University of Adelaide, Adelaide, SA, Australia

***Correspondence:**
P. Cmielewski
patricia.l.cmielewski@adelaide.edu.au

Cystic Fibrosis (CF) is caused by a defect in the CF transmembrane conductance regulator (*CFTR*) gene responsible for epithelial ion transport. Nasal potential difference (PD) measurement is a well established diagnostic technique for assessing the efficacy of therapies in CF patients and animal models. The aim was to establish a rapid nasal PD protocol in mice and quantify the efficacy of lentiviral (LV) vector-based *CFTR* gene therapy. Anaesthetised wild-type (WT) and CF mice were non-surgically intubated and nasal PD measurements were made using a range of buffer flow rates. Addition of the cAMP agonist, isoproterenol, to the buffer sequence was then examined. The optimised rapid PD technique was then used to assess CFTR function produced by second and third generation LV-*CFTR* vectors. V5 epitope tagged-CFTR in nasal tissue was identified by immunohistochemistry. When intubated, mice tolerated higher flow rates. Isoproterenol could discriminate between WT and CF mice. Improved chloride transport was observed for the second and third generation LV-CFTR vectors, with up to 60% correction of the cAMP-driven chloride response towards WT. V5-CFTR was located in ciliated epithelial cells. The rapid PD technique enables improved functional assessment of the bioelectrical ion transport defect for both current and potential CF therapies.

Keywords: gene therapy, lentival vector, potential difference measurement, CFTR, mouse models

INTRODUCTION

Cystic fibrosis (CF) is one of the most common autosomal recessive genetic disorders in the Caucasian population, with the majority of the mortality and morbidity due to lung disease. CF is caused by a defect in the CF transmembrane conductance regulator (*CFTR*) gene, which results in abnormal CFTR protein levels. CFTR is classified as an adenosine triphosphate (ATP)-binding cassette transporter, and transports chloride (Cl^-) and bicarbonate ions across the membranes of cells predominantly in the lungs, liver, pancreas, intestinal tract, reproductive tract and skin (Boucher, 2002; Davis, 2006; Quinton, 2008). The CFTR protein is primarily located on the apical surface of epithelial cell membranes, where the chloride ion channel transports salt and fluid across the epithelium to maintain surface hydration (i.e., transepithelial transport) (Riordan et al., 1989; Welsh et al., 1992).

CFTR electrolyte transport can be measured electrically as the transepithelial potential difference (PD). This technique involves using a sensitive high-impedance voltmeter to measure the voltage between a fluid-filled sensing electrode in the nose and a reference electrode placed elsewhere into the body (Knowles et al., 1981). The use of a fluid-filled electrode enables solutions that alter ion channel conductances to be introduced into the nasal cavity, and the resulting electrical responses related to specific ion channels can then be assessed.

As a consequence of the Cl^- defect in CF airways, a raised PD measurement can be used as a diagnostic tool (Middleton et al., 1994). The electrical characteristic of a CF airway is a greater negative (hyperpolarized) potential across the nasal airway at baseline, a large depolarization (more positive) in response to the sodium (Na^+) channel blocker amiloride, and a reduced or absent response to the effect of a chloride-free environment compared to normal and heterozygous/carriers for CF (Knowles et al., 1981). There is also an impaired response to Cl^- stimulation in the presence of the β-adrenergic agonist isoproterenol (Iso) in the nasal airways of CF patients (Wilschanski et al., 2006; Bienvenu et al., 2010), a finding also noted in the lower airways in both paediatric and adult CF populations (Davies et al., 2005).

The ability to accurately measure the PD *in vivo* is particularly important when assessing therapies that alter CFTR, such as airway gene therapies that deliver a correct copy of *CFTR* to airway cells (De Boeck et al., 2013). To determine the effectiveness of a lentiviral (LV) gene therapy in live intact CF mice, we have used a well-established transepithelial PD technique in the nasal airways, originally based on the method described by Parsons et al. (2000), and subsequently used in a longitudinal study to measure the persistence of CFTR lentiviral airway gene therapy (Cmielewski et al., 2014). A range of other LV gene therapy studies for CF have utilised PD measurements as an outcome measure (Limberis et al., 2002; Stocker et al., 2009; Alton et al., 2017; Reyne et al., 2021).

The PD method identifies defects in the Cl^- transport levels across nasal epithelia by delivering a range of Krebs-Ringer Buffers (KRB) in a multi-step process beginning with normal basal KRB, and then sequentially adding amiloride and then low chloride (LC) KRB under amiloride. It can be used to assess the differences between normal and CF CFTR channel function by measuring Na^+ hyperabsorption using baseline KRB and the response to the Na^+ channel blocker, amiloride. An electrical gradient produced by perfusing LC KRB is required to assess Cl^- movement across the airways, and the change or lack of change in PD can be a determinant of CFTR function.

CFTR can also regulate other membrane proteins such as the up-regulation of an alternate outwardly rectifying Cl^- channel (Egan et al., 1992; Gabriel et al., 1993) and the inwardly rectifying renal outer medullary potassium channel (Hryciw and Guggino, 2000). The introduction of cyclic adenosine monophosphate (cAMP) agonists, ATP or CFTR inhibitors in the perfusion fluid sequence can aid in not only distinguishing between CF and non-CF, but also quantify the success of a functional CFTR treatment (Rowe et al., 2011). However, the use of an increased number of KRBs means that fluid delivery to a mouse's nasal airways can accumulate both in the nasal passages and the lungs, disrupting nasal PD readings and causing respiratory difficulties. To attempt to mitigate these interferences we have previously used small volumes and slow flow rates. However, the result has been that each solution is slow to achieve a plateau, which typically takes up to 20 min per solution (e.g., three solutions can take up to 60 min). As a result, we cannot use as many perfusion choices as desired without dramatically increasing study time, and increasing the risk of adverse animal outcomes. Together, all of these issues can compromise the characterisation of channel function *in vivo*. An ideal system would allow more rapid perfusion flow rates to increase the number of KRB solutions that can be accommodated in a nasal PD measurement run, such as the β-agonist Iso, enabling assessment of CFTR function by cAMP-driven Cl^- transport without causing respiratory or anaesthesia issues.

This study had two objectives. Firstly, we examined whether the use of non-surgical intubation to maintain a patent airway throughout the PD procedure would allow higher flow rates and additional fluid perfusion solutions to be delivered, enabling improved characterisation. Secondly, we determined the ability to detect the functional effects of second and third generation LV-*CFTR* gene addition vectors in CF murine airways using this new rapid nasal PD protocol in mice.

METHODS

All animal studies were approved by the Animal Ethics Committee's of the University of Adelaide (M-2015–100, M-2015–101, M-2017–083) and the Women's and Children's Health Network, Adelaide (AE1007 and AE1008). We first compared our standard nasal PD perfusion flow rate with increased flow rates in intubated wild-type (WT) mice to determine the optimum flow rate. That optimal flow rate was then applied to measuring the nasal PD in WT and CF mice using our standard KRB solutions. The addition of the β-agonist, Iso, in the KRB sequence was then examined in both WT and CF mice, using the newly optimised intubation assisted rapid PD method, to assess the benefits provided by this additional perfusion solution.

The new rapid PD method was next tested by assessing the success of a second generation nasal LV-*CFTR* gene addition treatment in CF mice to correct the electrophysiological defect and determine its repeatability. The efficacy of a more clinically-relevant third generation LV-*CFTR* vector with and without an epitope tag was also examined.

Nasal Potential Difference

The PD measurement system was configured as previously described (**Supplementary Figure 1**) (Cmielewski et al., 2010; Cmielewski et al., 2014). Briefly, the end of a fine microloader pipette tip (Cat #5242 956.003, Eppendorf™, Germany) was inserted into one nostril of an anaesthetised mouse to a depth of 2.5–3 mm, and a fluid circuit was created by attaching the pipette tip to fine polyethylene tubing (PE-10, Cat # I-10338, SteriHealth, Australia) connected to agarose bridges (3% w/v in

TABLE 1 | Primer and V5 sequences used to PCR amplify the pCCL-EF1α-V5-CFTR vector.

V5-forward	ggatagcacc*agcggcggcggcggcagcggcggcagc*atgcagaggtcgcctctggaaaaggccag
V5-reverse	*cgccgccgc*tggtgctatccaggcccagcagcgggttcggaatcggtttgcc**catggtggc**ggtctctcacgacacctgaaatggaagaaaaaaactttgaaccactg

0.9% NaCl), and to calomel electrodes (Hg_2Cl_2 in 3 M KCl, Cole-Parmer Instruments, United States). The reference needle-electrode was inserted subcutaneously into the abdomen of the mouse. The resulting electrical signal was displayed in millivolts (mV) using an Iso-Millivolt meter (World Precision Instruments, United States) and recorded using a PASPort Sensor (Pasco Scientific, United States) connected to a laptop using DataStudio Version 10 (Pasco Scientific, United States).

Flow Rates

Normal C57Bl/6 wild-type (WT) and knock-out CF (*cftr*$^{(tm1unc)}$-Tg (FABp-CFTR)/1Jaw) mice (2–6 months of age) were anaesthetised with an intraperitoneal injection of a mix of medetomidine (1 mg/kg) and ketamine (75 mg/kg). To permit normal breathing during the increased rate of solution perfusion the mice were non-surgically intubated with an 20 G cannula (BD Insyte™ i. v. cannula) and fibre optic light as previously described (Cmielewski et al., 2017). Following all recovery procedures, anaesthesia was reversed using atipamezole (1 mg/kg), and mice were kept warm on a heating mat or in a pre-warmed incubator until fully recovered.

We first examined the feasibility of infusion rates of 10, 20 and 50 µl/min and compared these to our standard 1 µl/min in the same animal, using normal basal (B) and LC KRB to determine an optimal flow rate in WT mice (B, LC; n = 4). The sequence of infusion rates was performed in the same animal from 1 to 50 µl/min (n = 2) and in the reverse order from 50 to 1 µl/min (n = 2) to eliminate fluid bias.

The standard slow infusion rate (1 µl/min, non-intubated) was then compared to the optimal infusion rate (20 µl/min; see Results) in both WT and CF mice, using the addition of the Na^+ channel blocker amiloride (A) and the cAMP driven Iso to the fluid sequence (B, B + A, LC + A; n = 9). However, the length of anaesthesia and fluid overload that occurred when using the 1 µl/min infusion rate resulted in rejection of the nasal PD recordings due to poor signal quality. Therefore the final solution of LC + A + Iso was only compared at the higher infusion rate group in which all mice were intubated (B, B + A, LC + A, LC + A + Iso; n = 5–9). When PD measurements were repeated in an animal, a minimum gap of one week was used between procedures to enable the airway epithelium to recover from any physical disturbances that may have occurred due to previous placement of the recording/perfusion cannula.

Cloning of the V5 Epitope Tag Into the CCL-CFTR Vector

PCR amplification of the third generation lentiviral backbone, CCL-EF1α-CFTR, was performed using primers containing a Kozak sequence (bold), the V5 amino acid sequence (underlined), and a serine/glycine polypeptide linker (italics). The resulting vector contained an N-terminus V5-tagged CFTR whose expression was driven by the human elongation factor-alpha (EF1α) promoter. The V5 tag is used as a surrogate marker of CFTR as immunological detection of CFTR is generally very poor, whereas antibodies directed against the V5 epitope have high binding affinity and specificity (**Table 1**). The PCR parameters were: initial denaturation at 98°C for 40 s, followed by 18 cycles of 98°C for 20 s, 70–65°C (−0.3°C/cycle) for 20 s, 72°C for 5 min 30 s followed by a further 20 cycles of 98°C for 20 s, 65°C for 20 s, 72°C for 5 min 30 s, and a final elongation step of 72°C for 10 min. PCR product was fused using In-Fusion cloning to generate the pCCL-EF1α-V5-CFTR vector (designated CCL-V5-CFTR).

Vector Production and Titering

Three LV-CFTR vectors pseudotyped with the vesicular stomatitis virus carrying the glycoprotein G (VSV-G) were produced by a range of large or small scale production methods, utilising the transient transfection of HEK293T cells, depending on experimental needs.

For the repeatability experiment, a second generation HIV-1 based (WT 5′ LTR) LV-CFTR under the EF1α promoter was produced by calcium phosphate coprecipitation in large-scale multilayer cell factors with a five plasmid trans-activating regulatory protein (Tat) dependent system, as previously described (Rout-Pitt et al., 2018). LV vector was diluted in FreeStyle™ 293 Expression Medium (Cat # 12338018, Life Technologies Corp, United States). The titre was determined by transducing NIH 3T3 cells, followed by quantitative real time PCR (CFX, BioRad, Australia) of proviral genomic DNA obtained after 4 weeks of culturing the transduced cells to dilute out potential contaminating plasmid DNA (Anson et al., 2007).

For the comparison experiments, small-scale production of third generation LV, either with or without a V5 tag using a CCL backbone (partially deleted 5′ LTR fused to CMV enhancer/promoter) under the EF1α promoter was performed as previously described (Buckley et al., 2015). Transcription in third generation vectors is initiated by the chimeric CMV promoter within the viral LTR (Dull et al., 1998). A deletion in the 3′LTR of the third generation vector abolishes the probability of full-length viral mRNA being produced and packaged following initial transduction (Zufferey et al., 1998), a significant safety feature that is currently required for any clinical vector. This four plasmid, tat-independent system consisted of 50 µg transfer plasmid, 32.5 µg pMDLg/RRE (gag-pol), 17.5 µg pMD2. G (VSV-G env), and 17.5 µgpRSV-Rev. LV vector was resuspended in OptiMem (Cat # 31985070, Life Technologies Corp, United States). Vectors were titered using a p24 ELISA kit

(Cat # 080111, ZeptoMetrix, United States) as per manufacturer's instructions using dilutions of 10^{-8}.

Immunocytochemistry for V5

The presence of the V5 tag in the third generation CFTR vector was validated in cell culture via immunocytochemistry (ICC) prior to delivery to animals. HEK293T cells were transduced with VSV-G pseudotyped CCL-V5-CFTR lentivirus. Samples were fixed in 4% paraformaldehyde for 10 min at room temperature before being washed in PBS. Cells were permeabilised by incubation in 1% bovine serum albumin (BSA) in PBS containing 0.1% Triton-X 100 for 10 min at room temperature. Cells were washed in PBS and blocked with 1% BSA in PBS for 1 h at room temperature. Samples were incubated in rabbit anti-V5 antibody (1:600) (Cat # 13,202, Cell Signalling Technologies, United States) diluted in 1% BSA + PBS +0.1% Tween-20 (PBST) overnight at 4°C. Samples were washed with 0.1% PBST before being incubated in donkey anti-rabbit Alexa Fluor 488 (1:600) (Cat # ab150073, Abcam, United Kingdom) diluted in 1% BSA + 0.1% PBST for 1 h at room temperature. Cells were washed in 0.1% PBST before incubation in DAPI for 5 min followed by rinsing in 0.1% PBST. The presence of V5 immunofluorescence was confirmed using a Nikon Eclipse Ts2 microscope with NIS-Elements imaging software Version 5.20.00.

Nasal LV-CFTR Delivery

In all CFTR gene delivery studies, mice were anaesthetised as above and suspended by their front incisors and a single bolus of 4 µl 0.3% lysophosphatidylcholine in phosphate buffered saline (PBS) was pipetted into the right nostril. One hour later, 20 µl (2 × 10 µl aliquots) of LV-CFTR was delivered to the same nostril in the same manner. Anaesthesia was reversed, animals were allowed to recover, and the rapid PD method was tested at baseline (pre-LV delivery) and at least one week after LV-CFTR delivery.

A second generation, VSV-G pseudotyped LV vector expressing CFTR from the constitutively active EF1α physiological promoter was produced and resuspended in FreeStyle™ media and tested in CF mice (n = 9). The repeatability of this new rapid PD method was tested at baseline, one and two weeks after LV-CFTR delivery. We then examined the more clinically relevant CCL third generation LV vector resuspended in OptiMem. Vectors with and without a V5 epitope tag (n = 5) were tested to evaluate histological detection of the tag as a surrogate for CFTR presence. PD assessment was performed one week after nasal administration, and compared to baseline.

After the last PD measurement mice were humanely killed by carbon dioxide asphyxiation. Following decapitation the fur was removed and heads were placed into 10% formalin for at least 24 h, and the bone was decalcified with 25% EDTA at 37°C for 2–3 days. Samples were transferred to 70% ethanol and, once the lower jaw was removed, the heads were sliced into several standard locations (Mery et al., 1994; Kremer et al., 2007), paraffin embedded and 5 µm sections mounted onto 0.85% 3-aminopropyltriethoxysilane (Cat #A36487, Sigma-Merck, United States) coated glass microscope slides prior to V5 epitope immunostaining.

Immunohistochemistry for V5

Sections of mouse nasal samples and archival rat lungs treated with CCL-V5-CFTR lentivirus as a positive control (McIntyre et al., 2018; Reyne et al., 2021) were deparaffinised by immersion in xylene twice for 10 min. Slides were brought to water through decreasing concentrations of ethanol with a final rinse in distilled water. Antigen retrieval was performed by heating slides in a 10 mM sodium citrate buffer at pH 6.0 until boiling followed by simmering for 20 min. Once cooled to room temperature, slides were rinsed in 0.05% PBST, permeabilised in 0.3% Triton-X 100 in PBS for 10 min and again rinsed with 0.05% PBST. Sections were blocked for 1 h at room temperature with 1% BSA in PBS and then incubated with goat anti-V5 primary antibody (1:300) (Cat # ab95038, Abcam, United Kingdom) diluted in 1% BSA + 0.1% PBST overnight at 4°C. Tissue sections were rinsed in 0.05% PBST and incubated in donkey anti-goat Alexa Fluor 568 (1:400) (Cat # ab175704, Abcam, United Kingdom) made in 1% BSA + 0.1% PBST for 1 h in the dark. Samples were washed with 0.05% PBST, counterstained with DAPI for approximately 10 min, washed again, and mounted with ProLong™ Diamond antifade mounting media (Cat #P36961, Life Technologies, United States). Negative controls of mouse nasal tissue that did not receive the CCL-V5-CFTR vector were included, as well as reagent only, and secondary only antibody controls. Slides were visualised for the presence of V5 under an Olympus BX51 research-grade optical microscope DIC with AnalySIS imaging software, with ciliated cells identified based on their distinct morphology.

Statistics

Statistical analyses were performed using GraphPad Prism Version 8 (GraphPad Software Inc., United States) with statistical significance set at p = 0.05 and power ≥ 0.8. All data are expressed as mean ± SEM, unless stated elsewhere. Standard paired or unpaired t-tests were performed between pre- and post-data, or when there were two treatment groups, respectively. Multiple treatment groups were analysed by one-way analysis of variance (ANOVA) or repeated measures (RM ANOVA) as appropriate, with post-test multiple comparisons. If data failed normality, non-parametric methods were used.

RESULTS

Nasal Potential Difference Flow Rates

When intubated, the mice tolerated the higher flow rates (10, 20, 50 µl/min) without any incidents. For the higher flow rates there was no significant difference in PD measurements (**Figure 1**) for Basal, LC KRB, or the change in nasal PD (ΔPD) in normal mice under LC conditions, when compared to our standard infusion rate of 1 µl/min (n.s., RM ANOVA, n = 4).

The optimal flow rate for rapid and consistently stabilised PD recordings was the 20 µl/min infusion rate, which resulted in a

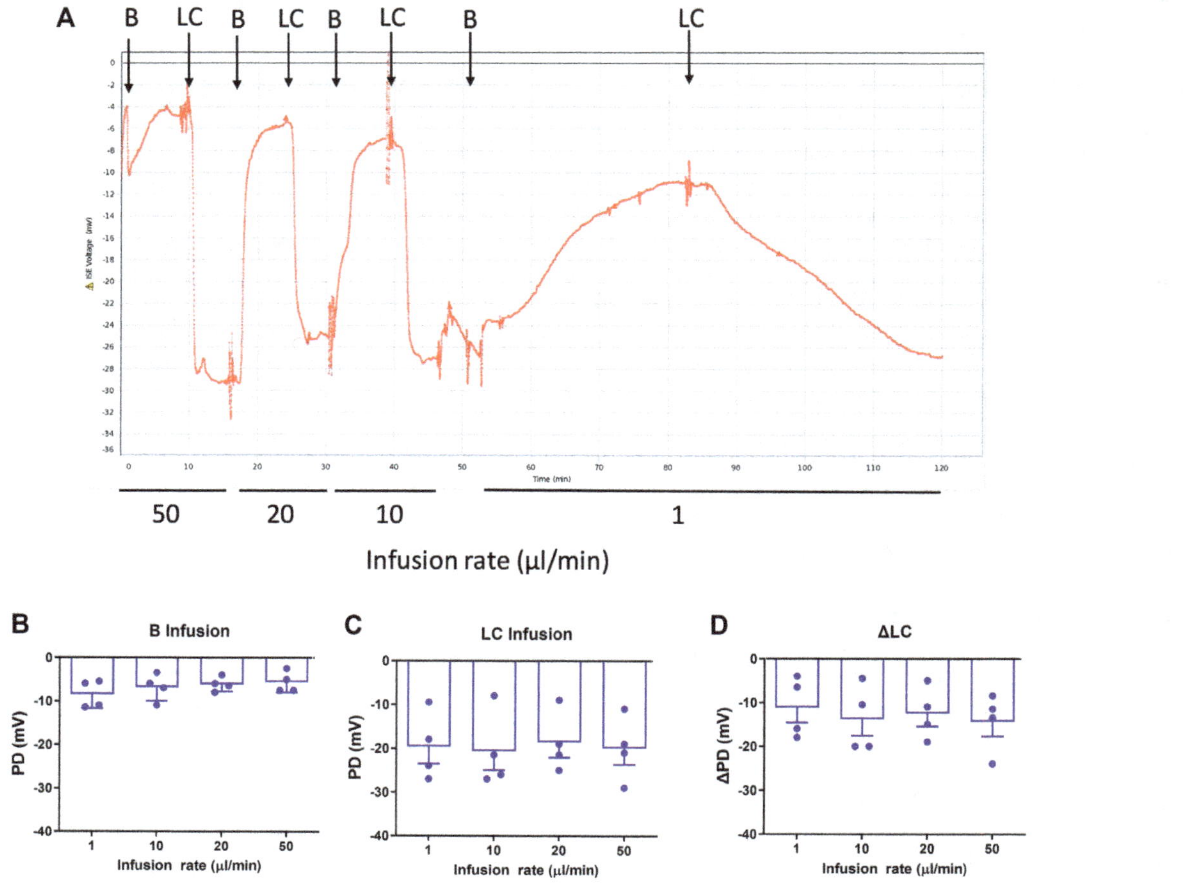

FIGURE 1 | Nasal PD measurements at different infusion rates in WT mice. **(A)** Typical nasal PD trace showing the reproducibility of the rapid PD method (here, alternating basal and low chloride perfusions) in the same animal. The mean response following **(B)** Basal (B), **(C)** Low chloride (LC) KRB and **(D)** the difference between LC and Basal (ΔLC), n.s. Dunnett's RM ANOVA, mean±SEM, $n = 4$.

typical mean reduction in PD assessment time for each solution to reach a stable plateau averaging from 16.4 min/solution (range of 12–32 min), to 6.5 min/solution (range of 5–12 min), i.e., 2.5 times faster. This reduction in time allowed for more KRB solutions to be added in the sequence without health or welfare issues related to potential morbidities associated with lengthy anaesthesia.

There was no significant difference in nasal PD when the 20 µl flow rate was compared to our standard 1 µl/min rate for both WT and CF mice with the addition of amiloride in the KRB sequence (**Figure 2**). When performed at the 20 µl flow rate the cAMP agonist isoproterenol could also be included in the KRB sequence for both WT (**Figure 3A**) and CF mice (**Figure 3B**) without any fluid overload issues or anaesthesia related morbidities. CF and WT mice displayed significantly different nasal ΔPD responses to the addition of amiloride in basal KRB ($p < 0.0001$; **Figure 3C**) and LC + A perfusion ($p < 0.0001$; **Figure 3D**). The addition of isoproterenol under the LC + A perfusion was also significantly different between CF and WT mice ($p < 0.01$; **Figure 3E**). These results demonstrate that the rapid method can characterise the altered nasal ion channel function in the CF animals.

Nasal LV-CFTR Delivery

Following the successful introduction of the β-adrenergic agonist, isoproterenol, to the KRB sequence, we next tested if our new rapid PD technique could detect whether *CFTR* gene delivery corrected the electrophysiological defect in CF mouse nasal airways towards a more normal phenotype, and whether the measurements were repeatable. Second generation LV-*CFTR* vector was diluted in FreeStyle™ Medium, and delivered at a titre of 5.3 x10^8 TU/ml. A typical nasal PD trace of a mouse that received LV-*CFTR* after 1 week is shown in **Figure 4A**. When compared to baseline there was a significant depolarisation in ΔPD response to amiloride one week after delivery of LV-*CFTR*, but this was not detected at week two (**Figure 4B**, $p < 0.05$, RM ANOVA, $n = 9$). In contrast, a significant hyperpolarisation (more negative response towards wildtype) to overall Cl^- transport was present after 2 weeks (**Figure 4C**, $p < 0.01$, RM ANOVA, $n = 9$), corresponding to an approximate 32% correction. Importantly, a significant hyperpolarisation to the isoproterenol cAMP driven Cl^-

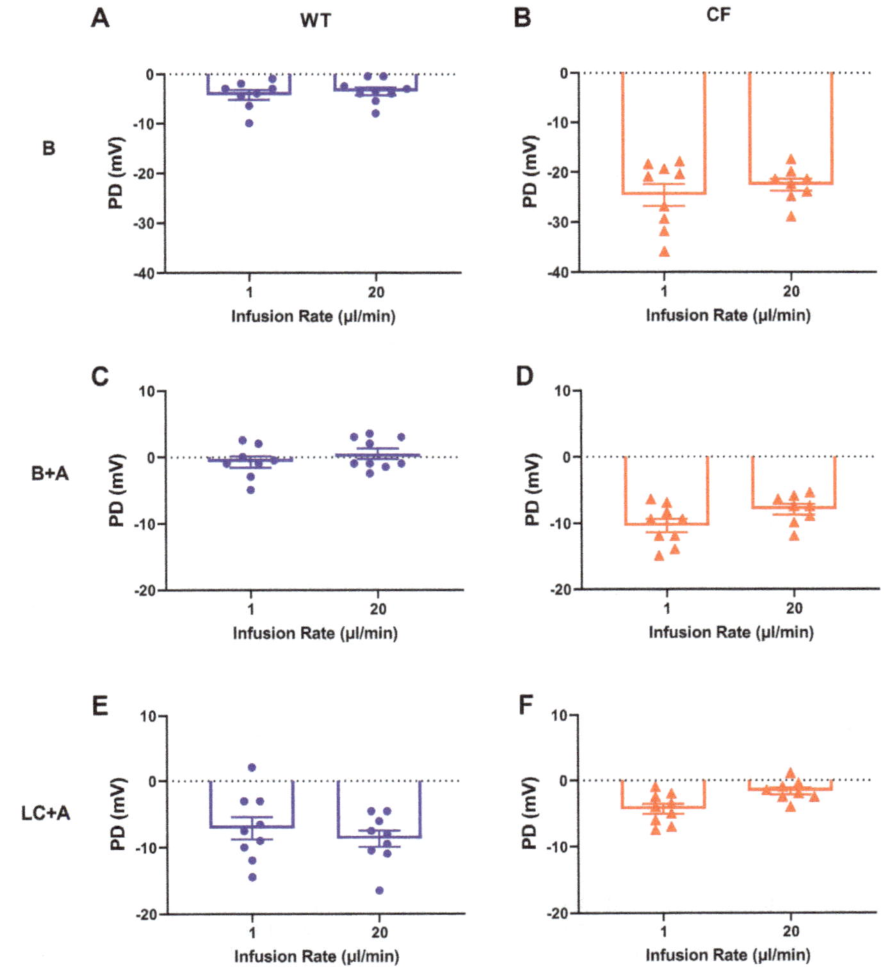

FIGURE 2 | Characteristic nasal PD response of **(A,C,E)** WT (blue circle) and **(B,D,F)** CF mice (red triangle) after 1 and 20 µl/min performed 1 week apart following an infusion of basal KRB **(top panels)**, basal + amiloride (B + A) **(middle panels)** and Low chloride + amiloride (LC + A) **(bottom panels)**. No significant difference (n.s.) between 1 vs. 20 µl/min infusion rate, paired t-test, mean±SEM, $n = 9$).

transport was present at both 1 and 2 weeks (**Figure 4D**, $p < 0.01$ and $p < 0.05$, respectively, RM ANOVA, $n = 9$), which corresponds to approximately 60% correction towards a normal wildtype bioelectrical functional response. These data suggest the chloride ion transport in CF mouse nasal airways was shifted towards a wildtype response following delivery of a second generation LV-*CFTR* vector.

Third Generation LV-CFTR Vectors

To move towards a gene therapy for human CF airway disease a more clinically relevant LV vector was developed. Third generation CCL-*CFTR* vectors were constructed with and without a V5 tag (~2.9×10^9 vp/ml).

There was no difference in the ΔPD to the sodium channel blocker amiloride for all constructs 1 week after LV-*CFTR* delivery compared to baseline (**Figure 5A**) as expected. At one week, there was a hyperpolarisation of the ΔPD chloride response in the presence of amiloride however this did not reach significance for both third generation LV vectors (**Figure 5B**, n. s, paired t-test, $n = 5$).

In the mice that received the third generation CCL-V5-*CFTR* vector, but not the CCL-*CFTR* vector, the addition of the β-agonist Iso in the KRB sequence resulted in a significant change towards a normal bioelectrical response (**Figure 5C**, $p < 0.05$, paired t-test, $n = 5$). Furthermore there was no significant difference between the CCL-*CFTR* and CCL-V5-*CFTR* versions (n. s, unpaired t-test, $n = 5$), suggesting that the V5 epitope does not compromise exogenous CFTR functionality.

Immunocytochemistry and Immunohistochemistry Validation and Detection of V5

Following cloning of the V5 epitope tag into the CCL-*CFTR* lentiviral vector, detection of the V5 tag was performed by ICC. HEK293T cells were transduced with the modified V5-containing lentiviral vector, and the V5 tag was clearly detected using a V5-specific antibody (**Figure 6A**). V5 was detected in ciliated cells in nasal histological sections in mice that received the third generation CCL-V5-*CFTR*

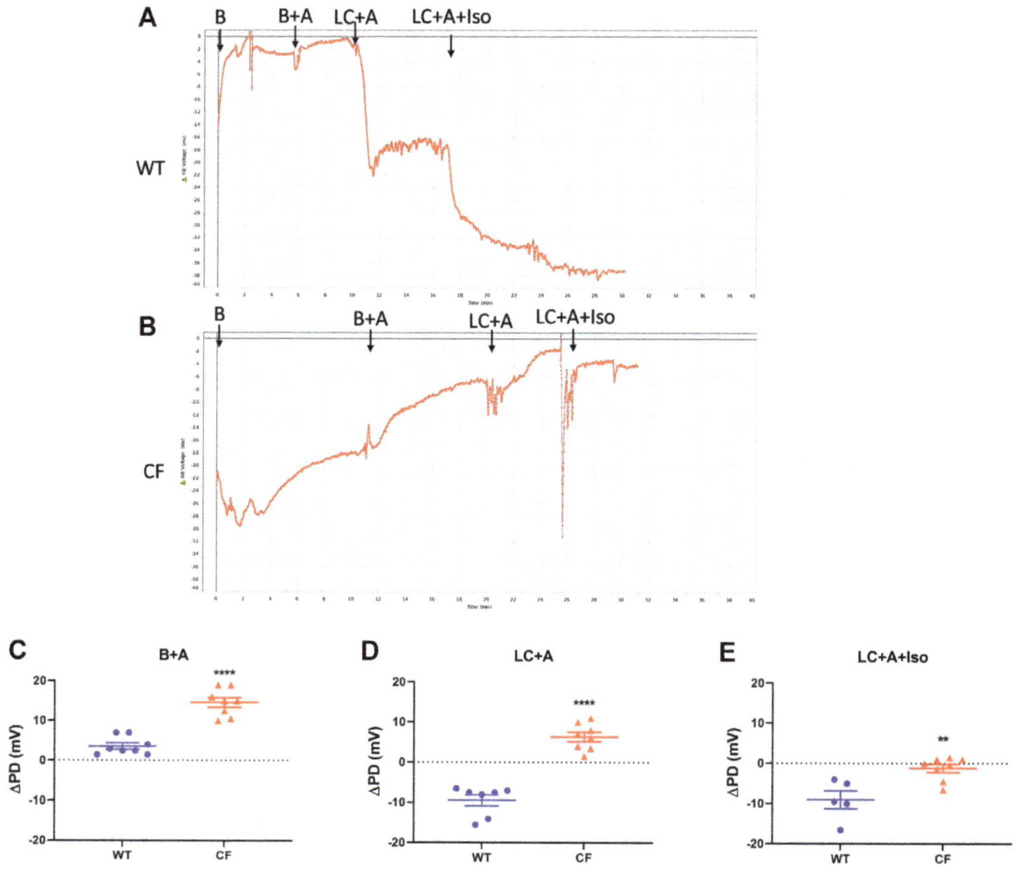

FIGURE 3 | Nasal PD trace of **(A)** WT and **(B)** CF mice following infusion of KRB basal (B), basal + amiloride (B + A), Low chloride + amiloride (LC + A) and Low chloride + amiloride + isoproterenol (LC + A + Iso). ΔPD in WT (blue circle) and CF (red triangle) mice after **(C)** the addition of amiloride (B + A), **(D)** Low chloride (LC + A) and **(E)** the agonist isoproterenol (LC + A + Iso) into the sequence at the 20 μl/min infusion rate (**$p < 0.01$, ****$p < 0.0001$, t-test, mean±SEM, n = 5–9).

vector, validating its suitability to be used as a surrogate marker for CFTR protein detection (**Figure 6B**). Archival samples of rat lung transduced with the same vector were used as a positive control for immunohistochemistry (IHC), as they contained V5 staining within several bronchioles (**Supplementary Figure 2**). There was no V5 detected in any negative control samples from untreated CF animals.

DISCUSSION

In this paper we describe a rapid nasal PD method in a CF mouse model, in conjunction with non-surgical lung intubation, which provides greatly improved nasal PD measurement capability compared to previously described techniques (Cmielewski et al., 2014). Use of this approach eliminated potential adverse effects due to fluid accumulation in the lungs, and improved animal PD assessment throughput four-fold.

In other studies a slow rate of fluid perfusion, in conjunction with intubation assisted by oxygen supplementation with the mouse at a 15° head down tilt angle, has shown to be successful, however their approach was limited due to anaesthesia constraints (MacDonald et al., 2008). Other researchers have also used buffer solutions containing compounds that cannot be used clinically, low buffer infusion rates that could restrict their timing/recording of solutions, and different anaesthetics and body orientations (da Cunha et al., 2016). In contrast, in the present study we ensured that all infusions came to a steady-state plateau for accurate PD measurement, and the faster infusion rate allowed for the overall anaesthesia time to be reduced.

The faster infusion rate also allowed for the inclusion of additional perfusion solutions to further discriminate specific changes in the bioelectrical defect responsible for CF. Use of the β-agonist isoproterenol in the perfusion sequence allowed for measurement of cAMP directed chloride transport. Isoproterenol KRB is a clinically relevant perfusion used for phenotyping CF patients and for measuring the success of new treatments such as CFTR modulators (Pranke et al., 2017). Our rapid PD technique was also highly reproducible, enabling the same animal to have multiple assessments over time, which is a prerequisite for testing and monitoring CFTR therapies such as gene or cell addition, new CFTR modulators, or new drug treatments. Together, all of our changes have improved the quality and speed of nasal PD assessment.

We also demonstrated successful gene correction of the electrophysiological bioelectrical defect in the nasal airways of CF mice using a LV-CFTR under the non-viral human physiological EF1α promoter. Although this new vector was applied at approximately 40x lower titre than our previous LV-CFTR vector

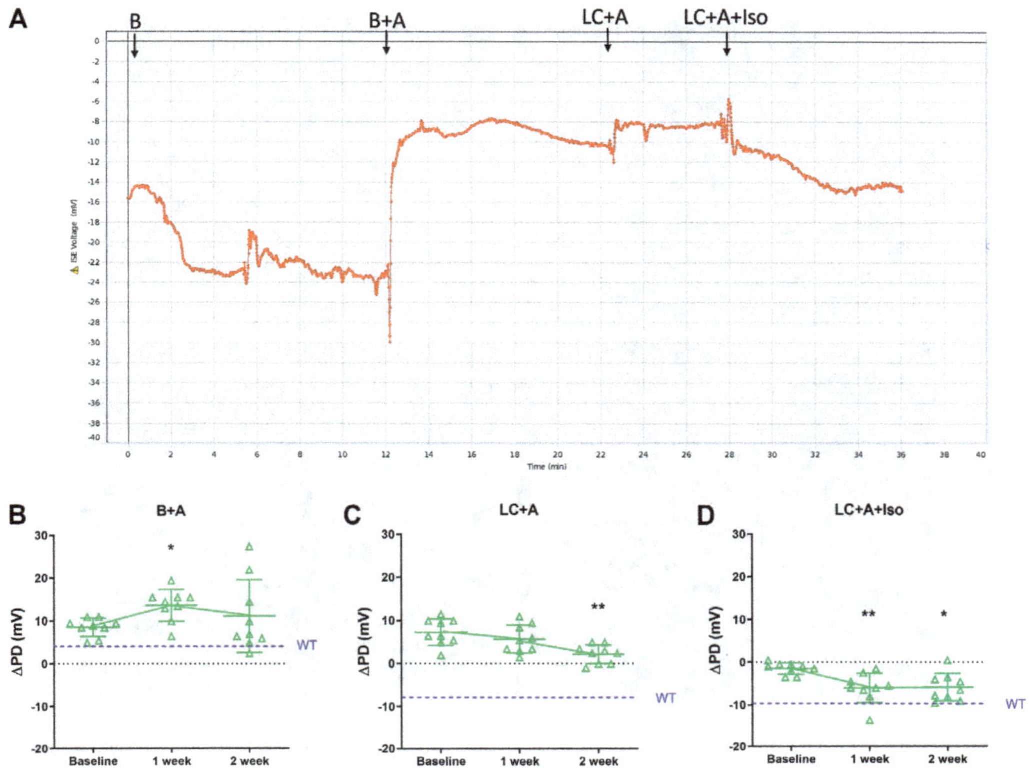

FIGURE 4 | (A) Nasal PD trace of a CFTR treated CF mouse following infusion of KRB basal (B), basal + amiloride (B + A), Low chloride + amiloride (LC + A) and Low chloride + amiloride + isoproterenol (LC + A + Iso). ΔPD in CF mice before (Baseline), 1 and 2 weeks after second generation LV-*CFTR* gene addition to nasal airways following **(B)** Basal + Amiloride (B + A), **(C)** Low chloride under amiloride (LC + A) and **(D)** LC + A and isoproterenol (Iso) in KRB at the 20 µl/min infusion rate (*$p < 0.05$, **$p < 0.01$, Mean±SD, Dunnett's RM ANOVA vs Baseline, $n = 9$). The ΔPD wildtype level (WT) designated by dashed blue line.

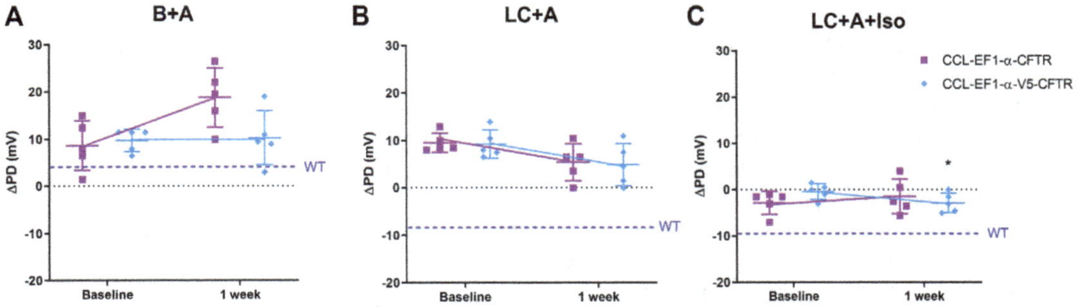

FIGURE 5 | Electrophysiological responses (ΔPD) in CF mice before (baseline) and 1 week after delivery of a third generation CCL-*CFTR* (purple square), or CCL-*CFTR* with V5 tag (light blue diamond) vectors. Gene addition to nasal airways following **(A)** Basal + Amiloride (B + A), **(B)** Low chloride under amiloride (LC + A) and **(C)** LC + A and isoproterenol (Iso) in KRB at the 20 µl/min infusion rate (*$p < 0.05$, Mean±SD, paired t-test vs baseline, $n = 5$; n.s., unpaired t-test, CCL-*CFTR* vs CCL-V5-*CFTR*, $n = 5$). The ΔPD wildtype level (WT) designated by dashed blue line.

driven by the simian virus 40 promoter (Cmielewski et al., 2014), the level of correction of the electrophysiological defect observed here could provide a therapeutic benefit. Importantly, the third generation lentiviral vector–with lower titre, non-viral internal promoter and improved safety profile–provided not only correction of the chloride defect in murine nasal airways, but is a more clinically relevant vector that may be useful for future human CFTR gene therapy trials (White et al., 2017; Marquez Loza et al., 2019).

We have confirmed for the first time in mice that the N-terminus epitope tagging with V5 did not affect CFTR function, and was used to successfully detect CFTR expressing cells in the desired airway regions, i.e., in mouse ciliated nasal epithelium. Third generation batch titres were slightly higher than the second generation, but this may be a consequence of the titering assay. The method of detection of viral titre for the third generation vector was based on total p24

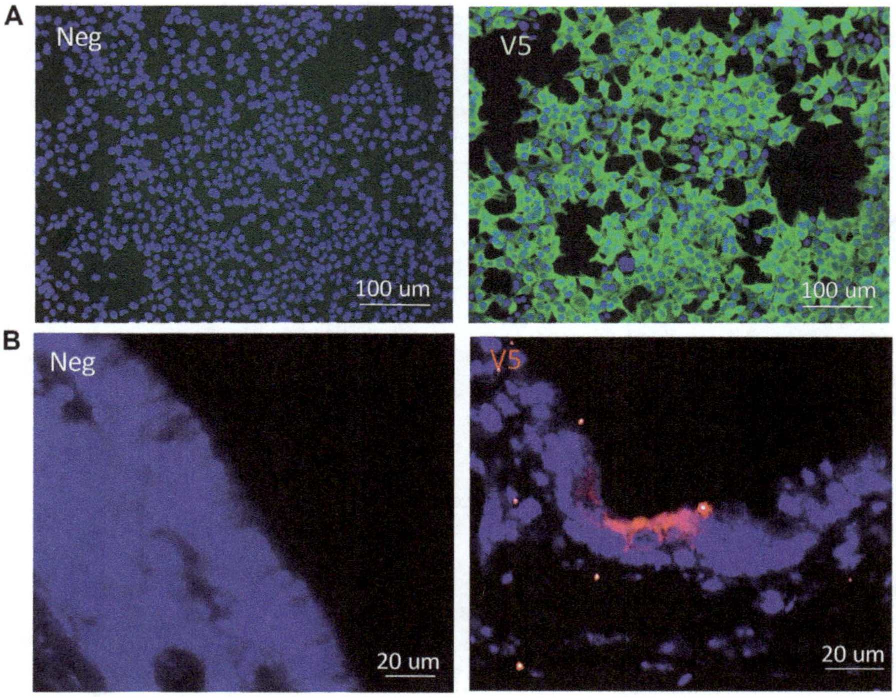

FIGURE 6 | Validation of the V5 tag following delivery of the CCL-V5-*CFTR* vector in **(A)** *in vitro* samples of HEK293T cells by ICC; **(B)** in mouse ciliated nasal epithelium using IHC. All merged images (DAPI blue, V5 green or red) with non-CFTR treated cells or CF animals as negative controls (neg) on left panels, V5 staining images on right panels.

antigen concentrations, which overestimates non-functional empty viral particles compared to the real-time PCR technique used for the second generation vector that quantifies functional vector particles. These newer vectors are now ready for upscaled production (McCarron et al., 2016) for use in larger rodents and other CF models.

A limitation of this study was the use of a smaller cohort of mice for the third generation LV vector validation experiments, which likely reduced the study power. To adapt this rapid PD method into larger CF species, such as the CF rat (Tuggle et al., 2014; McCarron et al., 2020) or other CF models, the coupling of non-surgical intubation with the faster infusion of greater fluid volumes must first be optimised to ensure it is well tolerated. This optimisation will likely differ between species.

Together these data demonstrate an advance in both LV vector development and *in vivo* techniques for the detection and functional assessment of the bioelectrical ion transport defect for current and potential CF therapies.

AUTHOR CONTRIBUTIONS

PC assisted in experimental design, performed all *in vivo* experimental procedures, histochemical analyses, interpretation, statistical analyses and wrote and edited manuscript. JD assisted in experimental design, performed LV vector development and production, immuno-cytochemistry and immuno-histochemistry techniques, assisted in interpretation and manuscript preparation and editing. MD and DP assisted in design, interpretation and manuscript preparation and editing.

ACKNOWLEDGMENTS

We acknowledge the support of Adelaide Microscopy services and AHMS histology services. We also thank Nathan Rout-Pitt for assistance in lentiviral vector production.

REFERENCES

Alton, E. W. F. W., Beekman, J. M., Boyd, A. C., Brand, J., Carlon, M. S., Connolly, M. M., et al. (2017). Preparation for a First-In-Man Lentivirus Trial in Patients with Cystic Fibrosis. *Thorax* 72, 137–147. doi:10.1136/thoraxjnl-2016-208406

Anson, D. S., McIntyre, C., Thomas, B., Koldej, R., Ranieri, E., Roberts, A., et al. (2007). Lentiviral-mediated Gene Correction of Mucopolysaccharidosis Type IIIA. *Genet. Vaccin. Ther* 5, 1. doi:10.1186/1479-0556-5-1

Bienvenu, T., Sermet-Gaudelus, I., Burgel, P.-R., Hubert, D., Crestani, B., Bassinet, L., et al. (2010). Cystic Fibrosis Transmembrane Conductance Regulator Channel Dysfunction in Non-cystic Fibrosis Bronchiectasis. *Am. J. Respir. Crit. Care Med.* 181, 1078–1084. doi:10.1164/rccm.200909-1434OC

Boucher, R. C. (2002). An Overview of the Pathogenesis of Cystic Fibrosis Lung Disease. *Adv. Drug Deliv. Rev.* 54, 1359–1371. doi:10.1016/s0169-409x(02)00144-8

Buckley, S. M. K., Delhove, J. M. K. M., Perocheau, D. P., Karda, R., Rahim, A. A., Howe, S. J., et al. (2015). *In Vivo* bioimaging with Tissue-specific Transcription

Factor Activated Luciferase Reporters. *Sci. Rep.* 5, 11842. doi:10.1038/srep11842

Cmielewski, P., Anson, D. S., and Parsons, D. W. (2010). Lysophosphatidylcholine as an Adjuvant for Lentiviral Vector Mediated Gene Transfer to Airway Epithelium: Effect of Acyl Chain Length. *Respir. Res.* 11, 84. doi:10.1186/1465-9921-11-84

Cmielewski, P., Donnelley, M., and Parsons, D. W. (2014). Long-term Therapeutic and Reporter Gene Expression in Lentiviral Vector Treated Cystic Fibrosis Mice. *J. Gene Med.* 16, 291–299. doi:10.1002/jgm.2778

Cmielewski, P., Farrow, N., Devereux, S., Parsons, D., and Donnelley, M. (2017). Gene Therapy for Cystic Fibrosis: Improved Delivery Techniques and Conditioning with Lysophosphatidylcholine Enhance Lentiviral Gene Transfer in Mouse Lung Airways. *Exp. Lung Res.* 43, 426–433. doi:10.1080/01902148.2017.1395931

da Cunha, M. F., Simonin, J., Sassi, A., Freund, R., Hatton, A., Cottart, C.-H., et al. (2016). Analysis of Nasal Potential in Murine Cystic Fibrosis Models. *Int. J. Biochem. Cel Biol.* 80, 87–97. doi:10.1016/j.biocel.2016.10.001

Davies, J. C., Davies, M., McShane, D., Smith, S., Chadwick, S., Jaffe, A., et al. (2005). Potential Difference Measurements in the Lower Airway of Children with and without Cystic Fibrosis. *Am. J. Respir. Crit. Care Med.* 171, 1015–1019. doi:10.1164/rccm.200408-1116OC

Davis, P. B. (2006). Cystic Fibrosis since 1938. *Am. J. Respir. Crit. Care Med.* 173, 475–482. doi:10.1164/rccm.200505-840OE

De Boeck, K., Kent, L., Davies, J., Derichs, N., Amaral, M., Rowe, S. M., et al. (2013). CFTR Biomarkers: Time for Promotion to Surrogate End-point. *Eur. Respir. J.* 41, 203–216. doi:10.1183/09031936.00057512

Dull, T., Zufferey, R., Kelly, M., Mandel, R. J., Nguyen, M., Trono, D., et al. (1998). A Third-Generation Lentivirus Vector with a Conditional Packaging System. *J. Virol.* 72, 8463–8471. doi:10.1128/JVI.72.11.8463-8471.1998

Egan, M., Flotte, T., Afione, S., Solow, R., Zeitlin, P. L., Carter, B. J., et al. (1992). Defective Regulation of Outwardly Rectifying Cl− Channels by Protein Kinase A Corrected by Insertion of CFTR. *Nature* 358, 581–584. doi:10.1038/358581a0

Gabriel, S. E., Clarke, L. L., Boucher, R. C., and Stutts, M. J. (1993). CFTR and Outward Rectifying Chloride Channels Are Distinct Proteins with a Regulatory Relationship. *Nature* 363, 263–266. doi:10.1038/363263a0

Hryciw, D. H., and Guggino, W. B. (2000). Cystic Fibrosis Transmembrane Conductance Regulator and the Outwardly Rectifying Chloride Channel: a Relationship between Two Chloride Channels Expressed in Epithelial Cells. *Clin. Exp. Pharmacol. Physiol.* 27, 892–895. doi:10.1046/j.1440-1681.2000.03356.x

Knowles, M., Gatzy, J., and Boucher, R. (1981). Increased Bioelectric Potential Difference across Respiratory Epithelia in Cystic Fibrosis. *N. Engl. J. Med.* 305, 1489–1495. doi:10.1056/NEJM198112173052502

Kremer, K. L., Dunning, K. R., Parsons, D. W., and Anson, D. S. (2007). Gene Delivery to Airway Epithelial Cellsin Vivo: a Direct Comparison of Apical and Basolateral Transduction Strategies Using Pseudotyped Lentivirus Vectors. *J. Gene Med.* 9, 362–368. doi:10.1002/jgm.1025

Limberis, M., Anson, D. S., Fuller, M., and Parsons, D. W. (2002). Recovery of Airway Cystic Fibrosis Transmembrane Conductance Regulator Function in Mice with Cystic Fibrosis after Single-Dose Lentivirus-Mediated Gene Transfer. *Hum. Gene Ther.* 13, 1961–1970. doi:10.1089/10430340260355365

MacDonald, K. D., McKenzie, K. R., Henderson, M. J., Hawkins, C. E., Vij, N., and Zeitlin, P. L. (2008). Lubiprostone Activates Non-CFTR-dependent Respiratory Epithelial Chloride Secretion in Cystic Fibrosis Mice. *Am. J. Physiology-Lung Cell Mol. Physiol.* 295, L933–L940. doi:10.1152/ajplung.90221.2008

Marquez Loza, L., Yuen, E., and McCray, P., Jr. (2019). Lentiviral Vectors for the Treatment and Prevention of Cystic Fibrosis Lung Disease. *Genes* 10, 218. doi:10.3390/genes10030218

McCarron, A., Cmielewski, P., Reyne, N., McIntyre, C., Finnie, J., Craig, F., et al. (2020). Phenotypic Characterization and Comparison of Cystic Fibrosis Rat Models Generated Using CRISPR/Cas9 Gene Editing. *Am. J. Pathol.* 190, 977–993. doi:10.1016/j.ajpath.2020.01.009

McCarron, A., Donnelley, M., McIntyre, C., and Parsons, D. (2016). Challenges of Up-Scaling Lentivirus Production and Processing. *J. Biotechnol.* 240, 23–30. doi:10.1016/j.jbiotec.2016.10.016

McIntyre, C., Donnelley, M., Rout-Pitt, N., and Parsons, D. (2018). Lobe-Specific Gene Vector Delivery to Rat Lungs Using a Miniature Bronchoscope. *Hum. Gene Ther. Methods* 29, 228 235. doi:10.1089/hgtb.2018.050

Mery, S., Gross, E. A., Joyner, D. R., Godo, M., and Morgan, K. T. (1994). Nasal Diagrams: a Tool for Recording the Distribution of Nasal Lesions in Rats and Mice. *Toxicol. Pathol.* 22, 353–372. doi:10.1177/019262339402200402

Middleton, P. G., Geddes, D. M., and Alton, E. W. (1994). Protocols for *In Vivo* Measurement of the Ion Transport Defects in Cystic Fibrosis Nasal Epithelium. *Eur. Respir. J.* 7, 2050–2056. doi:10.1183/09031936.94.07030442

Parsons, D. W., Hopkins, P. J., Bourne, A. J., Boucher, R. C., and Martin, A. J. (2000). Airway Gene Transfer in Mouse Nasal-Airways: Importance of Identification of Epithelial Type for Assessment of Gene Transfer. *Gene Ther.* 7, 1810–1815. doi:10.1038/sj.gt.3301317

Pranke, I. M., Hatton, A., Simonin, J., Jais, J. P., Le Pimpec-Barthes, F., Carsin, A., et al. (2017). Correction of CFTR Function in Nasal Epithelial Cells from Cystic Fibrosis Patients Predicts Improvement of Respiratory Function by CFTR Modulators. *Sci. Rep.* 7, 7375. doi:10.1038/s41598-017-07504-1

Quinton, P. M. (2008). Cystic Fibrosis: Impaired Bicarbonate Secretion and Mucoviscidosis. *The Lancet* 372, 415–417. doi:10.1016/S0140-6736(08)61162-9

Reyne, N., Cmielewski, P., McCarron, A., Delhove, J., Parsons, D., and Donnelley, M. (2021). Single-Dose Lentiviral Mediated Gene Therapy Recovers CFTR Function in Cystic Fibrosis Knockout Rats. *Front. Pharmacol.* 12, 682299. doi:10.3389/fphar.2021.682299

Riordan, J. R., Rommens, J., Kerem, B., Alon, N., Rozmahel, R., Grzelczak, Z., et al. (1989). Identification of the Cystic Fibrosis Gene: Cloning and Characterization of Complementary DNA. *Science* 245, 1066–1073. doi:10.1126/science.2475911

Rout-Pitt, N., McCarron, A., McIntyre, C., Parsons, D., and Donnelley, M. (2018). Large-scale Production of Lentiviral Vectors Using Multilayer Cell Factories. *J. Biol. Methods* 5, e90. doi:10.14440/jbm.2018.236

Rowe, S. M., Clancy, J. P., and Wilschanski, M. (2011). Nasal Potential Difference Measurements to Assess CFTR Ion Channel Activity. *Methods Mol. Biol.* 741, 69–86. doi:10.1007/978-1-61779-117-8_6

Stocker, A. G., Kremer, K. L., Koldej, R., Miller, D. S., Anson, D. S., and Parsons, D. W. (2009). Single-dose Lentiviral Gene Transfer for Lifetime Airway Gene Expression. *J. Gene Med.* 11, 861–867. doi:10.1002/jgm.1368

Tuggle, K. L., Birket, S. E., Cui, X., Hong, J., Warren, J., Reid, L., et al. (2014). Characterization of Defects in Ion Transport and Tissue Development in Cystic Fibrosis Transmembrane Conductance Regulator (CFTR)-knockout Rats. *PLoS One* 9, e91253, 2014. e91253. doi:10.1371/journal.pone.0091253

Welsh, M. J., Anderson, M. P., Rich, D. P., Berger, H. A., Denning, G. M., Ostedgaard, L. S., et al. (1992). Cystic Fibrosis Transmembrane Conductance Regulator: a Chloride Channel with Novel Regulation. *Neuron* 8, 821–829. doi:10.1016/0896-6273(92)90196-k

White, M., Whittaker, R., Gándara, C., and Stoll, E. A. (2017). A Guide to Approaching Regulatory Considerations for Lentiviral-Mediated Gene Therapies. *Hum. Gene Ther. Methods* 28, 163–176. doi:10.1089/hgtb.2017.096

Wilschanski, M., Dupuis, A., Ellis, L., Jarvi, K., Zielenski, J., Tullis, E., et al. (2006). Mutations in the Cystic Fibrosis Transmembrane Regulator Gene and In VivoTransepithelial Potentials. *Am. J. Respir. Crit. Care Med.* 174, 787–794. doi:10.1164/rccm.200509-1377OC

Zufferey, R., Dull, T., Mandel, R. J., Bukovsky, A., Quiroz, D., Naldini, L., et al. (1998). Self-inactivating Lentivirus Vector for Safe and Efficient *In Vivo* Gene Delivery. *J. Virol.* 72, 9873–9880. doi:10.1128/JVI.72.12.9873-9880.1998

10

Treatment of Cystic Fibrosis: From Gene- to Cell-Based Therapies

Katelin M. Allan[1,2], *Nigel Farrow*[3,4,5], *Martin Donnelley*[3,4,5], *Adam Jaffe*[1,2,6] *and Shafagh A. Waters*[1,2,6]*

[1]School of Women's and Children's Health, Faculty of Medicine, University of New South Wales, Sydney, Australia, [2]Molecular and Integrative Cystic Fibrosis Research Centre (miCF_RC), University of New South Wales and Sydney Children's Hospital, Sydney, Australia, [3]Respiratory and Sleep Medicine, Women's and Children's Health Network, Adelaide, Australia, [4]Robinson Research Institute, The University of Adelaide, Adelaide, Australia, [5]Adelaide Medical School, The University of Adelaide, Adelaide, Australia, [6]Department of Respiratory Medicine, Sydney Children's Hospital, Sydney, Australia

***Correspondence:**
Shafagh A. Waters
shafagh.waters@unsw.edu.au

Prognosis of patients with cystic fibrosis (CF) varies extensively despite recent advances in targeted therapies that improve CF transmembrane conductance regulator (CFTR) function. Despite being a multi-organ disease, extensive lung tissue destruction remains the major cause of morbidity and mortality. Progress towards a curative treatment strategy that implements a *CFTR* gene addition-technology to the patients' lungs has been slow and not yet developed beyond clinical trials. Improved delivery vectors are needed to overcome the body's defense system and ensure an efficient and consistent clinical response before gene therapy is suitable for clinical care. Cell-based therapy–which relies on functional modification of allogenic or autologous cells *ex vivo*, prior to transplantation into the patient–is now a therapeutic reality for various diseases. For CF, pioneering research has demonstrated proof-of-principle for allogenic transplantation of cultured human airway stem cells into mouse airways. However, applying a cell-based therapy to the human airways has distinct challenges. We review CF gene therapies using viral and non-viral delivery strategies and discuss current advances towards autologous cell-based therapies. Progress towards identification, correction, and expansion of a suitable regenerative cell, as well as refinement of pre-cell transplant lung conditioning protocols is discussed.

Keywords: cystic fibrosis, CFTR, gene therapy, cell-based therapy, therapeutic vectors, stem cells

CFTR CORRECTION STRATEGIES

Cystic fibrosis (CF) is an inherited, multi-organ disease caused by mutations in the CF transmembrane conductance regulator (*CFTR*) gene (Rowe et al., 2005). CF is progressive, with its major pathology impacting the lung, liver, pancreas and intestine. Mortality in CF patients is mostly due to respiratory failure (Elborn, 2016). The CFTR protein, an anion channel, is expressed in a diverse range of epithelial tissues (Riordan, 2008). CFTR dysfunction disrupts ion transport equilibrium, deregulating fluid absorption and secretion processes in epithelial tissue such as the

---

Abbreviations: AAV, adeno-associated virus; AAV2, adeno-associated virus serotype 2; AAV6, adeno-associated virus serotype 6; AECs, airway epithelial cells; ASO, antisense oligonucleotide; CF, cystic fibrosis; CFTR, cystic fibrosis transmembrane conductance regulator; CRISPR, clustered regularly interspaced short palindromic repeat; CRC, conditionally reprogrammed cell; iPSCs, induced pluripotent stem cells; IV, immunodeficiency virus; LNPs, lipid nanoparticles; LV, lentivirus vector; mRNA, messenger RNA; MSCs, mesenchymal stem cells; NMD, nonsense mediated decay; TALENs, transcription activator-like effector nucleases; ZFNs, zinc-finger nucleases

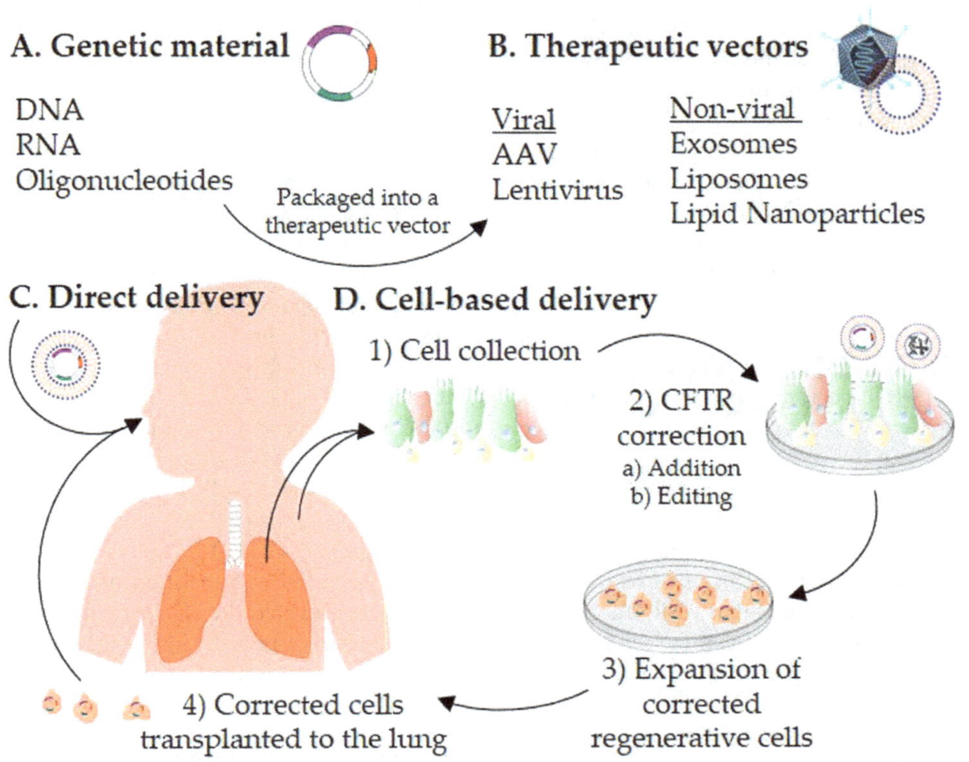

FIGURE 1 | Schematic representation of CFTR correction strategies for the treatment of cystic fibrosis. Genetic materials **(A)** are packaged into a therapeutic vector **(B)**. The therapeutic vector is delivered directly to the patient's lungs **(C)** or introduced into cells *ex vivo* **(D)**. For autologous cell-based therapy, 1) airway cells are isolated from the patient's respiratory tract or induced pluripotent stem cells are generated from the patient's skin fibroblasts or blood. 2) CFTR is corrected *in vitro* in the collected cells by a) addition or b) editing strategies. 3) The CFTR-corrected regenerative cells are expanded to reach a therapeutic dose, and then 4) transplanted back to repopulate the patient lung epithelium.

airways, resulting in mucus accumulation and recurrent bacterial infections (Ratjen et al., 2015). Symptomatic therapies such as airway clearance by physiotherapy, mucus thinning agents, antibiotics and anti-inflammatories remain crucial for the management of CF airways (Flume et al., 2007).

Recently, targeted therapies have been approved for CF treatment. These small molecule compounds modulate CFTR protein abundance and/or function at the apical epithelial cell membrane (Davies, 2015). A combination of three CFTR modulating small molecules–elexacaftor/tezacaftor/ivacaftor–is the most advanced targeted therapeutic approved for patients with one or two Phe508del-CFTR alleles–the most common *CFTR* mutation in the population. CFTR modulator therapies result in improved lung function and better quality of life for patients with CF (Davies et al., 2018). Yet, variable therapeutic response, inadequate long-term efficacy data, adverse effects and unavailability of modulators for the 10% of CF patients with mutations that produce little or no CFTR protein has rekindled great interest in the development of *CFTR* mutation-independent corrective strategies.

In vivo transfer of a functional copy of *CFTR* has been envisioned as a CF airway treatment since 1989 when the *CFTR* gene was identified as the cause of this multisystemic disease (Tsui et al., 1985; Wainwright et al., 1985). Gene therapy has received FDA approval for treatment of monogenic disorders (U.S. Food and Drug Administration. 2020) such as spinal muscular atrophy (Kariyawasam et al., 2018), coagulative disorders (Batty and Lillicrap 2019), and immunodeficiency diseases (Booth et al., 2019), but not yet for CF. Numerous research programs and clinical trials have been undertaken to explicate the most effective vector (viral or non-viral) to deliver *CFTR* to airway cells (Griesenbach et al., 2015). However, clinical efficacy of these vectors *in vivo* in humans has been insignificant and inconsistent in improving lung function (Alton et al., 2015a). The greatest barrier to enabling clinical translation of gene therapy for CF remains the lack of an effective delivery system to the lungs. A successful gene therapy system for restoration of CFTR function needs to navigate the complexities of the lung clearance and innate immunity defense functions that are further complicated in the CF airways due to increased mucus volume and viscosity (reviewed in (Donnelley and Parsons 2018)). Even if these obstacles are circumvented, heterogeneous and highly regulated CFTR expression in various cell types of the lung raises the question of the most appropriate cellular target.

One proposed strategy to deal with the challenges associated with *in vivo* delivery of *CFTR* to the airway cells is to correct the airway cells *ex vivo* followed by transplanting the corrected cells to repopulate the patient's lung with *CFTR*-corrected cells

(**Figure 1**). This approach is the basis of the first *ex vivo* hematopoietic stem cell gene therapy, Strimvelis, which was approved for treatment of adenosine deaminase-severe combined immunodeficiency (Stirnadel-Farrant et al., 2018). In this review, we will first describe alternative strategies to CFTR DNA therapy, and discuss the advances in the main groups of viral and non-viral vectors that have shown promise in CF therapy. The second part of this review will focus on recent progress in cell-based therapies, including the gene editing technologies that facilitate CFTR correction in *ex vivo* cells.

THERAPEUTIC GENETIC MATERIAL OTHER THAN DNA: RNA ADDITION AND REPAIR

The earliest efforts to deliver genetic material into diseased cells focused on directly introducing therapeutic *CFTR* DNA as an addition strategy to subsequently produce functional CFTR protein (reviewed in (Cooney et al., 2018)). A novel alternative to DNA therapeutics is based on addition of RNA. Since the functional site of messenger RNA (mRNA) is the cell cytoplasm, the challenge of nuclear translocation is eliminated (Hajj and Whitehead 2017).

Exogenous nucleic acids are susceptible to degradation by nucleases and can trigger an immune response upon cellular entry (Alexopoulou et al., 2001; Kariko et al., 2004). Therefore, current strategies utilize chemical modification of the nucleic acid bases to reduce immunogenicity and increase stability (Sahin et al., 2014; Pardi et al., 2015). Manufacturing and addition of modifications to RNA is easier than DNA, extending the usefulness of RNA therapy (Kuhn et al., 2012). Yet, repeat RNA administration remains necessary to sustain therapeutic levels of protein (Patel et al., 2019b). Successful delivery of chemically modified CFTR mRNA to patient-derived bronchial epithelial cells has demonstrated increased CFTR expression at the plasma membrane and rescue of chloride transport (Robinson et al., 2018). Aerosolized delivery of *in vitro* transcribed CFTR mRNA complexed with lipids to the lungs (Orphan drug MRT5005) is a therapeutic forerunner currently being tested in a phase 1/2 trial (NCT03375047) which has highly anticipated results for *in vivo* correction of CFTR.

In addition to direct RNA supplementation, an alternative therapeutic option is to alter the defective RNA to restore proper CFTR protein function. This can be achieved using antisense oligonucleotides (ASOs). ASOs are short synthetic oligonucleotides that are chemically modified to bind to target RNA, offering a tool for direct mRNA restoration (Oren et al., 2017). *In vivo* delivery of ASOs to the airway epithelium of mice initially resulted in no significant uptake (Griesenbach et al., 2006). It was postulated that this inefficiency was due to physical barriers to airway epithelial cell delivery (Griesenbach et al., 2006). Advances in RNA chemical modifications have been key to the development of a successful ASO-mediated therapy, with the accelerated FDA approval of eteplirsen (Exondys 51) being granted in 2016 for patients with Duchenne muscular dystrophy that have a mutation in the *dystrophin* gene which can be treated by exon 51 skipping (reviewed in (Bennett et al., 2017)). An ASO candidate for ASO-directed mRNA restoration, Eluforsen, binds to and restores the mRNA region encoding the Phe508 deletion (Beumer et al., 2019). In a phase 1 study, repeated administration of Eluforsen improved CFTR activity in patients homozygous for the Phe508 mutation (Sermet-Gaudelus et al., 2019) (NCT02564354). In the following phase 1b safety study with 70 enrolled participants Eluforsen was well-tolerated (NCT02532764), supporting the therapeutic translation of novel mRNA-based therapies for patients with CF. ASOs have also been tested for their ability to correct *CFTR* splicing mutations, which constitute 13% of disease-causing *CFTR* mutations, and result in no functional protein being produced (Igreja et al., 2016). Single-stranded DNA oligonucleotides designed to hybridize to pre-mRNA and modify aberrant splicing restored splicing in immortalized cells expressing the *CFTR* splicing mutation, c.2657 + 5G > A-*CFTR* (Igreja et al., 2016).

Although clinical translation of DNA or RNA therapy has been proven feasible, the efficient targeting and delivery of these genetic materials into the lung epithelium for treatment of CF remains exceedingly challenging.

THERAPEUTIC DELIVERY VECTORS

Nucleic acids are unable to cross the cell membrane because of their high negative charge, and therefore require assistance for intracellular delivery (reviewed in (Ni et al., 2019)). Numerous viral and non-viral delivery systems have been investigated for their ability to transfer genetic material–RNA (Therapeutic Genetic Material Other Than DNA: RNA Addition and Repair), DNA (this section) and gene editing system components (Gene Editing Technologies)–to the lung. The main groups of viral and non-viral vectors used in CF therapy and advances toward their clinical translation will be summarized below.

Viral Vectors for Airway Gene Therapy

Viral vector-mediated gene delivery systems take advantage of a virus's natural ability to evade the lung mucus barrier and transduce the airway by inserting their DNA into epithelial cells. The natural tropism of viral vectors enables preferential targeting of the airway progenitor cells–the basal cells–so that multi-lineage transgene expression can be achieved (Havenga et al., 2002). Other advantages and disadvantages of available vectors have been discussed in depth elsewhere (Miah et al., 2019). Here we briefly discuss the most commonly used vectors for CF.

Adeno-Associated Virus

In the early 2000s, human CF clinical trials tested aerosolized viral vectors, including AAV serotype 2 (AAV2). Based on delivery of CFTR complementary DNA (cDNA) to the human nasal cavity and lung, AAV was determined safe, but failed to demonstrate significant clinical benefit in restoration of lung function (Wagner et al., 2002; Flotte et al., 2003; Moss et al., 2004; Moss et al., 2007).

These findings have been attributed to issues regarding the packaging capacity of the AAV2 genome to encompass a CFTR expression cassette (Wu et al., 2010) and also low transduction efficiency of the airway epithelial cells (AECs) due to the limited binding of AAV2 to the apical surface of human airway epithelia (Zabner et al., 2000).

To overcome the packaging capacity limitation of AAV, a split AAV gene delivery approach can be implemented, wherein a large transgene is split across multiple separate AAV vectors (Patel et al., 2019a). As a means of screening for AAV serotypes that display airway tropism and permit efficient gene delivery to the human lung parenchyma, lung bud organoids–a model of lung parenchyma derived from human embryonic stem cells–have been utilized (Meyer-Berg et al., 2020). A 2020 study identified AAV2 and AAV serotype 6 (AAV6) as having the highly efficient transduction of the human lung parenchyma. Additionally, it was recently discovered that unlike other AAV serotypes, AAV6 is capable of efficiently diffusing through mucus in primary differentiated CF airway cultures (Duncan et al., 2018). Inhaled administration of AAV6 provided high-level transgene expression (mediating roughly 30% airway coverage) in a mouse model with airway mucus obstruction (Duncan et al., 2018). Yet, the high immunogenicity of AAV draws concern to the potential for participants of viral-based gene therapy clinical trials to acquire AAV immunity, and for potential preexisting immunity in some patients (reviewed in (Ronzitti et al., 2020). These are major concerns because immunity to AAV is likely to prevent repeat administration of AAV gene therapy to patients (George et al., 2020), therefore risking their eligibility for future AAV-based therapies. In 2020, the imlifidase (IdeS) enzyme was tested in rodents and non-human primates and successfully demonstrated inhibition of the host immune response to AAV resulting from preexisting immunity and following AAV gene therapy (Leborgne et al., 2020). If IdeS treatment in human patients were to enable repeat administration of AAV-based therapies, this could have big implications for the future course of AAV gene therapy. To improve the gradual decrease in *CFTR* expression due to the transient episomal expression nature of AAV, and avoid the need for repeat dosing of the AAV vector, Cooney and colleagues designed a novel integrating AAV-based *CFTR*-expressing vector (termed *piggyBac*/AAV), which demonstrated efficient transduction and persistent expression in primary human CF airway cells *in vitro* and in mouse airways *in vivo* (Cooney et al., 2015). A follow-up large animal study delivered aerosolized *piggyBac*/AAV-CFTR to CF pig airways and demonstrated phenotypic restoration of CFTR function (Cooney et al., 2019).

Lentivirus

In comparison to AAVs, lentivirus vectors (LV) have a larger packaging capacity (approximately 8 kb) which makes them more compatible for full length CFTR packaging (Castellani and Conese, 2010). Additionally, LVs can transduce and integrate into the genome of both dividing and non-dividing cells (Naldini, Blomer et al., 1996; Wang et al., 1999). Proof-of-principle that a lentiviral vector could correct the CFTR defect *in vivo* and provide persistent *CFTR* expression was first demonstrated in mouse airways (Limberis et al., 2002). This was followed by a demonstration of partially restored *in vivo* CFTR channel activity following aerosol delivery of Feline immunodeficiency virus (IV)-*CFTR* to CF pig airways (Cooney et al., 2016). More recently, insertion of a LacZ marker gene into airway basal cells via a LV vector produced persistent transgene expression and importantly, the basal cells successfully passed on the introduced gene to their daughter cells in a mouse airway (Farrow et al., 2018b). In support of a first-in-man CF trial, a simian IV-based lentiviral vector, pseudotyped with Sendai virus fusion protein and Hemagglutinin/Neuraminidase envelope proteins exhibited efficient transduction of human airway cells *in vitro* and murine lung epithelium *in vivo* (Alton et al., 2017).

Non-viral Vectors

Progression of viral vectors as a clinical therapy for CF remains contingent on demonstrating successful long-term transduction efficacy, the safety of delivery to the CF lung and the ability for repeat dosing (Donnelley and Parsons, 2018). Some of these barriers have necessitated the development of more cost-effective non-viral vectors to provide an increased safety profile and limitless genetic material packaging size, while obtaining more reproducible delivery outcomes. Non-viral vectors are naturally produced by the body and can also be engineered in the laboratory. Despite reduced immunogenicity, the transfection efficiency of non-viral vectors is still low compared to viral vectors. Specifically, unmodified non-viral vectors are rapidly cleared and have low accumulation in target tissues and cells (Takahashi et al., 2013; Smyth et al., 2015), thus new compounds are constantly engineered and investigated (Murphy et al., 2019).

Exosomes

Exosomes are naturally occurring nanoscale extracellular vesicles which, following their release from cells, facilitate intercellular communication by transporting material to neighboring or distant recipient cells (Doyle and Wang, 2019). Due to this ability to function as an endogenous intercellular cargo transfer system, they have been exploited as vehicles for the delivery of genetic material, and as such, are a promising vector for *in vivo* gene therapy. Exosomes have been demonstrated to deliver human CFTR mature glycoprotein, as well as CFTR mRNA, in both Chinese hamster ovarian cells (Gonzalez et al., 2012) and CFTR-deficient cells derived from CF patients (Vituret et al., 2016; Villamizar et al., 2019). In both models, CFTR channel function was shown to be corrected in exosome-recipient cells. Exosomes have similarly shown utility in delivering small interfering RNA in well-differentiated human AECs (Singh et al., 2020), suggesting value beyond gene transfer for the delivery of gene editing materials. These studies demonstrated the potential application of exosomes as vectors for CFTR transfer and functional correction of the genetic defect in human CF cells.

Liposomes

Liposomes are artificially created vesicles with a lipid bilayer membrane and an aqueous core (Akbarzadeh et al., 2013). In a single dose, dose-escalation phase 1/2a safety trial assessment of a liposomal mixture that included the cationic lipid mixture

(GL67A) complexed with *CFTR* complementary DNA, patients with CF showed improved lung function and no adverse effects (Alton et al., 2015b). This was followed by a double-blind, placebo-controlled multi-dose phase 2b trial (NCT01621867) that found that repeated administration of GL67A liposome significantly, yet modestly, stabilized lung function in the treatment group ($n = 62$) vs. placebo ($n = 54$) in CF adults or children aged 12 years or older enrolled in this trial (Alton et al., 2015a). Although this trial reached its primary efficacy endpoint (lung function improvement), the magnitude and variability in effect did not support progression to phase 3 trials. These results established for the first time a proof of principle that gene therapy was capable of favorably modulating CF lung function, with no safety concerns with repeat dosing. However, they also highlighted the need for more efficacious methods of gene delivery transport, such as viral vectors, before large-scale clinical translation can be achieved. Gene delivery systems likely face greater barriers in adults with established lung disease and irreversible fibrotic scarring in comparison to children, with less progressed lung disease. Strong reasoning to include children in gene therapy clinical trials has been given previously (Jaffe et al., 2006; Delhove et al., 2020) and may present the most rational avenue forward as a clinical target age.

Lipid Nanoparticles

Like liposomes, lipid nanoparticles (LNPs) are used to encapsulate and deliver therapeutic RNA formulations to the lung via intranasal or systemic routes. However, LNPs differ in their composition, often carrying cargo within a non-aqueous core (Kraft et al., 2014). Recent advances have focused on exploiting the dynamic structure of LNPs to engineer specialized formulations tailored to increase mucus penetrance (Nafee et al., 2018; Wan et al., 2018) and evade host immune detection (Vencken et al., 2019). This work climaxed in the successful LNP-mediated delivery of chemically modified CFTR mRNA to CF airway cells (Robinson et al., 2018). However, it has since been shown that LNPs only modestly increase CFTR expression in patient-derived human nasal epithelial cells (Villamizar et al., 2019). It is probable that the inefficiency of LNP delivery is due to endosome retention (Sahay et al., 2013), and as such, further work to engineer particles capable of escaping endosome retention is needed. Since CFTR expression in the epithelial airway is cell type specific (Plasschaert et al., 2018), further testing in *vitro* and *in vivo* models will be required before LNPs can be established as efficient and clinically relevant delivery systems.

CELL-BASED THERAPIES

Cell-based therapies offer an alternative therapeutic opportunity to *in vivo* gene therapy. This approach integrates advances in stem cell biology with the well-established platform of *in vitro* gene delivery and repair strategies. The exemplar for cell-based therapy is hematopoietic stem cell transplantation, which is successfully performed in over 50,0000 patients per year world-wide (Gratwohl and Niederwieser 2012). The safety of correcting a patient's cells *ex vivo* via a gene editing technology, before reintroducing them into the same patient (autologous transplantation), has been demonstrated in a clinical trial for hematological malignancies (Stadtmauer et al., 2020). Autologous cell therapy has also been used for treatment of epidermolysis bullosa (Eichstadt et al., 2019; Lwin et al., 2019; Marinkovich and Tang 2019), whilst treatment of insulin-dependent diabetes has shown success with transplant of allogenic islet cells (Kumagai et al., 2002; Yamada et al., 2011).

The efficacy of these regenerative cellular therapies has propagated investigation of cell-based therapy for CF. Yet, in the CF airways, the volume, viscosity and composition of the mucus that protects the airway from foreign particles and irritants is altered in such way that penetrating this barrier poses a great challenge. Successful clinical translation of a cell therapy approach will require regenerative cell 1) identification, 2) CFTR correction (addition or editing), 3) expansion, and 4) transplantation back into the patient's lungs (**Figure 1**). The remainder of this review will discuss the progress and challenges toward these milestones.

Identification of Suitable Regenerative Cells With Differentiation Capacity

One of the obstacles to cell-based therapy for CF is the identification of an optimal self-renewing cell that can also differentiate into the cells of the airway epithelium. In this review we discuss therapeutic perspectives of using adult tissue-resident basal stem cells, yet first we will briefly describe advances in the field using mesenchymal and induced pluripotent stem cells (iPSCs).

Mesenchymal stem cells (MSCs) are an allogenic source of cells that have been investigated for their application in CF cell-based therapy due to their immunomodulatory and anti-inflammatory properties (reviewed in (Caretti et al., 2019)). In favor of their potential for CF cell therapy, MSCs co-cultured with CF immortalized airway epithelial cells at air-liquid interface have demonstrated acquisition of an epithelial phenotype, and subsequent restoration of functional CFTR protein (Carbone et al., 2014; Carbone et al., 2018). However, there is concern over low engraftment levels of administered MSCs in the lung (Ortiz et al., 2003; Xu et al., 2007). Furthermore, recent studies suggest that MSCs function transiently to reduce inflammation via the secretion of extra-cellular vesicles such as exosomes (Zhu et al., 2014; Zulueta et al., 2018) that can be used for delivery of drugs or gene editing material (reviewed in (Almeida-Porada et al., 2020)). Exosomes derived from MSCs genetically engineered to carry a transcription activator protein have demonstrated success in targeting and activating CFTR transcription in primary human bronchial epithelial cells from patients with CF (Villamizar et al., 2021). Further *in vitro* and *in vivo* studies are needed before this approach is considered viable. Until then, there remains uncertainty surrounding the capacity of MSCs to effectively restore CFTR function in the respiratory epithelium.

iPSCs are routinely generated from skin or blood cells that are reprogrammed back into an embryonic-like pluripotent state. In addition, they are amenable to gene editing and expansion, thereby providing a large potential source of gene-corrected cells which upon differentiation into lung basal stem cells can be engrafted into the lung for therapeutic use. Two iPSC-derived cell populations have been isolated for the purpose of CF cell therapy: one- airway epithelial cells (AECs) or 2-basal stem cells. The strengths and limitations of both these will be discussed here briefly. Firstly, several reports have demonstrated successful directed differentiation of human iPSCs into AECs *in vitro* (Firth et al., 2014; Huang et al., 2014; Dye et al., 2015; Konishi et al., 2016; McCauley et al., 2017). The iPSC-derived AEC cultures are a heterogenous cell population containing limited numbers of basal cells with self-renewing capacity (McCauley et al., 2017). As such, transplanting AECs will only provide a short-term solution, even if engraftment of cells was successful. Therefore, although this method can generate ample AECs, transplantation of terminally differentiated AECs would not be an effective CF cell therapy.

More recently, iPSCs have been differentiated into basal cells, termed induced basal cells (iBCs) (Hawkins et al., 2020). These iBCs are functionally indistinct from native basal cells and have been shown *in vitro* to differentiate into a pseudostratified airway epithelium exhibiting CFTR activity (Hawkins et al., 2020). However, the rarer cell types of the epithelium such as the CFTR-expressing ionocytes, and brush cells, were not observed in *vitro* cultures of iBCs differentiated at air-liquid interface (Hawkins et al., 2020). Furthermore, the long-term effects of these manipulations are not well understood, and several questions regarding the *in vivo* competence of iBCs remain unanswered. For these reasons, development of additional screening assays similar to the dual fluorescent transporter assay used by Hawkins and colleagues will be necessary to verify the cellular phenotype and differentiation capacity of iBCs in comparison to their endogenous counterparts both *in vitro* and *in vivo* before clinical translation of iPSC-based CF cell therapy can be considered viable.

To improve the chances of successful cell transplantation to the lung, it is possible that tissue-resident adult stem cell from the lung itself would be a better suited candidate. For some time, there had been a lack of clarity as to the identity of airway stem cells. However, increased knowledge of stem cell biology together with the characterization of lung progenitor lineage has brought emerging consensus that basal cells are a stem cell or progenitor cell of the airway epithelium (Rock et al., 2009; Bertoncello, 2016). Importantly, basal cells have the capacity to differentiate into all the cell types of the pseudostratified airway epithelium, including the rare population of CFTR high-expressing ionocytes (Montoro et al., 2018; Plasschaert et al., 2018). This means that upon CFTR correction of basal cells, multi-lineage expression of the corrected CFTR could be achieved in the airway epithelium.

The existence of multiple progenitors with various differentiation capacities has been detected in human bronchial xenografts (Engelhardt et al., 1995). This is in concordance with reports that mouse tracheal basal cells comprise two molecularly distinct subpopulations of multipotent stem cells and committed secretory precursors (Hong et al., 2004; Watson et al., 2015). More recently, a single-cell RNA-seq study on human airway epithelial cells identified a heterogenous population of basal cells that include multipotent and secretory-primed subsets (Carraro et al., 2020). However, it remains unknown whether secretory-primed basal cells represent a transitory state of basal cells or a phenotypically stable state. The implication is that cell therapy approaches will have to account for basal cell subtypes when selecting a suitable cell to target.

Correcting CFTR in Regenerative Cells

Correction of CFTR *in vitro* in airway epithelial cells can be achieved by direct addition of genetic material as discussed in the sections above (Therapeutic Genetic Material Other Than DNA: RNA Addition and Repair and Therapeutic Delivery Vectors). An alternative to introducing new material is to correct the defective *CFTR* via gene editing.

Gene Editing Technologies

The advent of gene editing technologies has refueled excitement over gene therapy and is an area of vast development. The three major gene editing technologies are clustered regularly interspaced short palindromic repeat (CRISPR)–Cas-associated nucleases, programmable nucleases, such as zinc-finger nucleases (ZFNs) and transcription activator-like effector nucleases (TALENs). The first *in vivo* application of CRISPR/Cas9 was employed for a person with a mutation in the *CEP290* gene which causes retinal degeneration (Ledford, 2020). Clinical trials are also underway to evaluate these therapeutic approaches for treatment of cancer and sickle cell disease (Ernst et al., 2020). In the context of CF, emerging gene editing technologies hold the potential to repair specific *CFTR* gene mutations and restore their function, offering the ultimate opportunity for precision medicine. However, to date, gene editing technologies for CF remain in the preclinical realm.

The first study of CRISPR/Cas9 as a potential therapy for CF used site-specific knock-in of the correct *CFTR* sequence to robustly restore CFTR function in human intestinal stem cell organoids derived from patients homozygous for the Phe508del mutation (Schwank et al., 2013). This approach has since been implemented in cell culture by Ruan and colleagues to achieve greater than 20% repair of patient-derived induced pluripotent stem cells (iPSCs) (Ruan et al., 2019). Furthermore, in recent advancements, an AAV-delivered Cas9 gene editing platform facilitated correction of >30% Phe508del-*CFTR* in patient-derived airway basal cells, prior to transplantation to an *ex vivo* engraftment scaffold and near-normal levels of CFTR function were restored (Vaidyanathan et al., 2020). Considering reports that suggest as little as 4.7% of WT CFTR expression can lead to a milder CF phenotype (Ramalho et al., 2002), prospects for clinical translation are promising. However, a shortcoming of these gene editing technologies is that they are mutation specific. As such, different mutations must be individually corrected, with some being more amenable to this strategy than others.

CRISPR/Cas9 has successfully corrected *CFTR* splicing mutations (Sanz et al., 2017) and mutations leading to the formation of a premature termination codon that produce no functional CFTR protein (Erwood et al., 2020). As such, an approach for allele-specific editing has been outlined. Gene editing using Zinc finger nucleases (ZFNs) has also facilitated the correction of iPSC-derived CF AECs (Crane et al., 2015). Crane and colleagues showed that *CFTR*-corrected iPSCs, following induced differentiation *in vitro,* expressed functional CFTR protein (Crane et al., 2015). A similar study used ZFNs to correct Phe508del and demonstrated restored CFTR protein expression and function in air-liquid interface cultures established from the edited basal cells (Suzuki et al., 2020). TALEN technologies have also been used to restore normal CFTR expression and activity in organoids derived from Phe508del patient-derived iPSCs (Fleischer et al., 2020). The ability to achieve *CFTR* correction in additional stem/progenitor cells such as airway basal cells, either as primary airway basal cells or those derived from iPSCs, has specific relevance for progress toward cell-based therapies for CF.

Expansion of CFTR-Corrected Regenerative Cells That Retain Differentiation Capacity

Irrespective of which regenerative cell type or *in vitro* correction method is to be used, cell-based therapy will require large numbers of viable cells to repopulate the lung by replacing the CFTR defective endogenous AECs. Hayes and colleagues have estimated that 60 million regenerative cells will be required to treat a human patient with cystic fibrosis cell therapy (Hayes et al., 2019). However, procurement of basal lung epithelial cells via bronchial lavage, sputum collection or endobronchial biopsy provides only low cell numbers (Mou et al., 2012; Pollock et al., 2013; Butler et al., 2016). To overcome the issue of low initial cell numbers, extensive cell expansion will be required prior to implantation.

Bronchial basal cells have a limited lifespan (Ghosh et al., 2011) with differentiation capacity that decreases over time *in vitro* (Gentzsch et al., 2017). Various culture protocols for cell expansion have been adapted to overcome these limitations (reviewed in (Awatade et al., 2018)). The conditionally reprogrammed cell (CRC) methodology (Liu et al., 2012) is one approach to increase bronchial cell yield (Martinovich et al., 2017) and maintain differentiation potential for multiple passages (Lee et al., 2020). CF and non-CF bronchial basal cells have been expanded to a therapeutic dose of 60 million cells via a modified CRC method, albeit the frequency of regenerative cells having decreased to 20% by the time the therapeutic dose was reached (Hayes et al., 2019). Importantly, the bronchial basal cells were demonstrated to retain their differentiation potential from passages 2 to 15 using this approach (Hayes et al., 2019). Yet, further concern is raised by reports of *in vitro* basal cell expansion altering CFTR functional activity (Awatade et al., 2021) and differentiation cell-fate composition, leading to a reduced number of ciliated cells in expanded cells compared to freshly isolated cells (Eenjes et al., 2018). If expanded basal cells differentiate to pseudostratified epithelium with an altered cell type composition, this would have implications for their suitability for cell therapy, therefore necessitating further investigation.

Another challenge faced by cell expansion for the purpose of CF cell-based therapy is reports that differentiated cultures established from extended *in vitro* expansion of basal cells often have decreased CFTR ion transport function (Peters-Hall et al., 2018). Lee and colleagues report that although CRC expanded cells have increased CFTR ion transport compared to conventionally expanded cells, short-circuit current (a proxy for CFTR function) still decreased by passage three in CRC expanded cells (Lee et al., 2020). A better understanding of the impact of extended cell expansion on CFTR function is required.

Transplantation of CFTR-Corrected Regenerative Cells

Basal cells are located within the surface epithelium, adjacent to the basement membrane, and their differentiation leads to the cellular diversity of the airway epithelium. As such, if CFTR-corrected basal cells are to be the basis of a cell therapy, then they would need to be engrafted onto the basement membrane of the airway epithelium. This should replenish the airways with CFTR-corrected ciliated and secretory cells, and ionocytes. Meanwhile, the engrafted basal cells, corrected by integrating *CFTR* addition or mutation-specific gene editing, would retain their capacity for self-renewal to establish a long-term corrected cell population.

Studies of hematopoietic stem cell transplantation show that transplanted cells compete with endogenous bone marrow stroma cells (Abbuehl et al., 2017). Similar concerns have been raised for competition between endogenous and transplanted cells used to repair the lung epithelium. In a competitive repopulation assay, a mixed culture of CF and healthy (non-CF) basal cells were differentiated at air-liquid interface to generate a pseudostratified airway epithelium *in vitro* (Lee et al., 2020). Lee and colleagues found that non-CF cells outcompeted CF donor cells, suggesting that endogenous airway epithelial repair and regeneration is likely to hinder cell engraftment. However, more work is required to fully comprehend and address factors such as these which may impact stable integration of transplanted cells.

The innate barrier properties of the CF airway epithelium–the thick mucus layer and the ciliated pseudostratified multi-layered nature of the epithelial tissue–will likely make the delivery of the corrected basal cells to the basement membrane difficult. An effective cell delivery method will need to first overcome the mucus layer covering the epithelial surface. Whilst aerosolization of stem cell MSCs has demonstrated feasibility as a new method of cell delivery *in vivo* in rabbit airways (Kardia et al., 2014; Kardia et al., 2018; Halim et al., 2019), this technique has not been trialed using basal stem cells. Most studies of basal cell engraftment delivered via intratracheal instillation (Ghosh et al., 2017) or injection (Millerl et al., 2018) use rodent models (Ghosh et al., 2017; Miller et al., 2018). However, these animal models are limited in their capacity to accurately recreate human CF airway pathogenesis. Evidently further testing in appropriate *in vivo* animal models is required to determine an effective approach for cell delivery capable of overcoming the altered mucus barrier in CF. Yet, even if an optimal method is achieved, it is anticipated that disruption of the epithelial cell layer via conditioning or transient injury will be necessary to facilitate effective cell transplantation. Similar strategies have been successful for conditioning of the bone marrow prior to haemopoietic stem cell transplantation (Gyurkocza and Sandmaier, 2014).

Experimental evidence for successful donor cell engraftment in the lungs of animal models has been shown with various injury protocols. Following conditioning with naphthalene, both iPSCs (Miller et al., 2018) and airway basal cells (Ghosh et al., 2017) successfully transplant into mouse airways and persist for up to six weeks. Comparatively, partially stripping the AECs by treatment with polidocanol, an agent that creates a larger site for donor cell engraftment than naphthalene, has enabled basal cells to engraft into live mouse airways and the transplanted cells remained viable for at least three weeks (Farrow et al., 2018a). The long-term effect of these conditioning protocols upon cell engraftment is yet to be examined. In the context of CF, no ideal strategy has yet been developed. To injure the already inflamed and infected lungs of CF recipients might appear counterintuitive. The question remains: what is the optimal conditioning scenario that will cause minimal injury, whilst facilitating effective engraftment of corrected cells in sufficient numbers to restore lung function?

CONCLUSION

There are clear challenges to the successful translation of gene and cell therapies designed to correct the CFTR defect in the airways. Various novel viral and non-viral therapeutic vectors have advanced to clinical trials; however, no significant clinical benefit has been achieved. The greatest barrier to the success of these gene therapeutics is their delivery to the human airways. Overcoming this barrier will be central to ongoing research and paramount to the achievement of an efficacious *in vivo* CF gene therapy.

Cell-based therapies represent a promising alternative strategy wherein CFTR is corrected *ex vivo*. Yet, questions remain unanswered. Even if regenerative basal cells that are corrected via integrating *CFTR* addition or mutation-specific gene editing can efficaciously transplant at the basement membrane of the airway epithelium, how safe are these *ex vivo*-corrected cells? We know that reprogramming, expansion, and editing increases the probability of tumorigenicity (reviewed in (Berical et al., 2019)). Can basal cells only be expanded to the necessary therapeutic dose at the cost of preserving the transcriptome, epigenome, and differentiation capacity of these basal cells? Long-term investigations are needed to confirm transplanted basal cells are free from mutations, that they are stably engrafted and that CFTR function is retained. Future studies to investigate and improve the findings discussed in this review are required to validate the feasibility of cell-based therapy for treatment of CF.

Moreover, challenges will likely be met in transitioning gene- and cell-based therapies to clinical care. Discussions of the difficulties in developing and sustaining a successful business model for cell-based therapies, and the changes in clinical care necessary to make this potentially transformative therapeutic approach accessible to patients, are ongoing (Elverum and Whitman, 2019). As we continue to forge ahead in this era of personalized medicine, improvements to current CFTR modulator drugs will likely herald increased patient benefit. However, clinical translation of gene or cell-based therapies, though still an ambitious goal, offers future promise of a mutation-agnostic cure for CF.

AUTHOR CONTRIBUTIONS

SW was responsible for conception and design. KA wrote the initial draft, in consultation with and edited by SW, NF, and MD, with critical input from AJ. All authors approved the final manuscript.

REFERENCES

Abbuehl, J.-P., Tatarova, Z., Held, W., and Huelsken, J. (2017). Long-term engraftment of primary bone marrow stromal cells repairs niche damage and improves hematopoietic stem cell transplantation. *Cell Stem Cell* 21 (2), 241–255. doi:10.1016/j.stem.2017.07.004

Akbarzadeh, A., Rezaei-Sadabady, R., Davaran, S., Joo, S. W., Zarghami, N., Hanifehpour, Y., et al. (2013). Liposome: classification, preparation, and applications. *Nanoscale Res. Lett.* 8 (1), 102. doi:10.1186/1556-276x-8-102

Alexopoulou, L., Holt, A. C., Medzhitov, R., and Flavell, R. A. (2001). Recognition of double-stranded RNA and activation of NF-κB by Toll-like receptor 3. *Nature* 413 (6857), 732–738. doi:10.1038/35099560

Almeida-Porada, G., Atala, A. J., and Porada, C. D. (2020). Therapeutic mesenchymal stromal cells for immunotherapy and for gene and drug delivery. *Mol. Ther.—Methods Clin. Develop.* 16, 204–224. doi:10.1016/j.omtm.2020.01.005

Alton, E. W. F. W., Armstrong, D. K., Ashby, D., Bayfield, K. J., Bilton, D., Bloomfield, E. V., et al. (2015a). Repeated nebulisation of non-viral CFTR gene therapy in patients with cystic fibrosis: a randomised, double-blind, placebo-controlled, phase 2b trial. *Lancet Respir. Med.* 3 (9), 684–691. doi:10.1016/s2213-2600(15)00245-3

Alton, E. W. F. W., Beekman, J. M., Boyd, A. C., Brand, J., Carlon, M. S., Connolly, M. M., et al. (2017). Preparation for a first-in-man lentivirus trial in patients with cystic fibrosis. *Thorax* 72 (2), 137–147. doi:10.1136/thoraxjnl-2016-208406

Alton, E. W. F. W., Boyd, A. C., Porteous, D. J., Davies, G., Davies, J. C., Griesenbach, U., et al. (2015b). A phase I/IIa safety and efficacy study of nebulized liposome-mediated gene therapy for cystic fibrosis supports a multidose trial. *Am. J. Respir. Crit. Care Med.* 192 (11), 1389–1392. doi:10.1164/rccm.201506-1193le

Awatade, N. T., Wong, S. L., Capraro, A., Pandzic, E., Slapetova, I., Zhong, L., et al. (2021). Significant functional differences in differentiated Conditionally Reprogrammed (CRC)- and Feeder-free Dual SMAD inhibited-expanded human nasal epithelial cells. *J. Cyst. Fibros.* S1569-1993(20), 30951–30956. doi:10.1016/j.jcf.2020.12.019

Awatade, N. T., Wong, S. L., Hewson, C. K., Fawcett, L. K., Kicic, A., Jaffe, A., et al. (2018). Human primary epithelial cell models: promising tools in the era of cystic fibrosis personalized medicine. *Front. Pharmacol.* 9, 1429. doi:10.3389/fphar.2018.01429

Batty, P., and Lillicrap, D. (2019). Advances and challenges for hemophilia gene therapy. *Hum. Mol. Genet.* 28 (R1), R95–R101. doi:10.1093/hmg/ddz157

Bennett, C. F., Baker, B. F., Pham, N., Swayze, E., and Geary, R. S. (2017). Pharmacology of antisense drugs. *Annu. Rev. Pharmacol. Toxicol.* 57, 81–105. doi:10.1146/annurev-pharmtox-010716-104846

Berical, A., Lee, R. E., Randell, S. H., and Hawkins, F. (2019). Challenges facing airway epithelial cell-based therapy for cystic fibrosis. *Front. Pharmacol.* 10, 74. doi:10.3389/fphar.2019.00074

Bertoncello, I. (2016). Properties of adult lung stem and progenitor cells. *J. Cel. Physiol.* 231 (12), 2582–2589. doi:10.1002/jcp.25404

Beumer, W., Swildens, J., Leal, T., Noel, S., Anthonijsz, H., van der Horst, G., et al. (2019). Evaluation of eluforsen, a novel RNA oligonucleotide for restoration of CFTR function in *in vitro* and murine models of p.Phe508del cystic fibrosis. *PLoS One* 14 (6), e0219182. doi:10.1371/journal.pone.0219182

Booth, C., Romano, R., Roncarolo, M. G., and Thrasher, A. J. (2019). Gene therapy for primary immunodeficiency. *Hum. Mol. Genet.* 28 (R1), R15–R23. doi:10.1093/hmg/ddz170

Butler, C. R., Hynds, R. E., Gowers, K. H. C., Lee, D. D. H., Brown, J. M., Crowley, C., et al. (2016). Rapid expansion of human epithelial stem cells suitable for airway tissue engineering. *Am. J. Respir. Crit. Care Med.* 194 (2), 156–168. doi:10.1164/rccm.201507-1414oc

Carbone, A., Castellani, S., Favia, M., Diana, A., Paracchini, V., Di Gioia, S., et al. (2014). Correction of defective CFTR/EN aC function and tightness of cystic fibrosis airway epithelium by amniotic mesenchymal stromal (stem) cells. *J. Cel. Mol. Med.* 18 (8), 1631–1643. doi:10.1111/jcmm.12303

Carbone, A., Zefferino, R., Beccia, E., Casavola, V., Castellani, S., Di Gioia, S., et al. (2018). Gap junctions are involved in the rescue of CFTR-dependent chloride efflux by amniotic mesenchymal stem cells in coculture with cystic fibrosis CFBE41o- cells. *Stem Cell Int* 2018, 1203717. doi:10.1155/2018/1203717

Caretti, A., Peli, V., Colombo, M., and Zulueta, A. (2019). Lights and shadows in the use of mesenchymal stem cells in lung inflammation, a poorly investigated topic in cystic fibrosis. *Cells* 9 (1), 20. doi:10.3390/cells9010020

Carraro, G., Mulay, A., Yao, C., Mizuno, T., Konda, B., Petrov, M., et al. (2020). Single-cell reconstruction of human basal cell diversity in normal and idiopathic pulmonary fibrosis lungs. *Am. J. Respir. Crit. Care Med.* 202 (11), 1540–1550. doi:10.1164/rccm.201904-0792oc

Castellani, S., and Conese, M. (2010). Lentiviral vectors and cystic fibrosis gene therapy. *Viruses* 2 (2), 395–412. doi:10.3390/v2020395

Cooney, A. L., Abou Alaiwa, M. H., Shah, V. S., Bouzek, D. C., Stroik, M. R., Powers, L. S., et al. (2016). Lentiviral-mediated phenotypic correction of cystic fibrosis pigs. *JCI Insight* 1 (14), e88730. doi:10.1172/jci.insight.88730

Cooney, A. L., McCray, P. B., and Sinn, P. L. (2018). Cystic fibrosis gene therapy: looking back, looking forward. *Genes (Basel)* 9 (11), 538. doi:10.3390/genes9110538

Cooney, A. L., Singh, B. K., and Sinn, P. L. (2015). Hybrid nonviral/viral vector systems for improved piggyBac DNA transposon *in vivo* delivery. *Mol. Ther.* 23 (4), 667–674. doi:10.1038/mt.2014.254

Cooney, A. L., Thornell, I. M., Singh, B. K., Shah, V. S., Stoltz, D. A., McCray, P. B., et al. (2019). A novel AAV-mediated gene delivery system corrects CFTR function in pigs. *Am. J. Respir. Cel. Mol. Biol.* 61 (6), 747–754. doi:10.1165/rcmb.2019-0006oc

Crane, A. M., Kramer, P., Bui, J. H., Chung, W. J., Li, X. S., Gonzalez-Garay, M. L., et al. (2015). Targeted correction and restored function of the CFTR gene in cystic fibrosis induced pluripotent stem cells. *Stem Cel. Rep.* 4 (4), 569–577. doi:10.1016/j.stemcr.2015.02.005

Davies, J. C., Moskowitz, S. M., Brown, C., Horsley, A., Mall, M. A., McKone, E. F., et al. (2018). VX-659-Tezacaftor-Ivacaftor in Patients with Cystic Fibrosis and One or Two Phe508del Alleles. *N. Engl. J. Med.* 379 (17), 1599–1611. doi:10.1056/nejmoa1807119

Davies, J. C. (2015). The future of CFTR modulating therapies for cystic fibrosis. *Curr. Opin. Pulm. Med.* 21 (6), 579–584. doi:10.1097/mcp.0000000000000211

Delhove, J., Osenk, I., Prichard, I., and Donnelley, M. (2020). Public acceptability of gene therapy and gene editing for human use: a systematic review. *Hum. Gene Ther.* 31 (1-2), 20–46. doi:10.1089/hum.2019.197

Donnelley, M., and Parsons, D. W. (2018). Gene therapy for cystic fibrosis lung disease: overcoming the barriers to translation to the clinic. *Front. Pharmacol.* 9, 1381. doi:10.3389/fphar.2018.01381

Doyle, L. M., and Wang, M. Z. (2019). Overview of extracellular vesicles, their origin, composition, purpose, and methods for exosome isolation and analysis. *Cells* 8 (7), 727. doi:10.3390/cells8070727

Duncan, G. A., Kim, N., Colon-Cortes, Y., Rodriguez, J., Mazur, M., Birket, S. E., et al. (2018). An adeno-associated viral vector capable of penetrating the mucus barrier to inhaled gene therapy. *Mol. Ther.—Methods Clin. Develop.* 9, 296–304. doi:10.1016/j.omtm.2018.03.006

Dye, B. R., Hill, D. R., Ferguson, M. A., Tsai, Y. H., Nagy, M. S., Dyal, R., et al. (2015). *In vitro* generation of human pluripotent stem cell derived lung organoids. *Elife* 4, e05098. doi:10.7554/elife.05098

Eenjes, E., Mertens, T. C. J., Buscop-van Kempen, M. J., van Wijck, Y., Taube, C., Rottier, R. J., et al. (2018). A novel method for expansion and differentiation of mouse tracheal epithelial cells in culture. *Sci. Rep.* 8 (1), 7349. doi:10.1038/s41598-018-25799-6

Eichstadt, S., Barriga, M., Ponakala, A., Teng, C., Nguyen, N. T., Siprashvili, Z., et al. (2019). Phase 1/2a clinical trial of gene-corrected autologous cell therapy for recessive dystrophic epidermolysis bullosa. *JCI Insight* 4 (19), e130554. doi:10.1172/jci.insight.130554

Elborn, J. S. (2016). Cystic fibrosis. *The Lancet* 388 (10059), 2519–2531. doi:10.1016/s0140-6736(16)00576-6

Elverum, K., and Whitman, M. (2019). Delivering cellular and gene therapies to patients: solutions for realizing the potential of the next generation of medicine. *Gene Ther.* 27, 537–544. doi:10.1038/s41434-019-0074-7

Engelhardt, J. F., Schlossberg, H., Yankaskas, J. R., and Dudus, L. (1995). Progenitor cells of the adult human airway involved in submucosal gland development. *Development* 121 (7), 2031–2046.

Ernst, M. P. T., Broeders, M., Herrero-Hernandez, P., Oussoren, E., van der Ploeg, A. T., and Pijnappel, W. W. M. P. (2020). Ready for repair? Gene editing enters the clinic for the treatment of human disease. *Mol. Ther.—Methods Clin. Develop.* 18, 532–557. doi:10.1016/j.omtm.2020.06.022

Erwood, S., Laselva, O., Bily, T. M. I., Brewer, R. A., Rutherford, A. H., Bear, C. E., et al. (2020). Allele-specific prevention of nonsense-mediated decay in cystic fibrosis using homology-independent genome editing. *Mol. Ther.—Methods Clin. Develop.* 17, 1118–1128. doi:10.1016/j.omtm.2020.05.002

Farrow, N., Cmielewski, P., Donnelley, M., Rout-Pitt, N., Moodley, Y., Bertoncello, I., et al. (2018a). Epithelial disruption: a new paradigm enabling human airway stem cell transplantation. *Stem Cell Res Ther.* 9 (1), 153. doi:10.1186/s13287-018-0911-4

Farrow, N., Donnelley, M., Cmielewski, P., Roscioli, E., Rout-Pitt, N., McIntyre, C., et al. (2018b). Role of basal cells in producing persistent lentivirus-mediated airway gene expression. *Hum. Gene Ther.* 29 (6), 653–662. doi:10.1089/hum.2017.059

Firth, A. L., Dargitz, C. T., Qualls, S. J., Menon, T., Wright, R., Singer, O., et al. (2014). Generation of multiciliated cells in functional airway epithelia from human induced pluripotent stem cells. *Proc. Natl. Acad. Sci.* 111 (17), E1723–E1730. doi:10.1073/pnas.1403470111

Fleischer, A., Vallejo-Díez, S., Martín-Fernández, J. M., Sánchez-Gilabert, A., Castresana, M., Del Pozo, A., et al. (2020). iPSC-Derived Intestinal Organoids from Cystic Fibrosis Patients Acquire CFTR Activity upon TALEN-Mediated Repair of the p.F508del mutation. *Mol. Ther.—Methods Clin. Develop.* 17, 858–870. doi:10.1016/j.omtm.2020.04.005

Flotte, T. R., Zeitlin, P. L., Reynolds, T. C., Heald, A. E., Pedersen, P., Beck, S., et al. (2003). Phase I trial of intranasal and endobronchial administration of a recombinant adeno-associated virus serotype 2 (rAAV2)-CFTR vector in adult cystic fibrosis patients: a two-part clinical study. *Hum. Gene Ther.* 14 (11), 1079–1088. doi:10.1089/104303403322124792

Flume, P. A., O'Sullivan, B. P., Robinson, K. A., Goss, C. H., Mogayzel, P. J., Willey-Courand, D. B., et al. (2007). Cystic fibrosis pulmonary guidelines. *Am. J. Respir. Crit. Care Med.* 176 (10), 957–969. doi:10.1164/rccm.200705-664oc

Gentzsch, M., Boyles, S. E., Cheluvaraju, C., Chaudhry, I. G., Quinney, N. L., Cho, C., et al. (2017). Pharmacological rescue of conditionally reprogrammed cystic fibrosis bronchial epithelial cells. *Am. J. Respir. Cell Mol. Biol.* 56 (5), 568–574. doi:10.1165/rcmb.2016-0276ma

George, L. A., Ragni, M. V., Rasko, J. E. J., Raffini, L. J., Samelson-Jones, B. J., Ozelo, M., et al. (2020). Long-term follow-up of the first in human intravascular delivery of AAV for gene transfer: AAV2-hFIX16 for severe hemophilia B. *Mol. Ther.* 28 (9), 2073–2082. doi:10.1016/j.ymthe.2020.06.001

Ghosh, M., Ahmad, S., White, C. W., and Reynolds, S. D. (2017). Transplantation of airway epithelial stem/progenitor cells: a future for cell-based therapy. *Am. J. Respir. Cell. Mol. Biol.* 56 (1), 1–10. doi:10.1165/rcmb.2016-0181ma

Ghosh, M., Helm, K. M., Smith, R. W., Giordanengo, M. S., Li, B., Shen, H., et al. (2011). A single cell functions as a tissue-specific stem cell and theIn VitroNiche-forming cell. *Am. J. Respir. Cell Mol. Biol.* 45 (3), 459–469. doi:10.1165/rcmb.2010-0314oc

Gonzalez, G., Vituret, C., Di Pietro, A., Chanson, M., Boulanger, P., and Hong, S. S. (2012). Microparticle-mediated transfer of the viral receptors CAR and CD46, and the CFTR channel in a CHO cell model confers new functions to target cells. *PLoS One* 7 (12), e52326. doi:10.1371/journal.pone.0052326

Gratwohl, A., and Niederwieser, D. (2012). History of hematopoietic stem cell transplantation: evolution and perspectives. *Curr. Probl. Dermatol.* 43, 81–90. doi:10.1159/000335266

Griesenbach, U., Kitson, C., Escudero Garcia, S., Farley, R., Singh, C., Somerton, L., et al. (2006). Inefficient cationic lipid-mediated siRNA and antisense oligonucleotide transfer to airway epithelial cells *in vivo*. *Respir. Res.* 7, 26. doi:10.1186/1465-9921-7-26

Griesenbach, U., Pytel, K. M., and Alton, E. W. F. W. (2015). Cystic fibrosis gene therapy in the UK and elsewhere. *Hum. Gene Ther.* 26 (5), 266–275. doi:10.1089/hum.2015.027

Gyurkocza, B., and Sandmaier, B. M. (2014). Conditioning regimens for hematopoietic cell transplantation: one size does not fit all. *Blood* 124 (3), 344–353. doi:10.1182/blood-2014-02-514778

Hajj, K. A., and Whitehead, K. A. (2017). Tools for translation: non-viral materials for therapeutic mRNA delivery. *Nat. Rev. Mater.* 2 (10), 17056. doi:10.1038/natrevmats.2017.56

Halim, N. S. S., Ch'ng, E. S., Kardia, E., Ali, S. A., Radzi, R., and Yahaya, B. H. (2019). Aerosolised mesenchymal stem cells expressing angiopoietin-1 enhances airway repair. *Stem Cel. Rev. Rep.* 15 (1), 112–125. doi:10.1007/s12015-018-9844-7

Havenga, M. J. E., Lemckert, A. A. C., Ophorst, O. J. A. E., van Meijer, M., Germeraad, W. T. V., Grimbergen, J., et al. (2002). Exploiting the natural diversity in adenovirus tropism for therapy and prevention of disease. *J. virol.* 76 (9), 4612–4620. doi:10.1128/jvi.76.9.4612-4620.2002

Hawkins, F. J., Suzuki, S., Beermann, M. L., Barilla, C., Wang, R., Villacorta-Martin, C., et al. (2020). Derivation of airway basal stem cells from human pluripotent stem cells. *Cell Stem Cell* 28, 79–95. doi:10.1016/j.stem.2020.09.017

Hayes, D., Kopp, B. T., Hill, C. L., Lallier, S. W., Schwartz, C. M., Tadesse, M., et al. (2019). Cell therapy for cystic fibrosis lung disease: regenerative basal cell amplification. *Stem Cells Translational Med.* 8 (3), 225–235. doi:10.1002/sctm.18-0098

Hong, K. U., Reynolds, S. D., Watkins, S., Fuchs, E., and Stripp, B. R. (2004). *In vivo* differentiation potential of tracheal basal cells: evidence for multipotent and unipotent subpopulations. *Am. J. Physiology-Lung Cell Mol. Physiol.* 286 (4), L643–L649. doi:10.1152/ajplung.00155.2003

Huang, S. X. L., Islam, M. N., O'Neill, J., Hu, Z., Yang, Y.-G., Chen, Y.-W., et al. (2014). Efficient generation of lung and airway epithelial cells from human pluripotent stem cells. *Nat. Biotechnol.* 32 (1), 84–91. doi:10.1038/nbt.2754

Igreja, S., Clarke, L. A., Botelho, H. M., Marques, L., and Amaral, M. D. (2016). Correction of a cystic fibrosis splicing mutation by antisense oligonucleotides. *Hum. Mutat.* 37 (2), 209–215. doi:10.1002/humu.22931

Jaffe, A., Prasad, S. A., Larcher, V., and Hart, S. (2006). Gene therapy for children with cystic fibrosis--who has the right to choose?. *J. Med. Ethics* 32 (6), 361–364. doi:10.1136/jme.2005.012740

Kardia, E., Ch'ng, E. S., and Yahaya, B. H. (2018). Aerosol-based airway epithelial cell delivery improves airway regeneration and repair. *J. Tissue Eng. Regen. Med.* 12 (2), e995–e1007. doi:10.1002/term.2421

Kardia, E., Yusoff, N. M., Zakaria, Z., and Yahaya, B. (2014). Aerosol-based delivery of fibroblast cells for treatment of lung diseases. *J. Aerosol. Med. Pulm. Drug Deliv.* 27 (1), 30–34. doi:10.1089/jamp.2012.1020

Karikó, K., Ni, H., Capodici, J., Lamphier, M., and Weissman, D. (2004). mRNA is an endogenous ligand for Toll-like receptor 3. *J. Biol. Chem.* 279 (13), 12542–12550. doi:10.1074/jbc.m310175200

Kariyawasam, D., Carey, K. A., Jones, K. J., and Farrar, M. A. (2018). New and developing therapies in spinal muscular atrophy. *Paediatric Respir. Rev.* 28, 3–10. doi:10.1016/j.prrv.2018.03.003

Konishi, S., Gotoh, S., Tateishi, K., Yamamoto, Y., Korogi, Y., Nagasaki, T., et al. (2016). Directed induction of functional multi-ciliated cells in proximal airway epithelial spheroids from human pluripotent stem cells. *Stem Cell Rep.* 6 (1), 18–25. doi:10.1016/j.stemcr.2015.11.010

Kraft, J. C., Freeling, J. P., Wang, Z., and Ho, R. J. Y. (2014). Emerging research and clinical development trends of liposome and lipid nanoparticle drug delivery systems. *J. Pharm. Sci.* 103 (1), 29–52. doi:10.1002/jps.23773

Kuhn, A. N., Beiβert, T., Simon, P., Vallazza, B., Buck, J., Davies, B. P., et al. (2012). mRNA as a versatile tool for exogenous protein expression. *Curr. Gene Ther.* 12 (5), 347–361. doi:10.2174/156652312802762536

Kumagai, N., LaMattina, J. C., Kamano, C., Vagefi, P. A., Barth, R. N., O'Neil, J. J., et al. (2002). Vascularized islet cell transplantation in miniature Swine: islet-kidney allografts correct the diabetic hyperglycemia induced by total pancreatectomy. *Diabetes* 51 (11), 3220–3228. doi:10.2337/diabetes.51.11.3220

Leborgne, C., Barbon, E., Alexander, J. M., Hanby, H., Delignat, S., Cohen, D. M., et al. (2020). IgG-cleaving endopeptidase enables *in vivo* gene therapy in the presence of anti-AAV neutralizing antibodies. *Nat. Med.* 26 (7), 1096–1101. doi:10.1038/s41591-020-0911-7

Ledford, H. (2020). CRISPR treatment inserted directly into the body for first time. *Nature* 579 (7798), 185. doi:10.1038/d41586-020-00655-8

Lee, R. E., Miller, S. M., Mascenik, T. M., Lewis, C. A., Dang, H., Boggs, Z. H., et al. (2020). Assessing human airway epithelial progenitor cells for cystic fibrosis cell therapy. *Am. J. Respir. Cell Mol. Biol.* 63 (3), 374–385. doi:10.1165/rcmb.2019-0384oc

Limberis, M., Anson, D. S., Fuller, M., and Parsons, D. W. (2002). Recovery of airway cystic fibrosis transmembrane conductance regulator function in mice with cystic fibrosis after single-dose lentivirus-mediated gene transfer. *Hum. Gene Ther.* 13 (16), 1961–1970. doi:10.1089/10430340260355365

Liu, X., Ory, V., Chapman, S., Yuan, H., Albanese, C., Kallakury, B., et al. (2012). ROCK inhibitor and feeder cells induce the conditional reprogramming of epithelial cells. *Am. J. Pathol.* 180 (2), 599–607. doi:10.1016/j.ajpath.2011.10.036

Lwin, S. M., Syed, F., Di, W. L., Kadiyirire, T., Liu, L., Guy, A., et al. (2019). Safety and early efficacy outcomes for lentiviral fibroblast gene therapy in recessive dystrophic epidermolysis bullosa. *JCI Insight* 4 (11), e126243. doi:10.1172/jci.insight.126243

Martinovich, K. M., Iosifidis, T., Buckley, A. G., Looi, K., Ling, K. M., Sutanto, E. N., et al. (2017). Conditionally reprogrammed primary airway epithelial cells maintain morphology, lineage and disease specific functional characteristics. *Sci. Rep.* 7 (1), 17971. doi:10.1038/s41598-017-17952-4

Marinkovich, M. P., and Tang, J. Y. (2019). Gene therapy for epidermolysis bullosa. *J. Invest. Dermatol.* 139 (6), 1221–1226. doi:10.1016/j.jid.2018.11.036

McCauley, K. B., Hawkins, F., Serra, M., Thomas, D. C., Jacob, A., and Kotton, D. N. (2017). Efficient derivation of functional human airway epithelium from pluripotent stem cells via temporal regulation of wnt signaling. *Cell Stem Cell* 20 (6), 844–857. doi:10.1016/j.stem.2017.03.001

Meyer-Berg, H., Zhou Yang, L., Pilar de Lucas, M., Zambrano, A., Hyde, S. C., and Gill, D. R. (2020). Identification of AAV serotypes for lung gene therapy in human embryonic stem cell-derived lung organoids. *Stem Cell Res. Ther.* 11 (1), 448. doi:10.1186/s13287-020-01950-x

Miah, K. M., Hyde, S. C., and Gill, D. R. (2019). Emerging gene therapies for cystic fibrosis. *Expert Rev. Respir. Med.* 13 (8), 709–725. doi:10.1080/17476348.2019.1634547

Miller, A. J., Hill, D. R., Nagy, M. S., Aoki, Y., Dye, B. R., Chin, A. M., et al. (2018). *In Vitro* induction and in vivo engraftment of lung bud tip progenitor cells derived from human pluripotent stem cells. *Stem Cell Rep.* 10 (1), 101–119. doi:10.1016/j.stemcr.2017.11.012

Montoro, D. T., Haber, A. L., Biton, M., Vinarsky, V., Lin, B., Birket, S. E., et al. (2018). A revised airway epithelial hierarchy includes CFTR-expressing ionocytes. *Nature* 560 (7718), 319–324. doi:10.1038/s41586-018-0393-7

Moss, R. B., Rodman, D., Spencer, L. T., Aitken, M. L., Zeitlin, P. L., Waltz, D., et al. (2004). Repeated adeno-associated virus serotype 2 aerosol-mediated cystic fibrosis transmembrane regulator gene transfer to the lungs of patients with cystic fibrosis. *Chest* 125 (2), 509–521. doi:10.1378/chest.125.2.509

Moss, R. B., Milla, C., Colombo, J., Accurso, F., Zeitlin, P. L., Clancy, J. P., et al. (2007). Repeated aerosolized AAV-CFTR for treatment of cystic fibrosis: a randomized placebo-controlled phase 2B trial. *Hum. Gene Ther.* 18 (8), 726–732. doi:10.1089/hum.2007.022

Mou, H., Zhao, R., Sherwood, R., Ahfeldt, T., Lapey, A., Wain, J., et al. (2012). Generation of multipotent lung and airway progenitors from mouse ESCs and patient-specific cystic fibrosis iPSCs. *Cell Stem Cell* 10 (4), 385–397. doi:10.1016/j.stem.2012.01.018

Murphy, D. E., de Jong, O. G., Brouwer, M., Wood, M. J., Lavieu, G., Schiffelers, R. M., et al. (2019). Extracellular vesicle-based therapeutics: natural versus engineered targeting and trafficking. *Exp. Mol. Med.* 51 (3), 1–12. doi:10.1038/s12276-019-0223-5

Nafee, N., Forier, K., Braeckmans, K., and Schneider, M. (2018). Mucus-penetrating solid lipid nanoparticles for the treatment of cystic fibrosis: proof of concept, challenges and pitfalls. *Eur. J. Pharmaceutics Biopharmaceutics* 124, 125–137. doi:10.1016/j.ejpb.2017.12.017

Naldini, L., Blomer, U., Gallay, P., Ory, D., Mulligan, R., Gage, F. H., et al. (1996). *In vivo* gene delivery and stable transduction of nondividing cells by a lentiviral vector. *Science* 272 (5259), 263–267. doi:10.1126/science.272.5259.263

Ni, R., Feng, R., and Chau, Y. (2019). Synthetic approaches for nucleic acid delivery: choosing the right carriers. *Life (Basel)* 9 (3), 59. doi:10.3390/life9030059

Oren, Y. S., Pranke, I. M., Kerem, B., and Sermet-Gaudelus, I. (2017). The suppression of premature termination codons and the repair of splicing mutations in CFTR. *Curr. Opin. Pharmacol.* 34, 125–131. doi:10.1016/j.coph.2017.09.017

Ortiz, L. A., Gambelli, F., McBride, C., Gaupp, D., Baddoo, M., Kaminski, N., et al. (2003). Mesenchymal stem cell engraftment in lung is enhanced in response to bleomycin exposure and ameliorates its fibrotic effects. *Pnas* 100 (14), 8407–8411. doi:10.1073/pnas.1432929100

Pardi, N., Tuyishime, S., Muramatsu, H., Kariko, K., Mui, B. L., Tam, Y. K., et al. (2015). Expression kinetics of nucleoside-modified mRNA delivered in lipid nanoparticles to mice by various routes. *J. Controlled Release* 217, 345–351. doi:10.1016/j.jconrel.2015.08.007

Patel, A., Zhao, J., Duan, D., and Lai, Y. (2019a). Design of AAV vectors for delivery of large or multiple transgenes. *Methods Mol. Biol.* 1950, 19–33. doi:10.1007/978-1-4939-9139-6_2

Patel, A. K., Kaczmarek, J. C., Bose, S., Kauffman, K. J., Mir, F., Heartlein, M. W., et al. (2019b). Inhaled nanoformulated mRNA polyplexes for protein production in lung epithelium. *Adv. Mater.* 31 (8), e1805116. doi:10.1002/adma.201970053

Peters-Hall, J. R., Coquelin, M. L., Torres, M. J., LaRanger, R., Alabi, B. R., Sho, S., et al. (2018). Long-term culture and cloning of primary human bronchial basal cells that maintain multipotent differentiation capacity and CFTR channel function. *Am. J. Physiology-Lung Cell Mol. Physiol.* 315 (2), L313–L327. doi:10.1152/ajplung.00355.2017

Plasschaert, L. W., Žilionis, R., Choo-Wing, R., Savova, V., Knehr, J., Roma, G., et al. (2018). A single-cell atlas of the airway epithelium reveals the CFTR-rich pulmonary ionocyte. *Nature* 560 (7718), 377–381. doi:10.1038/s41586-018-0394-6

Pollock, K., Albares, L., Wendt, C., and Hubel, A. (2013). Isolation of fibroblasts and epithelial cells in bronchoalveolar lavage (BAL). *Exp. Lung Res.* 39 (3), 146–154. doi:10.3109/01902148.2013.781720

Ramalho, A. S., Beck, S., Meyer, M., Penque, D., Cutting, G. R., and Amaral, M. D. (2002). Five percent of normal cystic fibrosis transmembrane conductance regulator mRNA ameliorates the severity of pulmonary disease in cystic fibrosis. *Am. J. Respir. Cel. Mol. Biol.* 27 (5), 619–627. doi:10.1165/rcmb.2001-0004oc

Ratjen, F., Bell, S. C., Rowe, S. M., Goss, C. H., Quittner, A. L., and Bush, A. (2015). Cystic fibrosis. *Nat. Rev. Dis. Primers* 1, 15010. doi:10.1038/nrdp.2015.10

Riordan, J. R. (2008). CFTR function and prospects for therapy. *Annu. Rev. Biochem.* 77, 701–726. doi:10.1146/annurev.biochem.75.103004.142532

Robinson, E., MacDonald, K. D., Slaughter, K., McKinney, M., Patel, S., Sun, C., et al. (2018). Lipid nanoparticle-delivered chemically modified mRNA restores chloride secretion in cystic fibrosis. *Mol. Ther.* 26 (8), 2034–2046. doi:10.1016/j.ymthe.2018.05.014

Rock, J. R., Onaitis, M. W., Rawlins, E. L., Lu, Y., Clark, C. P., Xue, Y., et al. (2009). Basal cells as stem cells of the mouse trachea and human airway epithelium. *Proc. Natl. Acad. Sci.* 106 (31), 12771–12775. doi:10.1073/pnas.0906850106

Ronzitti, G., Gross, D. A., and Mingozzi, F. (2020). Human immune responses to adeno-associated virus (AAV) vectors. *Front. Immunol.* 11, 670. doi:10.3389/fimmu.2020.00670

Rowe, S. M., Miller, S., and Sorscher, E. J. (2005). Cystic fibrosis. *N. Engl. J. Med.* 352 (19), 1992–2001. doi:10.1056/nejmra043184

Ruan, J., Hirai, H., Yang, D., Ma, L., Hou, X., Jiang, H., et al. (2019). Efficient gene editing at major CFTR mutation loci. *Mol. Ther.—Nucleic Acids* 16, 73–81. doi:10.1016/j.omtn.2019.02.006

Sahay, G., Querbes, W., Alabi, C., Eltoukhy, A., Sarkar, S., Zurenko, C., et al. (2013). Efficiency of siRNA delivery by lipid nanoparticles is limited by endocytic recycling. *Nat. Biotechnol.* 31 (7), 653–658. doi:10.1038/nbt.2614

Sahin, U., Türeci, K. Ö., and Tureci, O. (2014). mRNA-based therapeutics—developing a new class of drugs. *Nat. Rev. Drug Discov.* 13 (10), 759–780. doi:10.1038/nrd4278

Sanz, D. J., Hollywood, J. A., Scallan, M. F., and Harrison, P. T. (2017). Cas9/gRNA targeted excision of cystic fibrosis-causing deep-intronic splicing mutations restores normal splicing of CFTR mRNA. *PLoS One* 12 (9), e0184009. doi:10.1371/journal.pone.0184009

Schwank, G., Koo, B.-K., Sasselli, V., Dekkers, J. F., Heo, I., Demircan, T., et al. (2013). Functional repair of CFTR by CRISPR/Cas9 in intestinal stem cell organoids of cystic fibrosis patients. *Cell Stem Cell* 13 (6), 653–658. doi:10.1016/j.stem.2013.11.002

Sermet-Gaudelus, I., Clancy, J. P., Nichols, D. P., Nick, J. A., De Boeck, K., Solomon, G. M., et al. (2019). Antisense oligonucleotide eluforsen improves CFTR function in F508del cystic fibrosis. *J. Cystic Fibrosis* 18 (4), 536–542. doi:10.1016/j.jcf.2018.10.015

Singh, B. K., Cooney, A. L., Krishnamurthy, S., and Sinn, P. L. (2020). Extracellular vesicle-mediated siRNA delivery, protein delivery, and CFTR complementation in well-differentiated human airway epithelial cells. *Genes (Basel)* 11 (4), 351. doi:10.3390/genes11040351

Smyth, T., Kullberg, M., Malik, N., Smith-Jones, P., Graner, M. W., and Anchordoquy, T. J. (2015). Biodistribution and delivery efficiency of unmodified tumor-derived exosomes. *J. Controlled Release* 199, 145–155. doi:10.1016/j.jconrel.2014.12.013

Stadtmauer, E. A., Fraietta, J. A., Davis, M. M., Cohen, A. D., Weber, K. L., Lancaster, E., et al. (2020). CRISPR-engineered T cells in patients with refractory cancer. *Science* 367 (6481), eaba7365. doi:10.1126/science.aba7365

Stirnadel-Farrant, H., Kudari, M., Garman, N., Imrie, J., Chopra, B., Giannelli, S., et al. (2018). Gene therapy in rare diseases: the benefits and challenges of developing a patient-centric registry for Strimvelis in ADA-SCID. *Orphanet. J. Rare Dis.* 13 (1), 49. doi:10.1186/s13023-018-0791-9

Suzuki, S., Crane, A. M., Anirudhan, V., Barillà, C., Matthias, N., Randell, S. H., et al. (2020). Highly efficient gene editing of cystic fibrosis patient-derived airway basal cells results in functional CFTR correction. *Mol. Ther.* 28 (7), 1684–1695. doi:10.1016/j.ymthe.2020.04.021

Takahashi, Y., Nishikawa, M., Shinotsuka, H., Matsui, Y., Ohara, S., Imai, T., et al. (2013). Visualization and *in vivo* tracking of the exosomes of murine melanoma B16-BL6 cells in mice after intravenous injection. *J. Biotechnol.* 165 (2), 77–84. doi:10.1016/j.jbiotec.2013.03.013

Tsui, L., Buchwald, M., Barker, D., Braman, J., Knowlton, R., Schumm, J., et al. (1985). Cystic fibrosis locus defined by a genetically linked polymorphic DNA marker. *Science* 230 (4729), 1054–1057. doi:10.1126/science.2997931

U.S. Food and Drug Administration (2020). *Approved cellular and gene therapy products* Retrieved from: https://www.fda.gov/vaccines-blood-biologics/cellular-gene-therapy-products/approved-cellular-and-gene-therapy-products ((October 21, 2020)

Vaidyanathan, S., Salahudeen, A. A., Sellers, Z. M., Bravo, D. T., Choi, S. S., Batish, A., et al. (2020). High-efficiency, selection-free gene repair in airway stem cells from cystic fibrosis patients rescues CFTR function in differentiated epithelia. *Cell Stem Cell* 26 (2), 161–171. doi:10.1016/j.stem.2019.11.002

Vencken, S., Foged, C., Ramsey, J. M., Sweeney, L., Cryan, S. A., MacLoughlin, R. J., et al. (2019). Nebulised lipid-polymer hybrid nanoparticles for the delivery of a therapeutic anti-inflammatory microRNA to bronchial epithelial cells. *ERJ Open Res.* 5 (2), 00161. doi:10.1183/23120541.00161-2018

Villamizar, O., Waters, S. A., Scott, T., Saayman, S., Grepo, N., Urak, R., et al. (2019). Targeted activation of cystic fibrosis transmembrane conductance regulator. *Mol. Ther.* 27 (10), 1737–1748. doi:10.1016/j.ymthe.2019.07.002

Villamizar, O., Waters, S. A., Scott, T., Grepo, N., Jaffe, A., and Morris, K. V. (2021). Mesenchymal Stem Cell exosome delivered Zinc Finger Protein activation of cystic fibrosis transmembrane conductance regulator. *J. Extracell. Vesicles* 10 (3), e12053. doi:10.1002/jev2.12053

Vituret, C., Gallay, K., Confort, M.-P., Ftaich, N., Matei, C. I., Archer, F., et al. (2016). Transfer of the cystic fibrosis transmembrane conductance regulator to human cystic fibrosis cells mediated by extracellular vesicles. *Hum. Gene Ther.* 27 (2), 166–183. doi:10.1089/hum.2015.144

Wagner, J. A., Nepomuceno, I. B., Messner, A. H., Moran, M. L., Batson, E. P., Dimiceli, S., et al. (2002). A phase II, double-blind, randomized, placebo-controlled clinical trial of tgAAVCF using maxillary sinus delivery in patients with cystic fibrosis with antrostomies. *Hum. Gene Ther.* 13 (11), 1349–1359. doi:10.1089/104303402760128577

Wainwright, B. J., Scambler, P. J., Schmidtke, J., Watson, E. A., Law, H.-Y., Farrall, M., et al. (1985). Localization of cystic fibrosis locus to human chromosome 7cen-q22. *Nature* 318 (6044), 384–385. doi:10.1038/318384a0

Wan, F., Nylander, T., Klodzinska, S. N., Foged, C., Yang, M., Baldursdottir, S. G., et al. (2018). Lipid shell-enveloped polymeric nanoparticles with high integrity of lipid shells improve mucus penetration and interaction with cystic fibrosis-related bacterial biofilms. *ACS Appl. Mater. Inter.* 10 (13), 10678–10687. doi:10.1021/acsami.7b19762

Wang, G., Slepushkin, V., Zabner, J., Keshavjee, S., Johnston, J. C., Sauter, S. L., et al. (1999). Feline immunodeficiency virus vectors persistently transduce nondividing airway epithelia and correct the cystic fibrosis defect. *J. Clin. Invest.* 104 (11), R55–R62. doi:10.1172/jci8390

Watson, J. K., Rulands, S., Wilkinson, A. C., Wuidart, A., Ousset, M., Van Keymeulen, A., et al. (2015). Clonal dynamics reveal two distinct populations of basal cells in slow-turnover airway epithelium. *Cell Rep.* 12 (1), 90–101. doi:10.1016/j.celrep.2015.06.011

Wu, Z., Yang, H., and Colosi, P. (2010). Effect of genome size on AAV vector packaging. *Mol. Ther.* 18 (1), 80–86. doi:10.1038/mt.2009.255

Xu, J., Woods, C. R., Mora, A. L., Joodi, R., Brigham, K. L., Iyer, S., et al. (2007). Prevention of endotoxin-induced systemic response by bone marrow-derived mesenchymal stem cells in mice. *Am. J. Physiology-Lung Cell Mol. Physiol.* 293 (1), L131–L141. doi:10.1152/ajplung.00431.2006

Yamada, K., Hirakata, A., Tchipashvili, V., Shimizu, A., Iwaki, H., Griesemer, A., et al. (2011). Composite islet-kidneys from single baboon donors cure diabetes across fully allogenic barriers. *Am. J. Transpl.* 11 (12), 2603–2612. doi:10.1111/j.1600-6143.2011.03733.x

Zabner, J., Seiler, M., Walters, R., Kotin, R. M., Fulgeras, W., Davidson, B. L., et al. (2000). Adeno-associated virus type 5 (AAV5) but not AAV2 binds to the apical surfaces of airway epithelia and facilitates gene transfer. *J. Virol.* 74 (8), 3852–3858. doi:10.1128/jvi.74.8.3852-3858.2000

Zhu, Y.-g., Feng, X.-m., Abbott, J., Fang, X.-h., Hao, Q., Monsel, A., et al. (2014). Human mesenchymal stem cell microvesicles for treatment ofEscherichia coliEndotoxin-induced acute lung injury in mice. *Stem Cells* 32 (1), 116–125. doi:10.1002/stem.1504

Zulueta, A., Colombo, M., Peli, V., Falleni, M., Tosi, D., Ricciardi, M., et al. (2018). Lung mesenchymal stem cells-derived extracellular vesicles attenuate the inflammatory profile of Cystic Fibrosis epithelial cells. *Cell Signal.* 51, 110–118. doi:10.1016/j.cellsig.2018.07.015

11

Harnessing the ECM Microenvironment to Ameliorate Mesenchymal Stromal Cell-Based Therapy in Chronic Lung Diseases

Linda Elowsson Rendin, Anna Löfdahl, Måns Kadefors, Zackarias Söderlund, Emil Tykesson, Sara Rolandsson Enes, Jenny Wigén and Gunilla Westergren-Thorsson*

Lung Biology Unit, Department of Experimental Medical Science, Lund University, Lund, Sweden

***Correspondence:**
Linda Elowsson Rendin
linda.elowsson_rendin@med.lu.se

It is known that the cell environment such as biomechanical properties and extracellular matrix (ECM) composition dictate cell behaviour including migration, proliferation, and differentiation. Important constituents of the microenvironment, including ECM molecules such as proteoglycans and glycosaminoglycans (GAGs), determine events in both embryogenesis and repair of the adult lung. Mesenchymal stromal/stem cells (MSC) have been shown to have immunomodulatory properties and may be potent actors regulating tissue remodelling and regenerative cell responses upon lung injury. Using MSC in cell-based therapy holds promise for treatment of chronic lung diseases such as idiopathic pulmonary fibrosis (IPF) and chronic obstructive pulmonary disease (COPD). However, so far clinical trials with MSCs in COPD have not had a significant impact on disease amelioration nor on IPF, where low cell survival rate and pulmonary retention time are major hurdles to overcome. Research shows that the microenvironment has a profound impact on transplanted MSCs. In our studies on acellular lung tissue slices (lung scaffolds) from IPF patients versus healthy individuals, we see a profound effect on cellular activity, where healthy cells cultured in diseased lung scaffolds adapt and produce proteins further promoting a diseased environment, whereas cells on healthy scaffolds sustain a healthy proteomic profile. Therefore, modulating the environmental context for cell-based therapy may be a potent way to improve treatment using MSCs. In this review, we will describe the importance of the microenvironment for cell-based therapy in chronic lung diseases, how MSC-ECM interactions can affect therapeutic output and describe current progress in the field of cell-based therapy.

Keywords: chronic objective pulmonary disease, MSC, extracellular matrix, artificial lung scaffolds, idiopathic pulmonary fibrosis

INTRODUCTION

Chronic lung diseases such as idiopathic pulmonary fibrosis (IPF) and chronic obstructive pulmonary disease (COPD) are life-threatening progressive lower respiratory diseases that are increasing world-wide. COPD alone is the 3rd cause of death, and complicated by co-morbidities such as cardiovascular disease and lung cancer (Sin et al., 2006). COPD patients are mainly treated with bronchodilators and inhaled corticosteroids to help reduce symptoms, however, disease

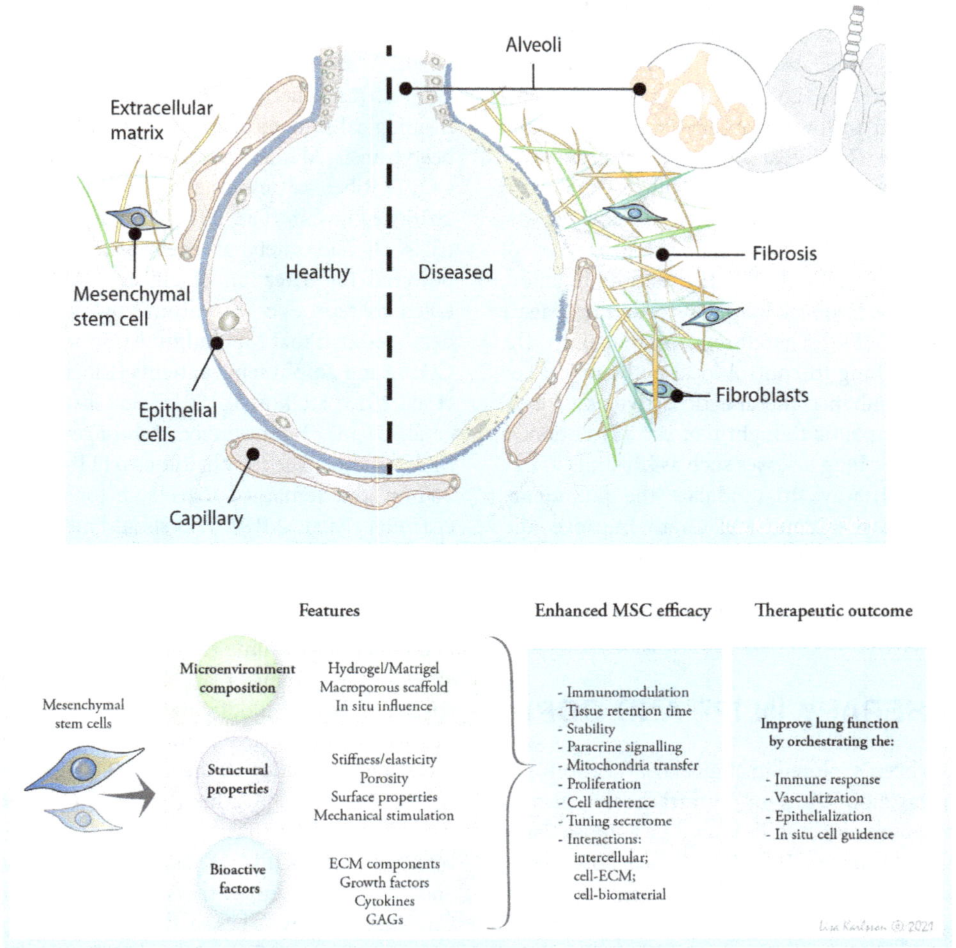

FIGURE 1 | The composition and mechanoelastic properties of ECM affect cell response and activity and therefore, moderating the microenvironment of therapeutic mesenchymal stem cells (MSC) may provide a novel approach to affect cell retention time, and improve therapeutic properties. Affecting the ECM *in situ* or providing an artificial microenvironment to enhance MSC therapeutic potential are future lines of research to affect the distorted lung tissue and reduce lung inflammation, and optimally heal emphysematic and fibrotic lesions to restore oxygen uptake.

progression is not halted (Yawn et al., 2021). The complex pathology exhibits a diverse spectrum of phenotypes with formation of fibrosis and/or emphysema and current treatment options involve only strategies to slow down the disease progression, and to improve quality of life (Negewo et al., 2015; Barrecheguren and Miravitlles, 2016). IPF, affecting 3 million people world-wide (Martinez et al., 2017) is also associated with cardiovascular comorbidities (Caminati et al., 2021) and share the risk factors of smoking and inhaled toxins with COPD. IPF, being a chronic fibrosing interstitial lung disease (ILD) with unknown etiology, is characterized by the histopathological pattern of usual interstitial pneumonia (UIP). The abnormal wound healing in response to epithelial distress results in exaggerated mesenchymal cell activities including build-up and turnover of ECM, causing the altered biomechanics and increased stiffness of the lung tissue. This ultimately disrupts gas exchange and lung function (Raghu et al., 2011). No treatment today affects the mortality associated with IPF to a great extent, but merely prolongs life, with patients still rarely exceeding 3–5 years after IPF diagnosis (Raghu et al., 2011). IPF is primarily treated with the antifibrotic drugs Nintedanib or Pirfenidone, which generate prolonged life-span, but treatment adherence is unfortunately low due to multiple side effects. Future treatment strategies include combining drugs to manage several activated cellular pathways that may differ between patients (Gao et al., 2021). Therefore stratifying patients in more detail may uncover novel therapeutic targets, which is reviewed in Trachalaki et al. (Trachalaki et al., 2021). The lack of curative treatments for both IPF and COPD therefore opts for new efficient strategies that not only affect disease severity but also inhibit progression or at best reverse the deterioration entirely and healing the lung. This is a priority for individual patients as well as for society (Hilberg et al., 2018), and the socioeconomic costs due to these diseases could be significantly reduced by minimizing prevalence and severity (Anees Ur and et al., 2020).

Common to both diseases is the structural remodeling of the lung tissue, resulting in impaired gas exchange that leads to decline in lung function. To date, the knowledge of the inherent capacity of the lung to repair is limited, but mesenchymal stromal cells (MSC) have been proposed to have a therapeutic potential due to their regenerative and immunomodulatory abilities in combination with their low immunogenicity attributed to low or absent human leukocyte antigen (HLA) expression (Lee et al., 2014). The structurally remodeled ECM may have a larger impact on cellular behavior in the local microenvironment than previously anticipated. An altered ECM actively affects the biomechanical properties of the lung tissue (Elowsson Rendin et al., 2019) and its function, creating an inherent vicious feedback loop that further propagate these diseases (**Figure 1**). Therefore, approaching the microenvironment of the lung to control local pathological cell responses that may also enhance therapeutic activities of local MSC, is an appealing therapeutic thought that can revolutionize treatment of serious chronic lung diseases such as IPF and COPD. This review elaborates on ways to modulate the pulmonary microenvironment of the therapeutic MSCs to improve and control efficacy of MSC treatment. This could mean providing an injectable cell-instructive artificial milieu (scaffold), or by directly affecting *in situ* environment of the injected MSC.

MSC BASED THERAPY IN IPF AND COPD

MSCbased therapy has been explored in clinical trials in both IPF and COPD using intravenous (i.v.) or intratracheal routes of administration of bone marrow, umbilical cord or adipose tissue derived MSC in a dosage range of 10^6–10^8 cells per dose, single dose or in some cases, up to 4 doses. Completed trials using primarily one dosage regimen show in COPD trials a safe profile and ameliorated clinical parameters in up to 50% of patients (Cruz and Rocco, 2020). In a small human trial in IPF, patients demonstrated that allogeneic MSC treatment is safe and tolerable upon applying a single injected dose of bone marrow derived MSC up to 200 x 10^6 cells (Glassberg et al., 2017). Similarly, low adverse effects were also shown when using placenta derived MSC (i.v. infusion) or adipose derived stromal cells from stromal vascular fraction (endobronchial infusion) in a phase 1b study in IPF patients (Tzouvelekis et al., 2013; Chambers et al., 2014). A recent study examined the efficacy of repeated i. v. administered MSC, showing improved lung function and 6°min walk test in patients with moderate to severe IPF(Averyanov et al., 2020). Collectively, pre-clinical studies demonstrate antifibrotic effects with MSC treatment, however, the long-term beneficial effects and feasibility of MSC as a therapeutic strategy in IPF patients are yet to be determined, where the few existing clinical trials demonstrate an acceptable safety profile. According to ClinicalTrials.gov, there are currently 5 clinical trials recruiting for stem cell treatment of pulmonary fibrosis. Of these, one is carried out at the University of North Carolina, Chapel Hill, United States, with the aim to evaluate safety and efficacy of infusing autologous lung spheroid stem cells derived from trans-bronchial biopsy specimens in IPF patients.

Several animal studies show promising results in treating pulmonary fibrosis with MSC or derivates thereof such as exosomes and extracellular vesicles (EVs), alleviating fibroblast activation and ECM deposition along with anti-inflammatory outcomes (Reddy et al., 2016; Mansouri et al., 2019; Gad et al., 2020; Wan et al., 2020). Pre-clinical studies on COPD demonstrate that MSCs reduce inflammation and improve histological lung structure (Cruz and Rocco, 2020), which have been translated into several human clinical trials for treatment of COPD(Ribeiro-Paes et al., 2011; Weiss et al., 2013; Stolk et al., 2016; de Oliveira et al., 2017; Armitage et al., 2018). These clinical trials all had safety as their primary endpoint and was not powered for detection of efficacy. Although the clinical trials failed to reproduce the promising pre-clinical results, they all demonstrated that MSC administration was well tolerated among COPD and emphysema patients (Ribeiro-Paes et al., 2011; Weiss et al., 2013; Stolk et al., 2016; de Oliveira et al., 2017; Armitage et al., 2018). Interestingly, Armitage et al. demonstrated that MSCs radiolabeled with indium-111 reached the lungs within 30 min and remained detectable for 24 h after administration (Armitage et al., 2018). This should mean that the effect of MSCs on damaged lung tissue and resident cells need to be rapid. Moreover, an increasing body of research suggests that the MSC therapeutic functions depend on the microenvironment encountered (Kusuma et al., 2017; Abreu et al., 2019; Islam et al., 2019; Abreu et al., 2020). Therefore, it is tempting to speculate that by modifying the microenvironment it would be possible to enhance the therapeutic time-frame for MSCs by increasing residency in the COPD lungs and thereby increasing the potency of the infused MSCs. Currently, there are three clinical trials recruiting patients to evaluate MSC for the treatment of COPD. A comprehensive overview of ongoing and completed human trials in IPF and COPD is searchable at ClinicalTrials.gov. These trials are encouraging and gives great hope to the scientific community to increase the therapeutic potential of MSC.

THE MECHANISM OF MSC

Anti-Inflammatory Function

MSCs are extensively explored as cell therapy candidates and are known for their potential to differentiate into multiple cell lineages, however their major therapeutic mechanism is from interactions via paracrine signaling and cell-cell contact (Murphy et al., 2013; Gao et al., 2016). MSCs have demonstrated both anti-inflammatory and anti-fibrotic capacity, which could be of importance for tissue repair and regeneration in chronic lung diseases (Cruz and Rocco, 2020). The observed anti-inflammatory properties of MSCs include effects on several cells of the immune system, including T-cells, B-cells, dendritic cells, monocytes, macrophages, and natural killer (NK) cells. For example, MSCs can suppress T-cell proliferation via Indoleamine-2,3dioxygenase (IDO) secretion, which mediates tryptophan depletion causing cellular stress in T cells (Meisel et al., 2004; Laing et al., 2019), or by inducing a switch toward a regulatory T-cell phenotype (Bartholomew et al., 2002; Benvenuto et al., 2007; Casiraghi et al., 2008). In an inflammatory setting, MSCs are able to direct macrophage polarization from a proinflammatory (M1) to an anti-inflammatory phenotype (M2). This occurs through feedback-loop involving MSC secreted prostaglandin E2 (PGE2) (reviewed in) (Prockop, 2013). In addition, MSCs are able to affect resident macrophages to reduce their secretion of pro-inflammatory mediators through a different negative feedback-loop, by secreting tumor necrosis factor (TNF)-α stimulated gene 6 (TSG-6) (Prockop, 2013).

While the anti-inflammatory effect of MSCs has been extensively used as a rationale for MSC-based therapy, their anti-fibrotic qualities could further motivate the use of MSC-based therapy in chronic diseases. In animal models of lung fibrosis, it has been shown that MSC administration can reduce the extent of fibrosis (reviewed in (Srour and Thébaud, 2015). Increased levels of the hepatocyte growth factor (HGF) has been linked to the anti-fibrotic properties of MSCs. *In vitro*, HGF inhibited epithelial-mesenchymal-transition (EMT) through inhibition of transforming growth factor β (TGF-β) signaling (Mias et al., 2009; Shukla et al., 2009). Interestingly, administration of MSC has been associated with changes in levels of ECM modifying enzymes such as metalloproteases (MMPs) and tissue inhibitor of metalloproteases (TIMPs), and the balance of these enzymes is important in both fibrosis and emphysema development (Mias et al., 2009; Moodley et al., 2009; Semedo et al., 2009).

Operating Neighboring Cells: Extracellular Vesicles

In addition to the secretion of anti-inflammatory and anti-fibrotic mediators, MSCs are also known to communicate with other cells by secretion of EVs (reviewed in (Farhat et al., 2019)). EVs are a heterogenous group of small lipid vesicles with cargoes containing mediators for intercellular communication such as proteins, microRNAs, and lipids (Thery and et al., 2018; van Niel et al., 2018). An increasing body of literature suggests that MSC-derived EVs possess immune regulatory functions (Farhat et al., 2019). MSC-derived EVs have been demonstrated to mitigate allergic hyperresponsiveness (Cruz et al., 2015), enhance M1 to M2 macrophage phenotype polarization, macrophage bioenergetics, and phagocytosis (Phinney et al., 2015; Jackson et al., 2016; Morrison et al., 2017), as well as to have an inhibitory effect on T-cell proliferation (Blazquez et al., 2014; Pachler et al., 2017; Mardpour et al., 2019). Moreover, MSC-derived EVs have been shown to decrease the influx of inflammatory cells in an *E. coli* endotoxin-induced acute lung injury model. This therapeutic effect was at least partly mediated through keratinocyte growth factor (KGF/FGF7)(Zhu et al., 2014). Interestingly, in an *E. coli*-induced acute lung injury rat model, it was demonstrated that EVs isolated from MSCs pre-exposed to IFN-g were more effective in attenuating lung injury compared to EVs isolated from naïve, non-exposed MSCs (Varkouhi et al., 2019). These data suggest that the EV cargo released by MSCs can vary significantly based on the microenvironment the cells have encountered.

Restore Cellular Function: Mitochondrial Transfer

Another possibility of MSCs potential in cell therapy is to use their mitochondria. The first evidence that MSCs have the capacity to transfer mitochondria to other cells was published in 2006 (Spees et al., 2006). In this study MSCs were able to restore the aerobic respiration in epithelial cells lacking functional mitochondria (Spees et al., 2006). Since then, it has been shown that MSCs can transfer mitochondria via EVs, microtubules, and tunneling nanotubes (TNTs) (Spees et al., 2006; Phinney et al., 2015; Morrison et al., 2017). For example, mitochondria transferred from MSCs to macrophages partly via TNTs, modulated macrophage phagocytosis both *in vitro* and *in vivo* (Jackson et al., 2016). MSC mitochondrial transfer has also been reported to reduce lung injury in a cigarette smoke-induced emphysema model (Li et al., 2014). Furthermore, Islam et al. reported that MSCs could protect against acute lung injury through mitochondrial transfer via Cx43-dependent alveolar attachment (Islam et al., 2012). Interestingly, Mahrouf-Yorgov et al. observed that MSCs had the capacity to sense, and subsequently engulf and degrade mitochondria from damaged cells. This process enhanced mitochondrial biogenesis and mitochondrial transfer by the MSCs (Mahrouf-Yorgov et al., 2017). Taken together, future directives using MSC based therapy in chronic lung diseases needs to consider the engraftment in the lung for therapeutic efficacy (Behnke et al., 2020).

THE INTRINSIC PROPERTIES OF THE LUNG-ECM

MSCs and other mesenchymal cells are the main producer of ECM. Interestingly, the role of the ECM is receiving increasing recognition as an important element in controlling cellular behavior during homeostasis and in disease progression (Deng et al., 2020). Apart from providing mechanical and structural support, the complex 3D structure of the ECM, consisting of glycoproteins, collagens, glycosaminoglycans (GAGs), proteoglycans, dictate cell migration, polarity, proliferation, differentiation, and survival, where the dynamics of the ECM molecules play a critical part (Wigén et al., 2019). Some proteins e.g., elastin fibers are stable over almost a lifetime (Shapiro et al., 1991), while certain collagens have a short turnaround, changing every day (Laurent, 1987). In the pulmonary interstitial layer, the major structural components are fibrillar collagens type I, III, IV, V, and XI (extensively reviewed by Laurent, 1987; Sherman 2015) that make up the core structure and contribute to the tensile strength, and elastin along with fibrillin contribute to the compliance of the tissue (Laurent, 1987; Sherman et al., 2015). This intricate meshwork of fibers is also composed of glycoproteins, GAGs, and proteoglycans providing the tissue with its viscoelastic properties. In the alveolar space, the epithelial and endothelial cells are anchored to a basement membrane primarily consisting of collagen type IV, laminins, and proteoglycans. Both in IPF and COPD the basement membrane and the interstitial layer are affected with altered structural properties affecting the biomechanics. In IPF, the alveolar basement membrane is fragmented and the interstitial layer is thickened, while in COPD, the ECM components are degraded and the structural properties are lost (Burgess et al., 2016)

Glycosaminoglycans and Growth Factors

While the most studied group of ECM molecules are the various collagens, lately however the family of proteoglycans have drawn large attention. Proteoglycans are proteins decorated with covalently attached linear polysaccharides, GAGs. The proteoglycans are heterogeneous molecules-both in terms of the core protein structure, as well as the chain length and chemical structure of the GAG side chains. These side chains strongly decide the physical properties of the proteoglycans. The main classes of proteoglycan-bound GAGs in the human lung are heparan sulfate/heparin (HS/hep) chondroitin/dermatan sulfate (CS/DS) and keratan sulfate (KS) (Papakonstantinou and Karakiulakis, 2009). A fourth type of GAG, hyaluronan (HA), is also prevalent in the lung, but is not bound to a core protein (Couchman and Pataki, 2012). All four types of GAGs contain disaccharide motifs, which are repeated throughout the polymer. For HS/hep, CS/DS and KS the disaccharide units can be modified by sulfation at various positions, giving rise to motifs/domains (Persson et al., 2020), which in turn are important for binding of specific mediators to be involved in chronic lung diseases such as TGF-b, HGF, and TNF-a (Esko et al., 2015). In this way the GAGs play an important role in interacting with growth factors, where the GAGs build gradients during embryonic development but also during tissue repair and delivering of growth factors to receptors. Interestingly, alterations in sulfation pattern, or induction of deacetylations and epimerizations in the GAG chains affect their role in tuning growth factor gradients, which alter cell activities (Wigén et al., 2019). In IPF, an increase in sulfation of both HS and CS/DS has been recognized in the border zone toward fibrotic lesions (Westergren-Thorsson et al., 2017). This may reflect an altered pulmonary landscape, navigating nearby cells toward regions of activated repair process, promoting a profibrotic phenotype.

ECM Bound Growth Factors

Arguably one of the most important interactions between cells is mediated through growth factors and cytokines. These factors travel large distances in the body to recruit and direct cells where they are needed. A largely overlooked process is how growth factors interact with the ECM via GAGs and how the ECM can increase or decrease the cell response to growth factors. Thus, the ECM serves as a reservoir for growth factors, which are slowly released over time. At the same time the growth factors bound to the ECM via the GAGs become protected from circulating proteases. Because of these properties, if the ECM is injured the release of growth factors will be instant, thus triggering an immediate cell response. For example, latent TGF-β (Saito et al., 2018) in the ECM become activated upon injury and is known to be one of the factors activating mesenchymal cells that in fibrosing diseases such as IPF lead to an over production of ECM. Another example of ECM bound factor is fibroblast growth factor (FGF)-2, which binds on a nanomolar level to HS (Ibrahimi et al., 2004). This GAG-growth factor complex increases the binding to the FGF receptor 1 and is crucial for adequate cell signaling (Yayon et al., 1991) and may be immunomodulatory factor in COPD (Tan et al., 2020). Therefore, the ECM and growth factor complexes works to fine-tune cell responses and control timing, making it an important target in the development of therapies in chronic lung diseases.

Cell-ECM Interaction

Even though lung cells derived from patients with chronic lung disease have shown to have inherent cellular features such as gene expression and proteomic profile (Hallgren et al., 2010; Woldhuis et al., 2020), the microenvironment of the tissue, however, appears to be the dominating factor in regulating cellular behavior, at least *in vitro* (Elowsson Rendin et al., 2019). It has been demonstrated that the pathological reconstructed ECM in IPF overrules intrinsic cellular characterizations, ultimately repr ogramming cells for fibrogenesis (Parker et al., 2014; Philp et al., 2018; Rodriguez et al., 2018). The wavy and aligned collagen structures of the ECM in distal IPF tissue alter migration patterns and cell morphology, creating elongated human lung fibroblasts with increased migratory speed (Tisler et al., 2020). Lung fibroblasts engrafted on fibrotic or emphysematous lung tissue readily adapt to surrounding structures and ECM niches of the lung with high morphological plasticity (Burgstaller et al., 2018). Non-cultured fibroblasts, isolated from lungs of IPF patients, demonstrated an altered genomic profile in comparison to healthy fibroblasts (Emblom-Callahan et al., 2010), as do epithelial cells when cultured on bronchial-ECM derived from COPD (Hedström et al., 2018). The positive feedback-loop created between cells and ECM is manifested quickly with marked differences in cellular activity, inducing a shift in the production of ECM proteins that steers the cellular response toward a continuous rebuild of fibrotic tissue with altered basement membrane structures (Elowsson Rendin et al., 2019). The constant changes in ECM composition during disease progression, resulting in pathological differences in lung architecture creates a disease specific proteomic change where the local microenvironment signals for continuous tissue reconstruction (Westergren-Thorsson et al., 2017; Åhrman et al., 2018).

The deformed lung tissue, caused by either excessive tissue repair or the lack thereof, also has an immense impact on the mechanical properties of the tissue, where mechanical forces sensed by surrounding cells activate mechanosensitive pathways (e.g., YAP/TAZ) and influence cell behavior (Asano et al., 2017; Haak et al., 2018). To maintain tissue homeostasis, the cells require anchoring to the ECM via integrin binding through which the cells sense the microenvironment and activate signaling transduction pathways, inducing mechanical and chemical intracellular signaling through the actin cytoskeleton (reviewed by Vogel, 2018 (Vogel, 2018)). Changes in the local mechanical properties create a mechanical gradient that affects cellular behavior such as migration, proliferation and differentiation. Integrins are also thought to be involved in growth factor signaling, acting synergistically with receptors for different growth factors. More specifically, the integrins are known to bind to Arg-Gly-Asp (RGD) motifs found predominantly on fibronectin (FN), but also in ECM proteins e.g., laminin, tenascin, and vitronectin (Widhe et al., 2016; Miron-Mendoza et al., 2017). Integrins are also the main receptors forming focal adhesions and are thought to be required for cell motility. The local microenvironment has been found to be decisive for the size and concentration of focal adhesions, which further impact on cell behavior (Wozniak et al., 2004; Costa et al., 2013).

MODULATING THE 3D ENVIRONMENT FOR TREATMENT

There are several *in vitro* studies showing how MSC are differently affected by the environment the cells encounter. Increasing research is focused on how to control the therapeutic effect of MSC, where one option being explored is by modulating the microenviroment *in situ* or by injectable biomaterials.

Hydrogel Encapsulation

Encapsulating MSC in injectable hydrogels is extensively explored to increase retention time and to modulate the cellular activity *in situ* (Farhat et al., 2019; Wong et al., 2020) by providing the cells with a 3D microenvironment that protects and promotes an anti-inflammatory and regenerative response, see outline in **Figure 1**. Techniques range from single cell encapsulation to larger scaffolds with macroporous structure (Kim et al., 2019). Efforts have been made to mimic the mechanical properties of the ECM to steer cellular behavior in health and disease (de Hilster et al., 2020; Pouliot et al., 2020). So far, hydrogels have been by far the most produced and studied substrate, where ECM-based hydrogels from murine, porcine and human tissues have been developed with different decellularization methods. In order to mimic the natural tissue when designing an artificial matrix, it is vital to maintain the components of the ECM, often measured as the GAG-DNA content ratio, as well as the viscoelastic properties (Uhl et al., 2020). Apart from hydrogels based on decellularized tissue, there are various natural, synthetic and hybrid (meaning combining natural, synthetic or ECM components) polymers that are being explored, including proteins, polysaccharides, recombinantly expressed peptides, and polyethylene glycol (Uhl et al., 2020). The advantage of hydrogels is that the structural properties can be easily modified through the crosslinking of the hydrophilic polymer chains. In addition, the biomaterial can be modulated by incorporating cell-instructive factors e.g. growth factors, RGD domains, and ECM proteins. Recombinantly produced biomaterials such as the elastin-like recombinamer polymer allows for the precise composition of structural and chemical properties, with gene technology introducing sequences for cell attachment and MMP degradation and at the same time exposing functional groups for binding of for example growth factors to promote or maintain the MSC therapeutic effect (Ibáñez-Fonseca et al., 2020). De Santis et al. recently demonstrated the functional outcome of a 3D bioprinted hybrid hydrogel combining decellularized lung tissue with alginate to form human airways containing primary human airway epithelial progenitor cells (De Santis et al., 2020). Transplanted in mice, the cells showed evidence of differentiation into mature epithelial cells. The hydrogel properties both had matched biomechanical properties and contained ECM instructive factors from the native lung tissue (De Santis et al., 2020). Hydrogels based on collagen type I, one of the major structural components of tissues, has been extensively explored in combination with other materials such as silk, a highly elastic protein, to improve the mechanical properties to mimic the viscoelastic properties of tissues (Sanz-Fraile et al., 2020). As discussed above, GAGs multiple functions in cell signaling and in tissue homeostasis and have been explored as biomaterials. CS that have modifiable functional groups for covalent and non-covalent bonding has been used for the development of injectable hydrogels to tune for different physical properties as well as release of therapeutic factors (Ornell et al., 2019).

Macroporous Scaffolds

In contrast to solid hydrogels, macroporous biomaterials or scaffolds introduces a more complex 3D environment, where the surface properties of the scaffold can be tuned to functionalize cell attachment, differentiation and migration, as well as to enhance cell diffusion to the scaffold.

In a recently published article, a collagen-based scaffold was developed with macroporous structures to mimic the distal lung tissue. The scaffold was functionalized with collagen binding HGF to enhance the regeneration of alveolar-like structures (Wang et al., 2020). When making a porous scaffold, pore size is often determined by changing the initial concentration of the reagents, which in turn changes the bulk stiffness. By adding an antifreezing agent (e.g., DMSO), pore size can be kept constant regardless of the initial concentration (Jiang et al., 2019). Jiang et al. could show that larger and stiffer pores induced an anti-inflammatory phenotype of macrophages (Jiang et al., 2019). Shamskhou et al. has shown that local delivery of IL-10 using a hyaluronan and heparin-based hydrogel system had an anti-inflammatory effect in bleomycin-treated mice (Shamskhou et al., 2019).

Pre-Conditioning of MSC to Enhance Therapeutic Effect

There are increasing evidence that MSC have a cellular memory, with sustained responses to preceding stimuli, which may influence the desired effect of MSC-based therapies (Yang et al., 2014). MSC cultured on substrates with different ECM molecules have been shown to affect the paracrine function of MSC. For example, De Lisio et al. showed that cell cultures on collagen reduced the gene expression of inflammatory factors in MSC compared to culturing on laminin (De Lisio et al., 2014). Preconditioning of the MSC prior to administration has also been investigated, where low doses of toxic or lethal factors or exposures to hypoxic or nutrient deprived environment triggered a beneficial effect of the cells with increased expression of immunomodulatory, anti-inflammatory and repair factors (Silva et al., 2018; Nonaka et al., 2020). In a recent study, lung-derived MSCs were biophysically preconditioned to modulate their paracrine signaling by culturing the cells in a natural microenvironment, on lung scaffolds, and subjecting them to cyclic stretch prior to being injected into a rat model for acute respiratory distress syndrome (ARDS). Compared to non-preconditioned MSCs, rats treated with biophysically preconditioned MSCs had an improvement in lung elastance and reduced amounts of inflammatory cytokines in the bronchoalveolar lavage fluid (Nonaka et al., 2020). In a recent study biophysical and biochemical cues were combined to explore the immunological effect of MSC. Bone marrow-derived MSC were encapsulated in alginate-based hydrogels with different stiffnesses and pre-cultured prior to exposure to the inflammatory cytokine TNF-α. MSC preconditioned in the softer hydrogel in combination with TNFα had an improved effect in controlling monocyte turnover (Wong et al., 2020). These studies demonstrate how intrinsic cues of the microenvironment impact cellular behavior that can be harnessed in improving the therapeutic potential of MSCs.

FUTURE DIRECTIONS

For MSC therapy to become an efficient alternative to current medicine in IPF and COPD, it is essential to ensure the functional outcome of the cells in the diseased tissue. One way is to control the microenvironment in which the cells are delivered. Recent advances have demonstrated that MSC actively interact and modify their pericellular environment, that there is an active interplay between the surrounding properties, both in terms of structural properties and chemical composition, thus will play a role in directing MSC function (Ferreira et al., 2018; Loebel et al., 2019). Several obstacles remain with current MSC therapy. Ensure long-term retention of the MSCs in the lung is one, although they do get trapped in pulmonary capillaries after systemic administration, they are considered cleared within 24 h (Wang et al., 2009). MSCs are also vulnerable to the inflammatory microenvironment, which affect their restorative potential (Silva et al., 2018). Therefore, we foresee a future, where we are able to increase the retention time in the organ and control the therapeutic effect of MSCs by providing a microenvironment that supports these properties. Research into the field of artificial scaffolds for medicinal purposes that can retain a particular therapeutic property is warranted to push forward this line of novel therapies for chronic lung diseases. Modifying the microenvironment *in situ* may hold difficulties in its approach in retaining tuned levels of cell mediators or in adapting specific ECM components in the location of transplanted MSC. Identifying key elements or biological properties of the ECM warrants further investigation as this would allow for more precise and directed manipulation of the pathological tissue *in situ*. The environmental responsiveness of the MSCs creates both challenges and opportunities in applying transplanted MSC as a cell-based therapy in lung diseases that are marked with massive structural and compositional tissue remodeling. Thus, pre-conditioning of MSC may hold a more transient approach in overcoming the powerful influential impact of surrounding tissue on cellular behavior, providing a more instant regenerative response.

The artificial scaffolds hold great promise in future therapeutic purposes as it can combine cell-instructive cues together with a supporting microenvironment, delicately designed in both structure and biomechanics, that together yield an optimal curative setting for MSC. The purpose of a controlled microenvironment is to create an interim support as well as *in situ* cell guidance over time as the scaffold is degraded and replaced with functional lung tissue. By providing structural support, we anticipate that both the MSC retention time will be greatly improved with remained activity and allowing endogenous cells to repopulate lost tissue area.

Altogether, harnessing the microenvironment holds promise to ameliorate future cell therapeutic regimens to be able to induce lung regeneration and healing of lung tissue in chronic lung diseases marked with massive structural remodeling like IPF and COPD.

AUTHOR CONTRIBUTIONS

All authors listed have made a substantial, direct, and intellectual contribution to the work and approved it for publication.

REFERENCES

Abreu, S. C., Hampton, T. H., Hoffman, E., Dearborn, J., Ashare, A., Singh Sidhu, K., et al. (2020). Differential effects of the cystic fibrosis lung inflammatory environment on mesenchymal stromal cells. *Am. J. Physiology-Lung Cell Mol. Physiol.* 319, L908–L925. doi:10.1152/ajplung.00218.2020

Abreu, S. C., Rolandsson Enes, S., Dearborn, J., Goodwin, M., Coffey, A., Borg, Z. D., et al. (2019). Lung inflammatory environments differentially alter mesenchymal stromal cell behavior. *Am. J. Physiology-Lung Cell Mol. Physiol.* 317, L823–L831. doi:10.1152/ajplung.00263.2019

Åhrman, E., Hallgren, O., Malmström, L., Hedström, U., Malmström, A., Bjermer, L., et al. (2018). Quantitative proteomic characterization of the lung extracellular matrix in chronic obstructive pulmonary disease and idiopathic pulmonary fibrosis. *J. Proteomics* 189, 23. doi:10.1016/j.jprot.2018.02.027

Anees Ur, R., Ahmad Hassali, M. A., Muhammad, S. A., Shah, S., Abbas, S., Hyder Ali, I. A. B, et al. (2020). The economic burden of chronic obstructive pulmonary disease (COPD) in the USA, Europe, and Asia: results from a systematic review of the literature. *Expert Rev. Pharmacoecon Outcomes Res.* 20, 661–672. doi:10.1080/14737167.2020.1678385

Armitage, J., Tan, D. B. A., Troedson, R., Young, P., Lam, K.-v., Shaw, K., et al. (2018). Mesenchymal stromal cell infusion modulates systemic immunological responses in stable COPD patients: a phase I pilot study. *Eur. Respir. J.* 51, 1702369. doi:10.1183/13993003.02369-2017

Asano, S., Ito, S., Takahashi, K., Furuya, K., Kondo, M., Sokabe, M., et al. (2017). Matrix stiffness regulates migration of human lung fibroblasts. *Physiol. Rep.* 5, e13281. doi:10.14814/phy2.13281

Averyanov, A., Koroleva, I., Konoplyannikov, M., Revkova, V., Lesnyak, V., Kalsin, V., et al. (2020). First-in-human high-cumulative-dose stem cell therapy in idiopathic pulmonary fibrosis with rapid lung function decline. *Stem Cell Transl Med* 9, 6–16. doi:10.1002/sctm.19-0037

Barrecheguren, M., and Miravitlles, M. (2016). COPD heterogeneity: implications for management. *Multidiscip Respir. Med.* 11, 14. doi:10.1186/s40248-016-0053-4

Bartholomew, A., Sturgeon, C., Siatskas, M., Ferrer, K., McIntosh, K., Patil, S., et al. (2002). Mesenchymal stem cells suppress lymphocyte proliferation *in vitro* and prolong skin graft survival *in vivo*. *Exp. Hematol.* 30, 42–48. doi:10.1016/s0301-472x(01)00769-x

Behnke, J., Kremer, S., Shahzad, T., Chao, C.-M., Böttcher-Friebertshäuser, E., Morty, R. E., et al. (2020). MSC based therapies-new perspectives for the injured lung. *Jcm* 9, 682. doi:10.3390/jcm9030682

Benvenuto, F., Ferrari, S., Gerdoni, E., Gualandi, F., Frassoni, F., Pistoia, V., et al. (2007). Human mesenchymal stem cells promote survival of T cells in a quiescent state. *Stem Cells* 25, 1753–1760. doi:10.1634/stemcells.2007-0068

Blazquez, R., Sanchez-Margallo, F. M., de la Rosa, O., Dalemans, W., Ã lvarez, V., Tarazona, R., et al. (2014). Immunomodulatory potential of human adipose mesenchymal stem cells derived exosomes on *in vitro* stimulated T cells. *Front. Immunol.* 5, 556. doi:10.3389/fimmu.2014.00556

Burgess, J. K., Mauad, T., Tjin, G., Karlsson, J. C., and Westergren-Thorsson, G. (2016). The extracellular matrix - the under-recognized element in lung disease?. *J. Pathol.* 240, 397–409. doi:10.1002/path.4808

Burgstaller, G., Sengupta, A., Vierkotten, S., Preissler, G., Lindner, M., Behr, J., et al. (2018). Distinct niches within the extracellular matrix dictate fibroblast function in (cell free) 3D lung tissue cultures. *Am. J. Physiology-Lung Cell Mol. Physiol.* 314, L708–L723. doi:10.1152/ajplung.00408.2017

Caminati, A., Madotto, F., Conti, S., Cesana, G., Mantovani, L., and Harari, S. (2021). The natural history of idiopathic pulmonary fibrosis in a large European population: the role of age, sex and comorbidities. *Intern. Emerg. Med.* doi:10.1007/s11739-021-02651-w

Casiraghi, F., Azzollini, N., Cassis, P., Imberti, B., Morigi, M., Cugini, D., et al. (2008). Pretransplant infusion of mesenchymal stem cells prolongs the survival of a semiallogeneic heart transplant through the generation of regulatory T cells. *J. Immunol.* 181, 3933–3946. doi:10.4049/jimmunol.181.6.3933

Chambers, D. C., Enever, D., Ilic, N., Sparks, L., Whitelaw, K., Ayres, J., et al. (2014). A phase 1b study of placenta-derived mesenchymal stromal cells in patients with idiopathic pulmonary fibrosis. *Respirology* 19, 1013–1018. doi:10.1111/resp.12343

Costa, P., Scales, T. M. E., Ivaska, J., and Parsons, M. (2013). Integrin-specific control of focal adhesion kinase and RhoA regulates membrane protrusion and invasion. *PLoS One* 8, e74659. doi:10.1371/journal.pone.0074659

Couchman, J. R., and Pataki, C. A. (2012). An introduction to proteoglycans and their localization. *J. Histochem. Cytochem.* 60, 885–897. doi:10.1369/0022155412464638

Cruz, F. F., Borg, Z. D., Goodwin, M., Sokocevic, D., Wagner, D. E., Coffey, A., et al. (2015). Systemic administration of human bone marrow-derived mesenchymal stromal cell extracellular vesicles AmelioratesAspergillusHyphal extract-induced allergic airway inflammation in immunocompetent mice. *Stem Cell Transl. Med.* 4, 1302–1316. doi:10.5966/sctm.2014-0280

Cruz, F. F., and Rocco, P. R. M. (2020). The potential of mesenchymal stem cell therapy for chronic lung disease. *Expert Rev. Respir. Med.* 14, 31–39. doi:10.1080/17476348.2020.1679628

de Hilster, R. H. J., Sharma, P. K., Jonker, M. R., White, E. S., Gercama, E. A., Roobeek, M., et al. (2020). Human lung extracellular matrix hydrogels resemble the stiffness and viscoelasticity of native lung tissue. *Am. J. Physiology-Lung Cell Mol. Physiol.* 318, L698–L704. doi:10.1152/ajplung.00451.2019

De Lisio, M., Jensen, T., Sukiennik, R. A., Huntsman, H. D., and Boppart, M. D. (2014). Substrate and strain alter the muscle-derived mesenchymal stem cell secretome to promote myogenesis. *Stem Cel Res. Ther.* 5, 74. doi:10.1186/scrt463

de Oliveira, H. G., Cruz, F. F., Antunes, M. A., de Macedo Neto, A. V., Oliveira, G. A., Svartman, F. M., et al. (2017). Combined bone marrow-derived mesenchymal stromal cell therapy and one-way endobronchial valve placement in patients with pulmonary emphysema: a phase I clinical trial. *STEM CELLS Translational Med.* 6, 962–969. doi:10.1002/sctm.16-0315

De Santis, M. M., Alsafadi, H. N., Tas, S., Bölükbas, D. A., Prithiviraj, S., Da Silva, I. A. N., et al. (2020). Extracellular-matrix-reinforced bioinks for 3D bioprinting human tissue. *Adv. Mater.* 33, 2005476. doi:10.1002/adma.202005476

Deng, Z., Fear, M. W., Suk Choi, Y., Wood, F. M., Allahham, A., Mutsaers, S. E., et al. (2020). The extracellular matrix and mechanotransduction in pulmonary fibrosis. *Int. J. Biochem. Cel Biol.* 126, 105802. doi:10.1016/j.biocel.2020.105802

Elowsson Rendin, L., Löfdahl, A., Åhrman, E., Müller, C., Notermans, T., Michaliková, B., et al. (2019). Matrisome properties of scaffolds direct fibroblasts in idiopathic pulmonary fibrosis. *Ijms* 20, 4013. doi:10.3390/ijms20164013

Emblom-Callahan, M. C., Chhina, M. K., Shlobin, O. A., Ahmad, S., Reese, E. S., Iyer, E. P. R., et al. (2010). Genomic phenotype of non-cultured pulmonary fibroblasts in idiopathic pulmonary fibrosis. *Genomics* 96, 134–145. doi:10.1016/j.ygeno.2010.04.005

J. D. Esko, H. P. James, A. Varki, R. D. Cummings, P. Stanley, R. J. Linhardt, et al. Editors (2015). in *Essentials of glycobiology*, 3rd edition. Cold Spring Harbor (NY): Cold Spring Harbor Laboratory Press, 493–502.

Farhat, W., Hasan, A., Lucia, L., Becquart, F., Ayoub, A., and Kobeissy, F. (2019). Hydrogels for advanced stem cell therapies: a biomimetic materials approach for enhancing natural tissue function. *IEEE Rev. Biomed. Eng.* 12, 333–351. doi:10.1109/RBME.2018.2824335

Ferreira, S. A., Motwani, M. S., Faull, P. A., Seymour, A. J., Yu, T. T. L., Enayati, M., et al. (2018). Bi-directional cell-pericellular matrix interactions direct stem cell fate. *Nat. Commun.* 9, 4049. doi:10.1038/s41467-018-06183-4

Gad, E. S., Salama, A. A. A., El-Shafie, M. F., Arafa, H. M. M., Abdelsalam, R. M., and Khattab, M. (2020). The anti-fibrotic and anti-inflammatory potential of bone marrow-derived mesenchymal stem cells and Nintedanib in bleomycin-induced lung fibrosis in rats. *Inflammation* 43, 123–134. doi:10.1007/s10753-019-01101-2

Gao, F., Chiu, S. M., Motan, D. A. L., Zhang, Z., Chen, L., Ji, H.-L., et al. (2016). Mesenchymal stem cells and immunomodulation: current status and future prospects. *Cell Death Dis* 7, e2062. doi:10.1038/cddis.2015.327

Gao, J., Kalafatis, D., Carlson, L., Pesonen, I. H. A., Li, C. X., Wheelock, Å., et al. (2021). Baseline characteristics and survival of patients of idiopathic pulmonary fibrosis: a longitudinal analysis of the Swedish IPF Registry. *Respir. Res.* 22, 40. doi:10.1186/s12931-021-01634-x

Glassberg, M. K., Minkiewicz, J., Toonkel, R. L., Simonet, E. S., Rubio, G. A., DiFede, D., et al. (2017). Allogeneic human mesenchymal stem cells in patients with idiopathic pulmonary fibrosis via intravenous delivery (AETHER). *Chest* 151, 971–981. doi:10.1016/j.chest.2016.10.061

Haak, A. J., Tan, Q., and Tschumperlin, D. J. (2018). Matrix biomechanics and dynamics in pulmonary fibrosis. *Matrix Biol.* 73, 64–76. doi:10.1016/j.matbio.2017.12.004

Hallgren, O., Nihlberg, K., Dahlbäck, M., Bjermer, L., Eriksson, L. T., Erjefält, J. S., et al. (2010). Altered fibroblast proteoglycan production in COPD. *Respir. Res.* 11, 55. doi:10.1186/1465-9921-11-55

Hedström, U., Hallgren, O., Öberg, L., DeMicco, A., Vaarala, O., Westergren-Thorsson, G., et al. (2018). Bronchial extracellular matrix from COPD patients induces altered gene expression in repopulated primary human bronchial epithelial cells. *Sci. Rep.* 8, 3502. doi:10.1038/s41598-018-21727-w

Hilberg, O., Bendstrup, E., Ibsen, R., Løkke, A., and Hyldgaard, C. (2018). Economic consequences of idiopathic pulmonary fibrosis in Denmark. *ERJ Open Res.* 4, 00045. doi:10.1183/23120541.00045-2017

Ibáñez-Fonseca, A., Santiago Maniega, S., Gorbenko del Blanco, D., Catalán Bernardos, B., Vega Castrillo, A., Álvarez Barcia, Á. J., et al. (2020). Elastin-like recombinamer hydrogels for improved skeletal muscle healing through modulation of macrophage polarization. *Front. Bioeng. Biotechnol.* 8, 413. doi:10.3389/fbioe.2020.00413

Ibrahimi, O. A., Zhang, F., Lang Hrstka, S. C., Mohammadi, M., and Linhardt, R. J. (2004). Kinetic model for FGF, FGFR, and proteoglycan signal transduction complex assembly†. *Biochemistry* 43, 4724–4730. doi:10.1021/bi0352320

Islam, D., Huang, Y., Fanelli, V., Delsedime, L., Wu, S., Khang, J., et al. (2019). Identification and modulation of microenvironment is crucial for effective mesenchymal stromal cell therapy in acute lung injury. *Am. J. Respir. Crit. Care Med.* 199, 1214–1224. doi:10.1164/rccm.201802-0356OC

Islam, M. N., Das, S. R., Emin, M. T., Wei, M., Sun, L., Westphalen, K., et al. (2012). Mitochondrial transfer from bone-marrow-derived stromal cells to pulmonary alveoli protects against acute lung injury. *Nat. Med.* 18, 759–765. doi:10.1038/nm.2736

Jackson, M. V., Morrison, T. J., Doherty, D. F., McAuley, D. F., Matthay, M. A., Kissenpfennig, A., et al. (2016). Mitochondrial transfer via tunneling nanotubes is an important mechanism by which mesenchymal stem cells enhance macrophage phagocytosis in the in vitro and in vivo models of ARDS. *Stem Cells* 34, 2210–2223. doi:10.1002/stem.2372

Jiang, S., Lyu, C., Zhao, P., Li, W., Kong, W., Huang, C., et al. (2019). Cryoprotectant enables structural control of porous scaffolds for exploration of cellular mechano-responsiveness in 3D. *Nat. Commun.* 10, 3491. doi:10.1038/s41467-019-11397-1

Kim, H., Bae, C., Kook, Y.-M., Koh, W.-G., Lee, K., and Park, M. H. (2019). Mesenchymal stem cell 3D encapsulation technologies for biomimetic microenvironment in tissue regeneration. *Stem Cell Res. Ther.* 10, 51. doi:10.1186/s13287-018-1130-8

Kusuma, G. D., Carthew, J., Lim, R., and Frith, J. E. (2017). Effect of the microenvironment on mesenchymal stem cell paracrine signaling: opportunities to engineer the therapeutic effect. *Stem Cell Development* 26, 617–631. doi:10.1089/scd.2016.0349

Laing, A. G., Fanelli, G., Ramirez-Valdez, A., Lechler, R. I., Lombardi, G., and Sharpe, P. T. (2019). Mesenchymal stem cells inhibit T-cell function through conserved induction of cellular stress. *PLoS One* 14, e0213170. doi:10.1371/journal.pone.0213170

Laurent, G. J. (1987). Dynamic state of collagen: pathways of collagen degradation *in vivo* and their possible role in regulation of collagen mass. *Am. J. Physiology-Cell Physiol.* 252, C1–C9. doi:10.1152/ajpcell.1987.252.1.C1

Lee, M., Jeong, S. Y., Ha, J., Kim, M., Jin, H. J., Kwon, S.-J., et al. (2014). Low immunogenicity of allogeneic human umbilical cord blood-derived mesenchymal stem cells *in vitro* and *in vivo*. *Biochem. Biophysical Res. Commun.* 446, 983–989. doi:10.1016/j.bbrc.2014.03.051

Li, X., Zhang, Y., Yeung, S. C., Liang, Y., Liang, X., Ding, Y., et al. (2014). Mitochondrial transfer of induced pluripotent stem cell-derived mesenchymal stem cells to airway epithelial cells attenuates cigarette smoke-induced damage. *Am. J. Respir. Cel Mol. Biol.* 51, 455–465. doi:10.1165/rcmb.2013-0529OC

Loebel, C., Mauck, R. L., and Burdick, J. A. (2019). Local nascent protein deposition and remodelling guide mesenchymal stromal cell mechanosensing and fate in three-dimensional hydrogels. *Nat. Mater.* 18, 883–891. doi:10.1038/s41563-019-0307-6

Mahrouf-Yorgov, M., Augeul, L., Da Silva, C. C., Jourdan, M., Rigolet, M., Manin, S., et al. (2017). Mesenchymal stem cells sense mitochondria released from damaged cells as danger signals to activate their rescue properties. *Cell Death Differ* 24, 1224–1238. doi:10.1038/cdd.2017.51

Mansouri, N., Willis, G. R., Fernandez-Gonzalez, A., Reis, M., Nassiri, S., Mitsialis, S. A., et al. (2019). Mesenchymal stromal cell exosomes prevent and revert experimental pulmonary fibrosis through modulation of monocyte phenotypes. *JCI Insight* 4, e128060. doi:10.1172/jci.insight.128060

Mardpour, S., Hamidieh, A. A., Taleahmad, S., Sharifzad, F., Taghikhani, A., and Baharvand, H. (2019). Interaction between mesenchymal stromal cell-derived extracellular vesicles and immune cells by distinct protein content. *J. Cel Physiol* 234, 8249–8258. doi:10.1002/jcp.27669

Martinez, F. J., Collard, H. R., Pardo, A., Raghu, G., Richeldi, L., Selman, M., et al. (2017). Idiopathic pulmonary fibrosis. *Nat. Rev. Dis. Primers* 3, 17074. doi:10.1038/nrdp.2017.74

Meisel, R., Zibert, A., Laryea, M., Göbel, U., Däubener, W., and Dilloo, D. (2004). Human bone marrow stromal cells inhibit allogeneic T-cell responses by indoleamine 2,3-dioxygenase-mediated tryptophan degradation. *Blood* 103, 4619–4621. doi:10.1182/blood-2003-11-3909

Mias, C. l., Lairez, O., Trouche, E., Roncalli, J. r., Calise, D., Seguelas, M.-H. l. n., et al. (2009). Mesenchymal stem cells promote matrix metalloproteinase secretion by cardiac fibroblasts and reduce cardiac ventricular fibrosis after myocardial infarction. *Stem Cells* 27, 2734–2743. doi:10.1002/stem.169

Miron-Mendoza, M., Graham, E., Manohar, S., and Petroll, W. M. (2017). Fibroblast-fibronectin patterning and network formation in 3D fibrin matrices. *Matrix Biol.* 64, 69–80. doi:10.1016/j.matbio.2017.06.001

Moodley, Y., Atienza, D., Manuelpillai, U., Samuel, C. S., Tchongue, J., Ilancheran, S., et al. (2009). Human umbilical cord mesenchymal stem cells reduce fibrosis of bleomycin-induced lung injury. *Am. J. Pathol.* 175, 303–313. doi:10.2353/ajpath.2009.080629

Morrison, T. J., Jackson, M. V., Cunningham, E. K., Kissenpfennig, A., McAuley, D. F., O'Kane, C. M., et al. (2017). Mesenchymal stromal cells modulate macrophages in clinically relevant lung injury models by extracellular vesicle mitochondrial transfer. *Am. J. Respir. Crit. Care Med.* 196, 1275–1286. doi:10.1164/rccm.201701-0170OC

Murphy, M. B., Moncivais, K., and Caplan, A. I. (2013). Mesenchymal stem cells: environmentally responsive therapeutics for regenerative medicine. *Exp. Mol. Med.* 45, e54. doi:10.1038/emm.2013.94

Negewo, N. A., Gibson, P. G., and McDonald, V. M. (2015). COPD and its comorbidities: impact, measurement and mechanisms. *Respirology* 20, 1160–1171. doi:10.1111/resp.12642

Nonaka, P. N., Falcones, B., Farre, R., Artigas, A., Almendros, I., and Navajas, D. (2020). Biophysically preconditioning mesenchymal stem cells improves treatment of ventilator-induced lung injury. *Archivos de Bronconeumología* 56, 179–181. doi:10.1016/j.arbres.2019.08.014

Ornell, K. J., Lozada, D., Phan, N. V., and Coburn, J. M. (2019). Controlling methacryloyl substitution of chondroitin sulfate: injectable hydrogels with tunable long-term drug release profiles. *J. Mater. Chem. B* 7, 2151–2161. doi:10.1039/c8tb03020k

Pachler, K., Ketterl, N., Desgeorges, A., Dunai, Z., Laner-Plamberger, S., Streif, D., et al. (2017). An in vitro potency assay for monitoring the immunomodulatory potential of stromal cell-derived extracellular vesicles. *Ijms* 18, 1413. doi:10.3390/ijms18071413

Papakonstantinou, E., and Karakiulakis, G. (2009). The 'sweet' and 'bitter' involvement of glycosaminoglycans in lung diseases: pharmacotherapeutic relevance. *Br. J. Pharmacol.* 157, 1111–1127. doi:10.1111/j.1476-5381.2009.00279.x

Parker, M. W., Rossi, D., Peterson, M., Smith, K., Sikström, K., White, E. S., et al. (2014). Fibrotic extracellular matrix activates a profibrotic positive feedback loop. *J. Clin. Invest.* 124, 1622–1635. doi:10.1172/JCI71386

Persson, A., Vorontsov, E., Larson, G., and Nilsson, J. (2020). Glycosaminoglycan domain mapping of cellular chondroitin/dermatan sulfates. *Sci. Rep.* 10, 3506. doi:10.1038/s41598-020-60526-0

Philp, C. J., Siebeke, I., Clements, D., Miller, S., Habgood, A., John, A. E., et al. (2018). Extracellular matrix cross-linking enhances fibroblast growth and protects against matrix proteolysis in lung fibrosis. *Am. J. Respir. Cel Mol. Biol.* 58, 594–603. doi:10.1165/rcmb.2016-0379OC

Phinney, D. G., Di Giuseppe, M., Njah, J., Sala, E., Shiva, S., St Croix, C. M., et al. (2015). Mesenchymal stem cells use extracellular vesicles to outsource mitophagy and shuttle microRNAs. *Nat. Commun.* 6, 8472. doi:10.1038/ncomms9472

Pouliot, R. A., Young, B. M., Link, P. A., Park, H. E., Kahn, A. R., Shankar, K., et al. (2020). Porcine lung-derived extracellular matrix hydrogel properties are dependent on pepsin digestion time. *Tissue Eng. C: Methods* 26, 332–346. doi:10.1089/ten.TEC.2020.0042

Prockop, D. J. (2013). Concise review: two negative feedback loops place mesenchymal stem/stromal cells at the center of early regulators of inflammation. *Stem Cells* 31, 2042–2046. doi:10.1002/stem.1400

Raghu, G., Collard, H. R., Egan, J. J., Martinez, F. J., Behr, J., Brown, K. K., et al. (2011). An official ATS/ERS/JRS/ALAT statement: idiopathic pulmonary fibrosis: evidence-based guidelines for diagnosis and management. *Am. J. Respir. Crit. Care Med.* 183, 788–824. doi:10.1164/rccm.2009-040GL

Reddy, M., Fonseca, L., Gowda, S., Chougule, B., Hari, A., and Totey, S. (2016). Human adipose-derived mesenchymal stem cells attenuate early stage of bleomycin induced pulmonary fibrosis: comparison with Pirfenidone. *Ijsc* 9, 192–206. doi:10.15283/ijsc16041

Ribeiro-Paes, J. T., Bilaqui, fnm., Greco, O. T., Ruiz, M. A., Marcelino, fnm., Stessuk, fnm., et al. (2011). Unicentric study of cell therapy in chronic obstructive pulmonary disease/pulmonary emphysema. *Copd* 6, 63–71. doi:10.2147/COPD.S15292

Rodriguez, L. R., Emblom-Callahan, M., Chhina, M., Bui, S., Aljeburry, B., Tran, L. H., et al. (2018). Global gene expression analysis in an *in vitro* fibroblast model of idiopathic pulmonary fibrosis reveals potential role for CXCL14/CXCR4. *Sci. Rep.* 8, 3983. doi:10.1038/s41598-018-21889-7

Saito, A., Horie, M., and Nagase, T. (2018). TGF-β signaling in lung health and disease. *Ijms* 19, 2460. doi:10.3390/ijms19082460

Sanz-Fraile, H., Amoros, S., Mendizabal, I., Galvez-Monton, C., Prat-Vidal, C., Bayes-Genis, A., et al. (2020). Silk-reinforced collagen hydrogels with raised multiscale stiffness for mesenchymal cells 3D culture. *Tissue Eng. A* 26, 358–370. doi:10.1089/ten.TEA.2019.0199

Semedo, P., Correa-Costa, M., Cenedeze, M. A., Malheiros, D. M. A. C., Antonia dos Reis, M., Shimizu, M. H., et al. (2009). Mesenchymal stem cells attenuate renal fibrosis through immune modulation and remodeling properties in a rat remnant kidney model. *Stem Cells* 27, A–N. doi:10.1002/stem.214

Shamskhou, E. A., Kratochvil, M. J., Orcholski, M. E., Nagy, N., Kaber, G., Steen, E., et al. (2019). Hydrogel-based delivery of Il-10 improves treatment of bleomycin-induced lung fibrosis in mice. *Biomaterials* 203, 52–62. doi:10.1016/j.biomaterials.2019.02.017

Shapiro, S. D., Endicott, S. K., Province, M. A., Pierce, J. A., and Campbell, E. J. (1991). Marked longevity of human lung parenchymal elastic fibers deduced from prevalence of D-aspartate and nuclear weapons-related radiocarbon. *J. Clin. Invest.* 87, 1828–1834. doi:10.1172/JCI115204

Sherman, V. R., Yang, W., and Meyers, M. A. (2015). The materials science of collagen. *J. Mech. Behav. Biomed. Mater.* 52, 22–50. doi:10.1016/j.jmbbm.2015.05.023

Shukla, M. N., Rose, J. L., Ray, R., Lathrop, K. L., Ray, A., and Ray, P. (2009). Hepatocyte growth factor inhibits epithelial to myofibroblast transition in lung cells via Smad7. *Am. J. Respir. Cell Mol Biol* 40, 643–653. doi:10.1165/rcmb.2008-0217OC

Silva, L. H. A., Antunes, M. A., Dos Santos, C. C., Weiss, D. J., Cruz, F. F., and Rocco, P. R. M. (2018). Strategies to improve the therapeutic effects of mesenchymal stromal cells in respiratory diseases. *Stem Cel Res Ther* 9, 45. doi:10.1186/s13287-018-0802-8

Sin, D. D., Anthonisen, N. R., Soriano, J. B., and Agusti, A. G. (2006). Mortality in COPD: role of comorbidities. *Eur. Respir. J.* 28, 1245–1257. doi:10.1183/09031936.00133805

Spees, J. L., Olson, S. D., Whitney, M. J., and Prockop, D. J. (2006). Mitochondrial transfer between cells can rescue aerobic respiration. *Proc. Natl. Acad. Sci.* 103, 1283–1288. doi:10.1073/pnas.0510511103

Srour, N., and Thébaud, B. (2015). Mesenchymal stromal cells in animal bleomycin pulmonary fibrosis models: a systematic review. *Stem Cell Transl Med* 4, 1500–1510. doi:10.5966/sctm.2015-0121

Stolk, J., Broekman, W., Mauad, T., Zwaginga, J. J., Roelofs, H., Fibbe, W. E., et al. (2016). A phase I study for intravenous autologous mesenchymal stromal cell administration to patients with severe emphysema. *QJM* 109, 331–336. doi:10.1093/qjmed/hcw001

Tan, Y., Qiao, Y., Chen, Z., Liu, J., Guo, Y., Tran, T., et al. (2020). FGF2, an immunomodulatory factor in asthma and chronic obstructive pulmonary disease (COPD). *Front. Cel Dev. Biol.* 8, 223. doi:10.3389/fcell.2020.00223

Thery, C., Witwer, K. W., Aikawa, E., Alcaraz, M. J., Anderson, J. D., Andriantsitohaina, R., et al. (2018). Minimal information for studies of extracellular vesicles 2018 (MISEV2018): a position statement of the International Society for Extracellular Vesicles and update of the MISEV2014 guidelines. *J. Extracell Vesicles* 7, 1535750. doi:10.1080/20013078.2018.1535750

Tisler, M., Alkmin, S., Chang, H.-Y., Leet, J., Bernau, K., Sandbo, N., et al. (2020). Analysis of fibroblast migration dynamics in idiopathic pulmonary fibrosis using image-based scaffolds of the lung extracellular matrix. *Am. J. Physiology-Lung Cell Mol. Physiol.* 318, L276–L286. doi:10.1152/ajplung.00087.2019

Trachalaki, A., Irfan, M., and Wells, A. U. (2021). Pharmacological management of Idiopathic Pulmonary Fibrosis: current and emerging options. *Expert Opin. Pharmacother.* 22, 191–204. doi:10.1080/14656566.2020.1822326

Tzouvelekis, A., Paspaliaris, V., Koliakos, G., Ntolios, P., Bouros, E., Oikonomou, A., et al. (2013). A prospective, non-randomized, no placebo-controlled, phase Ib clinical trial to study the safety of the adipose derived stromal cells-stromal vascular fraction in idiopathic pulmonary fibrosis. *J. Translational Med.* 11, 171. doi:10.1186/1479-5876-11-171

Uhl, F. E., Zhang, F., Pouliot, R. A., Uriarte, J. J., Rolandsson Enes, S., Han, X., et al. (2020). Functional role of glycosaminoglycans in decellularized lung extracellular matrix. *Acta Biomater.* 102, 231–246. doi:10.1016/j.actbio.2019.11.029

van Niel, G., D'Angelo, G., and Raposo, G. (2018). Shedding light on the cell biology of extracellular vesicles. *Nat. Rev. Mol. Cel Biol* 19, 213–228. doi:10.1038/nrm.2017.125

Varkouhi, A. K., Jerkic, M., Ormesher, L., Gagnon, S., Goyal, S., Rabani, R., et al. (2019). Extracellular vesicles from interferon-γ-primed human umbilical cord mesenchymal stromal cells reduce *Escherichia* coli-induced acute lung injury in rats. *Anesthesiology* 130, 778–790. doi:10.1097/ALN.0000000000002655

Vogel, V. (2018). Unraveling the mechanobiology of extracellular matrix. *Annu. Rev. Physiol.* 80, 353–387. doi:10.1146/annurev-physiol-021317-121312

Wan, X., Chen, S., Fang, Y., Zuo, W., Cui, J., and Xie, S. (2020). Mesenchymal stem cell-derived extracellular vesicles suppress the fibroblast proliferation by downregulating FZD6 expression in fibroblasts via micrRNA-29b-3p in idiopathic pulmonary fibrosis. *J. Cel Physiol.* 235, 8613–8625. doi:10.1002/jcp.29706

Wang, H., Cao, F., De, A., Cao, Y., Contag, C., Gambhir, S. S., et al. (2009). Trafficking mesenchymal stem cell engraftment and differentiation in tumor-bearing mice by bioluminescence imaging. *Stem Cells* 27, 1548–1558. doi:10.1002/stem.81

Wang, L., Zhao, Y., Yang, F., Feng, M., Zhao, Y., Chen, X., et al. (2020). Biomimetic collagen biomaterial induces *in situ* lung regeneration by forming functional alveolar. *Biomaterials* 236, 119825. doi:10.1016/j.biomaterials.2020.119825

Weiss, D. J., Casaburi, R., Flannery, R., LeRoux-Williams, M., and Tashkin, D. P. (2013). A placebo-controlled, randomized trial of mesenchymal stem cells in COPD. *Chest* 143, 1590–1598. doi:10.1378/chest.12-2094

Westergren-Thorsson, G., Hedström, U., Nybom, A., Tykesson, E., Åhrman, E., Hornfelt, M., et al. (2017). Increased deposition of glycosaminoglycans and altered structure of heparan sulfate in idiopathic pulmonary fibrosis. *Int. J. Biochem. Cel Biol.* 83, 27–38. doi:10.1016/j.biocel.2016.12.005

Widhe, M., Shalaly, N. D., and Hedhammar, M. (2016). A fibronectin mimetic motif improves integrin mediated cell biding to recombinant spider silk matrices. *Biomaterials* 74, 256–266. doi:10.1016/j.biomaterials.2015.10.013

Wigén, J., Elowsson-Rendin, L., Karlsson, L., Tykesson, E., and Westergren-Thorsson, G. (2019). Glycosaminoglycans: a link between development and regeneration in the lung. *Stem Cell Development* 28, 823–832. doi:10.1089/scd.2019.0009

Woldhuis, R. R., de Vries, M., Timens, W., van den Berge, M., Demaria, M., Oliver, B. G. G., et al. (2020). Link between increased cellular senescence and extracellular matrix changes in COPD. *Am. J. Physiology-Lung Cell Mol. Physiol.* 319, L48–L60. doi:10.1152/ajplung.00028.2020

Wong, S. W., Lenzini, S., Cooper, M. H., Mooney, D. J., and Shin, J.-W. (2020). Soft extracellular matrix enhances inflammatory activation of mesenchymal stromal cells to induce monocyte production and trafficking. *Sci. Adv.* 6, eaaw0158. doi:10.1126/sciadv.aaw0158

Wozniak, M. A., Modzelewska, K., Kwong, L., and Keely, P. J. (2004). Focal adhesion regulation of cell behavior. *Biochim. Biophys. Acta (Bba) - Mol. Cel Res.* 1692, 103–119. doi:10.1016/j.bbamcr.2004.04.007

Yang, C., Tibbitt, M. W., Basta, L., and Anseth, K. S. (2014). Mechanical memory and dosing influence stem cell fate. *Nat. Mater* 13, 645–652. doi:10.1038/nmat3889

Yawn, B. P., Mintz, M. L., and Doherty, D. E. (2021). GOLD in practice: chronic obstructive pulmonary disease treatment and management in the primary care setting. *Copd* 16, 289–299. doi:10.2147/COPD.S222664

Yayon, A., Klagsbrun, M., Esko, J. D., Leder, P., and Ornitz, D. M. (1991). Cell surface, heparin-like molecules are required for binding of basic fibroblast growth factor to its high affinity receptor. *Cell* 64, 841–848. doi:10.1016/0092-8674(91)90512-w

Zhu, Y.-g., Feng, X.-m., Abbott, J., Fang, X.-h., Hao, Q., Monsel, A., et al. (2014). Human mesenchymal stem cell microvesicles for treatment ofEscherichia coliEndotoxin-induced acute lung injury in mice. *Stem Cells* 32, 116–125. doi:10.1002/stem.1504

12

Single-Dose Lentiviral Mediated Gene Therapy Recovers CFTR Function in Cystic Fibrosis Knockout Rats

Nicole Reyne[1,2,3], Patricia Cmielewski[1,2,3], Alexandra McCarron[1,2,3], Juliette Delhove[1,2,3], David Parsons[1,2,3†] and Martin Donnelley[1,2,3†]*

[1]Adelaide Medical School, University of Adelaide, Adelaide, SA, Australia, [2]Respiratory and Sleep Medicine, Women's and Children's Hospital, North Adelaide, SA, Australia, [3]Robinson Research Institute, University of Adelaide, Adelaide, SA, Australia

***Correspondence:**
Nicole Reyne
nikki.reyne@adelaide.edu.au

†These authors share senior authorship

Cystic fibrosis (CF) is a genetic disease caused by mutations in the CF transmembrane conductance regulator (*CFTR*) gene, resulting in defective ion transport in the airways. Addition of a functioning *CFTR* gene into affected airway cells has the potential to be an effective treatment for lung disease. The therapeutic efficacy of airway gene transfer can be quantified in animal models by assessing ion transport in the treated nasal epithelium using the nasal potential difference (PD) measurement technique. The nasal PD technique is routinely used in CF mice, however when applied to a recently developed CF rat model those animals did not tolerate the initial nasal PD assessment, therefore the procedure was firstly optimised in rats. This study evaluated the effect of lentiviral (LV)-mediated *CFTR* airway gene delivery on nasal PD in a CFTR knockout rat model. LV gene vector containing the *CFTR* gene tagged with a V5 epitope tag (LV-V5-*CFTR*) was delivered to the nasal epithelium of CF rats, and one week later nasal PD was analysed. This study demonstrated for the first time that LV-V5-*CFTR* treatment produced a mean correction of 46% towards wild-type chloride response in treated CF rats. Transduced cells were subsequently identifiable using V5 immunohistochemical staining. These findings in the nose validate the use of airway gene therapy for future lung based experiments.

Keywords: cystic fibrosis, lentival vector, nasal potential difference (NPD), Rat, gene therapy

INTRODUCTION

Cystic fibrosis (CF) is a common, life-shortening, recessive genetic disorder, resulting from mutations in the cystic fibrosis transmembrane conductance regulator (*CFTR*) gene (Davis, 2006). CF affects multiple organs and despite symptomatic treatments and CFTR modulator therapies that improve quality of life it remains incurable, with lung disease the major cause of mortality (Carlon et al., 2017). The pathophysiology of CF results from a loss of CFTR chloride channel function and via its interaction with other ion channels such as the epithelial sodium channel (ENaC). Together these channels regulate chloride and sodium ion movement across the epithelial surface of many organs, maintaining osmolarity. In CF airways an imbalance of these ions creates altered movement of water, causing the mucus layer lining the airways to become dehydrated and vicious. The resulting viscous mucus is thick, difficult to clear, and the ideal environment for bacteria and other pathogens to grow. Thus, CF airways experience a continuous cycle of infection and inflammation, leading to permanent lung damage and ultimately respiratory failure (Chmiel et al., 2002).

Correcting CFTR dysfunction at the genetic level, by the addition of a functioning *CFTR* gene into affected airway cells, has the potential to be an effective treatment for CF lung disease. As CF is monogenic, addition of one correct copy of the *CFTR* gene into the cells should be sufficient to halt disease or prevent it if initiated early in life (Villate-Beitia et al., 2017). A range of viral and non-viral vectors can be used to facilitate the transfer of a gene to the airway epithelial cells. Lentiviral vectors (LV) are attractive vehicles as they can transduce dividing and non-dividing cells, integrate into the host genome providing long term expression, and generate little immune response (Castellani and Conese, 2010).

Our group has utilised a vesicular stomatitis virus type G (VSV-G) pseudotyped LV vector and two-step dosing procedure that involves conditioning the airways with lysophosphatidylcholine (LPC) prior to vector delivery. Using this approach, we have shown that nasal delivery of LV-*CFTR* can successfully correct CFTR function in a CF mouse model for up to 12 months after a single dose, and improves survival of the treated animals (Cmielewski et al., 2014). The nasal airway region is used because the ion transport defects in the CF mouse nasal airway epithelium closely resemble those of the human CF lung (Ferrari et al., 2002). Additionally, the nasal cavity is easily accessed, which makes it a suitable site to test ion transport function as a representation of the lower airways (Rowe et al., 2011). CF mouse models have predominantly been used in CF research, however they do not exhibit the human lung pathophysiology, so further lung investigations can be limited (McCarron et al., 2018; McCarron et al., 2020).

Nasal PD has been used as a CF diagnostic method in humans for over 25 years, as it is well tolerated (Knowles et al., 1981). It has been adapted for use in some CF animal models, particularly mice, to test the efficacy of various therapeutic strategies. A *CFTR* knockout (KO) rat model was recently developed by CRISPR/Cas9 gene editing as an alternative CF animal model for researchers (McCarron et al., 2020). Preliminary data from this model showed altered function of the nasal epithelial ion channels that is consistent with the CF profile (McCarron et al., 2020). Those preliminary nasal PD investigations were performed as non-recovery procedures due to rats displaying a heightened sensitivity to fluid in the airways and respiratory difficulties following the procedure, meaning that recovery was not possible. The initial nasal PD assessments in rats were performed in the same manner as for mice, with the animal hung by the dorsal incisors in a vertical position (Limberis et al., 2002). This orientation proved to be problematic, as all nasally delivered solutions collected in the lungs, resulting in respiratory distress. Other factors limiting the first nasal PD investigations in rats included the poor integrity of the existing nasal PD fluid delivery perfusion tubing arrangement. Therefore, the nasal PD measurement technique in rats needed to be optimised to achieve improved reliability so that the effect of treatments such as airway gene-addition therapy could be assessed.

In this study we firstly optimised the technique of performing nasal PD measurements in rats to test ion channel function. We then investigated whether a single dose of our LV-V5-*CFTR* vector delivered after conditioning with LPC recovers CFTR function in the nasal epithelium of CF KO rats.

METHODS

Animals

This project was conducted under the approval from the University of Adelaide Animal Ethics Committee (M-2017-056). All rats were maintained in conventional cages with a 12-h light/dark cycle. Food and water were provided *ad libitum*, with all rats receiving a 50:50 mix of normal and high fat (10%) rodent chow. CF rats received water containing 4.5% ColonLytley (Dendy Pharmaceuticals, Australia) to minimise CF related gut obstructions. Female and male CF KO rats (510X genotype) (McCarron et al., 2020) were used.

Nasal PD

Ion channel function was measured using a newly optimised nasal PD technique adapted from mouse protocols (Limberis et al., 2002; Cmielewski et al., 2010) and early CF rat characterisation studies (McCarron et al., 2020). Rats were anesthetized with 60–75 mg/kg of a mixture of ketamine (Ceva, Australia) and medetomidine 0.4 mg/kg (Ilium, Australia), delivered by intraperitoneal injection. Rats were then placed on a customised nasal PD platform, in the prone orientation. Upper incisors were hooked over a wire loop, resulting in their mouth being open, rather than vertical with an endotracheal tube as in the initial rat PD method.

Our old PD system was constructed using long thin polyethylene tubes and cut-down needles sealed with superglue or silicone sealant where connections were required. This perfusion tubing had poor integrity, with bubbles and blockages regularly interrupting the continuous electrical circuit, leading to erroneous PD readings. New perfusion lines (Instech, United States) were made using 25 ga tubing (#BTPE-25), PinPorts (#PNP3F25) and PinPort connectors (#PNP3M-50) designed for minimal dead space volumes, as well as three-way tubing connectors (#SCY25), to create an enclosed system that prevented bubble formation. A micropositioner provided fine tip positioning and firmly held the nasal cannula in place, thus limiting movement while the cannula sat in the nose. Excess perfusion fluid coming out of the nasal cavity and/or mouth was absorbed with tissue. A 15 ml centrifuge tube was placed under the neck to create a slight downwards bend of the head and nose tip to help prevent fluid from moving distally and entering the trachea. The cannula was inserted 4–7 mm into the nasal cavity, based on identification of the location of nasal respiratory epithelium using dissected rat heads (not shown) and comparison to rat nasal diagrams (Mery et al., 1994). The reference electrode inserted subcutaneously into the abdomen, and connected to calomel electrodes (Hg_2Cl_2 in 3 M KCl, Cole-Parmer Instruments, United States) (Limberis et al., 2002; Cmielewski et al., 2010).

The optimised nasal PD method was then tested in wild-type (WT) and CF KO rats. PD data was recorded using a optically isolated high-impedance millivolt meter (ISOMIL, World

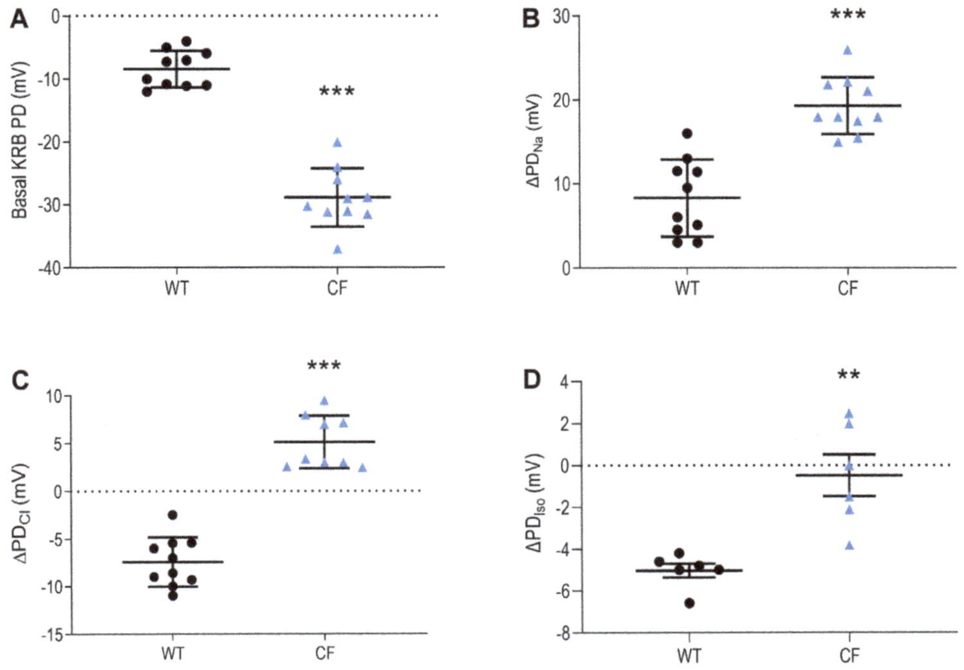

FIGURE 1 | Nasal PD measurements from WT and CF KO rats. Nasal PD measurements in WT and CF KO rats for **(A)** basal KRB **(B)** the ΔPD_{Na} **(C)** ΔPD_{Cl} and **(D)** ΔPD_{Iso} (n = 6–10 animals/group; $^{**}p \le 0.01$, $^{***}p \le 0.001$, unpaired t-test). Data represented as the mean –/+ SEM.

Precision Instruments) connected to an eight channel Powerlab, combined with Labchart software (Version 8, ADInstruments).

The nasal cavity was perfused at a rate of 10 µL/min with the following solutions: 1) normal Krebs-Ringer buffer (basal KRB), 2) KRB containing 100 µm amiloride, 3) low chloride KRB with 100 µm amiloride, and 4) low chloride KRB containing 100 µm of amiloride and 100 µm of isoproterenol. Each solution was perfused for 10–15 min until a plateau of 1–2 min was obtained. The change in PD (ΔPD) was calculated by subtracting the PD values at the plateau for each different solution. PD traces were rejected if they were non-responders.

Vector Production

This study employed a third generation, HIV-1 derived, VSV-G pseudotyped, *CFTR* gene vector with a V5 epitope tag located on the N-terminus. Gene expression was driven by the EF1α promoter (CCL-EF1α-V5-CFTR) The vector will be referred to as LV-V5-*CFTR*. LV vector was produced as described previously (Rout-Pitt et al., 2018). Briefly, HEK 293T cells seeded in 10-layer cell factories were transiently transfected using a five-plasmid system and calcium phosphate co-precipitation. Two days post-transfection the vector supernatant was harvested and purified by anion exchange chromatography, followed by ultracentrifugation. Vector was formulated in 0.1% heat-inactivated rat serum in 0.9% saline.

Vector Titre

The titre of the LV-V5-*CFTR* vector was determined by flow cytometric detection of V5 expressing-cells. HEK 293 T cells were transduced with a serially diluted (1:2,500–1:320,000) vector followed by collection 72 h post-transduction. Cells were fixed in 4% paraformaldehyde, permeabilized with ice cold 90% methanol, and resuspended to a concentration of 1×10^6 cell/mL for staining. Primary antibody rabbit anti-V5 Tag (#13202, Cell Signaling Technologies, United States) and secondary antibody goat anti-rabbit IgG (Alexa Fluor 568) (a11011, Invitrogen, United States of America) were added to the cells separately for 1 h and 30 min respectively at room temperature. Cells were washed between antibody staining and after, then resuspended in PBS. Cells were analysed using flow cytometry (LSRFortessa™; Becton Dickinson, United States). The proportion of V5-positive cells was used to calculate functional titre in transducing units per ml (TU/mL). A titre of 8×10^6 TU/ml was used for rat nasal dosing.

Nasal Vector Dosing

Rats were anaesthetised as described above. Lubricating eye ointment was placed onto the eyes to minimise drying. Rats were placed on a heating mat for the duration of the procedure and recovery period. Instillations were performed into the right nostril using a micropipette and thin gel tip (No: 5,242,956.003, Microloader, Eppendorf, Germany). Airway conditioning was performed with 2 × 5 µL aliquots of 0.3% LPC (#L4129 Sigma, United States), delivered 1 h prior to 2 × 10 µl aliquots of LV-V5-*CFTR* vector. Anaesthesia was reversed using 1 mg/kg atipamezole (Jurox, Australia). Baseline PD was performed at least one week before LV-*CFTR* delivery on the untreated nostril. One week after LV-*CFTR* delivery, PD measurement was performed on the treated

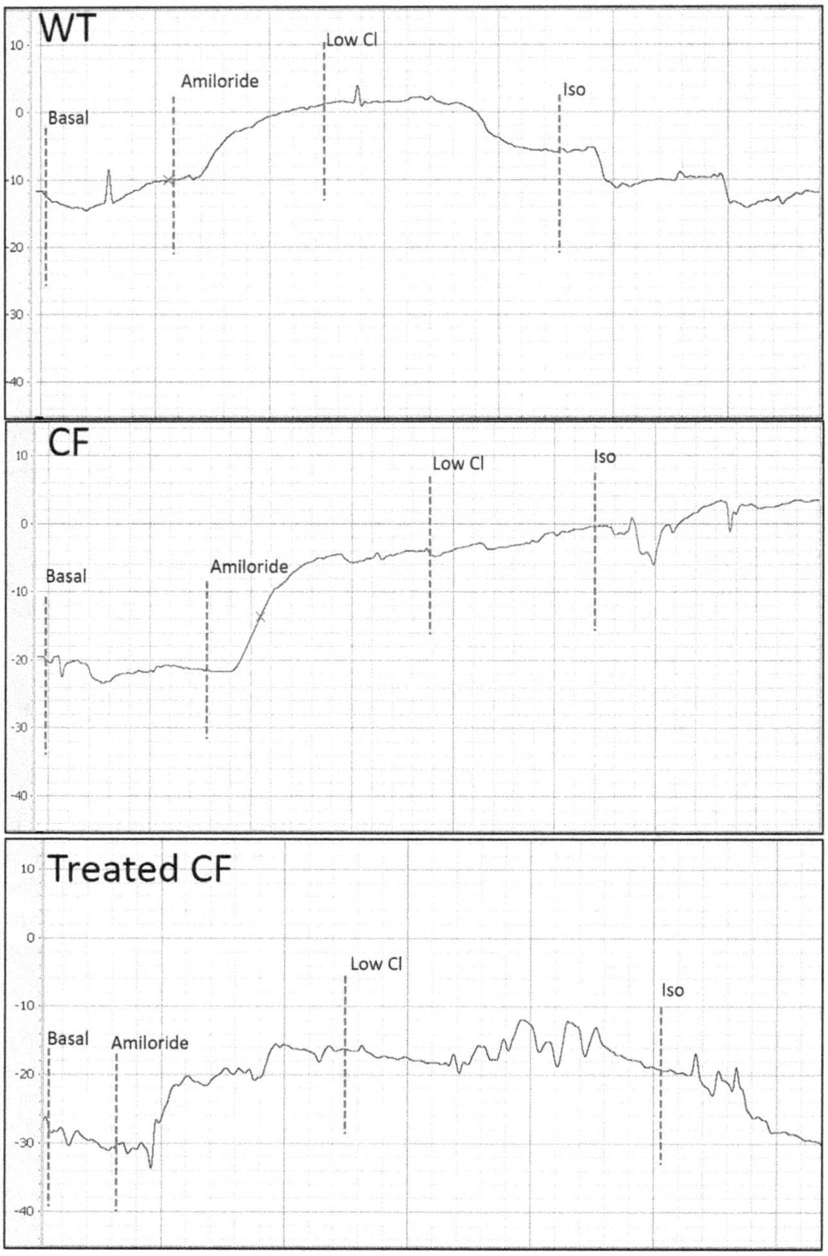

FIGURE 2 | Representative nasal PD tracing of WT, CF KO and treated CF KO rat. When compared to WT, CF KO rats demonstrate classic CF electrophysiological defects in nasal respiratory epithelium. Treated CF KO rats demonstrate a PD trace showing the corrected bioelectrical defect.

nostril. All PD tracings were interpreted by an experienced assessor blinded to the treatment.

Immunohistochemistry

Rats were humanely killed by intracardiac sodium pentobarbital overdose (300 mg/kg) while under anaesthetic. To examine the nasal passageways the heads were collected and immersion fixed in 10% neutral buffered formalin followed by decalcification in 25% EDTA (pH 7.4) for 7–14 days at 37°C. Heads were cut, paraffin-embedded, sectioned at 5–7 μm, and deparaffinised using standard histological procedures. Antigen retrieval was performed using 10 mM sodium citrate buffer (pH 6.0) for 20 min followed by permeabilisation in 0.3% Triton-X 100 in PBS for 10 min. Sections were blocked for 1 h at room temperature with 1% BSA in PBS and then incubated with goat anti-V5 primary antibody (1:300) (ab95038, Abcam) in 1% BSA + 0.05% Tween overnight at 4°C. Sections were rinsed and incubated in donkey anti-goat (IgG) Alexa Fluor 568 (1:400) (ab175704, Abcam) made in 1% BSA and 0.1% Tween incubated at room temperature for 1 h. Samples were washed with 0.1% Tween-PBS, counterstained with DAPI for approximately 10 min, washed, and mounted with ProLong^{TM} Diamond antifade mounting media (#P36961, Life Technologies, United States). Slides were visualised

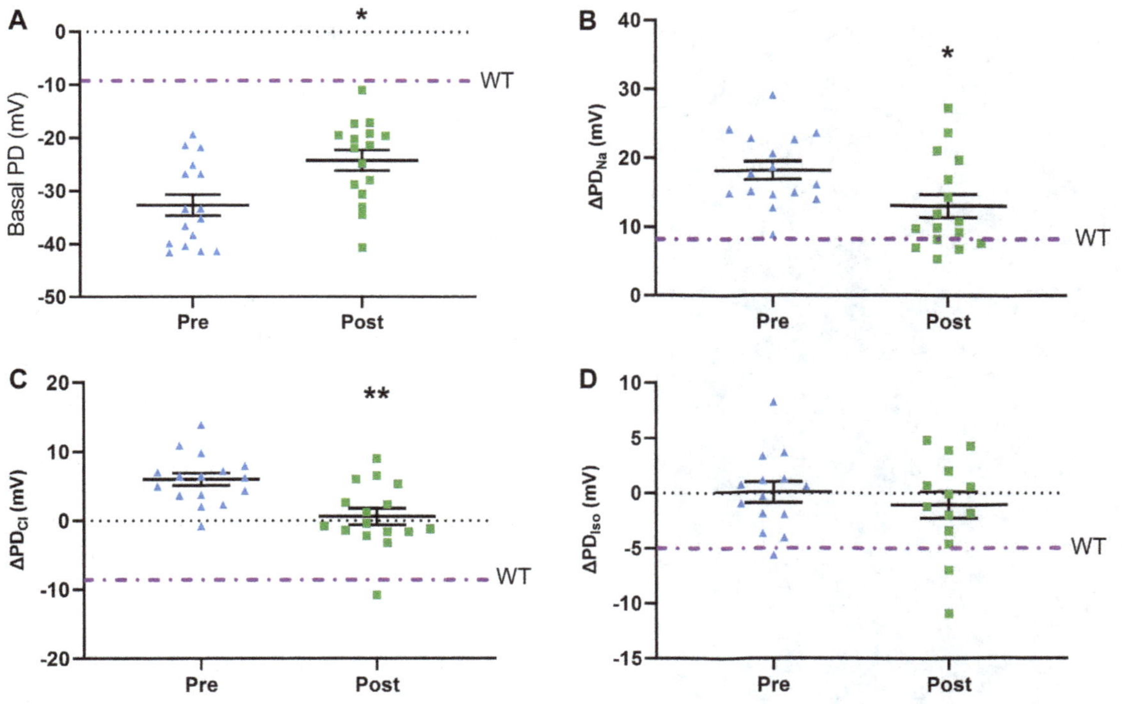

FIGURE 3 | Pre-treatment and post-treatment nasal PD results following LV-V5-*CFTR* vector delivery to nasal epithelium of CF KO rats. Nasal PD measurements in CF KO rats for **(A)** basal KRB **(B)** ΔPD_{Na} **(C)** ΔPD_{Cl}, and **(D)** ΔPD_{Iso}. Dot/dash line indicates the WT average ($^*p \leq 0.05$, $^{**}p \leq 0.01$, paired *t*-test; $n = 14–16$). Data represented as the mean with −/+ SEM.

for the presence of V5 staining using an Olympus BX51 Research grade optical microscope DIC with AnalySIS Life Sciences software.

Statistical Analysis

Statistical analysis was performed using Graphpad Prism V9.0 (GraphPad Software Inc.). Statistical significance was set at $p \leq 0.05$ and a statistical power greater than 0.80 was required. Paired t-tests were used to compare the treated and untreated nostril in each rat. In text values are reported as mean ±SD.

RESULTS

Nasal PD Assessment Was Optimized in Rats

To improve nasal PD assessments in rats we developed an optimised testing method. In the preliminary nasal PD studies (McCarron et al., 2020), rats readily inhaled the nasally delivered solutions into the lung, often leading to respiratory distress. This was a critical limitation, as rats could not be recovered from anaesthesia following the procedure. Several measures aimed at reducing that original procedure-associated complication were successfully trialed, including placing the rats in their naturally prone position, and absorbing the excess fluid from the nasal cavity. Using tubing with a smaller bore diameter reduced the volume of fluid in the system and enabled perfusion fluids to be rapidly changed, without excessive fluid delivery to the nose. Subsequently, rats did not show signs of respiratory distress and no mortality was associated with the nasal PD procedures.

Confirmation of WT and CF Rat Nasal PD Profiles

This study provides an improved characterisation of the airway bioelectric profile in our CF KO rats (McCarron et al., 2020), with the greater power revealing that there was a statistically significant difference in the isoproterenol response between WT and KO CF rats ($p \leq 0.01$, **Figure 1**). Under basal conditions, CF KO rats demonstrated a significant negative PD when compared to the WT rats. When the ENaC inhibitor amiloride was perfused, CF KO rats exhibited a more enhanced depolarisation response than WT rats, indicating increased luminal retention of sodium. Low chloride and isoproterenol solutions produced either no response or a small depolarisation in CF (whereas a hyperpolarisation was observed in WT rats) suggesting the absence of CFTR-mediated chloride transport.

Ion channel function can be restored in nasal epithelium of CF KO rats after treatment with LV-V5-CFTR

Figure 2 depicts representative PD traces from WT, CF KO and a treated CF KO rat, showing the correction of the bioelectrical in the treated CF KO rat.

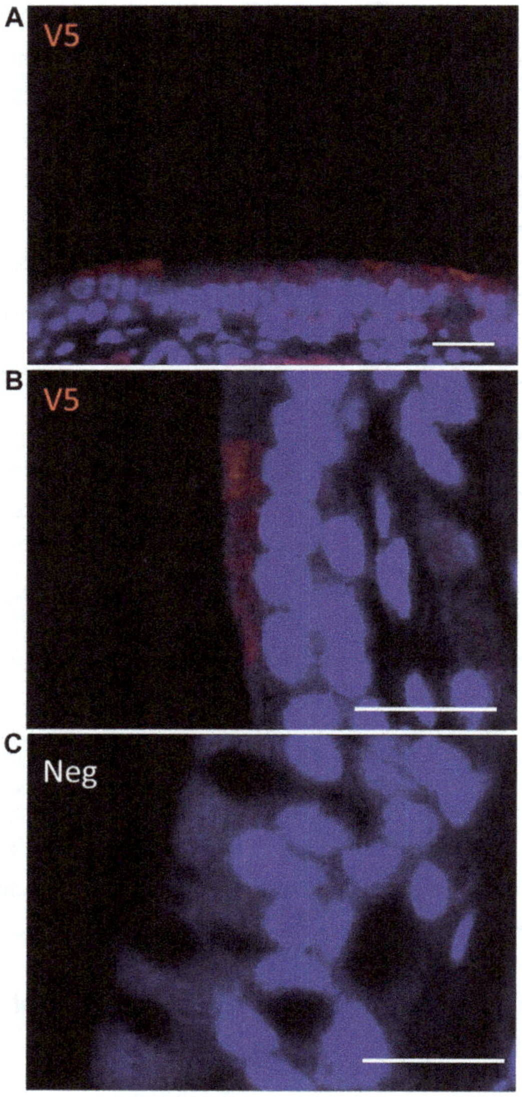

FIGURE 4 | Immunohistochemical detection of V5-*CFTR* in the rat nasal epithelium. **(A,B)** V5 IHC enables localisation of *CFTR* (red) in the right nostril (treated) one week after delivery of LV-V5-*CFTR*. **(C)** No staining was observed on the left (untreated) side of the rat nose. Scale bar 20 μm.

Seven days after delivery of LV-V5-*CFTR* to CF KO rats (n = 16), the basal KRB (−24.2 ± 7.8 mV) response exhibited a significantly smaller depolarisation compared to pre-treatment (−32.8 ± 7.9 mV), which was closer to a WT response ($p \leq 0.05$) (**Figure 3**). The amiloride response in treated (13.0 ± 6.7 mV) CF KO rats had an improvement of 51% toward the WT value when compared to the pre-treatment (18.2 ± 5.3 mV) ($p \leq 0.05$). Treated CF KO rats also showed a more negative low chloride response (0.6 ± 4.7 mV), which was significantly different from the pre-treatment response (5.9 ± 3.6 mV) ($p \leq 0.01$) (**Figure 3**). The isoproterenol response did not reach statistical significance between pre- and post-LV treatment (0.08 ± 3.6 and −1.5 ± 4.4 mV respectively).

Immunostaining with an anti-V5 antibody demonstrated the presence of the transgene in the right side (treated) of the nasal epithelium one week post-delivery, whereas no staining was observed in the left nostril (untreated). V5 positive staining was detected in the ciliated cells of the nasal epithelium (**Figure 4**).

DISCUSSION

Nasal PD measurement methods have been developed for use in mice, ferrets and pigs, and enable reliable repeated measurements in the same animal with low procedure-associated mortality (Beka and Leal, 2018; Kaza et al., 2017; Salinas et al., 2004). We have demonstrated that our newly optimised technique and equipment for conducting electrophysical measurements, can provide a reliable tool for evaluating airway gene therapy effects in CF rat nasal airways. The nasal PD baseline data collected from WT and CF KO rats confirmed that the CF KO rat displays a bioelectrical defect consistent with the CF profile (McCarron et al., 2020).

The nasal PD response to the low chloride gradient is used to both discriminate non-CF from CF animals (**Figure 2**), and more commonly to assess the response to therapeutics *in vivo* (Leonard et al., 2012). It has been suggested that a relatively small number of gene corrected airway cells (10%) can restore transepithelial chloride function to therapeutically significant levels, potentially providing dramatic improvements in pulmonary function (Johnson et al., 1992; Marquez Loza et al., 2019). Moreover, those CF patients with 'mild' mutations and residual CFTR function have less severe lung disease (Griesenbach et al., 2008) indicating that not all cells are required to be corrected. Our previous CF mouse study showed a 12–54% correction in PD towards WT CFTR function as assessed by chloride transport (Cmielewski et al., 2014), and in this present rat study, a mean of 46% correction was observed. The isoproterenol response did not reach statistical significance in this study, however larger studies or a higher level of correction may provide sufficient power to detect a difference. Importantly, this study showed for the first time that a single delivery of LV-V5-*CFTR* could achieve *in vivo* correction of nasal airway epithelium ion transport in a CF KO rat model.

CF epithelial ion transport is characterised by a greater hyperpolarisation (more negative) measurement of basal KRB due to the increased activity of ENaC, a large depolarisation in the presence of a sodium channel blocker, and a small or absent response to low chloride and isoproterenol solutions. Gene therapy efforts have focused on the correction of chloride function and some suggest that the direct interaction between CFTR and ENaC should be normalised for therapeutic outcomes (Johnson et al., 1995). Johnson et al. indicated with *in vitro* studies using ALI cultures that a majority of the cell monolayer is required to be expressing *CFTR* for ENaC transport to be corrected (Johnson et al., 1995), while another *in vitro* study suggested that 60% of ciliated cells may be enough to normalise sodium ion transport (Zhang et al., 2009). We noted there was a statistically significant mean correction of 51% towards WT in the amiloride response after LV vector treatment in CF rats. This may suggest that the sodium hyperabsorption defect present in CF rats may have been improved, however, further studies utilising Ussing chamber assessments are needed to link altered sodium absorption to the insertion of a functioning CFTR channel.

The HIV-1 virus-based vector system has been extensively modified to improve safety and efficacy for use in gene therapy (Milone and O'Doherty, 2018). While our previous *CFTR* airway gene-addition studies employed second generation LV vectors with internal viral promoters (e.g., SV40), for the first time this study used a third generation vector with an EF1α promoter, tagged with V5 for immunodetection. For these reasons this vector system is more appropriate for clinical application than those used in our previous mouse studies (Cmielewski et al., 2014). Importantly, the use of the V5 tag did not interfere with functionality of the CFTR protein, as demonstrated by significant correction of bioelectric defect as measured by nasal PD.

This study had some limitations. Firstly, it was designed to be a short-term assessment and did not investigate the ability to achieve long term correction of nasal ion transport. For gene therapy to be successful the expression of *CFTR* needs to be permanent and life long, and this study sets the stage for future long-term investigations in CF rats. Assessing persistence of gene expression over long durations in CF rats and the ability to re-dose if correction wanes are all next steps. Secondly, the total number of *CFTR* transduced cells was not quantified here, but in future studies where histological outcomes are not required the nasal epithelium could be removed, the cells dissociated and the V5 positive cell population quantified by flow cytometry. CFTR protein expression could also be further examined by Western blot. Thirdly, the use of a non-CFTR LV vector control could be employed to verify that the delivered *CFTR* gene was responsible for the effects observed here. Lastly, a CFTR inhibitor might be used to further discriminate CFTR function, although one study suggests that CFTRinh-172 does not have an effect in rats (Dreano et al., 2019).

In summary, using our optimised PD protocols we showed successful correction of the bioelectrical defect in our newly established CF KO rat model for the first time. Future studies will focus on assessing long-term CFTR correction, to help validate the effectiveness of this LV vector for translation to the clinic as a potential and fundamental treatment for CF lung disease.

AUTHOR CONTRIBUTIONS

NR redesigned and evaluated the nasal potential difference measurement system, and performed all animal studies including nasal potential difference recordings and assessments. NR performed all flow cytometry and immunohistochemistry, with oversight from AM and JD. Nasal potential difference traces were scored blinded by PC for confirmation. DP and MD assisted with study design, data interpretation and manuscript revision. All authors contributed to manuscript preparation.

ACKNOWLEDGMENTS

This study was supported by NHMRC GNT1160011 and a CFF Student Traineeship Award #REYNE20HO. We thank Nathan Rout-Pitt for assisting with vector production, University of Adelaide Laboratory Animal Services for assisting with animal husbandry, University of Adelaide Histological Services for preparing specimen slides, Adelaide Microscopy for use of the fluorescence microscope, and the University of South Australia for use of the flow cytometry facility. We thank Richard Boucher and Barbara Grubb (University of North Carolina at Chapel Hill) for their helpful discussions about the PD results from this study.

REFERENCES

Beka, M., and Leal, T. (2018). Nasal Potential Difference to Quantify Trans-epithelial Ion Transport in Mice. *JoVE (Journal of Visualized Experiments)* 4 (137), e57934. doi:10.3791/57934

Carlon, M. S., Vidović, D., and Birket, S. (2017). Roadmap for an Early Gene Therapy for Cystic Fibrosis Airway Disease. *Prenatal Diagn.* 37 (12), 1181–1190. doi:10.1002/pd.5164

Castellani, S., and Conese, M. (2010). Lentiviral Vectors and Cystic Fibrosis Gene Therapy. *Viruses* 2 (2), 395–412. doi:10.3390/v2020395

Chmiel, J. F., Berger, M., and Konstan, M. W. (2002). The Role of Inflammation in the Pathophysiology of CF Lung Disease. *Criai* 23 (1), 005–028. doi:10.1385/criai:23:1:005

Cmielewski, P., Anson, D. S., and Parsons, D. W. (2010). Lysophosphatidylcholine as an Adjuvant for Lentiviral Vector Mediated Gene Transfer to Airway Epithelium: Effect of Acyl Chain Length. *Respir. Res.* 11 (1), 1–11. doi:10.1186/1465-9921-11-84

Cmielewski, P., Donnelley, M., and Parsons, D. W. (2014). Long-term Therapeutic and Reporter Gene Expression in Lentiviral Vector Treated Cystic Fibrosis Mice. *J. Gene Med.* 16 (9-10), 291–299. doi:10.1002/jgm.2778

Davis, P. B. (2006). Cystic Fibrosis since 1938. *Am. J. Respir. Crit. Care Med.* 173 (5), 475–482. doi:10.1164/rccm.200505-840oe

Dreano, E., Bacchetta, M., Simonin, J., Galmiche, L., Usal, C., Slimani, L., et al. (2019). Characterization of two rat models of cystic fibrosis-KO and F508del CFTR-Generated by Crispr-Cas9. *Anim. Models Exp. Med.* 2 (4), 297–311. doi:10.1002/ame2.12091

Ferrari, S., Geddes, D. M., and Alton, E. W. F. W. (2002). Barriers to and New Approaches for Gene Therapy and Gene Delivery in Cystic Fibrosis. *Adv. Drug Deliv. Rev.* 54 (11), 1373–1393. doi:10.1016/s0169-409x(02)00145-x

Griesenbach, U., Smith, S. N., Farley, R., Singh, C., and Alton, E. W. F. W. (2008). Validation of Nasal Potential Difference Measurements in Gut-Corrected CF Knockout Mice. *Am. J. Respir. Cel Mol Biol* 39 (4), 490–496. doi:10.1165/rcmb.2007-0385oc

Johnson, L. G., Boyles, S. E., Wilson, J., and Boucher, R. C. (1995). Normalization of Raised Sodium Absorption and Raised Calcium-Mediated Chloride Secretion by Adenovirus-Mediated Expression of Cystic Fibrosis Transmembrane Conductance Regulator in Primary Human Cystic Fibrosis Airway Epithelial Cells. *J. Clin. Invest.* 95 (3), 1377–1382. doi:10.1172/jci117789

Johnson, L. G., Olsen, J. C., Sarkadi, B., Moore, K. L., Swanstrom, R., and Boucher, R. C. (1992). Efficiency of Gene Transfer for Restoration of Normal Airway Epithelial Function in Cystic Fibrosis. *Nat. Genet.* 2 (1), 21–25. doi:10.1038/ng0992-21

Kaza, N., Raju, S. V., Cadillac, J, M., Trombley, J. A., Rasmussen, L., Tang, L., et al. (2017). Use of Ferrets for Electrophysiologic Monitoring of Ion Transport. *Plos one* 12 (10), e0186984. doi:10.1371/journal.pone.0186984

Knowles, M., Gatzy, J., and Boucher, R. (1981). Increased Bioelectric Potential Difference across Respiratory Epithelia in Cystic Fibrosis. *N. Engl. J. Med.* 305 (25), 1489–1495. doi:10.1056/nejm198112173052502

Leonard, A., Lubamba, B., Dhooghe, B., Noel, S., Wallemacq, P., Lebecque, P., et al. (2012). Comparative Variability of Nasal Potential Difference Measurements in Human and Mice. *Ojrd* 02 (02), 43–56. doi:10.4236/ojrd.2012.22007

Limberis, M., Anson, D. S., Fuller, M., and Parsons, D. W. (2002). Recovery of Airway Cystic Fibrosis Transmembrane Conductance Regulator Function in Mice with Cystic Fibrosis after Single-Dose Lentivirus-Mediated Gene Transfer. *Hum. Gene Ther.* 13 (16), 1961–1970. doi:10.1089/10430340260355365

Marquez Loza, L., Yuen, E., and McCray, P. (2019). Lentiviral Vectors for the Treatment and Prevention of Cystic Fibrosis Lung Disease. *Genes* 10 (3), 218. doi:10.3390/genes10030218

McCarron, A., Cmielewski, P., Reyne, N., McIntyre, C., Finnie, J., Craig, F., et al. (2020). Phenotypic Characterization and Comparison of Cystic Fibrosis Rat Models Generated Using CRISPR/Cas9 Gene Editing. *Am. J. Pathol.* 190 (5), 977–993. doi:10.1016/j.ajpath.2020.01.009

McCarron, A., Donnelley, M., and Parsons, D. (2018). Airway Disease Phenotypes in Animal Models of Cystic Fibrosis. *Respir. Res.* 19 (1), 1–12. doi:10.1186/s12931-018-0750-y

McCarron, A., Parsons, D., and Donnelley, M. (2020). Animal and Cell Culture Models for Cystic Fibrosis: Which Model Is Right for Your Application?. *Am. J. Pathol.*, 191(2), 228–242. doi:10.1016/j.ajpath.2020.10.017

Mery, S., Gross, E. A., Joyner, D. R., Godo, M., and Morgan, K. T. (1994). Nasal Diagrams: a Tool for Recording the Distribution of Nasal Lesions in Rats and Mice. *Toxicol. Pathol.* 22 (4), 353–372. doi:10.1177/019262339402200402

Milone, M. C., and O'Doherty, U. (2018). Clinical Use of Lentiviral Vectors. *Leukemia* 32 (7), 1529–1541. doi:10.1038/s41375-018-0106-0

Rout-Pitt, N., McCarron, A., McIntyre, C., Parsons, D., and Donnelley, M. (2018). Large-Scale Production of Lentiviral Vectors Using Multilayer Cell Factories. *J. Biol. Methods* 5 (2), e90. doi:10.14440/jbm.2018.236

Rowe, S. M., Clancy, J. P., and Wilschanski, M. (2011). Nasal Potential Difference Measurements to Assess CFTR Ion Channel Activity, *Cystic Fibrosis*. Springer, 69–86. doi:10.1007/978-1-61779-117-8_6

Salinas, D. B., Pedemonte, N., Muanprasat, C., Finkbeiner, W. F., Nielson, D. W., and Verkman, A. S. (2004). CFTR Involvement in Nasal Potential Differences in Mice and Pigs Studied Using a Thiazolidinone CFTR Inhibitor. *Am. J. Physiology-Lung Cell Mol. Physiol.* 287 (5), L936–L943. doi:10.1152/ajplung.00354.2003

Villate-Beitia, I., Zarate, J., Puras, G., and Pedraz, J. L. (2017). Gene Delivery to the Lungs: Pulmonary Gene Therapy for Cystic Fibrosis. *Drug Dev. Ind. Pharm.* 43 (7), 1071–1081. doi:10.1080/03639045.2017.1298122

Zhang, L., Button, B., Gabriel, S. E., Burkett, S., Yan, Y., Skiadopoulos, M. H., et al. (2009). CFTR Delivery to 25% of Surface Epithelial Cells Restores Normal Rates of Mucus Transport to Human Cystic Fibrosis Airway Epithelium. *Plos Biol.* 7 (7), e1000155. doi:10.1371/journal.pbio.1000155

13

Adipose Stromal Cell-Secretome Counteracts Profibrotic Signals from IPF Lung Matrices

Gwenda F. Vasse[1,2,3,4‡], Lisette Van Os[4,5†‡], Marina De Jager[3], Marnix R. Jonker[4,5], Theo Borghuis[4,5], L. Tim Van Den Toorn[4,5], Pytrick Jellema[5], Eric S. White[6†], Patrick Van Rijn[1,2], Martin C. Harmsen[5], Irene H. Heijink[4,5,7], Barbro N. Melgert[3,4§] and Janette K. Burgess[2,4,5*§]*

[1]University of Groningen, University Medical Center Groningen, Department of Biomedical Engineering, Groningen, Netherlands, [2]University of Groningen, University Medical Center Groningen, W.J. Kolff Institute for Biomedical Engineering and Materials Science, Groningen, Netherlands, [3]University of Groningen, Department of Molecular Pharmacology, Groningen Research Institute for Pharmacy, Groningen, Netherlands, [4]University of Groningen, University Medical Center Groningen, Groningen Research Institute for Asthma and COPD (GRIAC), Groningen, Netherlands, [5]University of Groningen, University Medical Center Groningen, Department of Pathology and Medical Biology, Groningen, Netherlands, [6]Division of Pulmonary and Critical Care Medicine, University of Michigan Medical School, Ann Arbor, MI, United States, [7]University of Groningen, University Medical Center Groningen, Department of Pulmonology, Groningen, Netherlands

***Correspondence:**
Barbro N. Melgert
b.n.melgert@rug.nl
Janette K. Burgess
j.k.burgess@umcg.nl*

*[†]**Present address:**
Lisette Van Os,
ARTORG Center for Biomedical Engineering, University of Bern, Bern, Switzerland;
Eric S. White,
Boehringer Ingelheim Pharmaceuticals, Inc., Ridgefield, CT, United States*

[‡]These authors have contributed equally to this work and share first authorship

[§]These authors have contributed equally to this work and share last authorship

Introduction: Idiopathic pulmonary fibrosis (IPF) is a fibrotic lung disease characterized by excess deposition and altered structure of extracellular matrix (ECM) in the lungs. The fibrotic ECM is paramount in directing resident cells toward a profibrotic phenotype. Collagens, an important part of the fibrotic ECM, have been shown to be structurally different in IPF. To further understand the disease to develop better treatments, the signals from the ECM that drive fibrosis need to be identified. Adipose tissue-derived stromal cell conditioned medium (ASC-CM) has demonstrated antifibrotic effects in animal studies but has not been tested in human samples yet. In this study, the collagen structural integrity in (fibrotic) lung tissue, its interactions with fibroblasts and effects of ASC-CM treatment hereon were studied.

Methods: Native and decellularized lung tissue from patients with IPF and controls were stained for denatured collagen using a collagen hybridizing peptide. Primary lung fibroblasts were seeded into decellularized matrices from IPF and control subjects and cultured for 7 days in the presence or absence of ASC-CM. Reseeded matrices were fixed, stained and analyzed for total tissue deposition and specific protein expression.

Results: In both native and decellularized lung tissue, more denatured collagen was observed in IPF tissue compared to control tissue. Upon recellularization with fibroblasts, the presence of denatured collagen was equalized in IPF and control matrices, whereas total ECM was higher in IPF matrices than in the control. Treatment with ASC-CM resulted in less ECM deposition, but did not alter the levels of denatured collagen.

Discussion: Our data showed that ASC-CM can inhibit fibrotic ECM-induced profibrotic behavior of fibroblasts. This process was independent of collagen structural integrity. Our findings open up new avenues for ASC-CM to be explored as treatment for IPF.

Keywords: idiopathic pulmonary fibrosis (IPF), adipose tissue-derived stromal/stem cells (ASCs), decellularized lung matrices, denatured collagen, collagen hybridizing peptide, extracellular matrix (ECM), primary lung fibroblasts, conditioned medium

INTRODUCTION

Idiopathic pulmonary fibrosis (IPF) is a progressive and devastating lung disease with an estimated survival of less than 5 years after diagnosis. It is mainly characterized by excessive and imbalanced accumulation of extracellular matrix (ECM) proteins in the interstitium of lung tissue (Lederer and Martinez, 2018). ECM is a highly dynamic structure that is deposited and constantly remodeled by surrounding cells with fibroblasts and myofibroblasts being the most important producers of ECM proteins in the lung (Burgess et al., 2016; Burgstaller et al., 2017). In IPF, mainly myofibroblasts contribute to the dense ECM in characteristic fibroblastic foci (Raghu et al., 2011). Formation of these fibroblastic foci disrupts blood flow to alveolar septa, which leads to alveolar septa damage and thus a decreased gas exchange capacity (Yamaguchi et al., 2017).

Multiple ECM proteins such as fibronectin and periostin are known to be more abundant in lung tissue of patients with IPF (Naik et al., 2012; Lehtonen et al., 2016; Tomos et al., 2017; Kudo and Kii, 2018), but collagens are the most abundant. It is becoming increasingly evident that not only the amount, but also the folding and structural integrity of collagen, is different in fibrosis (Kristensen et al., 2014; Ricard-Blum et al., 2018). Collagen molecules are triple helical protein structures that can, depending on the fibrillar or non-fibrillar type of collagen, assemble into collagen fibrils and larger collagen fibers (Ricard-Blum, 2011; Chang and Buehler, 2014). In lung tissue from patients with IPF, collagen fibers are altered structurally: the fibers are thicker and more mature/organized as compared to collagen fibers in control lung tissue (Tjin et al., 2017). The recent introduction of a collagen hybridizing peptide has made advanced imaging of collagen remodeling on a molecular level possible (Li and Yu, 2013). This peptide specifically binds to a repeating triple-helical motif that is shared by all 28 collagen types. Upon collagen denaturation and/or partial degradation, improper folding of the triple helix exposes the triple-helical motif and allows the labeled peptide to hybridize with the denatured or structurally disrupted collagen (Li and Yu, 2013; Hwang et al., 2017a). Using this collagen hybridizing peptide, augmented levels of structurally disrupted collagen have been observed in lung tissue of mice with bleomycin-induced pulmonary fibrosis (Hwang et al., 2017a), but it is still unclear whether these molecular changes are also present in lung tissue from patients with IPF and whether these changes play a notable role in fibrotic responses.

Currently, only two drugs have been approved to treat IPF: pirfenidone and nintedanib. Although these two drugs can slow down disease progression in some patients, they do not improve long-term mortality and patients can suffer from severe side-effects (Spagnolo et al., 2015). As an alternative or addition to pharmacological approaches, stem cell-based therapies are being explored for the treatment of IPF. Adipose tissue-derived stromal cells (ASCs) have been tested experimentally for the treatment of various conditions, including IPF (Barczyk et al., 2015). A variety of studies showed attenuated, but not resolved, fibrosis after ASC treatment in bleomycin-induced lung fibrosis in mice and rats (Lee et al., 2014; Jiang et al., 2015; Tashiro et al., 2015; Rathinasabapathy et al., 2016; Reddy et al., 2016; Llontop et al., 2018; Felix et al., 2020). Similar results were achieved in other rat models of pulmonary fibrosis (Fikry et al., 2015; Chen et al., 2018; Zhang et al., 2019; Radwan et al., 2020). A phase Ib, non-randomized clinical trial in patients with IPF has shown that even though administration of ASCs was safe and hinted toward advantageous short-term effects, the long-term follow-up showed unaltered disease progression and survival rates (Tzouvelekis et al., 2013; Ntolios et al., 2018). Interestingly, the regenerative effect of ASCs lies not only with their differentiation capacity, but mostly in the soluble factors they produce (Salgado et al., 2010). The secretome of ASCs consists of various molecules involved in tissue regeneration, apoptosis, host cell proliferation and angiogenesis (Salgado et al., 2010; Blaber et al., 2012; Sabin and Kikyo, 2015). ASC-derived culture medium, also called ASC-conditioned medium (ASC-CM), can be used to administer only this secretome. The use of ASC-CM as opposed to ASCs themselves prevents any potential harmful effects of the ASCs, as ASCs respond to their environment and could react detrimentally in a profibrotic environment (Yan et al., 2007; Liu et al., 2018). ASC-CM has been shown to reduce lung injury in a bleomycin-induced pulmonary fibrosis rat model (Rathinasabapathy et al., 2016; Felix et al., 2020) and could therefore be an alternative for ASC treatment in IPF. Yet, to date no research has been reported on the possible modulating effect of ASC-CM in human (fibrotic) lungs.

Decellularized matrices can be employed to study the influence of human (fibrotic) lung ECM on cellular behavior, as well as the impact of soluble factors on these cell-matrix interactions. The decellularized matrices can be obtained by treating lungs with various chemicals in a multistep process, removing all cells but retaining the majority of the ECM composition and structure (Booth et al., 2012). Subsequent culturing of freshly isolated primary human lung cells in these scaffolds can provide important insights in the response and matrix remodeling behavior of these cells. Previously, it has been shown that IPF-derived decellularized matrices direct healthy lung fibroblasts toward a profibrotic phenotype (Booth et al., 2012; Parker et al., 2014), emphasizing the ability of ECM to modulate cell behavior and the importance of this constant two-way interaction in the fibrotic response.

In this study, we characterized collagen structural integrity in native and decellularized human lung tissue from control patients and patients with IPF, hypothesizing that collagen structural organization is more disrupted in IPF lungs compared to control lungs. Furthermore, primary human lung fibroblasts were seeded into control and IPF-derived decellularized lung matrices to study cell-ECM crosstalk in the presence or absence of ASC-derived conditioned medium. We hypothesized that upon recellularization, fibroblasts would be driven toward profibrotic behavior in the IPF lung ECM as opposed to the control lung ECM and that administration of ASC-CM would impair the fibrotic process.

MATERIALS AND METHODS

Human Lung Tissue

Human fibrotic lung tissue was collected with informed consent from patients with interstitial lung disease (ILD) undergoing lung transplantation at either the University Medical Center Groningen (UMCG) or at the Erasmus Medical Center Rotterdam. Human non-fibrotic control lung tissue was obtained at the UMCG from patients undergoing surgical resection for carcinoma. In tumor resections, histologically normal lung tissue was taken as far distally as possible from the tumor and assessed visually by a pathologist for the absence of abnormalities with a standard haematoxylin and eosin staining. All available donor characteristics are listed in **Table 1**. In Groningen, the study protocol was consistent with the Research Code of the University Medical Center Groningen (www.umcg.nl/EN/Research/Researchers/General/ResearchCode/Paginas/default.aspx) and the Dutch national ethical and professional guidelines ("Code of conduct; Dutch federation of biomedical scientific societies"; http://www.federa.org). The Medical Ethical Committee of the Erasmus Medical Center Rotterdam approved all protocols followed in that center.

Human lung tissue for decellularization was obtained from non-transplantable donors (control, non-fibrotic) and from explants of patients with IPF receiving a lung transplant at the University of Michigan Medical Center. These approaches were deemed exempt from oversight by The University of Michigan Institutional Review Board, as all tissues were de-identified and coming from deceased donors.

Sample Preparation

Pieces of native lung tissue were fixed in formalin, embedded in paraffin and cut into 5 μm sections using standard procedures. Prior to staining, sections were deparaffinized also using standard procedures. Decellularized lung tissue was prepared as described previously (Booth et al., 2012) and stored in PBS containing 1% penicillin-streptomycin (Gibco Laboratories, Grand Island, NE, United States) at 4°C. Decellularized and recellularized matrices (see below for details) were fixed, embedded in paraffin and sectioned at 4 μm for staining.

Cell Culture

Primary human lung fibroblasts were isolated from lung tissue of control individuals at the UMCG as described earlier (Krimmer et al., 2012). Cells were derived from three donor tissues. An overview of the donor characteristics is provided in **Table 1**. The fibroblasts were cultured in low glucose Dulbecco's Modified Eagle Medium (DMEM, Lonza, Basel, Switzerland) supplemented with 10% fetal bovine serum (FBS, Sigma, St. Louis, MI, United States), 100 U/ml penicillin, 100 μg/ml streptomycin (Pen/Strep, Gibco, Waltham, MA, United States) and 4 mM L-glutamine (Lonza, Basel, Switzerland). Cells were maintained in an incubator at 37°C and 5% CO_2.

TABLE 1 | Overview of lung tissue and lung fibroblast donor characteristics.

Donor	Diagnosis	Material	Gender	Age	Smoking status
1	x	Control fibroblasts	Male	65	Ex-smoker
2	x	Control fibroblasts	Female	65	Non-smoker
3	x	Control fibroblasts	Male	50	Non-smoker
4–7	N.A.	Control decellularized lung matrix	N.A.	N.A.	N.A.
8–11	IPF	IPF decellularized lung matrix	N.A.	N.A.	N.A.
12	NSIP	Fibrotic lung tissue	Male	61	Non-smoker
13	End-stage fibrosis NOS/NSIP	Fibrotic lung tissue	Male	53	Non-smoker
14	IPF	Fibrotic lung tissue	Male	61	Ex-smoker
15	IPF	Fibrotic lung tissue	Male	64	Non-smoker
16	IPF	Fibrotic lung tissue	Male	61	Ex-smoker
17	N.A.	Fibrotic lung tissue	N.A.	48	N.A.
18	Scleroderma-associated pulmonary fibrosis	Fibrotic lung tissue	N.A.	45	N.A.
19	Non-IPF	Fibrotic lung tissue	Male	N.A.	N.A.
20	Methotrexate induced pulmonary fibrosis	Fibrotic lung tissue	Male	61	N.A.
21	Scleroderma-associated pulmonary fibrosis	Fibrotic lung tissue	N.A.	N.A.	N.A.
22	N.A.	Fibrotic lung tissue	N.A.	N.A.	N.A.
23	Polymyositis-associated fibrosis	Fibrotic lung tissue	N.A.	N.A.	N.A.
24	IPF	Fibrotic lung tissue	Male	42	N.A.
25	SFTPA2 mutation-associated pulmonary fibrosis	Fibrotic lung tissue	Female	27	N.A.
26	x	Control lung tissue	N.A.	N.A.	N.A.
27	x	Control lung tissue	N.A.	N.A.	N.A.
28	x	Control lung tissue	N.A.	N.A.	N.A.
29	x	Control lung tissue	N.A.	N.A.	N.A.

Adipose tissue-derived stromal cells (ASCs) were isolated from liposuction-derived fat tissue as described before (Przybyt et al., 2013) and grown to confluency in the above-described supplemented DMEM in an incubator at 37°C and 5% CO_2. At confluency, ASC culture medium was changed to low glucose DMEM supplemented with 0.1% bovine serum albumin (BSA, A8806-5g, Sigma, St Louis, United States), 100 U/mL penicillin, 100 µg/ml streptomycin and 4 mM L-glutamine. Then, ASC conditioned media (ASC-CM) was prepared as reported previously (Spiekman et al., 2014). In short, media was aspirated from a confluent ASC layer after 24 h incubation, centrifuged and filtered using a 0.22 µm filter. ASC-CM was derived from cells below passage 8. ASC-CM was stored at −20°C until further use.

Matrix Recellularization

Primary human lung fibroblasts (**Table 1**) were seeded in IPF and control decellularized lung matrices by incubating all matrices together with the fibroblasts on a rotary mixer at 37°C for 24 h, at a concentration of 250.000 cells/matrix in low glucose DMEM supplemented with 0.1% BSA, 100 U/ml penicillin, 100 µg/ml streptomycin and 4 mM L-glutamine (further referred to as basal medium). Recellularized matrices were then separated for further experiments. The recellularized matrices were subsequently incubated in basal medium or in a 1:1 mix of basal medium and ASC-derived conditioned medium (ASC-CM) at 37°C and 5% CO_2. As we sought to investigate the effects of the fibrotic ECM and ASC-CM on fibroblast behavior in this study, FBS was omitted to prevent it from activating the fibroblasts and possibly masking any effects from the ECM or the ASC-CM on the cells. After 7 and 14 days, the recellularized matrices were formalin fixed and paraffin embedded for further analysis.

CHP Staining

Sections of native lung tissue and pieces of decellularized lung tissue were stained using collagen hybridizing peptide-Cy3 conjugate (R-CHP), according to the manufacturer's protocol (3Helix Inc., Salt Lake City, UT, United States). A working solution of 5 µM R-CHP in PBS was heated at 80°C for 5 min and subsequently cooled down in an ice bath for 15–90 s to prevent heat shock to the lung tissue upon addition. After adding the R-CHP working solution, the lung tissues were incubated overnight at 4°C. Decellularized lung tissues were incubated while gently shaking. After incubation, the samples were washed three times in PBS for 5 min (lung tissue sections) or 30 min (decellularized lung tissue). Decellularized lung tissue was subsequently kept in PBS and lung tissue sections were mounted using DePeX mounting medium (Serva, Heidelberg, Germany). Both sample types were stored at 4°C until further analysis.

Sections of recellularized matrices were stained using collagen hybridizing peptide-biotin conjugate (B-CHP), according to the manufacturer's instructions (3Helix Inc.). Endogenous peroxidases were blocked by incubating the slides for 30 min in PBS with 0.3% H_2O_2. The slides were then washed three times in PBS, followed by removal of endogenous biotin and avidin binding site using an Avidin/Biotin blocking kit (Agilent, Santa Clara, CA, United States). Subsequently, a working solution of 0.02 µM B-CHP was prepared and added to the slides as described above for R-CHP. After overnight incubation at 4°C and three PBS washes, the slides were incubated with streptavidin peroxidase (Agilent) (1:300) in PBS with 1% BSA and 2% human AB serum (Sigma-Aldrich, Zwijndrecht, Netherlands) for 1 h. After a PBS wash, color was developed by incubating 10 min with NovaRED (Vector Labs, Burlingame, CA, United States) followed by three washes in demi water and an eosin counterstain for 2 min. After dehydration, the slides were mounted in Tissue-Tek Coverslipping Film with the Sakura Tissue-Tek Film Coverslipper (Sakura, Japan).

Histology

Sections of native lung tissue and decellularized matrices were stained to visualize total collagen using a Masson's trichrome stain kit (Sigma-Aldrich) according to the instructions of the manufacturer. Sections of recellularized matrices were stained with haematoxylin and eosin staining through consecutive incubation in the following solutions at room temperature: haematoxylin (Merck, Kenilworth, United States) for 5 min, regular tap water for 5 min, eosin (Chroma, Bellows Falls, United States) for 2 min, washed twice in 96% ethanol and twice in 100% ethanol. After staining, the dehydrated slides were mounted in Tissue-Tek Coverslipping Film with the Sakura Tissue-Tek Film Coverslipper.

Microscopy and Image Analysis

R-CHP staining in decellularized lung tissue and native tissue sections was imaged and captured using a Leica SP2 confocal microscope. Per subject, at least three fields of view were acquired from one experimental replicate. Lung tissue had to cover more than 50% of the image, with focus on alveolar regions while avoiding large airways and blood vessels. Decellularized lung tissue had to cover 30% of the image. The mean grey value of each image was analyzed using Fiji (Schindelin et al., 2012). Masson's trichrome, H&E and B-CHP staining were imaged and captured using a NanoZoomer XR digital slide scanner (Hamamatsu, Japan). Whole sections were imaged and data were generated from all pixels in these images. Representative images in the figures show a magnified part of the whole section. The density and distribution of the stainings were quantified automated using Fiji. Color deconvolution vectors were optimized to separate double stainings accurately (Ruifrok et al., 2003). Total tissue surface area was measured in grayscale images. The number of pixels above the threshold was used to calculate the positive staining area, while the average staining intensity was based on the intensity of these pixels above the threshold. Thresholds were set to an intensity value where background is excluded. The total positive staining above the threshold was divided in three equal categories (weak, moderate and strong) according to the pixel intensities. Weak, moderate and strong intensity was calculated as a percentage of the total positive area. For the Masson Trichrome staining, additional quantification of the relative amount of collagen in the total image area was carried out by dividing the number of collagen-positive pixels by the total number of pixels within the image area. Images were processed in batches using macros. An overview of the image analysis process can be found in **Supplementary Figure 1**.

Statistical Analyses

Normality of the datasets was tested with a QQ plot as reported by Morgan (2017) and a Shapiro-Wilk test. QQ plots can be found in

Supplementary Figure 2. When normality was confirmed, the data were tested with an unpaired *t*-test or a two-way ANOVA with a post hoc test controlling for the false discovery rate (original FDR method of Benjamini and Hochberg). $p < 0.05$ was considered significant. Statistical analyses were performed in GraphPad Prism 8.0 (GraphPad Software, La Jolla, CA, United States).

RESULTS

Higher Levels of Denatured Collagen in Lung Tissue From Patients With Idiopathic Pulmonary Fibrosis

To examine the levels of denatured collagen (i.e. collagen structural integrity) in lung tissue from control subjects and patients with ILD (including IPF), we stained lung tissue sections with the Cy3-conjugated collagen hybridizing peptide (R-CHP). As a reference, the total amount of collagen (both intact and denatured) was visualized with Masson's trichrome stain (**Figure 1A**), indicating higher staining intensity and relative amount of collagen in the whole imaging area in ILDs compared to control tissues (**Figures 1C,E**). The staining intensity of total collagen was not different when comparing only the IPF lung tissues to the control lung tissue (**Figures 1A,D**), but the relative amount of collagen was higher in IPF tissue compared to control lung tissue (**Figure 1F**). The R-CHP staining visualized low levels of denatured collagen in control lung tissue (**Figure 1B**, left panel), but a wider spread and denser R-CHP signal was observed in lung tissue from patients with ILD and especially in IPF (**Figure 1B**, right panel). Quantification of the R-CHP signal indicated higher levels of denatured collagen in fibrotic lung tissue (**Figure 1G**) and especially in IPF lung tissue (**Figure 1H**), as compared to control lung tissue.

Preservation of Idiopathic Pulmonary Fibrosis-Related Higher Levels of Denatured Collagen After Decellularization

To verify whether the difference in collagen denaturation was preserved after decellularization of lung tissue, decellularized control and fibrotic lung tissue were also stained using the same collagen hybridizing peptide and Masson's trichrome stain. Decellularized lung tissue from patients with IPF had a higher amount of collagen, measured as percentage of the imaged area (**Figure 2D**), but did not show higher staining intensity of collagen when compared to control lung tissue (**Figures 2A,C**). However, more R-CHP signal was observed in decellularized lung tissue from patients with IPF (**Figure 2B**, right panel) than in control lung tissue (**Figure 2B**, left panel) and quantification confirmed higher levels of denatured collagen in IPF decellularized lung tissue compared to control (**Figure 2E**). The fibrotic decellularized lung tissue contained approximately twice as much signal as the control decellularized lung tissue, reflecting the pattern observed in the native lung tissue. This indicates that the collagen denaturation status is retained in decellularized lung tissue, confirming its suitability for studying cell-(IPF) matrix interactions.

Lung Fibroblasts Deposit More Extracellular Matrix When Seeded in Idiopathic Pulmonary Fibrosis-Derived Lung Matrices

Primary lung fibroblasts were seeded into the decellularized matrices and cultured for 7 days to investigate the effects of the altered matrix in IPF on cellular behavior. Total deposition of ECM by the lung fibroblasts was visualized by H&E staining of the recellularized tissue (**Figure 3A**). Before recellularization, unseeded matrices showed variable, but similar tissue staining, indicating the heterogeneity of IPF (**Supplementary Figure 3A**). After recellularization, more tissue staining and denser tissue areas, reflecting the characteristics of the fibrotic foci in IPF, were observed in the IPF matrix compared to the control matrix (**Figures 3A, 5B**). As the IPF matrix with cells showed both dense and more open tissue areas, illustrating the heterogeneous nature of the tissue response in IPF, the intensity distribution of the staining was analyzed. The outcome of this analysis provides an indication of the relative amount of dense tissue in a section: areas with higher staining intensity often consist of denser tissue. After recellularization, IPF matrices had proportionally more moderate intensity staining and less weak intensity staining than control matrices (**Figure 3B**), indicating that more dense tissue areas are present in recellularized IPF matrices than in control matrices. Comparable results were observed when extending the culture time up to 14 days (data not shown). Hence, lung fibroblasts remodel more ECM with more dense areas when seeded in IPF-derived lung matrices compared to control matrices.

Lung Fibroblasts Equalize the Levels of Denatured Collagen in Control and Idiopathic Pulmonary Fibrosis Lung Matrices

To assess if more ECM deposition and dense tissue areas in IPF matrices corresponded with an alteration in collagen denaturation status, the levels of denatured collagen after recellularization were visualized using a biotin-conjugated collagen hybridizing peptide (B-CHP) (**Figure 4A**; **Supplementary Figure 3B**). Interestingly, the differences in the level of denatured collagen seen between control and IPF matrices (**Figure 2**) were no longer evident after reseeding (**Figure 4B**). Still, more moderate and less weak CHP staining was detected in the recellularized IPF matrices compared to the recellularized control matrices (**Figure 4C**). This observation suggests that fibroblasts were able to remodel the degree of denatured collagen in both control and IPF matrices, but were less effective in doing so in the IPF matrices.

Periostin and Fibronectin Do Not Contribute to the Higher Levels of Extracellular Matrix Deposition

As no differences were observed in the levels of denatured collagen between control and IPF matrices after recellularization, we investigated whether the ECM

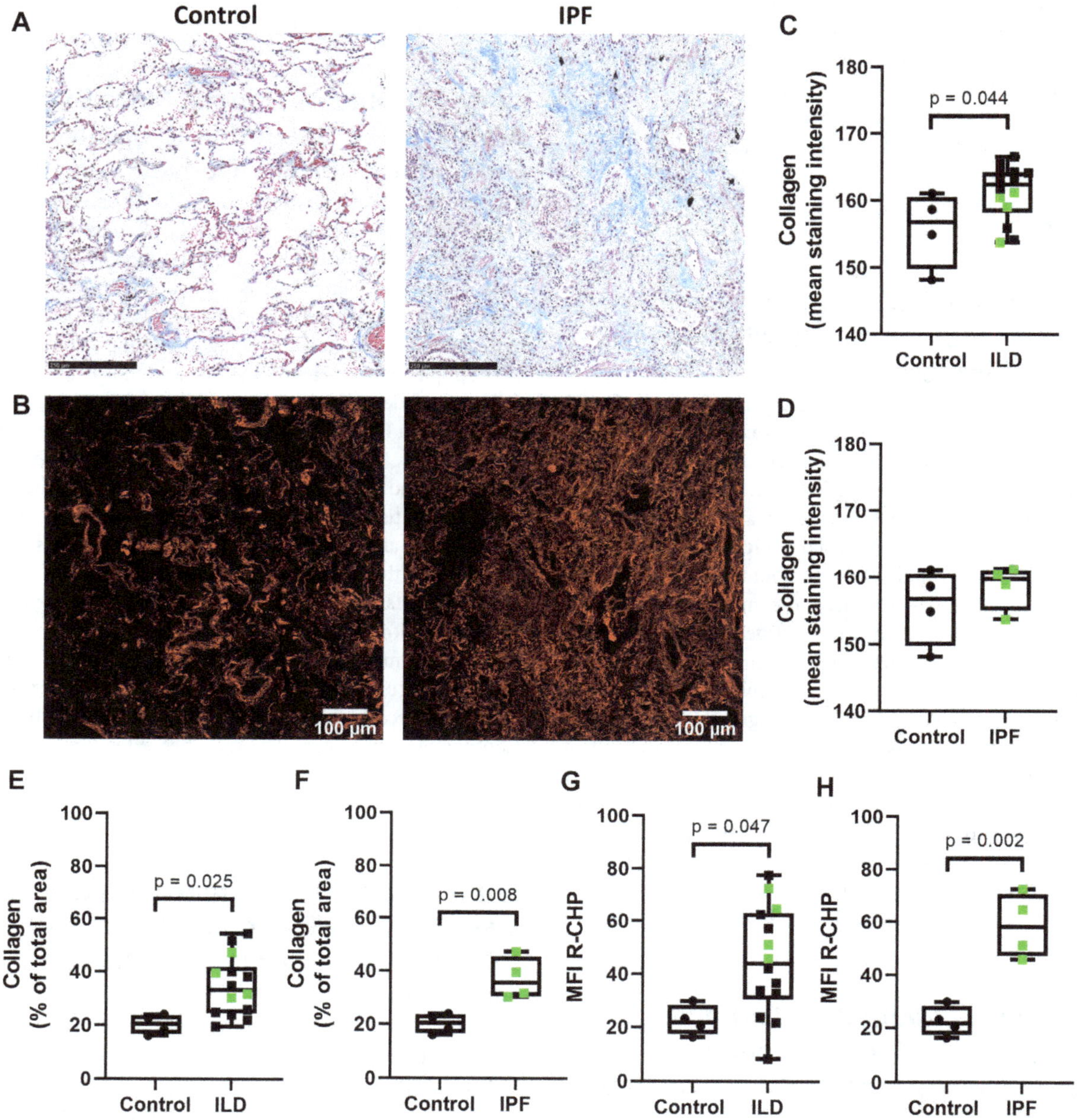

FIGURE 1 | Higher levels of denatured collagen in lung tissue from patients with IPF. Sections of lung tissue were stained using Masson's trichrome stain or Cy3-conjugated collagen hybridizing peptide (R-CHP). **(A)** Representative images of Masson's trichrome stain in control lung tissue (left panel) and lung tissue of a patient with idiopathic pulmonary fibrosis (IPF, right panel), showing collagen fibers in blue and cytoplasm in red. Magnified part of the whole tissue section. Scale bar = 250 µm. **(B)** Representative fluorescence images of the R-CHP signal in control lung tissue (left panel) and lung tissue of a patient with IPF (right panel), from the same patients as in **(A)**. **(C-F)** Quantification of Masson's trichrome staining, showing the mean staining intensity **(C,D)** and the relative amount of collagen in the whole imaging area **(E,F)**. Control lung tissue compared to ILD in general **(C,E)**, as well as specifically to IPF lung tissue [**(D,F)**, data from **(C,E)** partially repeated for visualization purposes]. **(G,H)** Quantification of the R-CHP signal, showing the average mean fluorescence intensity of at least three images per section. Control lung tissue compared to ILD in general **(G)**, as well as specifically to IPF lung tissue [**(H)**, data from **(G)** partially repeated for visualization purposes]. One experimental replicate per subject, sample size $n = 4$ (control) and $n = 14$ (ILD, including 4 lung tissues from patients with IPF). Data represented as min to max box-and-whiskers plots showing all points. Groups were compared using an unpaired *t*-test after assessing the normal distribution with use of a QQ plot and a Shapiro-Wilk normality test (**Supplementary Figure 2A**). $p < 0.05$ was considered significant.

proteins fibronectin or periostin were contributing to the higher levels of ECM in IPF matrices. However, periostin and fibronectin levels did not change in the recellularized IPF matrices when compared to recellularized control matrices (**Supplementary Figures 4, 5**). Thus, changes in the levels of periostin or fibronectin did not play a key role in regulating the altered matrix deposition in the IPF matrices observed in this study.

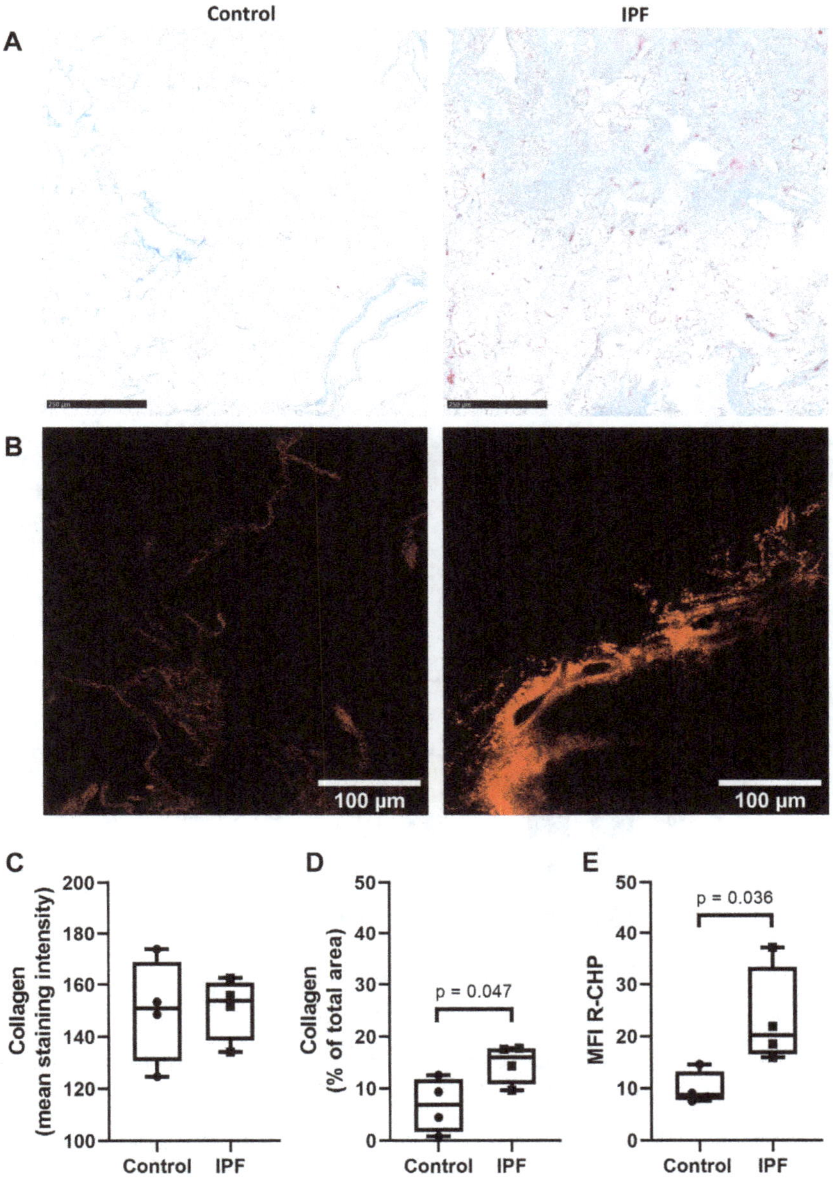

FIGURE 2 | Preservation of IPF-related difference in levels of denatured collagen after decellularization of lung tissue. Decellularized lung tissue was stained using Masson's trichrome staining or Cy3-conjugated collagen hybridizing peptide (R-CHP). **(A)** Representative images of Masson's trichrome stain in control lung tissue (left panel) and lung tissue of a patient with idiopathic pulmonary fibrosis (IPF, right panel), showing collagen fibers in blue and cytoplasm in red. Magnified part of the whole decellularized tissue section. Scale bar = 250 µm. **(B)** Representative fluorescence images of R-CHP signal in decellularized lung tissue from control patients (left panel) and from patients with idiopathic pulmonary fibrosis (IPF, right panel). **(C,D)** Quantification of the Masson's trichrome staining, showing the mean staining intensity **(C)** and the relative amount of collagen in the whole imaging area **(D)**. **(E)** Quantification of the R-CHP signal, showing the average mean fluorescence intensity of at least three images per decellularized lung tissue. One experimental replicate per subject, sample size n = 4 for both control and IPF decellularized lung matrices. Data represented as min to max box-and-whiskers plots showing all points. Groups were compared using an unpaired t-test after assessing the normal distribution with use of a QQ plot and a Shapiro-Wilk normality test (**Supplementary Figure 2A**). $p < 0.05$ was considered significant.

Adipose Tissue-Derived Stromal Cell Conditioned Medium Attenuates Extracellular Matrix Deposition by Lung Fibroblasts in Lung Matrices

To study the potential antifibrotic effect of ASC-CM in this human *in vitro* model of IPF, decellularized matrices were reseeded with primary human lung fibroblasts and incubated with or without ASC-CM for 7 days. The addition of ASC-CM clearly resulted in less total ECM in both control and IPF matrices, as visualized by an H&E staining (**Figure 5A**). Quantification indeed revealed a drop in mean staining intensity (p = 0.0002, **Figure 5B**), as well as changes in the staining intensity distribution between recellularized matrices in the presence and absence of ASC-CM (**Figure 5C**). ASC-CM treatment resulted in a shift from

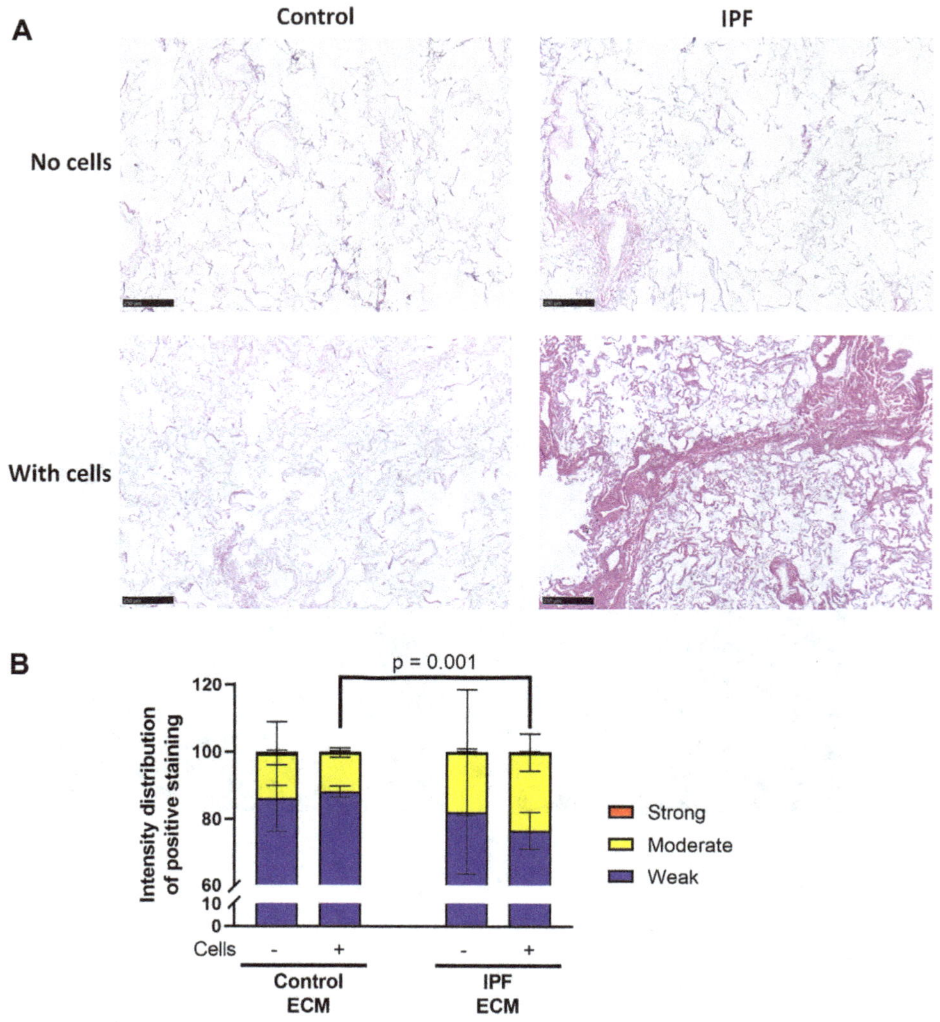

FIGURE 3 | More ECM deposition in IPF matrices upon recellularization compared to control matrices. Primary lung fibroblasts were seeded into decellularized matrices and cultured for 7 days. Sections of recellularized lung tissue were stained with haematoxylin (blue) and eosin (pink). **(A)** Representative images of the stained recellularized matrices, showing a magnified part of the image of the total tissue section. Scale bar = 250 μm. **(B)** Quantification of the intensity distribution of the staining. Groups were compared using a two-way ANOVA followed by the original FDR method of Benjamin and Hochberg post hoc test. $p < 0.05$ was considered significant. All matrices are derived from the same control and IPF donor, primary lung fibroblasts were obtained from three different control donors.

moderate intensity staining to weak intensity staining in both IPF and control matrices when compared to untreated reseeded matrices (**Figure 5C**). The higher levels of weak staining indicate that there is less dense tissue in the ASC-CM treated matrices compared to both IPF and control matrices without ASC-CM. Also, the significant differences in total tissue and relative amount of dense tissue areas between control and IPF recellularized matrices (shown in **Figure 3B**) were abolished by ASC-CM treatment. Thus, even though ECM deposition and tissue density were higher in recellularized IPF matrices compared to control matrices, the addition of ASC-CM neutralized the profibrotic signals provided to the fibroblasts by the ECM, thereby resulting in less ECM remodeling and lower tissue density to similar levels in control and IPF matrices.

Adipose Tissue-Derived Stromal Cell Conditioned Medium Does Not Influence the Levels of Denatured Collagen in Recellularized Lung Matrices

The levels of denatured collagen after ASC-CM treatment were assessed with a B-CHP staining. The representative images, mean staining intensity and the distribution of staining intensity did not show significant alterations in levels of denatured collagen upon ASC-CM treatment in comparison to recellularized matrices in the absence of ASC-CM (**Figure 6**). This indicates that addition of ASC-CM does not interfere with the collagen remodeling activity of primary lung fibroblasts. Similarly, the levels of periostin and fibronectin were also not altered by ASC-CM treatment (**Supplementary Figures 4, 5**).

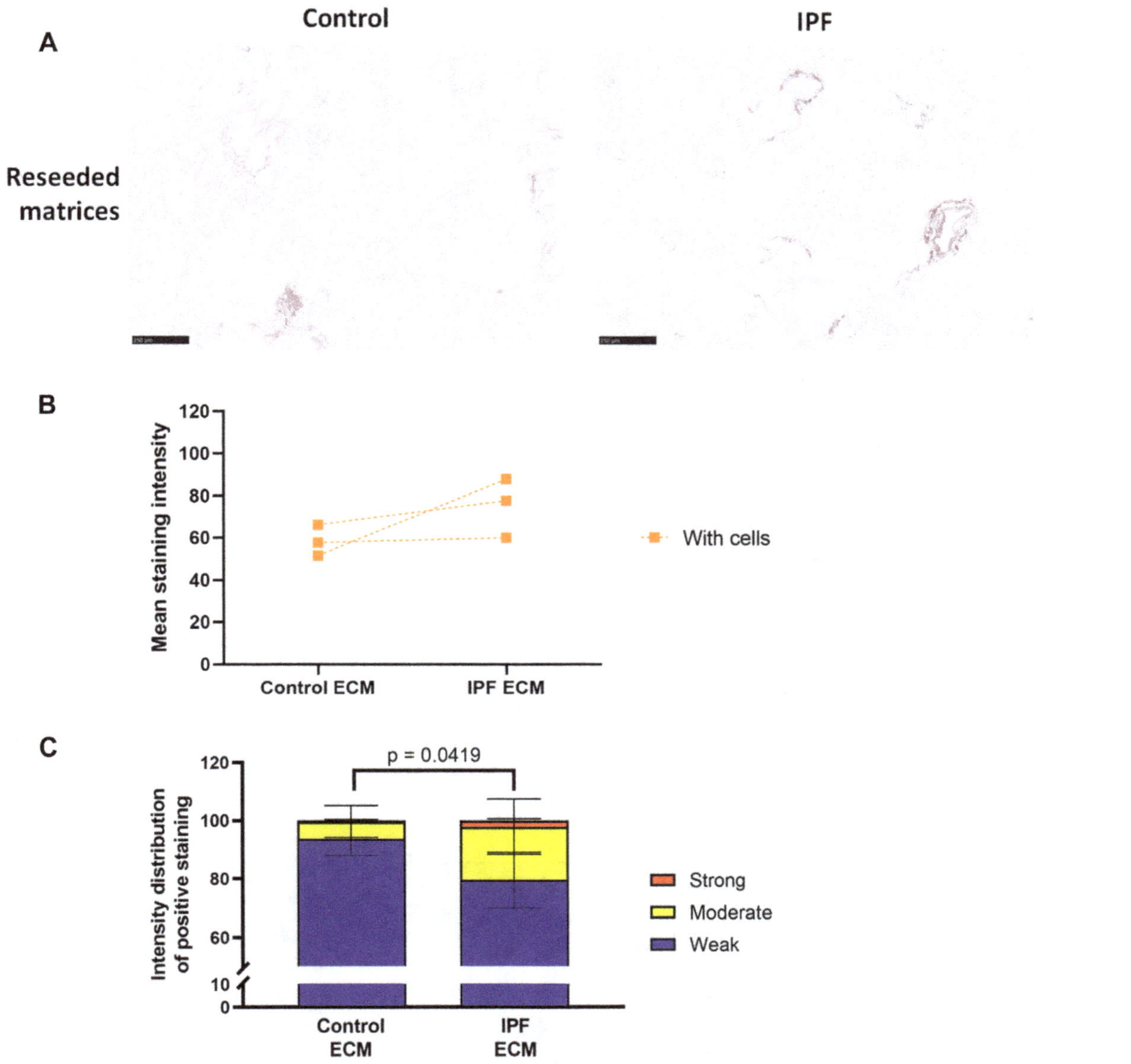

FIGURE 4 | Equal levels of denatured collagen in recellularized control and IPF matrices. Primary lung fibroblasts were seeded into decellularized matrices and cultured for 7 days. Sections of recellularized lung tissue were stained using collagen hybridizing peptide (B-CHP, brown) and an eosin counterstain (pink). **(A)** Representative images of the B-CHP stained recellularized matrices, showing a magnified part of the image of the total tissue section. Scale bar = 250 μm. **(B)** Quantification of the B-CHP staining, showing the mean staining intensity. Groups were compared using an unpaired *t* test after assessing the normal distribution with use of a QQ plot and a Shapiro-Wilk normality test (**Supplementary Figure 2A**). No significant differences were observed ($p > 0.05$). **(C)** Quantification of the intensity distribution of the B-CHP staining. Groups were compared using a two-way ANOVA followed by the original FDR method of Benjamini and Hochberg post hoc test. $p > 0.05$ was considered significant. All matrices are derived from the same control and IPF donor, primary lung fibroblasts were obtained from three different control donors ($n = 3$, dots connected per *n*).

DISCUSSION

In this study, we found that ASC-CM can inhibit IPF lung matrix-driven ECM deposition by primary human lung fibroblasts. While higher levels of denatured collagen were observed in both native and decellularized lung tissue from patients with IPF than in control lung tissue, this characteristic was independent of the factors driving the enhanced matrix deposition by lung fibroblasts in IPF matrices. Reseeding with human lung fibroblasts reversed the collagen denaturation status of the matrices, bringing the denatured collagen in both control and IPF matrices to comparable levels. We investigated the potential regulatory role of fibronectin and periostin within the matrices but found that these levels were not altered, making these proteins unlikely candidates as the factors responsible for the modulation of the fibroblast responses.

There is a lot of interest in the potential of stem cells as a therapeutic approach for lung regeneration in IPF. To date, the impact of these cells (or their bioactive secreted factors) on the interactions of resident cells with the fibrotic

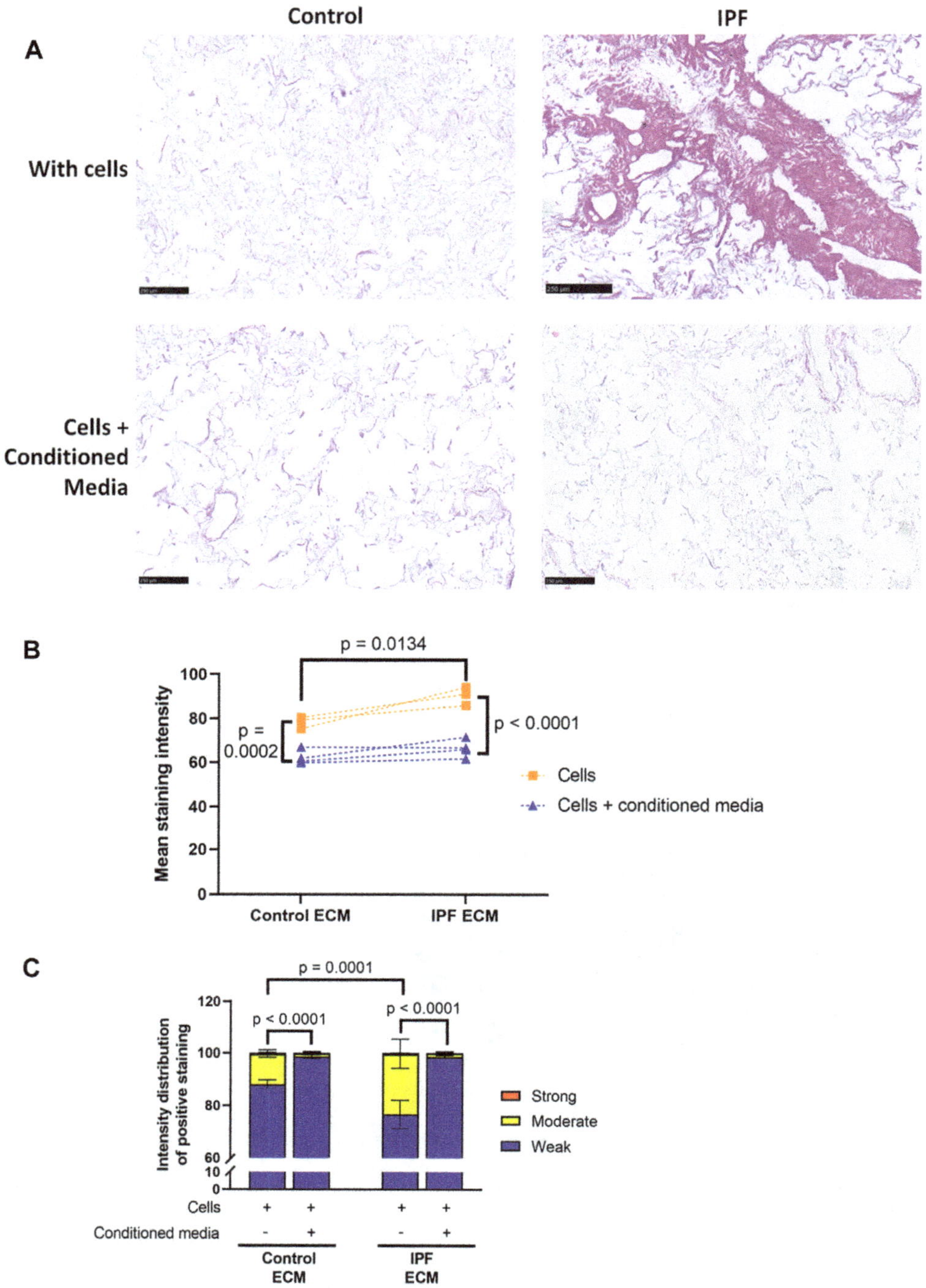

FIGURE 5 | Less ECM deposition in recellularized control and IPF matrices upon ASC-CM treatment. Primary lung fibroblasts were seeded into decellularized matrices and cultured in the absence or presence of ASC-CM for 7 days. Sections of recellularized lung tissue were stained with haematoxylin (blue) and eosin (pink). **(A)** Representative images of the stained recellularized matrices, showing a magnified part of the whole tissue section. Scale bar = 250 μm. **(B)** Quantification of the H&E staining, showing the mean staining intensity. **(C)** Quantification of the intensity distribution of the staining. Groups were compared using a two-way ANOVA followed by the original FDR method of Benjamini and Hochberg as a post-hoc test. $p < 0.05$ was considered significant. All matrices are derived from the same control and IPF donor, primary lung fibroblasts were obtained from three different control donors ($n = 3$, dots connected per n).

microenvironment, and more importantly vice versa, had not been elucidated yet. In light of this, we investigated whether ASC-CM could interfere with fibroblast-(IPF) matrix interactions and subsequent ECM deposition and remodeling. Although ASC-CM did not modulate levels of denatured collagen, fibronectin or periostin, it did result in less ECM deposition in both control and IPF-derived decellularized matrices, thus demonstrating an antifibrotic effect of the ASC-CM. The lack of influence on the denatured collagen may reflect the fact that cells establish an

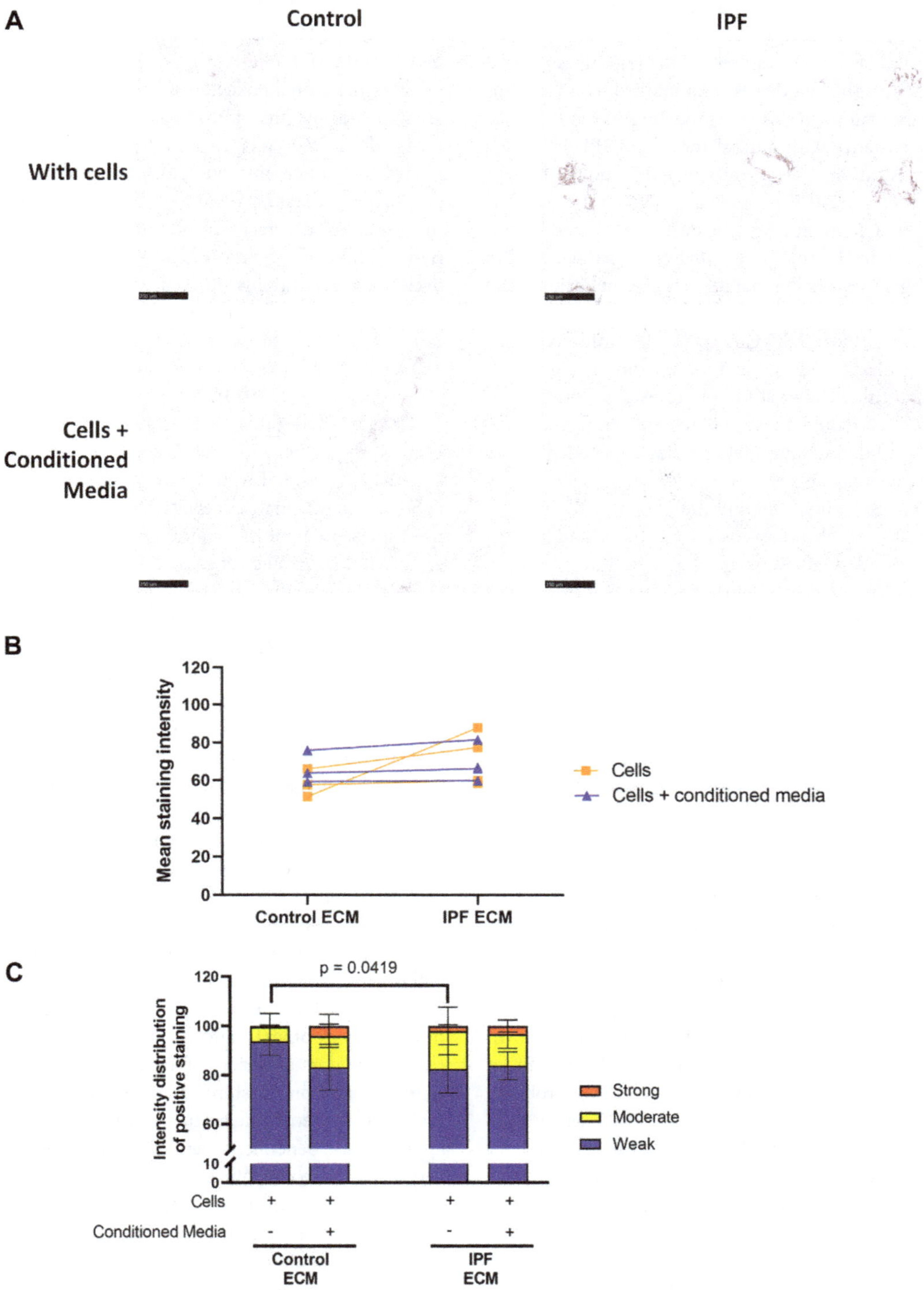

FIGURE 6 | Treatment with ASC-CM does not alter the levels of denatured collagen. Primary lung fibroblasts were seeded into decellularized matrices and cultured in the absence or presence of ASC-CM for 7 days. Sections of recellularized lung tissue were stained using collagen hybridizing peptide (B-CHP, brown) and an eosin counterstain (pink). Data of matrices with cells are repeated from **Figure 4** to allow for a clear comparison. **(A)** Representative images of the stained recellularized matrices showing a magnified part of the image of the total tissue section. Scale bar = 250 µm. **(B)** Quantification of the B-CHP staining, showing the mean staining intensity. **(C)** Quantification of the intensity distribution of the B-CHP staining. Groups were compared using a two-way ANOVA followed by the original FDR method of Benjamini and Hochberg as a post-hoc test. $p < 0.05$ was considered significant. All matrices are derived from the same control and IPF donor, primary lung fibroblasts were obtained from three different control donors (n = 3, dots connected per n).

equilibrium achieving a certain degree of spatial arrangement within the collagen structural organization and that further collagen remodeling is not required. Further investigation, beyond the scope of this study, is required to confirm this hypothesis. The abrogation of tissue remodeling induced by the ASC-CM is in accordance with animal models of IPF, in which ASC-CM administration also attenuated lung fibrosis (Rathinasabapathy et al., 2016; Felix et al., 2020). Of note, it is of interest that ASC-CM treatment not only contributed to less total ECM deposition in IPF matrices, but also to a similar level in control matrices, again suggesting that there is an equilibrium state for the collagen fiber organization that the cells seek to achieve. These data illustrate that ASC-CM generally inhibits ECM deposition by fibroblasts, independent of the fibrotic status of the ECM. Although this *in vitro* study indicates that conditioned media from stem cells could have a therapeutic effect in IPF, extensive (clinical) validation and safety studies are needed before considering clinical application.

As this study aimed at investigating the effects of the fibrotic ECM and ASC-CM on fibroblast behavior, the standard cell culture media were adapted. Regular FBS in culture medium can activate fibroblasts and was therefore omitted, as it could have masked any effects from the ECM or the ASC-CM that we sought to investigate. Therefore, fibroblasts were cultured in the matrices in cell culture medium with 1% BSA instead of FBS. However, H&E staining of the matrices indicated that no fibroblasts were left in our matrices after 7 days incubation. A limitation of our study could be that this 1% BSA-containing medium was not an optimal culture condition for the fibroblasts. However, our results illustrate that the fibroblasts were able to remodel their microenvironment during the period they were present in the lung matrices.

The secretome of ASCs consists of a multitude of factors, which are involved in different processes such as cell proliferation and angiogenesis (Salgado et al., 2010; Kapur and Katz, 2013). This is the main advantage of ASC-CM: instead of administering a single factor that could potentially inhibit fibrosis, multiple factors are administered that can have synergistic effects. We have shown previously that our ASC-CM inhibits TGF-β1-induced differentiation of human dermal fibroblasts to myofibroblasts (Spiekman et al., 2014). In the current study, IPF ECM induced a profibrotic phenotype in lung fibroblasts, as measured by higher levels of ECM deposition. ASC-CM treatment inhibited this profibrotic phenotype, allowing less ECM deposition in its presence. Interestingly, in recent studies, ASCs in culture were stimulated with either pro-inflammatory factors or a specific microRNA (miR-146a) resulting in a CM that was more anti-inflammatory, pro-angiogenic or aided in homing of immune cells to tumors (Domenis et al., 2018; Li et al., 2019; Waters et al., 2019). To further enhance the antifibrotic properties of ASC-CM, addition of specific factors to ASC cultures to precondition these cells could be an option.

To investigate the effect of ECM on the remodeling behavior of fibroblasts, we visualized collagen denaturation in IPF and control matrices. The presence of higher levels of structurally disrupted collagen in lung tissue from patients with IPF indicates that even though there is excessive accumulation of collagen, collagen degradation is still taking place at the molecular level. This is, to our knowledge, the first study to examine the degree of collagen denaturation in human lung tissues. Interestingly, the comparable levels of denatured collagen in IPF and control matrices after cell seeding indicate that fibroblasts were able to repair or remove excess denatured collagen found in IPF lung matrices. The cells sensed their microenvironment and remodeled this as such to a defined level that was equivalent across the two different starting matrices. In contrast to our observations regarding cellular remodeling of denatured collagen, cellular responses to decellularized scaffolds differed between fibrotic and nonfibrotic matrices. We found that fibrotic matrix stimulated fibroblasts to produce and deposit more ECM, confirming the feedback loop in fibrotic matrices that has been observed previously (Booth et al., 2012; Parker et al., 2014).

Decellularized (lung) matrices are gaining attention in tissue engineering as *in vitro* models to study cellular behavior (Gilpin and Wagner, 2018; Taylor et al., 2018). However, it is important to keep in mind that decellularization protocols can affect the mechanical and morphological properties of the ECM (Petersen et al., 2012; Hwang et al., 2017b). The collagen hybridizing peptide used in this study has previously been applied to show that decellularizing agents can induce collagen denaturation (Hwang et al., 2017b). In this study, we could not investigate the effect of our decellularization protocol on the absolute levels of denatured collagen, as the native and decellularized lung tissues were not derived from the same patient and processed differently. Nonetheless, we did observe that the relative difference in levels of denatured collagen between lung tissue from patients with IPF and controls was comparable in native and decellularized lung tissue. The preservation of this IPF-related difference in levels of denatured collagen emphasizes that decellularized lung tissue is suitable for *in vitro* models studying cellular responses to this denatured collagen.

A major asset of our study is the use of human materials. Although bleomycin-induced pulmonary fibrosis is currently the most accepted model to investigate IPF, the different etiology, disease development, and especially the spontaneous fibrosis resolution after a period of time, are quite different from the human condition (Tashiro et al., 2017). Hence, by using human materials, we represent human disease specifically. However, this approach also generates several challenges. IPF is associated with a very heterogeneous pattern, with both control and fibrotic areas being recognized within lung tissue of the same patient (Travis et al., 2002; DePianto et al., 2015). This likely contributes to the significant variation in levels of denatured collagen observed between IPF samples. Interpatient variability in disease severity could also contribute to this variation (Raghu et al., 2011). In liver fibrosis, collagen hybridizing peptide staining has recently been suggested to have value in quantitatively assessing disease severity and predicting the need for liver transplantation (Jaramillo et al., 2020).

In conclusion, this study has shown that levels of denatured collagen are higher in lung tissue from patients with IPF than from control patients and that this difference is preserved in decellularized lung tissue. After recellularization, IPF ECM drives fibroblasts toward profibrotic behavior, which can be counteracted by administration of ASC-CM. These findings further confirm in a human *in vitro* model that the use of ASC-CM may be a promising approach to stop fibrotic ECM from directing profibrotic behavior in fibroblasts in IPF.

AUTHOR CONTRIBUTIONS

GV, LO, PR, MH, BM, and JB conceived and designed the study. GV, LO, MDJ, MRJ, TB, LT, and PJ performed the experiments. MH provided the ASCs, EW provided the decellularized lung matrices. GV, MRJ, and TB executed the image analysis. GV and LO analyzed and interpreted the data and wrote the initial draft of the manuscript. PR, MH, EW, IH, BM, and JB interpreted the results and thoroughly reviewed the manuscript. All authors read and approved the final manuscript.

ACKNOWLEDGMENTS

The authors would like to acknowledge Henk Moorlag for embedding and sectioning the recellularized lung matrices.

REFERENCES

Barczyk, M., Schmidt, M., and Mattoli, S. (2015). Stem Cell-Based Therapy in Idiopathic Pulmonary Fibrosis. *Stem Cel. Rev. Rep.* 11, 598–620. doi:10.1007/s12015-015-9587-7

Blaber, S. P., Webster, R. A., Hill, C. J., Breen, E. J., Kuah, D., Vesey, G., et al. (2012). Analysis of *In Vitro* Secretion Profiles from Adipose-Derived Cell Populations. *J. Translational Med.* 10, 172. doi:10.1186/1479-5876-10-172

Booth, A. J., Hadley, R., Cornett, A. M., Dreffs, A. A., Matthes, S. A., Tsui, J. L., et al. (2012). Acellular Normal and Fibrotic Human Lung Matrices as a Culture System forIn VitroInvestigation. *Am. J. Respir. Crit. Care Med.* 186, 866–876. doi:10.1164/rccm.201204-0754OC

Burgess, J. K., Mauad, T., Tjin, G., Karlsson, J. C., and Westergren-Thorsson, G. (2016). The Extracellular Matrix - the Under-recognized Element in Lung Disease? *J. Pathol.* 240, 397–409. doi:10.1002/path.4808

Burgstaller, G., Oehrle, B., Gerckens, M., White, E. S., Schiller, H. B., and Eickelberg, O. (2017). The Instructive Extracellular Matrix of the Lung: Basic Composition and Alterations in Chronic Lung Disease. *Eur. Respir. J.* 50, 1601805. doi:10.1183/13993003.01805-2016

Chang, S.-W., and Buehler, M. J. (2014). Molecular Biomechanics of Collagen Molecules. *Mater. Today* 17, 70–76. doi:10.1016/j.mattod.2014.01.019

Chen, S., Cui, G., Peng, C., Lavin, M. F., Sun, X., Zhang, E., et al. (2018). Transplantation of Adipose-Derived Mesenchymal Stem Cells Attenuates Pulmonary Fibrosis of Silicosis via Anti-inflammatory and Anti-apoptosis Effects in Rats. *Stem Cel. Res. Ther.* 9. doi:10.1186/s13287-018-0846-9

DePianto, D. J., Chandriani, S., Abbas, A. R., Jia, G., N'Diaye, E. N., Caplazi, P., et al. (2015). Heterogeneous Gene Expression Signatures Correspond to Distinct Lung Pathologies and Biomarkers of Disease Severity in Idiopathic Pulmonary Fibrosis. *Thorax.* 70, 48–56. doi:10.1136/thoraxjnl-2013-204596

Domenis, R., Cifù, A., Quaglia, S., Pistis, C., Moretti, M., Vicario, A., et al. (2018). Pro Inflammatory Stimuli Enhance the Immunosuppressive Functions of Adipose Mesenchymal Stem Cells-Derived Exosomes. *Sci. Rep.* 8. doi:10.1038/s41598-018-31707-9

Felix, R. G., Bovolato, A. L. C., Cotrim, O. S., Leão, P. D. S., Batah, S. S., Golim, M. A., et al. (2020). Adipose-derived Stem Cells and Adipose-Derived Stem Cell-Conditioned Medium Modulate *In Situ* Imbalance between Collagen I- and Collagen V-Mediated IL-17 Immune Response Recovering Bleomycin Pulmonary Fibrosis. *Histol. Histopathol.* 35, 289–301. doi:10.14670/HH-18-152

Fikry, E. M., Safar, M. M., Hasan, W. A., Fawzy, H. M., and El-Denshary, E.-E. -D. S. (2015). Bone Marrow and Adipose-Derived Mesenchymal Stem Cells Alleviate Methotrexate-Induced Pulmonary Fibrosis in Rat: Comparison with Dexamethasone. *J. Biochem. Mol. Toxicol.* 29, 321–329. doi:10.1002/jbt.21701

Gilpin, S. E., and Wagner, D. E. (2018). Acellular Human Lung Scaffolds to Model Lung Disease and Tissue Regeneration. *Eur. Respir. Rev.* 27, 180021. doi:10.1183/16000617.0021-2018

Hwang, J., Huang, Y., Burwell, T. J., Peterson, N. C., Connor, J., Weiss, S. J., et al. (2017a). *In Situ* Imaging of Tissue Remodeling with Collagen Hybridizing Peptides. *ACS Nano* 11, 9825–9835. doi:10.1021/acsnano.7b03150

Hwang, J., San, B. H., Turner, N. J., White, L. J., Faulk, D. M., Badylak, S. F., et al. (2017b). Molecular Assessment of Collagen Denaturation in Decellularized Tissues Using a Collagen Hybridizing Peptide. *Acta Biomater.* 53, 268–278. doi:10.1016/j.actbio.2017.01.079

Jaramillo, C., Guthery, S. L., Lowichik, A., Stoddard, G., Kim, T., Li, Y., et al. (2020). Quantitative Liver Fibrosis Using Collagen Hybridizing Peptide to Predict Native Liver Survival in Biliary Atresia: A Pilot Study. *J. Pediatr. Gastroenterol. Nutr.* 70, 87–92. doi:10.1097/MPG.0000000000002505

Jiang, H., Zhang, J., Zhang, Z., Ren, S., and Zhang, C. (2015). Effect of Transplanted Adipose-Derived Stem Cells in Mice Exhibiting Idiopathic Pulmonary Fibrosis. *Mol. Med. Rep.* 12, 5933–5938. doi:10.3892/mmr.2015.4178

Kapur, S. K., and Katz, A. J. (2013). Review of the Adipose Derived Stem Cell Secretome. *Biochimie* 95, 2222–2228. doi:10.1016/j.biochi.2013.06.001

Krimmer, D. I., Burgess, J. K., Wooi, T. K., Black, J. L., and Oliver, B. G. G. (2012). Matrix Proteins from Smoke-Exposed Fibroblasts Are Pro-proliferative. *Am. J. Respir. Cel. Mol. Biol.* 46, 34–39. doi:10.1165/rcmb.2010-0426OC

Kristensen, J. H., Karsdal, M. A., Genovese, F., Johnson, S., Svensson, B., Jacobsen, S., et al. (2014). The Role of Extracellular Matrix Quality in Pulmonary Fibrosis. *Respiration* 88, 487–499. doi:10.1159/000368163

Kudo, A., and Kii, I. (2018). Periostin Function in Communication with Extracellular Matrices. *J. Cel. Commun. Signal.* 12, 301–308. doi:10.1007/s12079-017-0422-6

Lederer, D. J., and Martinez, F. J. (2018). Idiopathic Pulmonary Fibrosis. *N. Engl. J. Med.* 378, 1811–1823. doi:10.1056/NEJMra1705751

Lee, S. H., Lee, E. J., Lee, S. Y., Kim, J. H., Shim, J. J., Shin, C., et al. (2014). The Effect of Adipose Stem Cell Therapy on Pulmonary Fibrosis Induced by Repetitive Intratracheal Bleomycin in Mice. *Exp. Lung Res.* 40, 117–125. doi:10.3109/01902148.2014.881930

Lehtonen, S. T., Veijola, A., Karvonen, H., Lappi-Blanco, E., Sormunen, R., Korpela, S., et al. (2016). Pirfenidone and Nintedanib Modulate Properties of Fibroblasts and Myofibroblasts in Idiopathic Pulmonary Fibrosis. *Respir. Res.* 17, 14. doi:10.1186/s12931-016-0328-5

Li, M., Zeng, L., Liu, S., Dangelmajer, S., Kahlert, U. D., Huang, H., et al. (2019). Transforming Growth Factor-β Promotes Homing and Therapeutic Efficacy of Human Mesenchymal Stem Cells to Glioblastoma. *J. Neuropathol. Exp. Neurol.* 78, 315–325. doi:10.1093/jnen/nlz016

Li, Y., and Yu, S. M. (2013). Targeting and Mimicking Collagens via Triple Helical Peptide Assembly. *Curr. Opin. Chem. Biol.* 17, 968–975. doi:10.1016/j.cbpa.2013.10.018

Liu, J., Ren, J., Su, L., Cheng, S., Zhou, J., Ye, X., et al. (2018). Human Adipose Tissue-Derived Stem Cells Inhibit the Activity of Keloid Fibroblasts and Fibrosis in a Keloid Model by Paracrine Signaling. *Burns* 44, 370–385. doi:10.1016/j.burns.2017.08.017

Llontop, P., Lopez-Fernandez, D., Clavo, B., Afonso Martín, J. L., Fiuza-Pérez, M. D., García Arranz, M., et al. (2018). Airway Transplantation of Adipose Stem Cells Protects against Bleomycin-Induced Pulmonary Fibrosis. *J. Investig. Med.* 66, 739–746. doi:10.1136/jim-2017-000494

Morgan, C. J. (2017). Use of Proper Statistical Techniques for Research Studies with Small Samples. *Am. J. Physiology-Lung Cell Mol. Physiol.* 313, L873–L877. doi:10.1152/ajplung.00238.2017

Naik, P. K., Bozyk, P. D., Bentley, J. K., Popova, A. P., Birch, C. M., Wilke, C. A., et al. (2012). Periostin Promotes Fibrosis and Predicts Progression in Patients with Idiopathic Pulmonary Fibrosis. *Am. J. Physiology-Lung Cell Mol. Physiol.* 303, L1046–L1056. doi:10.1152/ajplung.00139.2012

Ntolios, P., Manoloudi, E., Tzouvelekis, A., Bouros, E., Steiropoulos, P., Anevlavis, S., et al. (2018). Longitudinal Outcomes of Patients Enrolled in a Phase Ib Clinical Trial of the Adipose-Derived Stromal Cells-Stromal Vascular Fraction in Idiopathic Pulmonary Fibrosis. *Clin. Respir. J.* 12, 2084–2089. doi:10.1111/crj.12777

Parker, M. W., Rossi, D., Peterson, M., Smith, K., Sikström, K., White, E. S., et al. (2014). Fibrotic Extracellular Matrix Activates a Profibrotic Positive Feedback Loop. *J. Clin. Invest.* 124, 1622–1635. doi:10.1172/JCI71386

Petersen, T. H., Calle, E. A., Colehour, M. B., and Niklason, L. E. (2012). Matrix Composition and Mechanics of Decellularized Lung Scaffolds. *Cells Tissues Organs.* 195, 222–231. doi:10.1159/000324896

Przybyt, E., Krenning, G., Brinker, M. G., and Harmsen, M. C. (2013). Adipose Stromal Cells Primed with Hypoxia and Inflammation Enhance Cardiomyocyte Proliferation Rate *In Vitro* through STAT3 and Erk1/2. *J. Translational Med.* 11, 39. doi:10.1186/1479-5876-11-39

Radwan, S. M., Ghoneim, D., Salem, M., Saeed, M., Saleh, Y., Elhamy, M., et al. (2020). Adipose Tissue-Derived Mesenchymal Stem Cells Protect against Amiodarone-Induced Lung Injury in Rats. *Appl. Biochem. Biotechnol.* 191, 1027–1041. doi:10.1007/s12010-020-03227-8

Raghu, G., Collard, H. R., Egan, J. J., Martinez, F. J., Behr, J., Brown, K. K., et al. (2011). An Official ATS/ERS/JRS/ALAT Statement: Idiopathic Pulmonary Fibrosis: Evidence-Based Guidelines for Diagnosis and Management. *Am. J. Respir. Crit. Care Med.* 183, 788–824. doi:10.1164/rccm.2009-040GL

Rathinasabapathy, A., Bruce, E., Espejo, A., Horowitz, A., Sudhan, D. R., Nair, A., et al. (2016). Therapeutic Potential of Adipose Stem Cell-Derived Conditioned Medium against Pulmonary Hypertension and Lung Fibrosis. *Br. J. Pharmacol.* 173, 2859–2879. doi:10.1111/bph.13562

Reddy, M., Fonseca, L., Gowda, S., Chougule, B., Hari, A., and Totey, S. (2016). Human Adipose-Derived Mesenchymal Stem Cells Attenuate Early Stage of Bleomycin Induced Pulmonary Fibrosis: Comparison with Pirfenidone. *Ijsc* 9, 192–206. doi:10.15283/ijsc16041

Ricard-Blum, S., Baffet, G., and Théret, N. (2018). Molecular and Tissue Alterations of Collagens in Fibrosis. *Matrix Biol.* 68-69 (69), 122–149. doi:10.1016/j.matbio.2018.02.004

Ricard-Blum, S. (2011). The Collagen Family. *Cold Spring Harbor Perspect. Biol.* 3, a004978. doi:10.1101/cshperspect.a004978

Ruifrok, A. C., Katz, R. L., and Johnston, D. A. (2003). Comparison of Quantification of Histochemical Staining by Hue-Saturation-Intensity (HSI) Transformation and Color-Deconvolution. *Appl. Immunohistochem. Mol. Morphol.* 11, 85–91. doi:10.1097/00129039-200303000-00014

Sabin, K., and Kikyo, N. (2016). Microvesicles as Mediators of Tissue Regeneration. In *Translating Regenerative Medicine To the Clinic*, 215–224. doi:10.1016/B978-0-12-800548-4.00014-0

Salgado, A. J., Reis, R. L., Sousa, N. J., and Gimble, J. M. (2010). Adipose Tissue Derived Stem Cells Secretome: Soluble Factors and Their Roles in Regenerative Medicine. *Curr. Stem Cel. Res. Ther.* 5, 103–110. doi:10.2174/157488810791268564

Schindelin, J., Arganda-Carreras, I., Frise, E., Kaynig, V., Longair, M., Pietzsch, T., et al. (2012). Fiji: An Open-Source Platform for Biological-Image Analysis. *Nat. Methods* 9, 676–682. doi:10.1038/nmeth.2019

Spagnolo, P., Sverzellati, N., Rossi, G., Cavazza, A., Tzouvelekis, A., Crestani, B., et al. (2015). Idiopathic Pulmonary Fibrosis: an Update. *Ann. Med.* 47, 15–27. doi:10.3109/07853890.2014.982165

Spiekman, M., Przybyt, E., Plantinga, J. A., Gibbs, S., Van Der Lei, B., and Harmsen, M. C. (2014). Adipose Tissue-Derived Stromal Cells Inhibit TGF-B1-Induced Differentiation of Human Dermal Fibroblasts and Keloid Scar-Derived Fibroblasts in a Paracrine Fashion. *Plast. Reconstr. Surg.* 134, 699–712. doi:10.1097/PRS.0000000000000504

Tashiro, J., Elliot, S. J., Gerth, D. J., Xia, X., Pereira-Simon, S., Choi, R., et al. (2015). Therapeutic Benefits of Young, but Not Old, Adipose-Derived Mesenchymal Stem Cells in a Chronic Mouse Model of Bleomycin-Induced Pulmonary Fibrosis. *Translational Res.* 166, 554–567. doi:10.1016/j.trsl.2015.09.004

Tashiro, J., Rubio, G. A., Limper, A. H., Williams, K., Elliot, S. J., Ninou, I., et al. (2017). Exploring Animal Models that Resemble Idiopathic Pulmonary Fibrosis. *Front. Med.* 4, 118. doi:10.3389/fmed.2017.00118

Taylor, D. A., Sampaio, L. C., Ferdous, Z., Gobin, A. S., and Taite, L. J. (2018). Decellularized Matrices in Regenerative Medicine. *Acta Biomater.* 74, 74–89. doi:10.1016/j.actbio.2018.04.044

Tjin, G., White, E. S., Faiz, A., Sicard, D., Tschumperlin, D. J., Mahar, A., et al. (2017). Lysyl Oxidases Regulate Fibrillar Collagen Remodelling in Idiopathic Pulmonary Fibrosis. *DMM Dis. Model. Mech.* 10, 1301–1312. doi:10.1242/dmm.030114

Tomos, I. P., Tzouvelekis, A., Aidinis, V., Manali, E. D., Bouros, E., Bouros, D., et al. (2017). Extracellular Matrix Remodeling in Idiopathic Pulmonary Fibrosis. It Is the 'bed' that Counts and Not 'the Sleepers'. *Expert Rev. Respir. Med.* 11, 299–309. doi:10.1080/17476348.2017.1300533

Travis, W. D., King, T. E., Bateman, E. D., Lynch, D. A., Capron, F., Center, D., et al. (2002). American Thoracic Society/European Respiratory Society International Multidisciplinary Consensus Classification of the Idiopathic Interstitial Pneumonias. *Am. J. Respir. Crit. Care Med.* 165, 277–304. doi:10.1164/ajrccm.165.2.ats01

Tzouvelekis, A., Paspaliaris, V., Koliakos, G., Ntolios, P., Bouros, E., Oikonomou, A., et al. (2013). A Prospective, Non-randomized, No Placebo-Controlled, Phase Ib Clinical Trial to Study the Safety of the Adipose Derived Stromal Cells-Stromal Vascular Fraction in Idiopathic Pulmonary Fibrosis. *J. Translational Med.* 11, 171. doi:10.1186/1479-5876-11-171

Waters, R., Subham, S., Pacelli, S., Modaresi, S., Chakravarti, A. R., and Paul, A. (2019). Development of MicroRNA-146a-Enriched Stem Cell Secretome for Wound-Healing Applications. *Mol. Pharmaceutics* 16, 4302–4312. doi:10.1021/acs.molpharmaceut.9b00639

Yamaguchi, M., Hirai, S., Tanaka, Y., Sumi, T., Miyajima, M., Mishina, T., et al. (2017). Fibroblastic Foci, Covered with Alveolar Epithelia Exhibiting Epithelial-Mesenchymal Transition, Destroy Alveolar Septa by Disrupting Blood Flow in Idiopathic Pulmonary Fibrosis. *Lab. Invest.* 97, 232–242. doi:10.1038/labinvest.2016.135

Yan, X., Liu, Y., Han, Q., Jia, M., Liao, L., Qi, M., et al. (2007). Injured Microenvironment Directly Guides the Differentiation of Engrafted Flk-1+ Mesenchymal Stem Cell in Lung. *Exp. Hematol.* 35, 1466–1475. doi:10.1016/j.exphem.2007.05.012

Zhang, Y., Jiang, X., and Ren, L. (2019). Optimization of the Adipose-Derived Mesenchymal Stem Cell Delivery Time for Radiation-Induced Lung Fibrosis Treatment in Rats. *Sci. Rep.* 9, 1–10. doi:10.1038/s41598-019-41576-5

14

Ellagic Acid Attenuates BLM-Induced Pulmonary Fibrosis *via* Inhibiting Wnt Signaling Pathway

Xiaohe Li[1,2†], Kai Huang[1†], Xiaowei Liu[1,2†], Hao Ruan[1,2†], Ling Ma[1,2], Jingjing Liang[1,2], Yunyao Cui[1,2], Yanhua Wang[1], Shuyang Wu[1], Hailong Li[1], Yuli Wei[1], Zeping Li[1,2], Jingjing Gao[2], Bo Yang[3], Xiaoping Li[3], Guang Yang[1], Honggang Zhou[1,2*] and Cheng Yang[1,2*]*

[1]State Key Laboratory of Medicinal Chemical Biology, College of Pharmacy and Tianjin Key Laboratory of Molecular Drug Research, Nankai University, Tianjin, China, [2]Tianjin Key Laboratory of Molecular Drug Research, Tianjin International Joint Academy of Biomedicine, Tianjin, China, [3]Department of Thoracic Surgery, Tianjin First Central Hospital, Tianjin, China

***Correspondence:**
Guang Yang
Guang.yang@nankai.edu.cn
Honggang Zhou
honggang.zhou@nankai.edu.cn
Cheng Yang
cheng.yang@nankai.edu.cn

†These authors have contributed equally to this work and share first authorship

Idiopathic pulmonary fibrosis is a progressive lung disease with high mortality and limited therapy that is characterized by epithelial cell damage and fibroblast activation. Ellagic acid is a natural polyphenol compound widely found in fruits and nuts that has multiple pharmacological activities. In this study, we explored the potential effects and mechanisms of Ellagic acid on pulmonary fibrosis *in vivo* and *in vitro*. *In vivo* studies showed that Ellagic acid significantly alleviated bleomycin (BLM)-induced pulmonary fibrosis in mice. *In vitro* experiments indicated that Ellagic acid could suppress Wnt signaling and attenuate Wnt3a-induced myofibroblast activation and the phosphorylation of Erk2 and Akt. Further studies showed that Ellagic acid could induce autophagy formation in myofibroblasts mainly by suppressing mTOR signaling and promoting apoptosis of myofibroblasts. *In vivo* experiments revealed that Ellagic acid significantly inhibited myofibroblast activation and promoted autophagy formation. Taken together, our results show that Ellagic acid effectively attenuates BLM-induced pulmonary fibrosis in mice by suppressing myofibroblast activation and promoting autophagy and apoptosis of myofibroblasts by inhibiting the Wnt signaling pathway.

Keywords: pulmonary fibrosis, ellagic acid, myofibroblasts, autophagy, apoptosis, wnt

INTRODUCTION

Idiopathic pulmonary fibrosis is a progressive, fatal and age-associated disease, and the average survival time of IPF patients is only 2–5 years after diagnosis (Directors and Committie, 2000; Thannickal et al., 2004; Mora et al., 2017). In Europe and North America, the incidence range is 3–9 cases per 100,000 per year (Hutchinson et al., 2015). Although the pathogenesis is not completely

---

Abbreviations: BLM, Bleomycin; IPF, Idiopathic pulmonary fibrosis; ECM, Extracellular matrix; EA, Ellagic acid; mTOR, mammalian target of rapamycin; BCL2, B-cell lymphoma-2; TFEB, Transcription factor EB; PPF, Primary pulmonary fibroblasts; Mlg, Mouse lung fibroblasts cell; DMEM, dulbecco's modified eagle medium; NIH-3T3, Mouse embryonic fibroblasts cell line; FBS, Fetal bovine serum; CQ, Chloroquine; Baf A1, Bafilomycin A1; PMSF, Phenylmethylsulfonyl fluoride; PEI, Polyethylenimine; FVC, forced vital capacity; Cydn, dynamic compliance; Ri, inspiratory resistance; Re, expiratory resistance; Pf, fibrosis area pixel; Pw, total lung pixel; H-E, Hematoxylin-eosin; TGF-β, Transforming growth factor β; Fn, Fibronectin; Col 1, Collagen I; α-SMA, α-smooth muscle actin; LC3, Microtubules associated protein 1 light chain 3; MMP, Matrix metalloproteinase.

understood, many researchers believe that myofibroblast activation, autophagy and apoptosis are essential factors in fibrotic progression (Wynn, 2011).

The Wnt/β-catenin signal transduction pathway is essential for adult life and could control a myriad of biological phenomena throughout development (Clevers and Nusse, 2012). Wnt signaling also plays an essential role in fibrotic disease, and inhibiting this pathway could suppress fibrotic progression (Distler et al., 2019). In lung epithelial cells and fibroblasts, β-catenin is overexpressed under fibrotic conditions (Baarsma and Konigshoff, 2017). Many studies have revealed that Wnt ligands induce fibroblast activation and collagen synthesis and that blocking Wnt/β-catenin signaling attenuates BLM-induced pulmonary fibrosis (Konigshoff et al., 2008). Overactive fibroblasts can produce abundant extracellular matrix (ECM) proteins and inducing apoptosis of overactive fibroblasts is regarded as an effective method to alleviate fibrotic diseases (Hosseinzadeh et al., 2018). In breast cancer cells, blockade of Wnt signaling significantly induces cellular apoptosis (Bilir et al., 2013). Hence, inhibiting fibroblast activation and promoting myofibroblast apoptosis could attenuate pulmonary fibrosis by suppressing Wnt/β-catenin signaling.

There is an intimate relationship between autophagy and pulmonary fibrosis. The three main types of autophagy are chaperone-mediated autophagy, microautophagy and macroautophagy (Rubinsztein et al., 2007). Here, we focus on macroautophagy (hereafter referred to as autophagy), and the autophagic pathway is the catabolic mechanism for cytoplasmic organelles and degrading long-lived cellular proteins (Levine and Kroemer, 2008). Recent studies indicate that disruption of the beclin1-BCL2 complex is an effective mechanism to promote autophagy formation, which prevents premature ageing and improves the health span of mammals (Fernandez et al., 2018). Insufficient autophagy might result in the senescence of pulmonary epithelial cells and the activation of myofibroblasts in pulmonary fibrosis (Araya et al., 2013), and autophagy was inhibited in IPF patients (Patel et al., 2012). In lung epithelial cells, bleomycin could induce pulmonary fibrosis in mice by impeding TFEB-mediated autophagic flux (Wang et al., 2018). AMPK-dependent activation of autophagy enhances collagen turnover to deactivate myofibroblasts, which attenuates BLM-induced pulmonary fibrosis (Rangarajan et al., 2018). mTOR is a key regulator of growth in animals, regulating the balance of apoptosis and autophagy when cells are exposed to physiological stimulation and is also the downstream Wnt signal (Park et al., 2019). Sirolimus, a mTOR (mammalian target of rapamycin) inhibitor, attenuates BLM-induced pulmonary fibrosis in rats (Simler et al., 2002). Therefore, inhibiting Wnt/mTOR signaling could promote autophagy formation, and this is an effective method to attenuate pulmonary fibrosis.

Ellagic acid (EA) is generated by hydrolysis of complex polyphenolic compounds named ellagitannins and is found in a wide variety of fruits and nuts, such black currants, grapes, raspberries, and strawberries (De Ancos et al., 2000; Priyadarsini et al., 2002). Ellagic acid has shown multiple protective effects during fibrotic diseases such as liver fibrosis, pancreatic fibrosis and cardiac fibrosis (Buniatian, 2003; Suzuki et al., 2009; Lin et al., 2019). Ellagic acid promoted apoptosis and autophagy and suppressed Wnt/β-catenin and mTOR pathways in tumour cells (Li et al., 2005; Edderkaoui et al., 2008; Duan et al., 2019). In addition, previous studies have reported that Ellagic acid could attenuate BLM-induced pulmonary fibrosis in rats (Thresiamma and Kuttan, 1997; Saba et al., 2013), but the therapeutic effect of BLM-induced pulmonary fibrosis in mice and its mechanism are not clear. In our studies, we demonstrated that Ellagic acid could alleviate BLM-induced pulmonary fibrosis in mice mainly by inhibiting fibroblast activation and inducing myofibroblast autophagy and apoptosis, and its main mechanism is regulating the Wnt pathway.

METHODS AND MATERIALS

BLM-Induced Animal Model of Pulmonary Fibrosis

Fifty 7- to 8-week-old male C57BL/6J mice were purchased from Charles River (Beijing, China). All mice were housed and cared for in a pathogen-free facility at Nankai University. The mice were acclimatized in a room with constant temperature (25 ± 2°C) and relative humidity (60 ± 2%) and allowed free access to food and water. All animal experiments were approved by the Animal Care and Use Committee (IACUC) at Nankai University (Permit No. SYXK 2014-0003). The mice were randomly divided into five groups (n = 10 per group): Control, BLM, Pirfenidone-treated (200 mg/kg), Low-Ellagic acid-treated (10 mg/kg), and High-Ellagic acid-treated (20 mg/kg) groups. Pirfenidone was purchased from Dalian Meilun Biotechnology (Dalian, China), Ellagic acid was purchased from Macklin Biochemical (Shanghai, China). The mice were orally exposed to Ellagic acid, pirfenidone and water once a day for 7–13 days. For BLM administration, mice were anesthetized and then intratracheally injected with bleomycin (Nippon Kayaku Co., Ltd., Tokyo, Japan) at a dose of 2 U/kg body weight for analysis of the fibrotic response. The sham-operated group received intratracheal injections of the same amount of saline. The drug administration group were administered daily from the seventh day of modeling to the 13th day. Mice were sacrificed on day 14. In brief, after anesthetized, the hearts were perfused with PBS through the right ventricle until lungs cleared of blood, and then the right lung tissues were isolated for hydroxyproline assay (three lung lobes) and western blot assay (one lung lobe), the left lung tissues were inflated with 0.5 ml of 10% neutral buffered formalin and went through histology assay.

The Isolation of Primary Pulmonary Fibroblasts (PPF) and Cell Culture

A mouse lung fibroblast cell line (Mlg), mouse embryonic fibroblast cell line (NIH-3T3) (kindly supplied by Professor Wen Ning, Nankai University) were cultured in DMEM (Solarbio, Beijing, China) supplemented with 10% fetal bovine serum (FBS, Biological Industries, Israel) and antibiotics (100 mg/ml streptomycin and 100 U/ml penicillin G) in a 37°C atmosphere of 95% humidified air and 5% CO_2. Primary pulmonary fibroblasts (PPFs) were isolated from NaCl- and BLM-treated

TABLE 1 | The list of primary antibodies.

Antibody	Company and Item No.	Antibody	Company and Item No.
GAPDH	Affinity, AF7021	P62	Proteintech, 8420-1-AP
β-tubulin	Affinity, T0023	Atg16L1	CST, 8089T
β-catenin	CST, 8480T	LC3A/B	CST, 12741S
p-β-catenin (s33/37/Thr41)	CST, 9561T	mTOR	Abcam, ab32028
p-β-catenin (Thr41/Ser45)	CST, 9565T	p-mTOR (S2448)	Abcam, ab109268
α-SMA	Affinity, BF9212	S6 ribosomal protein (S6RP)	Affinity, AF7831
Collagen I	Affinity, AF7001	p-S6 ribosomal protein (S235/S236)	CST, 4858T
Fibronectin	Affinity, AF5335	Caspase3	CST, 9662S
Akt	SANTA CRUZ, sc-56878	Cleaved-Caspase3	CST, 9664T
p-Akt (Ser473)	SANTA CRUZ, sc-514032	Caspase9	CST, 9009T
Erk1/2	SANTA CRUZ, sc-514302	Cleaved-Caspase9	CST, 9504T
p-Erk1/2 (Thr202/Thy204)	SANTA CRUZ, sc-81492		

C57BL/6J mice as mentioned earlier (Ning et al., 2004). Briefly, the lungs were lavaged three times with 1 ml of PBS, digested with 2.5 mg/ml diepase II (Roche, United States), and 2.5 mg/ml collagenase Type 4 (Worthington, United States) for 30 min at 37°C and then centrifuged. The cell pellet was resuspended in DMEM containing 10% FBS and cultured in 5% CO_2 at 37°C in a humidified atmosphere. PPF cells at passages two to five were used for various assays. Chloroquine (Klionsky et al.) was purchased from Macklin (Shanghai, China), and bafilomycin A1 (Baf A1) was purchased from Cayman Chemical (Wuhan, China).

Western Blot

Lung tissue and cell samples were homogenized in RIPA lysis (Beyotime Biotechnology, Shanghai, China) buffer with PMSF and NaF (phosphatase inhibitor; added when extracting the phosphorylating protein) and then centrifuged (10,000 rpm, 10 min) to obtain supernatants. The total protein concentration was measured by a BCA Protein Assay kit (Beyotime Biotechnology, Shanghai, China). The secondary antibodies were goat anti-rabbit IgG-HRP (Abcam, Share, United Kingdom) and goat anti-mouse IgG-HRP (Abcam, Share, United Kingdom). The relative density of each band was analyzed by ImageJ. The following primary antibodies were used:

Quantitative Real-Time PCR (qRT-PCR)

Total RNA was extracted using TRIzol Reagent (Invitrogen, Carlsbad, CA, United States). cDNA was obtained from total RNA through reverse transcription. qRT-PCR was performed by using SYBR GreenER qPCR SuperMix Universal (Invitrogen, Carlsbad, CA, United States) according to the manufacturer's protocols. The relative quantification of gene expression (a-SMA, Collagen I, Fibronectin, Cyclin D1, MMP7, and Wisp1) was measured relative to the endogenous reference gene β-actin using the comparative CT method in the experiment. Sequences of the specific primer sets are as follows:

Hematoxylin-Eosin (H and E) and Masson Staining

Left lungs were fixed in 10% formalin for 24 h and embedded in paraffin. Then, lung sections (5 μm) were prepared and stained with hematoxylin-eosin or Masson's trichrome with commercial kits according to the manufacturers' instructions (Solarbio, Beijing, China). The digitized images of the slides were collected using an upright microscope (Leica DM1000, Germany). Quantification of pulmonary fibrosis was performed as described previously (Jiang et al., 2004). In brief, Masson staining slides were examined under high power (×10 objective), and five random fields per specimen were captured. Then, digitized images were opened in Image-Pro Plus Version 6.0 (Media Cybernetics, Inc., United States), and the software selection tool was used to select the entire lung tissue area and automatically calculate the total pixel (Pw) of the region. Then, the same method was used to calculate the total pixel (Pf) of the fibrosis region, fibrosis ratio = fibrosis area pixel (Pf)/total lung pixel (Pw).

GFP-LC3 and Cherry-GFP-LC3 Transfections and Immunofluorescence

GFP-LC3B (mouse) and Cherry-GFP-LC3B (mouse) plasmids were transfected into NIH-3T3 cells using PEI according to the supplier's protocol (Sino Biological Inc., Beijing, China). Cells were fixed in 4% paraformaldehyde for 20 min, washed with PBS, permeabilized with 0.2% Triton X-100 in PBS, blocked with 5% BSA and incubated with α-SMA antibodies. Cells were washed with PBS, and FITC was used for immunofluorescence visualization. Next, tissues were incubated with anti- α-SMA and anti-Col1 antibodies overnight at 4°C and then with secondary FITC- or rhodamine (TRITC)-labelled antibodies for 30 min. Fluorescein (FITC)-conjugated AffiniPure goat anti-mouse IgG (H + L) and rhodamine (TRITC)-conjugated Affinipure goat anti-rabbit IgG (H + L) were purchased from Jackson ImmunoResearch (Pennsylvania, Unites States). Nuclei were stained with DAPI (Solarbio, Beijing, China), and cells and tissues were photographed with a TCS SP8 confocal microscope (Leica).

Dual Luciferase Assay

TCF/LEF promoters were cloned into the pGL4.49 luciferase reporter vector, and NIH-3T3 cells were transfected with luciferase reporter plasmids using PEI. Renilla-luciferase was used as an internal control. Cells were treated 18 h after transfection with a series of EAs for 8 h. Cells were harvested,

TABLE 2 | The list of gene primers.

Gene	Forward primer sequence	Reverse primer sequence
α-SMA (NM_007392.2)	GCTGGTGATGATGCTCCCA	GCCCATTCCAACCATTACTCC
Fn (NM_010233.1)	GTGTAGCACAACTTCCAATTACGAA	GGAATTTCCGCCTCGAGTCT
Col1 a1 (NM_007742.3)	CCAAGAAGACATCCCTGAAGTCA	TGCACGTCATCGCACACA
Cyclin D1 (NM_007631)	GCGTACCCTGACACCAATCT	CAGGTCTCCTCCGTCTTGAG
Wisp1 (NM_018865)	CAGCACCACTAGAGGAAACGA	CTGGGCACATATCTTACAGCATT
β-actin (NM_007393.3)	AGGCCAACCGTGAAAAGATG	AGAGCATAGCCCTCGTAGATGG

and the luciferase activity of cell lysates was determined using a luciferase assay system (Promega, United States) as described by the manufacturer. Total light emission was measured using a GloMax®-Multi Detection System (Promega, United States).

Immunohistochemistry

The tissue sections were pre-treated in a microwave, blocked and incubated using a series of antibodies, and stained with DAB and hematoxylin. The results were captured using a microscope (Nikon, Japan). The method of counting the positive area is as follows: 1) Using ImageJ to open a picture, click "Image" and "type", change "RGB Color" to "RGB stack"; 2) Click "Image", drop down and click "adjust", change the B and W in the "Default" column to "Red"; 3) adjust the upper and lower pulleys to select the positive signal area, click "set", click "ok"; 4) Then, click "analyze", click "set measurement", choose "area fraction"; 5) Begin to count positive results, click "Control + M" on the keyboard, the number of "the% Aera" is the result.

Flow Cytometric Analysis of Apoptosis

NaCl-PPF or PPF-BLM cells/ml (1×10^6) were seeded into six-well plates and left for 24 h in an incubator to resume exponential growth. The extent of apoptosis was measured using an annexinV-FITC apoptosis detection kit (Beyotime, Shanghai, China) as described by the manufacturer's instructions. Cells were exposed to the drug and incubated for 24 h. Then, they were collected and washed with PBS twice, and gently resuspended in annexin-V binding buffer and incubated with annexinV-FITC/PI in the dark for 15 min. The number of apoptotic cells was detected by CytoFLEX S (Beckman Coulter, United States).

Hydroxyproline Assay

The collagen contents in the right lungs of mice were measured with a conventional hydroxyproline method (Taylor et al., 2002). In brief, the right lungs were dried and acid-hydrolyzed, the residue was filtered, and the pH value was adjusted to 6.5–8.0. Hydroxyproline analysis was performed using chloramine-T spectrophotometric absorbance as previously described.

Evaluation of Pulmonary Function

C57BL/6J mice were administered BLM (2 U/kg) on day 0; orally exposed to Ellagic acid, pirfenidone and water once a day for days 7–13; and finally, sacrificed on day 14. After the mice were anesthetized, we carefully cut the neck skin with a scalpel (trying not to bleed, otherwise it would affect the experimental data of lung functions) and subsequently used the surgical line to fix the cannula. The mice were transferred into the plethysmography chamber, and functions were analyzed using the Anires2005 system (Biolab, Beijing, China). This system automatically calculates and displays pulmonary function parameters, including forced vital capacity (FVC), dynamic compliance (Cydn), inspiratory resistance (Ri) and expiratory resistance (Re).

Statistical Analysis

Statistical analyses was performed using GraphPad Prism 6.0 software. One statistical approach that was One-way ANOVA with Greenhouse-Geisser correction followed by Dunnett's multiple comparisons test was used to calculate the significance of the differences between group means, and all data expressed as mean ± (Standard Error of Mean) SEM, $^*p < 0.05$, $^{**}p < 0.01$, $^{***}p < 0.001$, and NS: nonsignificant (one-way ANOVA).

RESULTS

Ellagic Acid Attenuates BLM-Induced Pulmonary Fibrosis in Mice

To determine the therapeutic impact of Ellagic acid on pulmonary fibrosis in mice, a BLM-induced pulmonary fibrosis mouse model was established, and mice were treated with Ellagic acid after exposure to BLM. Pirfenidone is one of the listed drugs for the treatment of IPF and was used as a positive drug. We treated C57BL/6 J mice with Ellagic acid (10 mg/kg, 20 mg/kg) from day 7 to day 13 after administrating BLM, and mice were sacrificed on day 14. Hematoxylin-eosin and Masson staining results indicated that Ellagic acid improved alveolar structure distortion and decreased the fibrotic percent (**Figures 1A,B**). The dead ratio of mice sharply increased and reached up to 60% when the mice were exposed to BLM, and Ellagic acid was able to increase the survival percentage of mice (**Figure 1C**). In addition, in the right lung tissue, Ellagic acid reduced the level of hydroxyproline (**Figure 1D**). Lung functions are a key indicator of treatment efficiency in clinical trials. Ellagic acid has positive impacts on lung functions such as forced vital capacity (FVC), dynamic compliance (Cydn), expiratory resistance (Re), and inspiratory resistance (Ri) (**Figures 1E–H**). These data indicate that Ellagic acid effectively attenuated BLM-induced pulmonary fibrosis in mice and that the therapeutic effect of Ellagic acid was better than that of the positive drug pirfenidone.

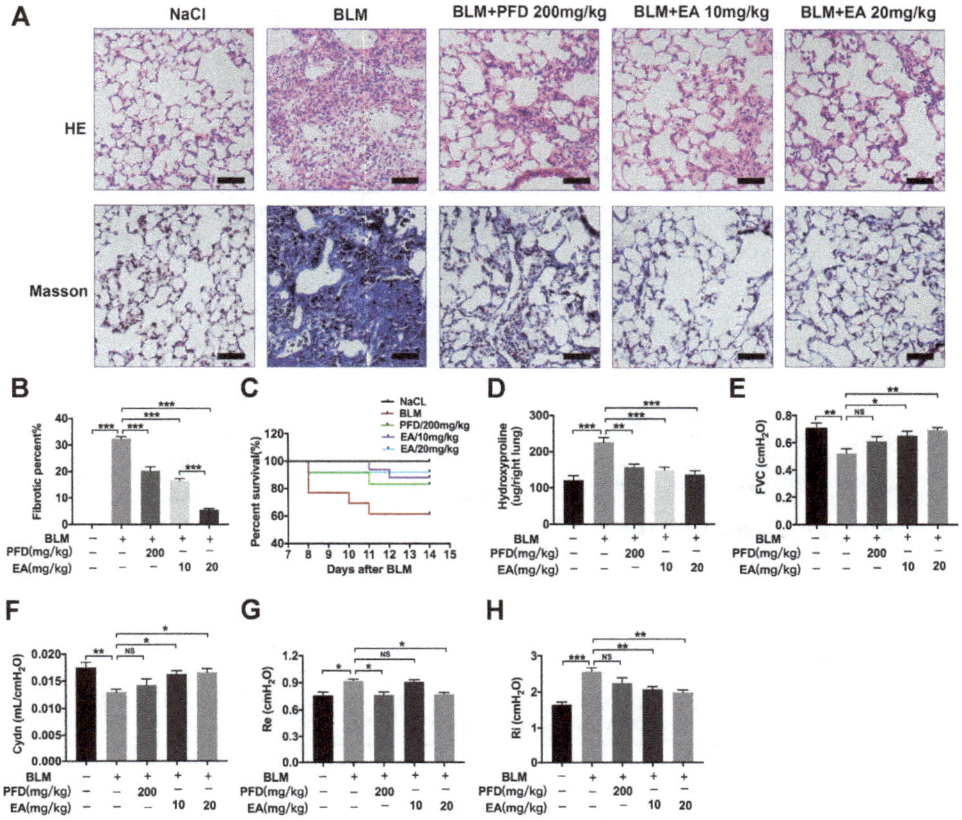

FIGURE 1 | Ellagic acid attenuates BLM-induced pulmonary fibrosis in mice. Ellagic acid (10 mg/kg, 20 mg/kg) and pirfenidone (200 mg/kg) were given orally once a day from day 7–13 after BLM treatment and lungs were harvested on day 14 **(A)** Representative images of hematoxylin-eosin (H and E) and Masson staining of lung tissue sections. Scale bars: 50 μm **(B)** Percentages of fibrotic area in each group **(C)** Percentages of surviving mice were plotted from day 7–13 after BLM treatment **(D)** Hydroxyproline contents in right lung tissues **(E–H)** Parameters of lung function such as forced vital capacity (FVC), dynamic compliance (Cydn), expiratory resistance (Re) and inspiratory resistance (Ri). Data (**Figures 1B–H**) are means ± Standard Error of Mean, $n = 6$, $^{*}p < 0.05$, $^{**}p < 0.01$, $^{***}p < 0.001$, and NS: nonsignificant (one-way ANOVA).

Ellagic Acid Inhibits the Wnt Signaling Pathway

Ellagic acid could attenuate Wnt signaling in other disease models, such as brain injury, HBP carcinomas and skin photoaging (Anitha et al., 2013; Liu et al., 2017; Moon et al., 2018), but whether Ellagic acid inhibits Wnt signaling in pulmonary fibrosis has not been definitely proven. Hence, we explored the effect of Ellagic acid on canonical Wnt signaling in pulmonary fibroblasts. We tested the ability of Ellagic acid to inhibit β-catenin/TCF reporter activity, which was measured with reporter genes harboring TCF/LEF-binding sites. Ellagic acid dose-dependently inhibited Wnt3a-induced TOPFlash activity in NIH-3T3 cells (**Figure 2A**) and inhibited the expression of Wnt signaling target genes, including CyclinD1 and Wisp1 in NaCl-PPF cells (**Figures 2B,C**). Further investigations indicated that Ellagic acid increased the ratio of phospho-β-catenin (Ser33/37/Thr41 and Thr41/Ser45) to β-catenin (**Figures 2D–F**). *In vivo* experiments also indicated that Wnt3a and β-catenin were overexpressed in lung tissues at day 7 and day 14 after BLM treatment and Ellagic acid inhibited the overexpression of Wnt3a and β-catenin (**Supplementary Figure S1**). We further tested the expression of β-catenin in BLM-PPF cells and the result was consistent with that of *in vivo* (**Supplementary Figure S2**). Therefore, these data demonstrate that Ellagic acid suppresses the canonical Wnt signaling pathway.

Ellagic Acid Suppresses Wnt3a-Induced Fibroblast Activation and ECM Accumulation by Regulating the Phosphorylation of Erk and Akt

We further explored whether Ellagic acid could decrease Wnt3a-induced myofibroblast activation and ECM production and its underlying mechanism. The results indicate that Ellagic acid could significantly decrease Wnt3a-induced Col 1 expression in Mlg cells and NaCl-PPF cells (**Figures 3A,B**). The immunofluorescence results also revealed that Ellagic acid suppressed Wnt3a-induced expression of α-SMA in Mlg and NaCl-PPF cells (**Figures 3C,D**). Ellagic acid also downregulated Wnt3a-induced mRNA levels of α-SMA, Col1 a1 and Fn in Mlg and NaCl-PPF cells

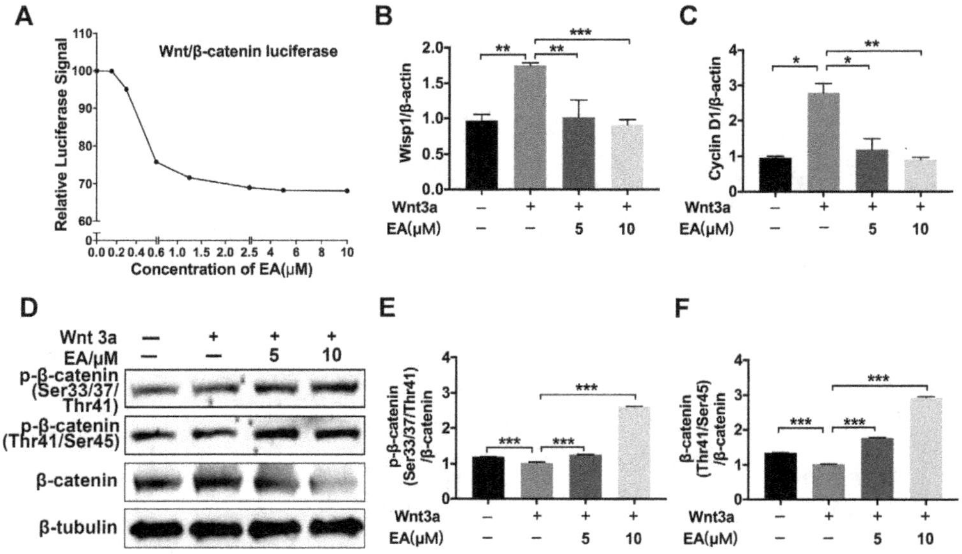

FIGURE 2 | Ellagic acid inhibits Wnt/β-catenin signaling pathway **(A)** NIH-3T3 cells were transfected with the TOPFlash plasmids. After 18 h of transfection, the cells were treated with Wnt3a (100 ng/ml) and/or Ellagic acid at various concentrations for 8 h and then lyzed for luciferase assays **(B,C)** NaCl-PPF cells were incubated with Ellagic acid (5 μM, 10 μM) and/or Wnt3a (100 ng/ml) for 12 h to analyze the mRNA levels of Wisp1 and Cyclin D1 by using quantitative real-time PCR **(D)** NaCl-PPF cells were treated with Ellagic acid (5 μM, 10 μM) and/or Wnt3a (100 ng/ml) for 4 h, p-β-catenin (Ser33/37/Thr41) and p-β-catenin (Thr41/Ser45) were detected by Western blot. Densitometric analyses were shown beside. Data (**Figures 2B–F**) are means ± Standard Error of Mean, $n = 3$, $^{*}p < 0.05$, $^{**}p < 0.01$, $^{***}p < 0.001$, and NS: nonsignificant (one-way ANOVA). β-tubulin was used as a loading control.

(**Figures 3E,F**). To further explore the mechanism, we detected whether Ellagic acid could affect downstream Wnt signaling. Since Wnt3a activates the proliferation of fibroblast cells via activation of both the Erk and Akt pathways (Yun et al., 2005; Kim et al., 2007), we further confirmed that Ellagic acid significantly decreased the Wnt3a-induced proportions of p-Erk1 (Thr202)/Erk1, p-Erk2 (Tyr204)/Erk2, and p-Akt (Ser473)/Akt in Mlg cells (**Figure 3G**), and BLM-PPF (BLM-primary pulmonary fibroblasts) cells incubated with Ellagic acid also showed similar results (**Figure 3H**). These results show that Ellagic could significantly decrease Wnt3a-induced pulmonary fibroblast activation and ECM production by inhibiting the activation of Erk1 (Thr202), Erk2 (Tyr204), and Akt (Ser475) in pulmonary fibroblasts.

Ellagic Promotes Pulmonary Fibroblast Autophagy by Inhibiting the Wnt-mTOR Signaling Pathway

The Wnt pathway is a well-known pathway and involves the regulation of autophagy (Ma et al., 2005; Semenov et al., 2007; Saiki et al., 2011). To explore whether Ellagic acid impacts autophagy and downstream Wnt signaling (mTOR signaling), we established a cellular model of inhibitory autophagy. p62 protein accumulation suggests that autophagy activity was decreased (Katsuragi et al., 2015). The two autophagy inhibitors, Chloroquine (CQ) and Bafilomycin a1 (Baf a1), could increase the expression levels of p62 (**Supplementary Figure S3**), and Ellagic acid significantly downregulated CQ and Baf A1-induced p62 protein expression in Mlg cells (**Figures 4A,B**). GFP-LC3B and mCherry-GFP-LC3B plasmids were used to detect autophagic flux. LC3B, its N terminus with a fluorescent protein such as GFP (GFP-LC3B), has been used to monitor autophagy through fluorescence microscopy, and the number of green puncta in cells indicated the quantity of GFP-LC3B puncta (Klionsky et al., 2016). A method that is designed to detect autophagy flux on the use of a tandem monomeric mCherry-GFP-tagged LC3B, and the number of green puncta and yellow puncta after merging mCherry and GFP indicated the quantity of autophagosomes and autolysosomes, respectively, (Klionsky et al., 2016). Our results showed that Ellagic acid increased Wnt3a-induced GFP-LC3B puncta in NIH-3T3 cells (**Figure 4C**). To corroborate these findings, we used mCherry-GFP-LC3B reporters to measure the formation of autophagosomes ($Cherry^{+}$ GFP^{+} signal) and autolysosomes ($Cherry^{+}$ GFP^{-}signal) in NIH3T3 cells. As expected, Ellagic acid treatment significantly increased Wnt3a-induced $Cherry^{+}$ GFP^{-}puncta (autolysosomes) (**Figure 4D**). In addition, we found that Ellagic acid promoted the expression of autophagy-related proteins such as Atg16 L, Beclin1, and LC3-II (LC3 lipidation) (**Figure 4E**). The mTOR pathway is the downstream Wnt signaling pathway and is related to autophagy formation, so we examined the protein expression of mTOR and S6RP (S6 ribosomal protein) and their phosphorylation by Western blot. Our studies revealed that the administration of Ellagic acid reduced phosphorylation levels of mTOR (S2248) and S6RP (S235/

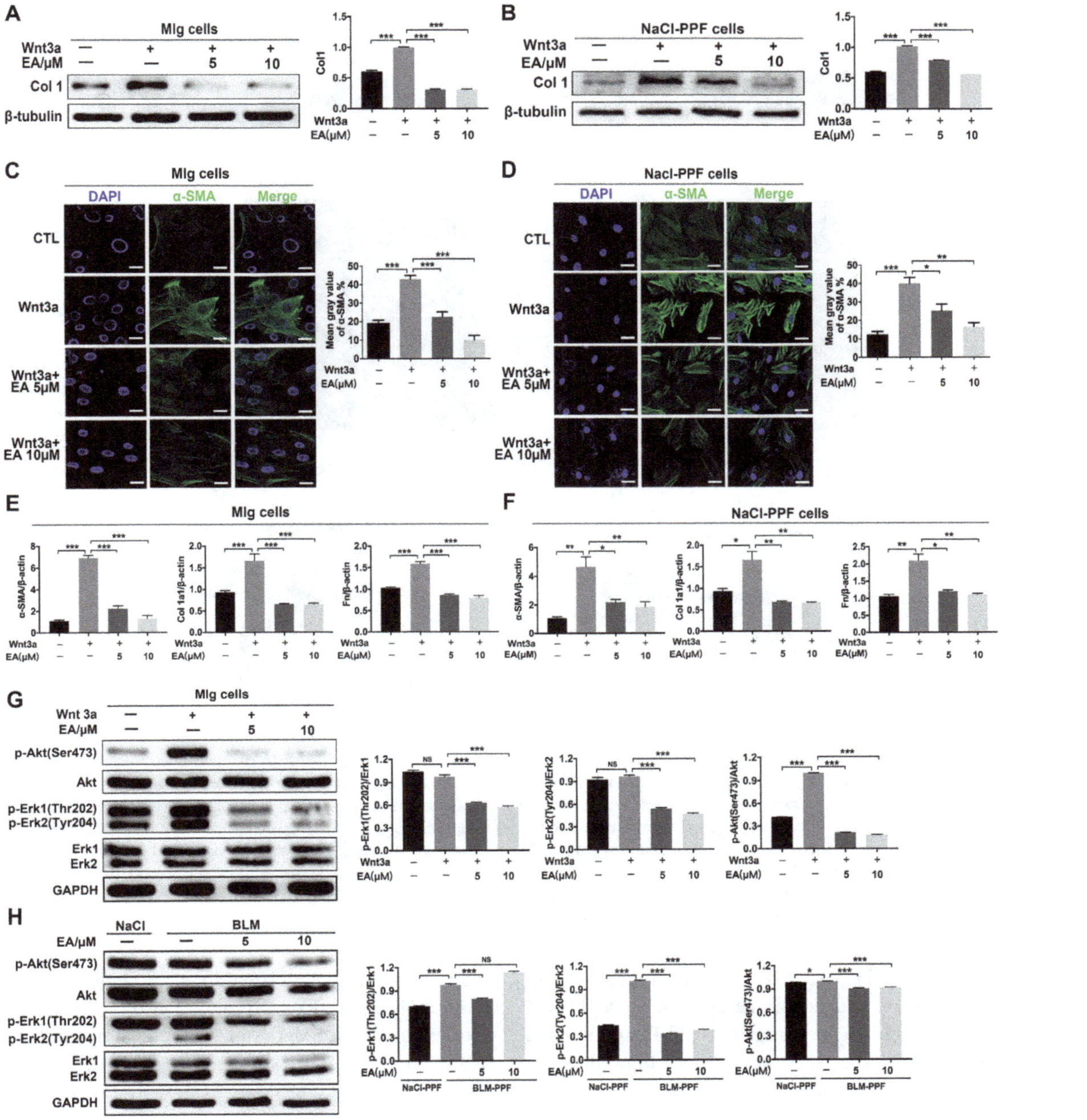

FIGURE 3 | Ellagic acid decreases Wnt3a-induced pulmonary fibroblasts activation and ECM accumulation **(A,B)** Mlg and NaCl-PPF cells were exposed to Wnt3a (100 ng/ml) and/or Ellagic acid (5 μM, 10 μM) 24 h to detect expression level of Col1 by using Western blot. Densitometric analyses were shown beside **(C,D)** Mlg and NaCl-PPF cells were exposed to Wnt3a (100 ng/ml) and/or Ellagic acid (5 μM, 10 μM) 24 h to detect the α-SMA expression level by immunofluorescence, the analyses of mean gray value were shown beside **(E,F)** Wnt3a (100 ng/ml) and/or Ellagic acid (5 μM, 10 μM) were incubated with Mlg and NaCl-PPF cells for 12 h, and cell lysate was used to analyze the mRNA levels of α-SMA, Col1 and Fn by using quantitative real-time PCR($n = 3$) **(G,H)** Mlg and NaCl-PPF cells were exposed to Wnt3a (100 ng/ml) and/or Ellagic acid (5 μM, 10 μM) for 12 h, BLM-PPF cells were treated with Ellagic acid (5 μM, 10 μM) for 12 h to evaluate protein expression levels of p-Akt (Ser473), Akt, p-Erk1/2 (Thr202/Tyr204)and Erk1/2 by western blot. Densitometric analyses were shown beside. Data (**Figures 4A–H**) are means ± Standard Error of Mean, $n = 3$, $^{*}p < 0.05$, $^{**}p < 0.01$, $^{***}p < 0.001$, and NS: nonsignificant (one-way ANOVA). β-tubulin or GAPDH was used as a loading control.

S236) in BLM-PPF cells (**Figure 4F**). Therefore, these data suggest that Ellagic acid induced autophagy formation by suppressing the Wnt-mTOR signaling pathway in pulmonary fibroblasts.

Ellagic Acid Promotes the Apoptosis of Pulmonary Myofibroblasts

To detect whether Ellagic acid contributed to apoptosis, we analyzed the number of apoptotic cells using flow cytometry. BLM-PPF cells

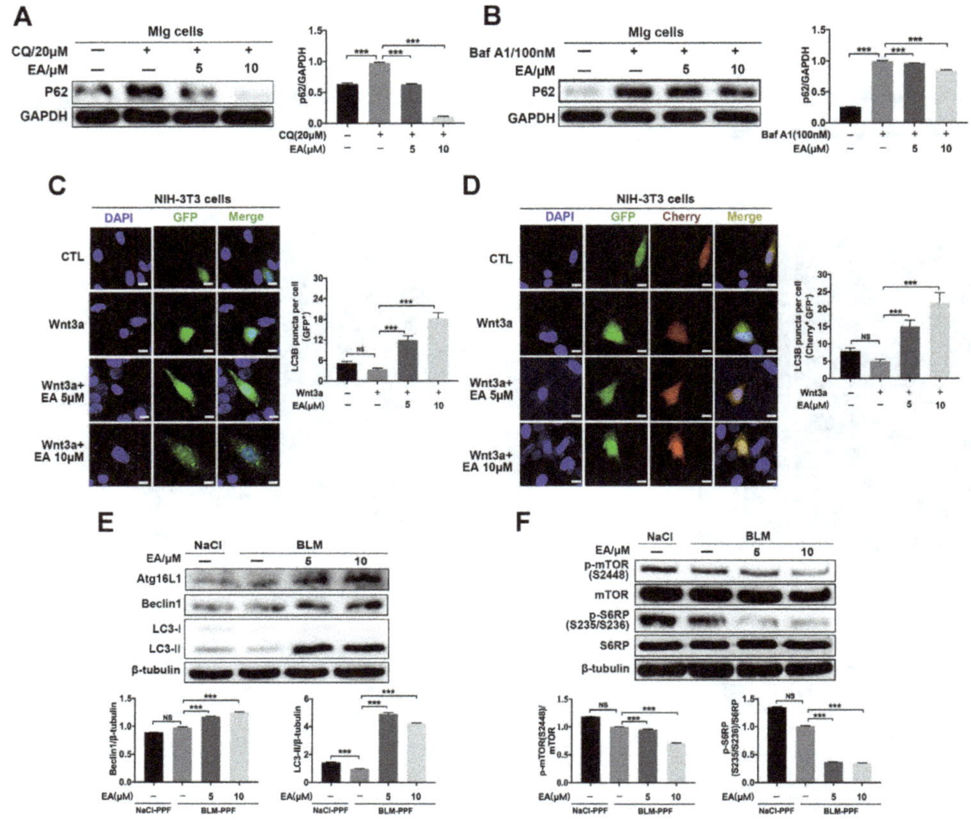

FIGURE 4 | Ellagic acid promotes pulmonary fibroblast autophagy mainly via inhibiting Wnt-mTOR signaling pathway **(A,B)** Mlg cells were exposed to CQ (20 μM) and Baf A1 (100 nM) with or without Ellagic acid (5 μM, 10 μM) to analyze the p62 expression level by using western blot. Densitometric analyses were shown beside **(C,D)** The plasmids of GFP-LC3B and mCherry-GFP-LC3B were transfected to NIH3T3 cells with PEI, and these cells were subsequently exposed to Ellagic acid (5 μM, 10 μM) and/or Wnt3a (100 ng/ml) for 12 h. DNA was counterstained with DAPI (blue). Quantitative analyses are showed beside. Scale bars: 50 μm **(E)** BLM-PPF cells were treated with Ellagic acid (5 μM, 10 μM) for 24 h, and the Atg16L1, Beclin1 and LC3-II/I expression levels were detected by Western blot. Densitometric analyses were shown below **(F)** BLM-PPF cells were treated with Ellagic acid (5 μM, 10 μM) for 12 h, and protein expression levels of mTOR, S6RP and their phosphorylation were detected by Western blot. Densitometric analyses were shown below. Data are means ± Standard Error of Mean, $n = 3$, $^{*}p < 0.05$, $^{**}p < 0.01$, $^{***}p < 0.001$, and NS: nonsignificant (one-way ANOVA). β-tubulin or GAPDH were used as a loading control.

were exposed to Ellagic acid to analyze the number of apoptosis cells by using flow cytometry, and double negative (not add PI and Annex-V-FITC staining) and single negative (add PI and not add Annex-V-FITC staining) were important tests to draw the gate. Treatment with Ellagic acid resulted in an increase in annexin V^+/PI^-cells (early apoptosis) but no change in Annexin V^+/PI^+ (late apoptosis) or annexin V^-/PI^+ cells (necrosis) (**Figure 5A**). In addition, caspase proteins are tightly related to cellular apoptosis. Our experiments indicated that Ellagic acid increased the expression of cleaved caspase-9 and cleaved caspase-3 in PPF cells (**Figure 5B**) and Wnt3a-induced the expression of cleaved caspase-9 in Mlg cells (**Figure 5C**). Hence, Ellagic acid could promote the apoptosis of pulmonary myofibroblasts.

Ellagic Attenuates BLM-Induced Fibroblast Activation and ECM Accumulation *in vivo*

The mice were treated with Ellagic acid on day 7 to day 13, and we employed immunohistochemistry to identify that Ellagic acid had a negative impact on the expression of α-SMA, Col 1 and Fn in lung sections, which were equal to the results of the positive drug pirfenidone (**Figure 6A**). Our immunofluorescence results also showed inhibitory expression of α-SMA and Col1 in lung sections (**Figures 6B,C**). In addition, we used a tissue homogenizer to lyse lung tissues, and α-SMA, LC3-1I/II, p-mTOR, and mTOR protein levels were analyzed by using Western blotting. Ellagic acid decreased α-SMA expression and the ratio of p-mTOR/mTOR and increased the ratio of LC3-II/LC3-I (**Figure 6D**). Together, these data identified that Ellagic acid significantly inhibited myofibroblast activation and mTOR signaling and promoted autophagy formation *in vivo*.

DISCUSSION

Idiopathic pulmonary fibrosis is a chronic, fatal lung disease, and many IPF patients experience respiratory failure (Mora et al., 2017). The importance of the Wnt signaling pathway has been identified in pulmonary fibrosis, and the main reason is that aberrant Wnt signaling could induce fibroblast activation and ECM production (Morrisey, 2003; Baarsma et al., 2011). When

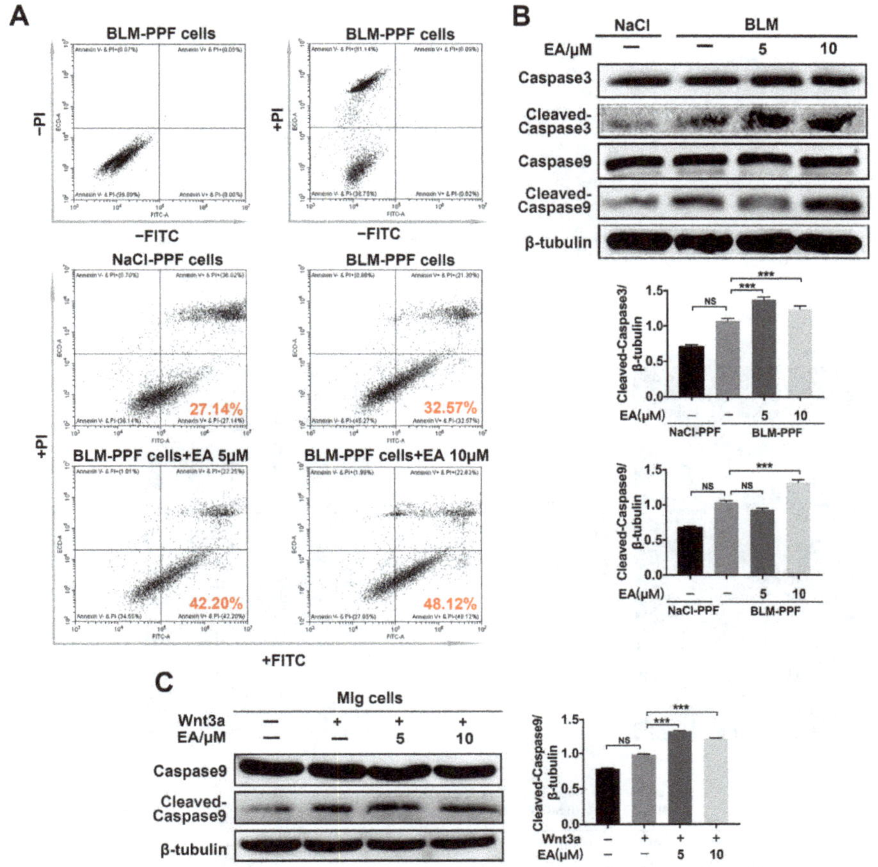

FIGURE 5 | Ellagic acid promotes the apoptosis of pulmonary myofibroblasts **(A)** BLM-PPF cells incubated with Ellagic acid (5 μM, 10 μM) and/or Wnt3a (100 ng/ml) for 24 h, and Annexin V/PI staining was subsequently performed to estimate early, late apoptosis and necrosis by flow cytometry **(B)** BLM-PPF cells were treated with Ellagic acid (5 μM, 10 μM) for 24 h, Lysates were immunoblotted for Caspase3, Cleaved-Caspase3, Caspase9 and Cleaved-Caspase9. Densitometric analyses were shown below **(C)** Mlg cells were treated with Ellagic acid (5 μM, 10 μM) and/or Wnt3a (100 ng/ml) for 24 h, Lysates were immunoblotted for Caspase9 and Cleaved-Caspase9. Densitometric analysis were shown beside. Data in **(B,C)** are means ± Standard Error of Mean, $n = 3$, $^{***}p < 0.001$, and NS: nonsignificant (one-way ANOVA). β-tubulin was used as a loading control.

Wnt signaling is abnormally activated, β-catenin is translocated into the nucleus to upregulate related target genes such as Cyclin D1, MMP7, and Wisp1 (Crawford et al., 1999; Konigshoff et al., 2009; Zhang et al., 2012). In our studies, Ellagic acid inhibited the Wnt/β-catenin signaling pathway by decreasing the expression of Cyclin D1, MMP7, Wisp1, and nuclear β-catenin and increasing the phosphorylation of β-catenin.

Collagen, a main component of extracellular protein, maintains the basic structure of the lung. However, there are overactivated fibroblasts and overexpressed ECM proteins in fibroblastic foci, and inhibiting this condition could effectively attenuate pulmonary fibrosis (Snijder et al., 2019). Excessive ECM proteins result in the formation of lung scars, which might accelerate the decline in force vital capacity (Bates et al., 2007; King et al., 2011). Previous studies showed that Wnt ligands promoted fibroblast activation and collagen synthesis (Konigshoff et al., 2008) and increased the phosphorylation levels of Akt and Erk (Yun et al., 2005; Kim et al., 2007). Therefore, there is an effective method to inhibit fibroblast activation and ECM accumulation by downregulating Wnt3a-induced activation of Akt and Erk. Our experimental results revealed that Ellagic acid significantly inhibited fibroblast activation and ECM production by decreasing the translation and transcription levels of α-SMA, Col 1 and Fn *in vivo or in vitro*, and the underlying mechanism was mainly the inhibitory Wnt/Akt and Erk signaling.

Insufficient autophagy plays an essential role in the pathogenesis of IPF. Many researchers focus on fibroblast activation because selected autophagy could promote collagen turnover (Rangarajan et al., 2018). The PB1 domain of the p62 protein is involved in the degradation of polyubiquitinated, misfolded, aggregated proteins and dysfunctional organelles by regulating autophagy formation in mammalian cells (Moscat and Diaz-Meco, 2009). Our studies showed that Ellagic acid could increase the expression of p62 in pulmonary fibroblasts. LC3-II, a processed form of LC3, is localized in the membrane of autophagosomes and is regarded as a powerful marker for autophagosomes (Kabeya et al., 2000). During the formation of early autophagosomes, some complexes formed by LC3-II and other autophagy-related proteins are required (Tanida et al., 2004). In addition, Atg16 L[1] and beclin1 are essential factors in autophagic flux and its biological function (Matsushita et al., 2007; Wirawan et al., 2012). In BLM primary pulmonary fibroblasts, Ellagic acid

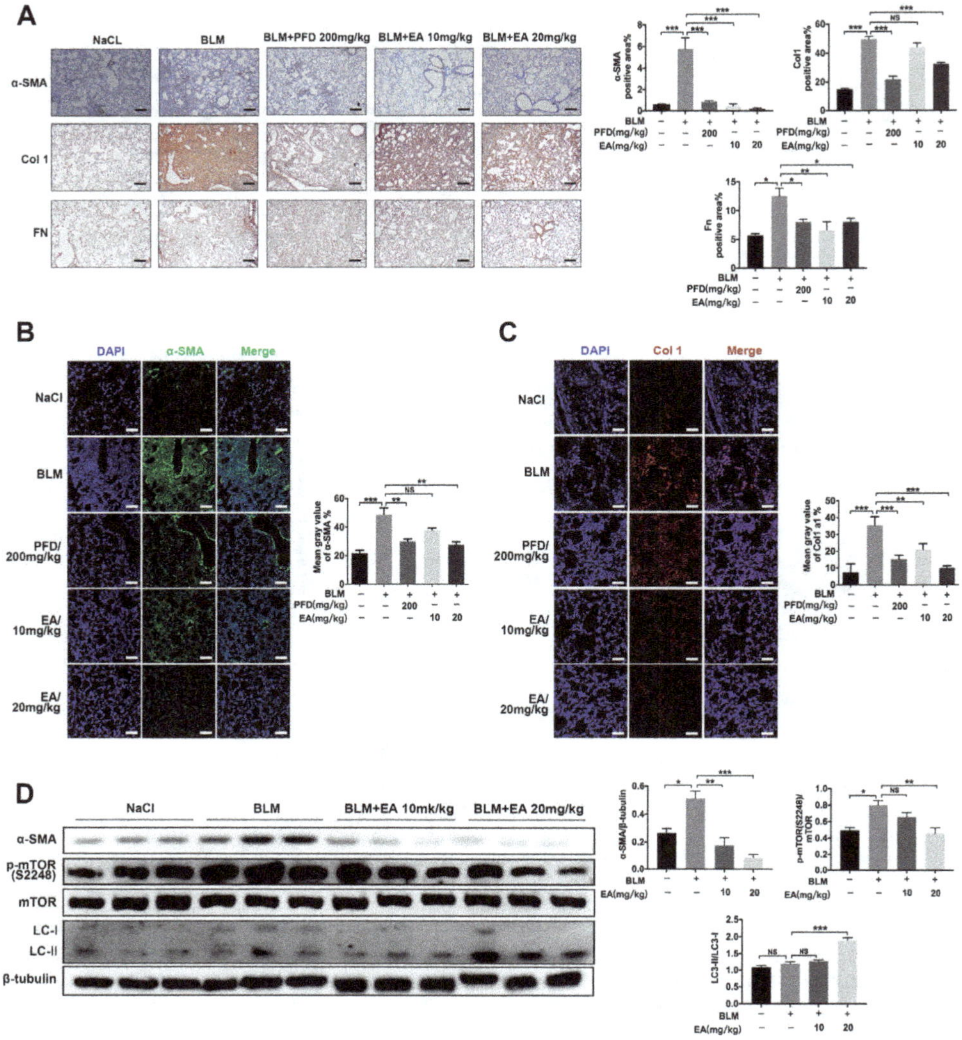

FIGURE 6 | Ellagic acid attenuates BLM-induced fibroblasts activation and ECM accumulation *in vivo*. The mice were treated with Ellagic acid (10 mg/kg, 20 mg/kg) from day 7–13 after administrating BLM **(A)** Immunohistochemistry was used to analyze the expression levels of α-SMA, Col1 and Fn ($n = 3$). Quantitative analysis was shown beside. Scale bars: 50 μm **(B–C)** The expression levels of α-SMA and Col1 were detected by immunofluorescence in lung sections. The analyses of mean gray value were shown beside. Scale bars: 50 μm **(D)** Lung homogenization was used to analysis the α-SMA, LC3-II/I and *p*-mTOR (S2248), mTOR expression levels by Western blot ($n = 6$). Densitometric analyses were shown beside. Data in **(A,D)** are means ± Standard Error of Mean, $^{*}p < 0.05$, $^{**}p < 0.01$, $^{***}p < 0.001$, and NS: nonsignificant (one-way ANOVA). β-tubulin was used as a loading control.

treatment increased LC3-II, Atg16 L[1] and beclin1 expression. The mTOR pathway also plays an important role in regulating balanced growth and autophagy in response to environmental stress, and this signal is regulated by Wnt signaling (Yang and Guan, 2007). Interestingly, our results showed that Ellagic acid significantly inhibited Wnt3a-induced activation of mTOR signaling in pulmonary fibroblasts. Hence, Ellagic acid could induce autophagy, and this process might be regulated by the Wnt/mTOR signaling pathway in pulmonary fibrosis. Inhibition of autophagy (by knockout of Atg3, Atg5, Atg7 and mutation of Atg1, Atg13, vsp34) suppresses the induction of apoptosis (Nezis et al., 2010; Rubinstein et al., 2011; Young et al., 2012). Autophagy can degrade catalase and promote necrotic cell death (Yu et al., 2006). In chronic lymphocytic leukaemia cells, downregulating the Wnt signaling pathway promoted cell apoptosis (Lu et al., 2011). Ellagic acid induced apoptosis by increasing the number of early apoptotic cells and promoting the activation of Caspase3 and Caspase9 in Mlg and PPF cells.

In conclusion, we identified that Ellagic acid alleviated BLM-induced pulmonary function and improved lung function in mice. *In vitro* experiments revealed that Ellagic acid could inhibit fibroblast activation and ECM production and promote myofibroblast autophagy and apoptosis by downregulating the Wnt signaling pathway. Ellagic acid also inhibited myofibroblast activation and promoted autophagy formation *in vivo*. Therefore, our studies support for the use of Ellagic acid as a candidate compound for anti-pulmonary fibrosis drugs and provide more potential therapeutic options for IPF patients.

AUTHOR CONTRIBUTIONS

Conception and design: CY, HZ, GY; Collection and assembly of data: XHL, KH, XWL, LM, YC and YHW; Data analysis and interpretation: JL, SW, HL, YLW, ZL; Data revision: HR; Manuscript writing: XHL, JG, BY and XPL. All authors read and approved the final manuscript.

ACKNOWLEDGMENTS

Thanks to Professor Wen Ning for her generous offer of MLG and NIH-3T3.

REFERENCES

Anitha, P., Priyadarsini, R. V., Kavitha, K., Thiyagarajan, P., and Nagini, S. (2013). Ellagic acid coordinately attenuates Wnt/β-catenin and NF-κB signaling pathways to induce intrinsic apoptosis in an animal model of oral oncogenesis. *Eur. J. Nutr.* 52, 75–84. doi:10.1007/s00394-011-0288-y

Araya, J., Kojima, J., Takasaka, N., Ito, S., Fujii, S., Hara, H., et al. (2013). Insufficient autophagy in idiopathic pulmonary fibrosis. *Am. J. Physiology-Lung Cell Mol. Physiol.* 304, L56–L69. doi:10.1152/ajplung.00213.2012

Baarsma, H. A., and Königshoff, M. (2017). 'WNT-er is coming': WNT signalling in chronic lung diseases. *Thorax* 72, 746–759. doi:10.1136/thoraxjnl-2016-209753

Baarsma, H. A., Spanjer, A. I., Haitsma, G., Engelbertink, L. H., Meurs, H., Jonker, M. R., et al. (2011). Activation of WNT/beta-catenin signaling in pulmonary fibroblasts by TGF-beta(1) is increased in chronic obstructive pulmonary disease. *PLoS One* 6, e25450. doi:10.1371/journal.pone.0025450

Bates, J. H. T., Davis, G. S., Majumdar, A., Butnor, K. J., and Suki, B. (2007). Linking parenchymal disease progression to changes in lung mechanical function by percolation. *Am. J. Respir. Crit. Care Med.* 176, 617–623. doi:10.1164/rccm.200611-1739oc

Bilir, B., Kucuk, O., and Moreno, C. S. (2013). Wnt signaling blockage inhibits cell proliferation and migration, and induces apoptosis in triple-negative breast cancer cells. *J. Translational Med.* 11, 280. doi:10.1186/1479-5876-11-280

Buniatian, G. H. (2003). Stages of activation of hepatic stellate cells: effects of ellagic acid, an inhibiter of liver fibrosis, on their differentiation in culture. *Cell Prolif* 36, 307–319. doi:10.1046/j.1365-2184.2003.00287.x

Clevers, H., and Nusse, R. (2012). Wnt/β-Catenin signaling and disease. *Cell.* 149, 1192–1205. doi:10.1016/j.cell.2012.05.012

Crawford, H. C., Fingleton, B. M., Rudolph-Owen, L. A., Goss, K. J. H., Rubinfeld, B., Polakis, P., et al. (1999). The metalloproteinase matrilysin is a target of β-catenin transactivation in intestinal tumors. *Oncogene* 18, 2883–2891. doi:10.1038/sj.onc.1202627

De Ancos, B., González, E. M., and Cano, M. P. (2000). Ellagic acid, vitamin C, and total phenolic contents and radical scavenging capacity affected by freezing and frozen storage in raspberry fruit. *J. Agric. Food Chem.* 48, 4565–4570. doi:10.1021/jf0001684

Directors, and Committie (2000). American Thoracic Society. Idiopathic pulmonary fibrosis: diagnosis and treatment. International consensus statement. American Thoracic Society (ATS), and the European Respiratory Society (ERS). *Am. J. Respir. Crit. Care Med.* 161, 646–664. doi:10.1164/ajrccm.161.2.ats3-00

Distler, J. H. W., Györfi, A.-H., Ramanujam, M., Whitfield, M. L., Königshoff, M., and Lafyatis, R. (2019). Shared and distinct mechanisms of fibrosis. *Nat. Rev. Rheumatol.* 15, 705–730. doi:10.1038/s41584-019-0322-7

Duan, J., Zhan, J.-C., Wang, G.-Z., Zhao, X.-C., Huang, W.-D., and Zhou, G.-B. (2019). The red wine component ellagic acid induces autophagy and exhibits anti-lung cancer activity *in vitro* and *in vivo*. *J. Cel Mol Med.* 23, 143–154. doi:10.1111/jcmm.13899

Edderkaoui, M., Odinokova, I., Ohno, I., Gukovsky, I., Go, V. L. W., Pandol, S. J., et al. (2008). Ellagic acid induces apoptosis through inhibition of nuclear factor kB in pancreatic cancer cells. *Wjg* 14, 3672–3680. doi:10.3748/wjg.14.3672

Fernández, Á. F., Sebti, S., Wei, Y., Zou, Z., Shi, M., Mcmillan, K. L., et al. (2018). Disruption of the beclin 1-BCL2 autophagy regulatory complex promotes longevity in mice. *Nature* 558, 136–140. doi:10.1038/s41586-018-0162-7

Hosseinzadeh, A., Javad-Moosavi, S. A., Reiter, R. J., Yarahmadi, R., Ghaznavi, H., and Mehrzadi, S. (2018). Oxidative/nitrosative stress, autophagy and apoptosis as therapeutic targets of melatonin in idiopathic pulmonary fibrosis. *Expert Opin. Ther. Targets* 22, 1049–1061. doi:10.1080/14728222.2018.1541318

Hutchinson, J., Fogarty, A., Hubbard, R., and Mckeever, T. (2015). Global incidence and mortality of idiopathic pulmonary fibrosis: a systematic review. *Eur. Respir. J.* 46, 795–806. doi:10.1183/09031936.00185114

Jiang, D., Liang, J., Hodge, J., Lu, B., Zhu, Z., Yu, S., et al. (2004). Regulation of pulmonary fibrosis by chemokine receptor CXCR3. *J. Clin. Invest.* 114, 291–299. doi:10.1172/jci16861

Kabeya, Y., Mizushima, N., Ueno, T., Yamamoto, A., Kirisako, T., Noda, T., et al. (2000). LC3, a mammalian homologue of yeast Apg8p, is localized in autophagosome membranes after processing. *EMBO J.* 19, 5720–5728. doi:10.1093/emboj/19.21.5720

Katsuragi, Y., Ichimura, Y., and Komatsu, M. (2015). p62/SQSTM1 functions as a signaling hub and an autophagy adaptor. *FEBS J.* 282, 4672–4678. doi:10.1111/febs.13540

Kim, S.-E., Lee, W.-J., and Choi, K.-Y. (2007). The PI3 kinase-Akt pathway mediates Wnt3a-induced proliferation. *Cell Signal.* 19, 511–518. doi:10.1016/j.cellsig.2006.08.008

King, T. E., Jr., Pardo, A., and Selman, M. (2011). Idiopathic pulmonary fibrosis. *The Lancet* 378, 1949–1961. doi:10.1016/s0140-6736(11)60052-4

Klionsky, D. J., Abdelmohsen, K., Abe, A., Abedin, M. J., Abeliovich, H., Acevedo Arozena, A., et al. (2016). Guidelines for the use and interpretation of assays for monitoring autophagy. *Autophagy* 12, 1–222. doi:10.1080/15548627.2016.11392643rd edition

Königshoff, M., Kramer, M., Balsara, N., Wilhelm, J., Amarie, O. V., Jahn, A., et al. (2009). WNT1-inducible signaling protein-1 mediates pulmonary fibrosis in mice and is upregulated in humans with idiopathic pulmonary fibrosis. *J. Clin. Invest.* 119, 772–787. doi:10.1172/JCI33950

Konigshoff, M., Balsara, N., Pfaff, E. M., Kramer, M., Chrobak, I., Seeger, W., et al. (2008). Functional Wnt signaling is increased in idiopathic pulmonary fibrosis. *PLoS One* 3, e2142. doi:10.1371/journal.pone.0002142

Levine, B., and Kroemer, G. (2008). Autophagy in the pathogenesis of disease. *Cell* 132, 27–42. doi:10.1016/j.cell.2007.12.018

Li, T. M., Chen, G. W., Su, C. C., Lin, J. G., Yeh, C. C., Cheng, K. C., et al. (2005). Ellagic acid induced p53/p21 expression, G1 arrest and apoptosis in human bladder cancer T24 cells. *Anticancer Res.* 25, 971–(979.)

Lin, C., Wei, D., Xin, D., Pan, J., and Huang, M. (2019). Ellagic acid inhibits proliferation and migration of cardiac fibroblasts by down-regulating expression of HDAC1. *J. Toxicol. Sci.* 44, 425–433. doi:10.2131/jts.44.425

Liu, Q. S., Li, S. R., Li, K., Li, X., Yin, X., and Pang, Z. (2017). Ellagic acid improves endogenous neural stem cells proliferation and neurorestoration through Wnt/beta-catenin signaling *in vivo* and *in vitro*. *Mol. Nutr. Food Res.* 61. doi:10.1002/mnfr.201600587

Lu, D., Choi, M. Y., Yu, J., Castro, J. E., Kipps, T. J., and Carson, D. A. (2011). Salinomycin inhibits Wnt signaling and selectively induces apoptosis in chronic lymphocytic leukemia cells. *Proc. Natl. Acad. Sci. USA* 108, 13253–13257. doi:10.1073/pnas.1110431108

Ma, L., Chen, Z., Erdjument-Bromage, H., Tempst, P., and Pandolfi, P. P. (2005). Phosphorylation and functional inactivation of TSC2 by Erk. *Cell* 121, 179–193. doi:10.1016/j.cell.2005.02.031

Matsushita, M., Suzuki, N. N., Obara, K., Fujioka, Y., Ohsumi, Y., and Inagaki, F. (2007). Structure of Atg5·Atg16, a complex essential for autophagy. *J. Biol. Chem.* 282, 6763–6772. doi:10.1074/jbc.m609876200

Moon, N. R., Kang, S., and Park, S. (2018). Consumption of ellagic acid and dihydromyricetin synergistically protects against UV-B induced photoaging, possibly by activating both TGF-β1 and wnt signaling pathways. *J. Photochem. Photobiol. B: Biol.* 178, 92–100. doi:10.1016/j.jphotobiol.2017.11.004

Mora, A. L., Rojas, M., Pardo, A., and Selman, M. (2017). Erratum: emerging therapies for idiopathic pulmonary fibrosis, a progressive age-related disease. *Nat. Rev. Drug Discov.* 16, 810. doi:10.1038/nrd.2017.225

Morrisey, E. E. (2003). Wnt signaling and pulmonary fibrosis. *Am. J. Pathol.* 162, 1393–1397. doi:10.1016/s0002-9440(10)64271-x

Moscat, J., and Diaz-Meco, M. T. (2009). p62 at the crossroads of autophagy, apoptosis, and cancer. *Cell* 137, 1001–1004. doi:10.1016/j.cell.2009.05.023

Nezis, I. P., Shravage, B. V., Sagona, A. P., Lamark, T., Bjørkøy, G., Johansen, T., et al. (2010). Autophagic degradation of dBruce controls DNA fragmentation in nurse cells during late *Drosophila melanogaster* oogenesis. *J. Cel Biol* 190, 523–531. doi:10.1083/jcb.201002035

Ning, W., Li, C.-J., Kaminski, N., Feghali-Bostwick, C. A., Alber, S. M., Di, Y. P., et al. (2004). Comprehensive gene expression profiles reveal pathways related to the pathogenesis of chronic obstructive pulmonary disease. *Proc. Natl. Acad. Sci.* 101, 14895–14900. doi:10.1073/pnas.0401168101

Park, Y.-L., Kim, H.-P., Cho, Y.-W., Min, D.-W., Cheon, S.-K., Lim, Y. J., et al. (2019). Activation of WNT/β-catenin signaling results in resistance to a dual PI3K/mTOR inhibitor in colorectal cancer cells harboringPIK3CAmutations. *Int. J. Cancer* 144, 389–401. doi:10.1002/ijc.31662

Patel, A. S., Lin, L., Geyer, A., Haspel, J. A., An, C. H., Cao, J., et al. (2012). Autophagy in idiopathic pulmonary fibrosis. *PLoS One* 7, e41394. doi:10.1371/journal.pone.0041394

Priyadarsini, K. I., Khopde, S. M., Kumar, S. S., and Mohan, H. (2002). Free radical studies of ellagic acid, a natural phenolic antioxidant. *J. Agric. Food Chem.* 50, 2200–2206. doi:10.1021/jf011275g

Rangarajan, S., Bone, N. B., Zmijewska, A. A., Jiang, S., Park, D. W., Bernard, K., et al. (2018). Author Correction: metformin reverses established lung fibrosis in a bleomycin model. *Nat. Med.* 24, 1627. doi:10.1038/s41591-018-0170-z

Rubinstein, A. D., Eisenstein, M., Ber, Y., Bialik, S., and Kimchi, A. (2011). The autophagy protein Atg12 associates with antiapoptotic Bcl-2 family members to promote mitochondrial apoptosis. *Mol. Cel* 44, 698–709. doi:10.1016/j.molcel.2011.10.014

Rubinsztein, D. C., Gestwicki, J. E., Murphy, L. O., and Klionsky, D. J. (2007). Potential therapeutic applications of autophagy. *Nat. Rev. Drug Discov.* 6, 304–312. doi:10.1038/nrd2272

Saba, Khan, S., Parvez, S., Chaudhari, B., Ahmad, F., Anjum, S., et al. (2013). Ellagic acid attenuates bleomycin and cyclophosphamide-induced pulmonary toxicity in Wistar rats. *Food Chem. Toxicol.* 58, 210–219. doi:10.1016/j.fct.2013.03.046

Saiki, S., Sasazawa, Y., Imamichi, Y., Kawajiri, S., Fujimaki, T., Tanida, I., et al. (2011). Caffeine induces apoptosis by enhancement of autophagy via PI3K/Akt/mTOR/p70S6K inhibition. *Autophagy* 7, 176–187. doi:10.4161/auto.7.2.14074

Semenov, M. V., Habas, R., Macdonald, B. T., and He, X. (2007). SnapShot: noncanonical wnt signaling pathways. *Cell* 131, 1378. doi:10.1016/j.cell.2007.12.011

Simler, N. R., Howell, D. C. J., Marshall, R. P., Goldsack, N. R., Hasleton, P. S., Laurent, G. J., et al. (2002). The rapamycin analogue SDZ RAD attenuates bleomycin-induced pulmonary fibrosis in rats. *Eur. Respir. J.* 19, 1124–1127. doi:10.1183/09031936.02.00281602

Snijder, J., Peraza, J., Padilla, M., Capaccione, K., and Salvatore, M. M. (2019). Pulmonary fibrosis: a disease of alveolar collapse and collagen deposition. *Expert Rev. Respir. Med.* 13, 615–619. doi:10.1080/17476348.2019.1623028

Suzuki, N., Masamune, A., Kikuta, K., Watanabe, T., Satoh, K., and Shimosegawa, T. (2009). Ellagic acid inhibits pancreatic fibrosis in male Wistar Bonn/Kobori rats. *Dig. Dis. Sci.* 54, 802–810. doi:10.1007/s10620-008-0423-7

Tanida, I., Ueno, T., and Kominami, E. (2004). LC3 conjugation system in mammalian autophagy. *Int. J. Biochem. Cel Biol.* 36, 2503–2518. doi:10.1016/j.biocel.2004.05.009

Taylor, M. D., Roberts, J. R., Hubbs, A. F., Reasor, M. J., and Antonini, J. M. (2002). Quantitative image analysis of drug-induced lung fibrosis using laser scanning confocal microscopy. *Toxicol. Sci.* 67, 295–302. doi:10.1093/toxsci/67.2.295

Thannickal, V. J., Flaherty, K. R., Martinez, F. J., and Lynch, J. P., 3rd (2004). Idiopathic pulmonary fibrosis: emerging concepts on pharmacotherapy. *Expert Opin. Pharmacother.* 5, 1671–1686. doi:10.1517/14656566.5.8.1671

Thresiamma, K. C., and Kuttan, R. (1997). Effect of antioxidants on lung fibrosis induced in rats. *J. Clin. Biochem. Nutr.* 22, 125–129. doi:10.3164/jcbn.22.125

Wang, K., Zhang, T., Lei, Y., Li, X., Jiang, J., Lan, J., et al. (2018). Identification of ANXA2 (annexin A2) as a specific bleomycin target to induce pulmonary fibrosis by impeding TFEB-mediated autophagic flux. *Autophagy* 14, 269–282. doi:10.1080/15548627.2017.1409405

Wirawan, E., Lippens, S., Vanden Berghe, T., Romagnoli, A., Fimia, G. M., Piacentini, M., et al. (2012). Beclin1: a role in membrane dynamics and beyond. *Autophagy* 8, 6–17. doi:10.4161/auto.8.1.16645

Wynn, T. A. (2011). Integrating mechanisms of pulmonary fibrosis. *J. Exp. Med.* 208, 1339–1350. doi:10.1084/jem.20110551

Yang, Q., and Guan, K.-L. (2007). Expanding mTOR signaling. *Cell Res.* 17, 666–681. doi:10.1038/cr.2007.64

Young, M. M., Takahashi, Y., Khan, O., Park, S., Hori, T., Yun, J., et al. (2012). Autophagosomal membrane serves as platform for intracellular death-inducing signaling complex (iDISC)-mediated caspase-8 activation and apoptosis. *J. Biol. Chem.* 287, 12455–12468. doi:10.1074/jbc.m111.309104

Yu, L., Wan, F., Dutta, S., Welsh, S., Liu, Z., Freundt, E., et al. (2006). Autophagic programmed cell death by selective catalase degradation. *Proc. Natl. Acad. Sci.* 103, 4952–4957. doi:10.1073/pnas.0511288103

Yun, M.-S., Kim, S. E., Jeon, S. H., Lee, J. S., and Choi, K. Y. (2005). Both ERK and Wnt/-catenin pathways are involved in Wnt3a-induced proliferation. *J. Cel Sci.* 118, 313–322. doi:10.1242/jcs.01601

Zhang, J., Gill, A. J. M., Issacs, J. D., Atmore, B., Johns, A., Delbridge, L. W., et al. (2012). The Wnt/β-catenin pathway drives increased cyclin D1 levels in lymph node metastasis in papillary thyroid cancer. *Hum. Pathol.* 43, 1044–1050. doi:10.1016/j.humpath.2011.08.013

15

Breaching the Delivery Barrier: Chemical and Physical Airway Epithelium Disruption Strategies for Enhancing Lentiviral-Mediated Gene Therapy

Alexandra McCarron[1,2,3], Nigel Farrow[1,2,3], Patricia Cmielewski[1,2,3], Emma Knight[4,5], Martin Donnelley[1,2,3†] and David Parsons[1,2,3†]*

[1]Adelaide Medical School, University of Adelaide, Adelaide, SA, Australia, [2]Robinson Research Institute, University of Adelaide, Adelaide, SA, Australia, [3]Department of Respiratory and Sleep Medicine, Women's and Children's Hospital, Adelaide, SA, Australia, [4]School of Public Health, University of Adelaide, Adelaide, SA, Australia, [5]South Australian Health and Medical Research Institute, Adelaide, SA, Australia

***Correspondence:**
Alexandra McCarron
alexandra.mccarron@adelaide.edu.au

†These authors share senior authorship

The lungs have evolved complex physical, biological and immunological defences to prevent foreign material from entering the airway epithelial cells. These mechanisms can also affect both viral and non-viral gene transfer agents, and significantly diminish the effectiveness of airway gene-addition therapies. One strategy to overcome the physical barrier properties of the airway is to transiently disturb the integrity of the epithelium prior to delivery of the gene transfer vector. In this study, chemical (lysophosphatidylcholine, LPC) and physical epithelium disruption using wire abrasion were compared for their ability to improve airway-based lentiviral (LV) vector mediated transduction and reporter gene expression in rats. When *luciferase* expression was assessed at 1-week post LV delivery, LPC airway conditioning significantly enhanced gene expression levels in rat lungs, while a long-term assessment in a separate cohort of rats at 12 months revealed that LPC conditioning did not improve gene expression longevity. In rats receiving physical perturbation to the trachea prior to gene delivery, significantly higher *LacZ* gene expression levels were found when compared to LPC-conditioned or LV-only control rats when evaluated 1-week post gene transfer. This proof-of-principle study has shown that airway epithelial disruption strategies based on physical perturbation substantially enhanced LV-mediated airway gene transfer in the trachea.

Keywords: lentiviral vector, gene therapy, airway, epithelium, rat

INTRODUCTION

Airway gene-addition therapy is currently under development for treatment of a range of hereditary and acquired pulmonary disorders. Of particular interest is the development of a gene therapy to treat airway disease caused by the genetic disorder cystic fibrosis. Gene-addition therapy employs a vector (non-viral or viral) to deliver wild-type gene copies to the relevant airway cells, with the ultimate goal of correcting the disease pathophysiology that results from the defective gene. While gene vectors can be readily delivered into the lung airways, physical, anatomical, and immune barriers have evolved to protect the host airway cells against airborne pathogens. These natural defences are also directed towards gene transfer vectors, thus limiting gene transduction in the airway epithelium.

Major hurdles to efficient viral-vector mediated gene transfer include a polarised epithelium, paucity of viral receptors on the apical membrane, and the presence of airway tight-junctions that prevent vectors from accessing receptors located on the basolateral side (Copreni et al., 2004). One way to overcome these barriers is to perform epithelial perturbation prior to, or in conjunction with gene transfer vector delivery. Perturbation methods act to disrupt tight-junction integrity, allowing vector particles access to basolateral receptors, thus enhancing vector-mediated gene transfer (Johnson et al., 2000; Pickles, 2004; Kim et al., 2016). Epithelial perturbation can also potentially expose cells for transduction that are not in direct contact with the airway lumen, particularly the basal cells, which function as tissue-specific stem cells (Rock et al., 2009).

To achieve basolateral access, airway conditioning with a chemical "tight-junction opener" can be employed to increase paracellular permeability. Airway conditioning with compounds including ethylene glycol tetraacetic acid (EGTA) (Chu et al., 2001), perfluorochemicals (Li et al., 2007), sodium caprate (Gregory et al., 2003), and sulphur dioxide inhalation (Johnson et al., 2000) have proven effective for disrupting tight-junctions and increasing viral-vector mediated gene transfer in proof-of-principle animal studies (Castellani and Conese, 2010). Another compound that has been investigated extensively for this purpose is lysophosphatidylcholine (LPC) (Limberis et al., 2002; Koehler et al., 2005; Cmielewski et al., 2010; Cao et al., 2013; Cmielewski et al., 2014). LPC is a natural component of lung surfactant that can be used to transiently open cellular tight-junctions when applied to the airway surface. A two-step dosing regimen employing LPC conditioning prior to the delivery of a HIV-1-derived lentiviral (LV) vector pseudotyped with the vesicular stomatitis virus glycoprotein (VSV-G) has proven effective at increasing airway gene transfer in mouse nasal airways (Cmielewski et al., 2010; Cmielewski et al., 2014), but has not yet been assessed in rat lower airways.

Chemical conditioning approaches have disadvantages when it comes to performing LV-mediated gene transfer. LV vectors are highly fragile due to the presence of an outer lipid envelope (Bandeira et al., 2012) and can be inactivated upon contact with conditioning agents such as LPC. Although two separate administrations–one to deliver the conditioning compound, and then a second to deliver the vector after the chemical effect occurs–can be used to enable LV vectors to take advantage of this delivery enhancement effect, this two-step process increases procedure time and complexity. Additionally, transduction may be variable as there is no guarantee that the conditioning compound and the vector will localise to the same regions (Flotte et al., 2007).

An alternative strategy to disrupt the integrity of the airway epithelium is *via* physical perturbation techniques. An early airway gene therapy study employing an adenoviral vector demonstrated that externally applied mechanical injury to the airway epithelium *via* use of fine forceps is a simple and effective way to produce strong reporter gene expression in the trachea of mice. Mechanical perturbation also resulted in high levels of basal cell transduction as this technique removed the superficial transduction-resistant columnar cells thus exposing underlying basal cells to the vector (Pickles et al., 1996). While early studies validated the potential efficacy of a physical perturbation strategy, it has not been investigated further for pre-clinical development, likely due to the perceived impracticalities of performing controlled airway-surface perturbation in animal models. To our knowledge there are no reports of physical airway injury being used in combination with LV vectors for *in vivo* gene delivery.

In this study, physical airway epithelium perturbation was explored as a strategy to improve *in vivo* gene transfer levels in the trachea of rats and this method was compared to standard LPC-conditioning and a perturbation-free LV-only control group. Additionally, we provide the first evidence of the effectiveness of LPC conditioning and LV vector delivery in rat lungs over both short-term (1-week) and long-term (12-month) durations.

MATERIALS AND METHODS

Multiple treatment groups were employed in this project. The first study assessed whether LPC had an effect on short- and long-term gene expression levels. In this study, rats received LPC conditioning or a PBS-sham treatment, followed by a HIV-1 derived EF1α-3XFLAG-fLuc-F2A-eGFP vector (LV-FLAG-Luc-GFP) vector. In one cohort (n = 6 per group) *luciferase* expression was measured 1-week following gene delivery, and in a separate cohort (n = 12 per group) expression was measured 12-months after LV delivery. To investigate and compare airway epithelial disruption strategies, separate groups of rats received either no epithelial disruption (control group), physical perturbation, or standard 0.1% LPC conditioning, followed by delivery of a HIV-1-MPSV-nlsLacZ vector (LV-LacZ) (n = 6 per group). Gene expression levels were assessed 1-week post gene transfer in this cohort of animals, as it was expected that the damaged airway epithelium would be largely regenerated and that gene expression would be readily apparent by this stage (Shimizu et al., 1994; Pickles et al., 1996).

Lentiviral Vector Production

LV vector was produced using previously described methods (Rout-Pitt et al., 2018; McCarron et al., 2019). The bicistronic LV-FLAG-Luc-GFP vector expressed firefly *luciferase* and enhanced *green fluorescent protein* (eGFP) genes under control of the EF1α promoter, together with three epitope FLAG tags. The LV-LacZ vector construct expressed a nuclear-localised β-*galactosidase* gene directed by the MPSV (myeloproliferative sarcoma virus) promoter. LV-FLAG-Luc-GFP was titered by quantifying the proportion of GFP positive cells using flow cytometry (McCarron et al., 2019). The titre of the LV-LacZ vector was determined using real-time quantitative PCR as previously described (Anson et al., 2007).

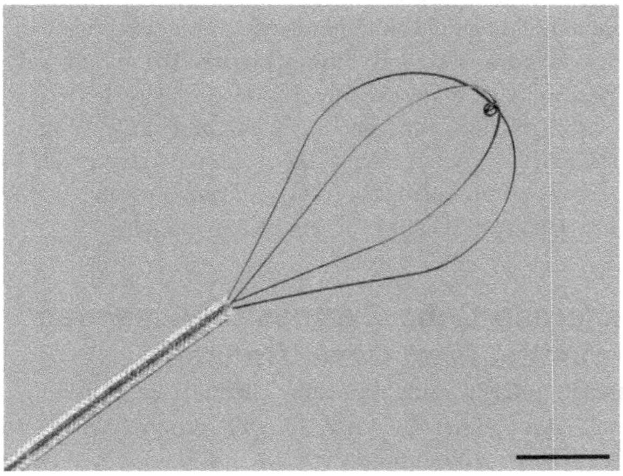

FIGURE 1 | Flexible wire basket used to physically perturb the tracheal airway epithelium. The basket is 1 cm in diameter at full expansion and 1.5 cm in length. Scale bar = 5 mm.

Animals

All animal procedures were approved by the University of Adelaide Animal Ethics Committee under applications M-2016–086 and M-2019–061. Female and male Sprague Dawley rats aged >8 weeks were used. For all LV-dosing procedures, rats were anaesthetised with medetomidine (0.4 mg/kg) and ketamine (60 mg/kg) by intraperitoneal injection. Following anaesthesia, the rats were non-surgically intubated with a 16-gauge intravenous cannula (Terumo, SR-FF1651, Japan) acting as an endotracheal (ET) tube, positioned with the tip just past the vocal cords so that the majority of the tracheal tissue was exposed to the conditioning or perturbation and LVvector. Rats that received physical airway perturbation were given subcutaneous administration of meloxicam (1 mg/kg) for precautionary pain relief. After procedure completion anaesthesia was reversed with atipamezole (1 mg/kg).

Intratracheal Administration of LPC and Lentiviral Vector

Animals were placed in a supine position and received either 25 µL of 0.1% LPC (Sigma-Aldrich, L4129, USA) or PBS. Fluid was administered to the trachea *via* the ET tube using a gel-loading pipette tip that was lengthened with fine polyethylene tubing marked to reach the distal tip of the ET tube. LV vector delivery was performed either without any pre-treatment or one hour following LPC conditioning (or PBS-sham) as this is the time when LPC epithelial tight-junction opening effects are apparent (Cmielewski et al., 2010). LV-FLAG-Luc-GFP (1×10^9 TU/mL) or LV-LacZ (2×10^9 TU/mL) were delivered to the trachea in two aliquots of 25 µL (50 µL total per animal).

Physical Epithelial Perturbation

With the intubated animal in the supine position, a pliable wire-basket (NCircle® Nitinol Tipless Stone Extractor NTSE-022115-UDH, Cook Medical, USA; **Figure 1**) was fed in the retracted position down the ET tube to approximately the carina (based on an average trachea length measurement). The basket was then extended, fully expanded, and drawn up and down the trachea (approximately 10 times per animal) for 30 seconds followed by withdrawal. Two 25 µL aliquots of LV-LacZ (2×10^9 TU/mL) were delivered *via* the ET tube within ten minutes of the perturbation event.

Bioluminescence Imaging (BLI)

Either 1-week or 12-months following LV-FLAG-Luc-GFP delivery rats were anaesthetised with 2.5% inhaled isoflurane. Once unconscious, 200 µL of 15 mg/mL D-luciferin (Cayman Chemicals, United States) was delivered to the nostrils as a bolus. Each animal was imaged in the supine position (IVIS Lumina XRMS *in vivo* imaging system, PerkinElmer, United States) while maintained with 1.5–2% isoflurane. Animals were imaged with an automatic exposure at 5-minute intervals for up to 15 minutes post D-luciferin delivery. The animals were then humanely killed with intraperitoneal delivery of sodium pentobarbital (150–300 mg/kg). The trachea and lungs were immediately excised and imaged separately in a petri dish containing PBS. Bioluminescence flux (photons/second) was measured using the contour tool (Living Image, version 4.7.2, PerkinElmer, United States).

Assessment of LacZ Gene Expression

Animals were humanely killed by carbon dioxide asphyxiation and the airway tissues harvested for LacZ staining. Tissues were fixed in 4% PFA and stained for β-galactosidase (LacZ) activity using X-gal as previously described (Cmielewski et al., 2017). Following X-gal staining, the trachea was cut and opened longitudinally, and separated into two halves. *En face* images of the tissue were acquired with a Nikon SMZ1500 stereo microscope; DigiLite 3.0 MP Camera and TC capture software (Tucsen Photonics, China). Illumination intensity was not altered between samples. Tracheas were subsequently paraffin-embedded, sectioned at 5 µM, and counterstained with nuclear fast red. Histology images were captured with a Nikon Eclipse E400 microscope, DS-Fi2-U3 camera and NIS-elements D software (version 5.20.00).

Immunohistochemistry

X-gal stained sections were deparaffinised and subjected to heat-mediated antigen retrieval in sodium citrate buffer (10 mM sodium citrate, 0.05% Tween 20, pH 6.0) at 95–100°C for 20 minutes. A peroxidase blocking step was performed using 3% hydrogen peroxide followed by permeabilisation with 0.3% Triton X-100 for 10 minutes. Protein blocking was performed with 10% goat serum in PBS. Primary and secondary antibodies were diluted in 1% bovine serum albumin and 0.1% Triton X-100 in PBS. Sections were probed with rabbit anti-cytokeratin 5 antibody (Abcam, ab52635, UK) (1:400 dilution) and were incubated overnight at 4°C. Tissues were washed and subsequently incubated with goat anti-rabbit IgG HRP (Abcam, ab97051, UK) (1:500 dilution) for 1 hour at room temperature followed by staining with 3,3′-Diaminobenzidine.

Digital Quantification of LacZ Staining in en Face Trachea Images

The amount of LacZ staining in the *en face* images of the trachea was quantified using a custom-written script in Matlab (R2020a, MathWorks) that calculated the area of the trachea that was the specific shade of blue/green of LacZ-positive cells. Briefly, images were converted from the RGB to HSV colour space, and separate thresholds were applied to the hue ($0.45 < H < 0.6$) and saturation ($s > 0.4$) channels. The value channel was not used because the illumination across the sample was uneven and did not help discriminate the transduced cells. A binary mask was created from the regions of the image that satisfied both criteria. The mask area was converted from pixels into mm.

Statistical Analyses

Statistical analyses were performed using either R v4.0.0 (Team, 2020) or GraphPad Prism v8 (GraphPad Software, Inc.). Statistical significance was set at $p \leq 0.05$. For the short-term study, comparisons of flux between PBS and LPC groups were performed using Welch two sample t-tests on log-transformed data. To compare flux between the PBS and LPC treatments for the long-term study, a hurdle regression model was fitted using the *hurdle* function in the *pscl* package in R (Zeileis et al., 2008). The hurdle regression model is a two-part model; a binary logit model to distinguish between the positive counts and those below the detection limit (assigned the value 100), and a zero-truncated negative binomial model for the positive counts. Treatment (PBS, LPC) was fitted as the regressor in both parts of the model. Differences between the groups were assessed using a Wald Chi-Squared test. The LacZ staining area measurements from the *en face* images was analysed using a one-way ANOVA with Tukey's multiple comparisons test.

RESULTS

Animal Procedures

Chemical and physical airway perturbation techniques were well-tolerated by the rats with all animals surviving the procedures. Animal weight, health and wellbeing characteristics were assessed daily for the duration of the study using a score-based animal monitoring system, with no significant effects on animal health noted. Expected transient weight loss was similar in all experimental groups (LPC, physical and LV-only), irrespective of whether airway perturbation was performed (data not shown).

Luciferase Gene Expression Assessed 1-week Post Gene Transfer

In the short-term assessment, rats received either PBS or LPC conditioning and were imaged 1-week following a single LV gene delivery. Bioluminescence was predominantly observed in the lungs *in vivo*, with only one animal exhibiting signal in the trachea region (**Figure 2**). Statistical analysis of the *in vivo* data revealed that LPC conditioning resulted in significantly higher flux when compared to animals that received the PBS sham treatment (**Figure 4A**). Upon excision of the tissues and subsequent imaging, bioluminescence was observed in the trachea (**Figure 3A**) and lungs (**Figure 3B**) of all animals. Analysis of the *ex vivo* data indicated that there was no difference in flux between the LPC and PBS conditioned groups for the trachea, while the excised lungs revealed that LPC airway conditioned rats had significantly greater flux levels (**Figure 4A**), regardless of the sex of the animals.

Luciferase Gene Expression Assessed 12-months Post Gene Transfer

In the long-term study assessing chemical conditioning, few animals from either the LPC or PBS group had detectable levels of *in vivo* bioluminescence at the 12-month time point (data not shown), therefore statistical comparisons could not be performed on this data. *Ex vivo* imaging of the trachea also revealed insufficient animals with bioluminescence present to perform statistical analysis. Imaging of the *ex vivo* lungs showed that close to half the animals from both LPC and PBS groups had values recorded at the limit of bioluminescence detection. Additionally, the flux levels measured in the *ex vivo* lungs at 12 months were substantially lower compared to the animals imaged at 1-week post-delivery. *Ex vivo* lung imaging revealed that there was no significant difference in flux between LPC conditioned and PBS-sham animals' 12-months following LV-delivery (**Figure 4B**).

Tracheal LacZ Gene Expression Following Chemical Conditioning and Physical Perturbation

En face observations of the trachea revealed different levels of LacZ staining as a result of the perturbation or conditioning method used. Visually, rats that received physical perturbation prior to LV-delivery demonstrated greatly enhanced LacZ staining in the trachea when compared to rats that received LPC conditioning or LV vector-only (**Figure 5**). Interestingly, one animal in the physical perturbation group exhibited much lower staining levels compared to the others, indicative of potential variability with this technique. The transduction patterns observed as a result of physical perturbation were not uniform in appearance. Striated regions of increased staining over the intercartilaginous ligaments were apparent in all specimens, possibly reflecting the presence of cilia-rich zones that overlay the ligament segments in rats (Oliveira et al., 2003) and preferential transduction of ciliated cells by the VSV-G pseudotyped LV gene transfer vector. Varying LacZ staining patterns and strong expression were observed in animals that received physical perturbation (**Figures 6A–F**). Notably, rats in the LPC and LV-only groups demonstrated the highest levels of staining in the proximal trachea (**Supplementary Figure S1**), likely due to unintentional ET tube-induced epithelial damage in this region, providing further support for the effectiveness of physical perturbation in boosting airway gene transfer.

Digital quantification of the blue-green coloured regions in the *en face* trachea images demonstrated significantly greater levels of

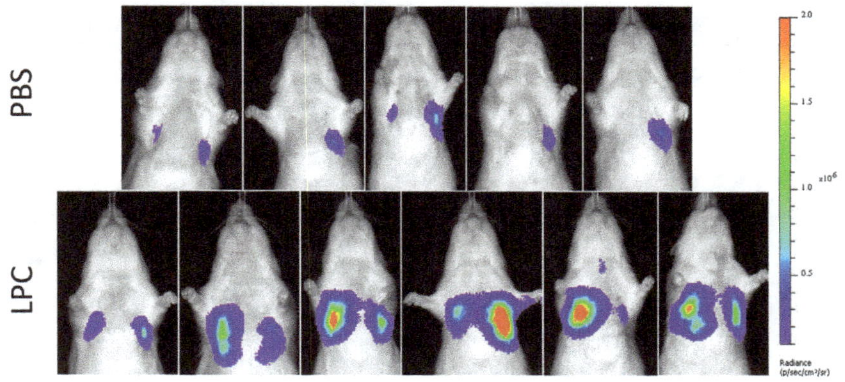

FIGURE 2 | *In vivo* bioluminescence images acquired 1-week following LV-FLAG-Luc-GFP delivery in PBS-sham and LPC conditioned rats. Localisation of bioluminescence *in vivo* was predominantly in the lung region in both PBS and LPC pre-treated animals.

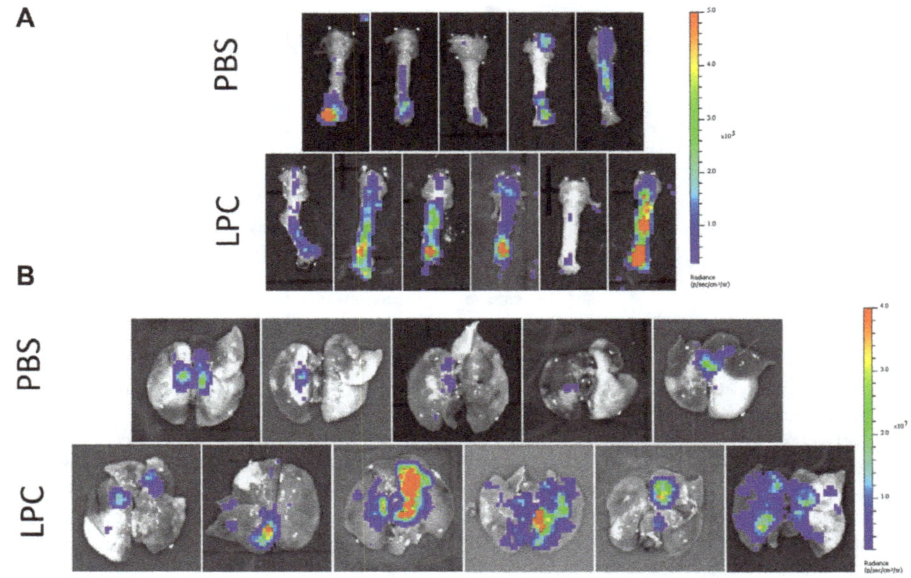

FIGURE 3 | *Ex vivo* bioluminescence images acquired 1-week following LV-FLAG-Luc-GFP delivery in PBS-sham and LPC conditioned rats. *Ex vivo* images of **(A)** the trachea and **(B)** lungs following removal of the trachea.

LacZ staining in the physical perturbation group, when compared to LPC conditioned and LV vector-only control rats (**Figure 7**). The physical damage group demonstrated more than a 1000-fold increase in the area of LacZ staining when compared to the control group. There was no statistically significant difference in staining area between LPC conditioned rats and controls that received only LV vector with no epithelial disruption prior to delivery.

Histological Observations Arising From Physical Perturbation

A range of different cell types were transduced as a result of performing physical perturbation prior to LV vector delivery. LacZ-positive ciliated and non-ciliated cells were observed in the tracheal epithelium (**Figures 8A,B**) and immunohistochemical staining for cytokeratin 5 confirmed the presence of transduced basal cells (**Figure 9**). Cells within the lamina propria were also transduced, including suspected macrophages (**Figure 8C**) and regions of connective tissue (**Figure 8D**). Histologically, the tracheal tissue demonstrated evidence of repair processes caused by damage to the epithelium and surrounding areas. Most regions of the tracheal epithelium had fully regenerated by 1-week post treatment, consistent with the timing observed in previous studies (Shimizu et al., 1994; Pickles et al., 1996). However, occasionally areas of epithelium were found to still be undergoing repair, as indicated by an attenuated appearance, lack of cilia and rounding of the columnar cells (**Figure 8E**), or in other regions, proliferation of connective tissue (**Figure 8F**). Goblet cell hyperplasia was also apparent at the carina and

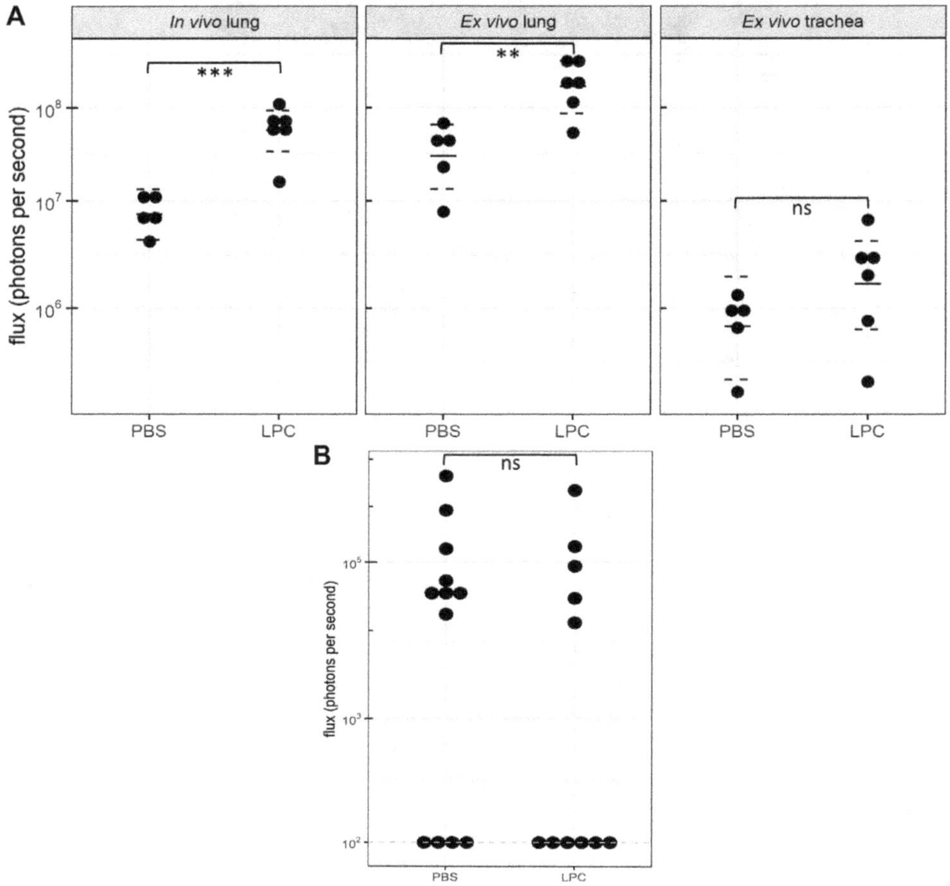

FIGURE 4 | Bioluminescence flux (log scale) acquired 1-week and 12 months following LV-FLAG-Luc-GFP delivery in PBS-sham and LPC conditioned rats. **(A)** *In vivo* and *ex vivo* bioluminescence flux acquired 1-week post gene transfer. Statistical analyses of the *in vivo and ex vivo* lung data revealed significant differences in flux between PBS and LPC conditioned groups, with $p = 0.0002$ and $p = 0.005$, respectively. Statistical analysis of the *ex vivo* trachea indicated there was no significant difference in flux between LPC and PBS groups, $p = 0.2$. The plot shows the estimated median and 95% confidence intervals. $n = 5$-6 animals per group, Welch two sample *t*-test, ns = not significant, $^{**}p \leq 0.01$, $^{***}p \leq 0.001$. **(B)** *Ex vivo* lung bioluminescence flux acquired 12 months following gene transfer. The dashed line indicates the limit of detection of the IVIS machine (10^2). No significant difference in flux was observed between animals in the PBS and LPC groups, $p = 0.6$. $n = 11$–12 animals per group, Wald Chi-squared test, ns = not significant.

upper bronchi of two animals (**Figure 8G**). Interestingly, many of these hyperplastic goblet cells appeared to be LacZ-positive (**Figure 8H**).

DISCUSSION

Gene-addition therapy is a promising option for treatment of certain pulmonary diseases, but there are still many challenges to successful translation to the clinic. Adequate delivery of therapeutic agents to cells of the airway epithelium remains one of the greatest challenges to achieving effective lung-based genetic therapies, including gene-addition and gene editing strategies. The lung has evolved mechanisms to resist invasion by foreign bodies, with the airway epithelium acting as a physical barrier that significantly reduces the efficacy of airway gene transfer. Many viral vectors used for airway gene therapies have a natural tropism toward receptors located on the basolateral membrane and thus produce limited transduction *via* the apical surface when applied to an intact airway epithelium.

To overcome inefficient transduction, strategies have been employed to disrupt the integrity of the airway epithelium prior to gene delivery, allowing the vector access to basolateral membrane-located receptors, and to cells that are not in direct contact with the airway lumen such as basal cells (Pickles, 2004). Given our recent generation of two cystic fibrosis rat models (McCarron et al., 2020), the work reported here employed normal rats to develop and assess chemical and physical airway perturbation methods. In these studies, the trachea was used a surrogate for the lower conducting airways, as it is easily accessible for physical perturbation techniques and the cellular architecture is similar to human lower airways (Mercer et al., 1994).

In this work, the effectiveness of LPC conditioning was assessed for the first time in rat airways. While mouse studies have shown enhanced gene expression when using LPC conditioning prior to LV gene transfer (Cmielewski et al., 2014; Cmielewski et al., 2017), its effects in rat airways were

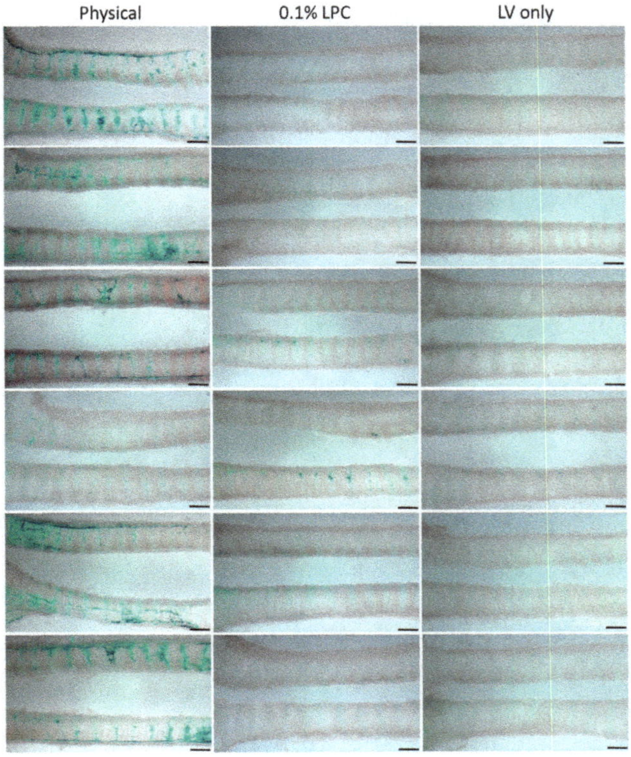

FIGURE 5 | Comparison of *en face* LacZ staining using physical perturbation, chemical conditioning with 0.1% LPC, or LV vector-only assessed 1-week post gene transfer. Images show the trachea from each individual animal longitudinally cut into two sections to reveal the LacZ staining present within the lumen. The images display the middle portion of the trachea and are oriented to show the proximal trachea on the right. $n = 6$ rats per group. Scale bar = 1.5 mm.

unknown. In this study, gene expression levels were found to be significantly increased in the lungs of rats that received LPC conditioning when assessed 1-week post vector delivery. Upon *in vivo* imaging, only one animal exhibited bioluminescence signal within the trachea, but following excision of the tissues and subsequent *ex vivo* imaging, bioluminescence was observed in the trachea of all animals, albeit at varying levels. When imaged *ex vivo* the flux emitted from the trachea was substantially lower than the *ex vivo* lung, therefore the low bioluminescence in combination with the need to detect the signal through the overlying skin and tissue may explain the lack of tracheal bioluminescence upon *in vivo* imaging. Notably, when the trachea was excised and imaged, LPC did not appear to enhance bioluminescence flux when compared to the PBS-sham group.

Long-term gene expression was assessed in a separate cohort of rats, which revealed that *luciferase* gene expression persisted in the lungs of some animals for up to 12 months following a single LV-delivery, irrespective of whether LPC airway conditioning was performed. These two studies indicate that while LPC conditioning initially improves transduction levels in the lungs, it does not increase the longevity of gene expression, suggesting that basal cell transduction was not substantially enhanced with use of LPC. Nevertheless, it is likely that basal cells, or other known lung stem cell types (e.g., club cells, alveolar type II cells), were transduced in animals from both LPC and PBS-sham groups, as the duration of gene expression exceeds the four month lifespan of terminally differentiated tracheal-bronchial epithelium described in adult rodents (Rawlins and Hogan, 2006).

While LV-mediated gene transfer demonstrated persistent *luciferase* gene expression in a proportion of rats, many individuals from both the LPC conditioning and PBS-sham groups had undetectable flux by 12 months. The lack of gene expression observed at the 12 month time point could potentially be attributed to transgene silencing (Ellis, 2005), alternatively, loss of gene-expressing cells with natural cell-turnover may explain this observation. We do not have data that can explain why some individuals responded better than others, though this phenomenon is consistently observed in airway gene therapy animal studies. Possible factors include but are not limited to, the proportion of basal cells transduced, varying host immune responses to the vector and formulation, size of the animal (which dictates the surface area to vector volume ratio), vector-fluid dynamics and animal respiration rate/depth, which can result in variable gene vector distribution within the airways, and the amount of time that the vector is in contact with the airway surface. An improved understanding of the basis of these variable individual responses to airway gene-addition therapy would provide significant value for progressing to clinical trials.

In the second study employing LV-LacZ vector, physical perturbation of the airway epithelium resulted in very high levels of gene transduction in the trachea when compared to animals receiving LPC chemical conditioning or LV vector-only. Moreover, LPC conditioning did not significantly enhance tracheal LacZ expression above the control (LV-only) group, consistent with the short-term bioluminescence study where LPC use did not result in a significant increase in tracheal flux when compared with the PBS-sham group. However, it is important to note that the LPC conditioning protocol used here had been previously established for mice, therefore the concentration or volume employed may not have been optimal for rats.

As with many viral receptors, the VSV-G receptor (low-density lipoprotein) is located on the basolateral surface, and transduction *via* the apical surface is typically low level (Finkelshtein et al., 2013). While the mechanisms here are not fully understood, it is likely that physical perturbation increases gene transfer *via* two potential routes: 1) disruption of the integrity of the epithelial tight-junctions allowing the gene transfer vector entry to epithelial cells *via* basolateral receptors, or 2) removal of transduction-resistant columnar cells and exposure of more susceptible cell types on the basement membrane (e.g., basal cells). In this study, physical damage was confirmed to produce basal cell transduction. Additionally, both *en face* and histological examination revealed distinct clusters of LacZ-positive cells, reminiscent of basal cell clonal expansion observed in previous studies of induced regeneration following polidocanol epithelial stripping (Mitomo et al., 2010; Farrow et al., 2018). These clusters suggest

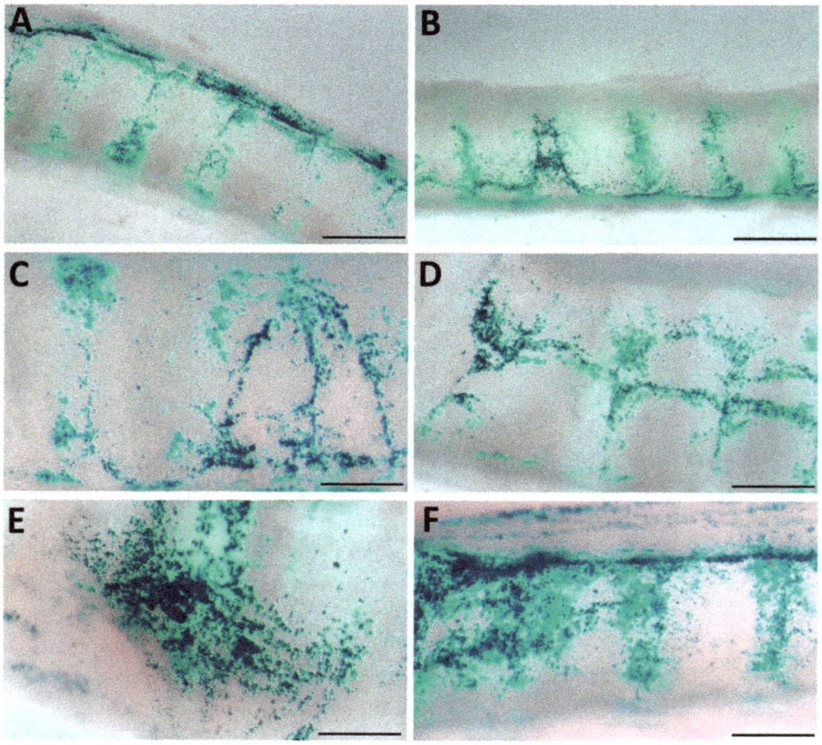

FIGURE 6 | Physical perturbation reveals varying patterns of LacZ staining. **(A, B)** LacZ staining is increased in the areas overlying the inter-cartilage segments **(C–F)** Basket-induced perturbation creates regions of strong staining. High magnification images were acquired from the samples shown in **Figure 5** and indicate staining patterns present in multiple animals. Scale bars A, B = 1.5 mm; C-F = 0.75 mm.

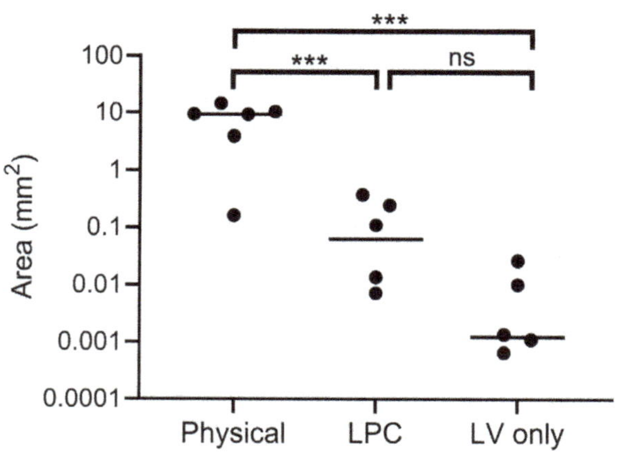

FIGURE 7 | Quantification of LacZ staining area (log scale) from *en face* trachea images shown in **Figure 5**. Physical perturbation had a significantly greater area of tracheal LacZ staining after 1-week when compared to LPC conditioned ($p = 0.001$) and LV vector-only control animals ($p = 0.0008$). There was no significant difference in the area of LacZ staining between LPC conditioned animals and those that received only LV vector ($p = 0.1$). The plot indicates the median. $n = 6$ animals per group, one-way ANOVA with Tukey's post-hoc test, ns = not significant, $^{***}p \leq 0.001$. Note that two animals are not observable on the plot as the quantified area was zero.

that one or more basal stem cells have been transduced and subsequently differentiated into a LacZ expressing pseudostratified epithelium, consistent with previous studies showing the timing of epithelial regeneration in rat airways following mechanical injury (Shimizu et al., 1994). However, further work including lineage tracing studies would be necessary to confirm this hypothesis. Alternatively, it is possible that clusters of LacZ-expressing cells may be due to strong focal damage or repetitive contact with the basket, making these areas more susceptible to LV-transduction.

Physical perturbation of the airway surface may provide gene transfer vectors with improved access to basal cells. An airway gene-addition therapy that transduces only the terminally differentiated airway surface cells could result in an inevitable waning of transgene expression with normal cell turnover, and the need for vector readministration. While repeated administration is unlikely to be completely avoided, multiple deliveries of a viral-based gene therapy is undesirable as immune responses may be elicited thus reducing the efficacy of subsequent doses (Sinn et al., 2009; Mitomo et al., 2010). Basal cells are multipotent stem cells of the conducting airways and have the capacity for self-renewal, clonal expansion, and the ability to differentiate into epithelial cells types to maintain homeostasis and repair following injury (Hong et al., 2004; Rock

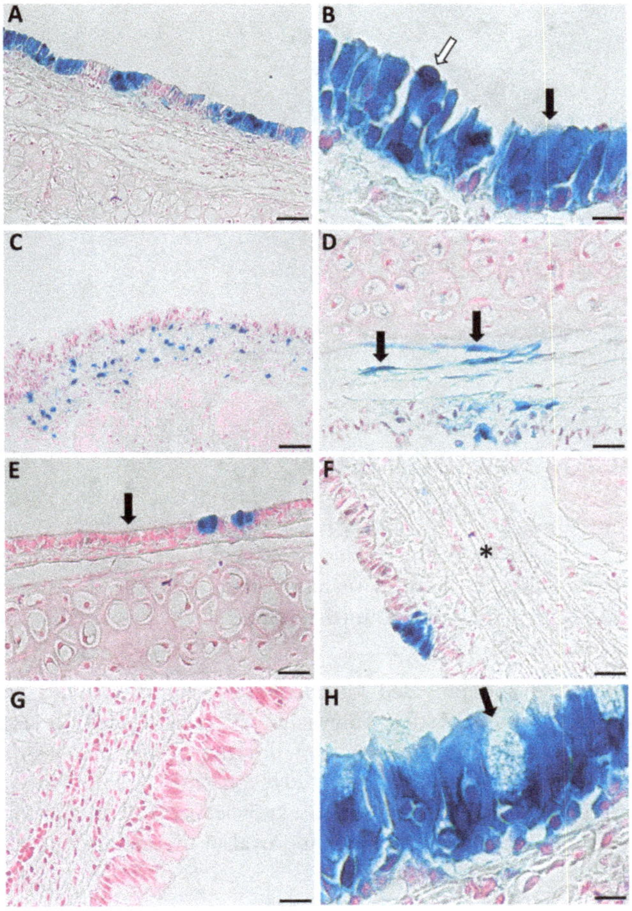

FIGURE 8 | Histological observations in the tracheal epithelium of rats that received physical perturbation prior to LV-LacZ vector delivery assessed 1-week post gene transfer. **(A)** LacZ staining was discontinuous throughout the tracheal epithelium with some areas of intense staining observed. **(B)** A range of LacZ-positive surface epithelial cell types were noted including ciliated (black arrow) and non-ciliated (white arrow) cells. Transduced regions were noted within the lamina propria including **(C)** suspected macrophages and **(D)** connective tissue. While most of the tissue demonstrated full regeneration, some regions showed **(E)** a flattened epithelial layer lacking pseudostratification, while other regions demonstrated **(F)** connective tissue proliferation (fibrosis) in response to healing (denoted by asterisk). **(G)** Goblet cell hyperplasia was found at the carina of two animals with **(H)** a proportion of these goblet cells exhibiting LacZ staining. Goblet cells were identified by a distinct goblet shape and granules filled with mucus. Images are shown from selected animals. Nuclear fast red counterstain. Scale bar = 10 μM.

et al., 2009; Rock et al., 2010; Hogan et al., 2014). Successful transduction of basal cells has the ability to produce enduring gene expression, as the gene-corrected progeny will repopulate the surface epithelium following natural cell turnover. It is therefore desirable to develop an airway gene-addition therapy that not only produces efficient gene transfer but can also transduce basal cells (Cao et al., 2018; Farrow et al., 2018).

Following use of physical perturbation, cells within some regions of the tracheal lamina propria appeared to be transduced. While a certain degree of epithelial injury was expected, these findings suggest that in some areas the physical perturbation extended too far into the airway surface, likely due to forces produced by the wire basket or repetitive contact. Goblet cell hyperplasia was also noted in some animals, a protective response that can occur as a result of mucosal surface irritation (Herbert et al., 2018). Notably, the animals that displayed goblet cell hyperplasia had many LacZ-positive goblet cells within these regions, suggesting that intact basal cells were transduced and subsequently differentiated into goblet cells upon epithelial regeneration. Our previous short-term assessments have shown that VSV-G pseudotyped LV vectors rarely transduce goblet cells (Limberis et al., 2002; Farrow et al., 2018), so their presence further indicates likely expansion and differentiation of transduced basal cells.

One major benefit of physical perturbation noted in this study is the ability to achieve high transduction levels from a relatively small number of LV particles per animal (1×10^8 TU). By using physical epithelial disruption methods to improve gene transfer efficacy, the LV titres required to achieve therapeutic levels of gene correction could be reduced, thus improving the feasibility of an *in vivo* gene therapy approach. Moreover, such reductions in vector titre would provide the benefits of lower LV production time and cost, as well as lessened immune responses. The advantages of physical perturbation could also be applied to improving the efficacy of other lung-based genetic therapies including delivery of gene editing machinery, nanoparticle-based gene transfer systems, and stem cell-transplantation strategies. For instance, airway engraftment of transplanted cells could be facilitated *via* use of physical perturbation methods rather than chemical agents, which have previously been employed pre-clinically to achieve epithelial disruption (King et al., 2020), but have disadvantages such as toxicity and poor delivery control.

While the results of this tracheal physical perturbation study provide promising proof-of-principle data, the target for cystic fibrosis airway gene-addition therapy will be the lower conducting airways, as this is where disease pathophysiology occurs. Accordingly, further pre-clinical work in rats is needed to assess the feasibility of this approach in the lower airways, with our previously established rat bronchoscopy methods offering a potential option for enabling access to these small airways for perturbation. Our minimally invasive miniature bronchoscope technique provides access to at least the fourth generation of branching in an adult rat, therefore perturbation-devices could be guided *via* the bronchoscope working channel to the small airways (McIntyre et al., 2018). In addition to rat studies, investigations using larger animals such as pigs or sheep will be necessary to identify the features of a perturbation device that would be considered safe and effective for human clinical use.

Histological assessment of the airway tissue immediately post-damage, and the time-course of epithelial regeneration following physical perturbation, will also provide value for understanding the mechanisms that result in improved gene transfer with this approach. Future studies should aim to establish more refined techniques to improve control and reduce the intensity of the perturbation, so that off-target cell transduction and disruption to the subepithelial tissue is minimised. Ultimately, a careful balance between safety, tolerability, and efficacy aspects will be critical in pursuing this type of physical perturbation approach for human

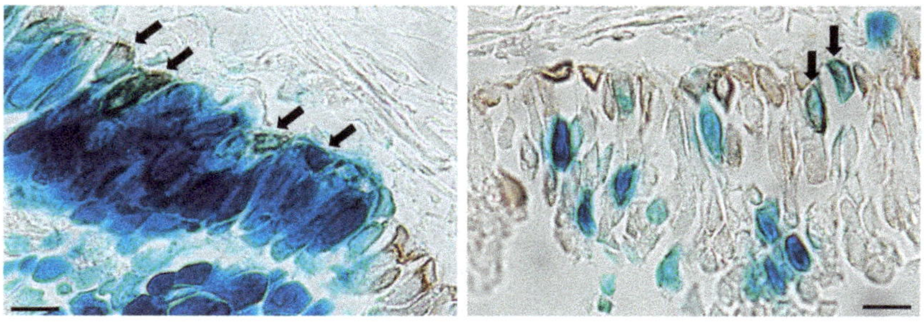

FIGURE 9 | Immunohistochemical detection of basal cells in rats that received physical perturbation prior to LV-LacZ vector delivery assessed 1-week post gene transfer. Basal cells were identified by immunohistochemical staining with anti-cytokeratin 5 antibody as shown by brown staining. Examples of transduced basal cells are indicated by arrows. Scale bar = 10 μM.

airway gene therapy clinical trials. In the interim however, there remains considerable research value in developing physical perturbation approaches for pre-clinical investigation.

In summary, although LPC conditioning initially increased gene expression levels in rat lungs, it did not appear to improve reporter gene expression longevity. Even without conditioning, a proportion of rats had measurable flux present in the lungs 12 months following dosing, indicating that a single LV delivery can provide persistent gene expression, albeit at low levels. Physical perturbation to the trachea immediately prior to LV-mediated gene transfer resulted in a 1000-fold increase in LacZ staining when compared to animals that did not receive any airway perturbation, demonstrating that this approach can provide significant benefit for improving gene transfer efficacy and warrants further development and investigation.

AUTHOR CONTRIBUTIONS

AM contributed to study design, data collection, analysis and interpretation, and manuscript drafting. NF contributed to study conception and provided knowledge. PC contributed to data collection and provided knowledge. EK contributed to data analysis, data interpretation, and drafting of the manuscript. MD and DP contributed to study conception, data analysis and interpretation, provision of knowledge, and manuscript drafting. All authors gave final approval of the manuscript.

ACKNOWLEDGMENTS

The authors thank Nicole Reyne for assistance with animal work and Professor John Finnie for guidance in histology interpretation. Assistance was also provided by the University of Adelaide Laboratory Animal Services, Histology Services, and Adelaide Microscopy.

REFERENCES

Anson, D. S., McIntyre, C., Thomas, B., Koldej, R., Ranieri, E., Roberts, A., et al. (2007). Lentiviral-mediated Gene Correction of Mucopolysaccharidosis Type IIIA. *Genet. Vaccin. Ther.* 5, 1. doi:10.1186/1479-0556-5-1

Bandeira, V., Peixoto, C., Rodrigues, A. F., Cruz, P. E., Alves, P. M., Coroadinha, A. S., et al. (2012). Downstream Processing of Lentiviral Vectors: Releasing Bottlenecks. *Hum. Gene Ther. Methods* 23, 255–263. doi:10.1089/hgtb.2012.059

Cao, H., Machuca, T. N., Yeung, J. C., Wu, J., Du, K., Duan, C., et al. (2013). Efficient Gene Delivery to Pig Airway Epithelia and Submucosal Glands Using Helper-dependent Adenoviral Vectors. *Mol. Ther. - Nucleic Acids* 2, e127. doi:10.1038/mtna.2013.55

Cao, H., Ouyang, H., Grasemann, H., Bartlett, C., Du, K., Duan, R., et al. (2018). Transducing Airway Basal Cells with a Helper-dependent Adenoviral Vector for Lung Gene Therapy. *Hum. Gene Ther.* 29, 643–652. doi:10.1089/hum.2017.201

Castellani, S., and Conese, M. (2010). Lentiviral Vectors and Cystic Fibrosis Gene Therapy. *Viruses* 2, 395–412. doi:10.3390/v2020395

Chu, Q., St. George, J. A., Lukason, M., Cheng, S. H., Scheule, R. K., and Eastman, S. J. (2001). EGTA Enhancement of Adenovirus-Mediated Gene Transfer to Mouse Tracheal Epitheliumin Vivo. *Hum. Gene Ther.* 12, 455–467. doi:10.1089/104303401300042348

Cmielewski, P., Anson, D. S., and Parsons, D. W. (2010). Lysophosphatidylcholine as an Adjuvant for Lentiviral Vector Mediated Gene Transfer to Airway Epithelium: Effect of Acyl Chain Length. *Respir. Res.* 11, 84. doi:10.1186/1465-9921-11-84

Cmielewski, P., Donnelley, M., and Parsons, D. W. (2014). Long-term Therapeutic and Reporter Gene Expression in Lentiviral Vector Treated Cystic Fibrosis Mice. *J. Gene Med.* 16, 291–299. doi:10.1002/jgm.2778

Cmielewski, P., Farrow, N., Devereux, S., Parsons, D., and Donnelley, M. (2017). Gene Therapy for Cystic Fibrosis: Improved Delivery Techniques and Conditioning with Lysophosphatidylcholine Enhance Lentiviral Gene Transfer in Mouse Lung Airways. *Exp. Lung Res.* 43, 426–433. doi:10.1080/01902148.2017.1395931

Copreni, E., Penzo, M., Carrabino, S., and Conese, M. (2004). Lentivirus-mediated Gene Transfer to the Respiratory Epithelium: a Promising Approach to Gene Therapy of Cystic Fibrosis. *Gene Ther.* 11, 67–75. doi:10.1038/sj.gt.3302372

Ellis, J. (2005). Silencing and Variegation of Gammaretrovirus and Lentivirus Vectors. *Hum. Gene Ther.* 16, 1241–1246. doi:10.1089/hum.2005.16.1241

Farrow, N., Donnelley, M., Cmielewski, P., Roscioli, E., Rout-Pitt, N., McIntyre, C., et al. (2018). Role of Basal Cells in Producing Persistent Lentivirus-Mediated Airway Gene Expression. *Hum. Gene Ther.* 29, 653–662. doi:10.1089/hum.2017.059

Finkelshtein, D., Werman, A., Novick, D., Barak, S., and Rubinstein, M. (2013). LDL Receptor and its Family Members Serve as the Cellular Receptors for Vesicular Stomatitis Virus. *Proc. Natl. Acad. Sci.* 110, 7306–7311. doi:10.1073/pnas.1214441110

Flotte, T. R., Ng, P., Dylla, D. E., McCray, P. B., Jr., Wang, G., Kolls, J. K., et al. (2007). Viral Vector-Mediated and Cell-Based Therapies for Treatment of Cystic Fibrosis. *Mol. Ther.* 15, 229–241. doi:10.1038/sj.mt.6300002

Gregory, L. G., Harbottle, R. P., Lawrence, L., Knapton, H. J., Themis, M., and Coutelle, C. (2003). Enhancement of Adenovirus-Mediated Gene Transfer to the Airways by DEAE Dextran and Sodium Caprate In Vivo. *Mol. Ther.* 7, 19–26. doi:10.1016/s1525-0016(02)00021-7

Herbert, R. A., Janardhan, K. S., Pandiri, A. R., Cesta, M. F., and Miller, R. A. (2018). "Chapter 22 - Nose, Larynx, and Trachea," in *Boorman's Pathology of the Rat*. Second Edition. Editor AW. Suttie (Boston: Academic Press), 391–435.

Hogan, B. L. M., Barkauskas, C. E., Chapman, H. A., Epstein, J. A., Jain, R., Hsia, C. C. W., et al. (2014). Repair and Regeneration of the Respiratory System: Complexity, Plasticity, and Mechanisms of Lung Stem Cell Function. *Cell Stem Cell* 15, 123–138. doi:10.1016/j.stem.2014.07.012

Hong, K. U., Reynolds, S. D., Watkins, S., Fuchs, E., and Stripp, B. R. (2004). Basal Cells Are a Multipotent Progenitor Capable of Renewing the Bronchial Epithelium. *Am. J. Pathol.* 164, 577–588. doi:10.1016/S0002-9440(10)63147-1

Johnson, L. G., Olsen, J. C., Naldini, L., and Boucher, R. C. (2000). Pseudotyped Human Lentiviral Vector-Mediated Gene Transfer to Airway Epithelia In Vivo. *Gene Ther.* 7, 568–574. doi:10.1038/sj.gt.3301138

Kim, N., Duncan, G. A., Hanes, J., and Suk, J. S. (2016). Barriers to Inhaled Gene Therapy of Obstructive Lung Diseases: A Review. *J. Controlled Release* 240, 465–488. doi:10.1016/j.jconrel.2016.05.031

King, N. E., Suzuki, S., Barillà, C., Hawkins, F. J., Randell, S. H., Reynolds, S. D., et al. (2020). Correction of Airway Stem Cells: Genome Editing Approaches for the Treatment of Cystic Fibrosis. *Hum. Gene Ther.* 31, 956–972. doi:10.1089/hum.2020.160

Koehler, D. R., Frndova, H., Leung, K., Louca, E., Palmer, D., Ng, P., et al. (2005). Aerosol Delivery of an Enhanced Helper-dependent Adenovirus Formulation to Rabbit Lung Using an Intratracheal Catheter. *J. Gene Med.* 7, 1409–1420. doi:10.1002/jgm.797

Li, J., Bonneau, L., Zimmerman, J., and Weiss, D. (2007). Perfluorochemical (PFC) Liquid Enhances Recombinant Adenovirus Vector-Mediated Viral Interleukin-10 (AdvIL-10) Expression in Rodent Lung. *J. Inflamm.* 4, 9. doi:10.1186/1476-9255-4-9

Limberis, M., Anson, D. S., Fuller, M., and Parsons, D. W. (2002). Recovery of Airway Cystic Fibrosis Transmembrane Conductance Regulator Function in Mice with Cystic Fibrosis after Single-Dose Lentivirus-Mediated Gene Transfer. *Hum. Gene Ther.* 13, 1961–1970. doi:10.1089/10430340260355365

McCarron, A., Cmielewski, P., Reyne, N., McIntyre, C., Finnie, J., Craig, F., et al. (2020). Phenotypic Characterization and Comparison of Cystic Fibrosis Rat Models Generated Using CRISPR/Cas9 Gene Editing. *Am. J. Pathol.* 190, 977–993. doi:10.1016/j.ajpath.2020.01.009

McCarron, A., Donnelley, M., McIntyre, C., and Parsons, D. (2019). Transient Lentiviral Vector Production Using a Packed-Bed Bioreactor System. *Hum. Gene Ther. Methods* 30, 93–101. doi:10.1089/hgtb.2019.038

McIntyre, C., Donnelley, M., Rout-Pitt, N., and Parsons, D. (2018). Lobe-Specific Gene Vector Delivery to Rat Lungs Using a Miniature Bronchoscope. *Hum. Gene Ther. Methods* 29, 228–235. doi:10.1089/hgtb.2018.050

Mercer, R. R., Russell, M. L., Roggli, V. L., and Crapo, J. D. (1994). Cell Number and Distribution in Human and Rat Airways. *Am. J. Respir. Cell Mol. Biol.* 10, 613. doi:10.1165/ajrcmb.10.6.8003339

Mitomo, K., Griesenbach, U., Inoue, M., Somerton, L., Meng, C., Akiba, E., et al. (2010). Toward Gene Therapy for Cystic Fibrosis Using a Lentivirus Pseudotyped with Sendai Virus Envelopes. *Mol. Ther.* 18, 1173–1182. doi:10.1038/Mt.2010.13

Oliveira, M. J. R., Pereira, A. S., Guimarães, L., Grande, N. R., Moreira de Sá, C., and Aguas, A. P. (2003). Zonation of Ciliated Cells on the Epithelium of the Rat Trachea. *Lung* 181, 275–282. doi:10.1007/s00408-003-1030-1

Pickles, R. J. (2004). Physical and Biological Barriers to Viral Vector-Mediated Delivery of Genes to the Airway Epithelium. *Proc. Am. Thorac. Soc.* 1, 302–308. doi:10.1513/pats.200403-024MS

Pickles, R. J., Barker, P. M., Ye, H., and Boucher, R. C. (1996). Efficient Adenovirus-Mediated Gene Transfer to Basal but Not Columnar Cells of Cartilaginous Airway Epithelia. *Hum. Gene Ther.* 7, 921–931. doi:10.1089/hum.1996.7.8-921

Rawlins, E. L., and Hogan, B. L. (2006). Epithelial Stem Cells of the Lung: Privileged Few or Opportunities for Many? *Development* 133, 2455–2465. doi:10.1242/dev.02407

Rock, J. R., Onaitis, M. W., Rawlins, E. L., Lu, Y., Clark, C. P., Xue, Y., et al. (2009). Basal Cells as Stem Cells of the Mouse Trachea and Human Airway Epithelium. *Proc. Natl. Acad. Sci.* 106, 12771. doi:10.1073/pnas.0906850106

Rock, J. R., Randell, S. H., and Hogan, B. L. M. (2010). Airway Basal Stem Cells: a Perspective on Their Roles in Epithelial Homeostasis and Remodeling. *Dis. Models Mech.* 3, 545–556. doi:10.1242/dmm.006031

Rout-Pitt, N., McCarron, A., McIntyre, C., Parsons, D., and Donnelley, M. (2018). Large-scale Production of Lentiviral Vectors Using Multilayer Cell Factories. *J. Biol. Methods* 5, e90. doi:10.14440/jbm.2018.236

Shimizu, T., Nishihara, M., Kawaguchi, S., and Sakakura, Y. (1994). Expression of Phenotypic Markers during Regeneration of Rat Tracheal Epithelium Following Mechanical Injury. *Am. J. Respir. Cell Mol Biol* 11, 85–94. doi:10.1165/ajrcmb.11.1.7517145

Sinn, P. L., Burnight, E. R., and McCray, P. B., Jr. (2009). Progress and Prospects: Prospects of Repeated Pulmonary Administration of Viral Vectors. *Gene Ther.* 16, 1059–1065. doi:10.1038/gt.2009.87

Team, R. C. (2020). *A Language and Environment for Statistical Computing.* Vienna, Austria: R Foundation for Statistical Computing. *2012* [Online]. Available at: https://www.r-project.org/ (Accessed November 20th, 2020).

Zeileis, A., Kleiber, C., and Jackman, S. (2008). Regression Models for Count Data in R. *J. Stat. Softw.* 27, 1–25. doi:10.18637/jss.v027.i08

16

Dissecting the Role of Mesenchymal Stem Cells in Idiopathic Pulmonary Fibrosis: Cause or Solution

Anna Valeria Samarelli[1,2†], Roberto Tonelli[1,2,3†], Irene Heijink[4], Aina Martin Medina[5], Alessandro Marchioni[1,2], Giulia Bruzzi[1,2], Ivana Castaniere[1,2,3], Dario Andrisani[1,2,3], Filippo Gozzi[1,2,3], Linda Manicardi[1,2], Antonio Moretti[1,2], Stefania Cerri[1,2], Riccardo Fantini[2], Luca Tabbì[2], Chiara Nani[2], Ilenia Mastrolia[6], Daniel J. Weiss[7], Massimo Dominici[8‡] and Enrico Clini[1,2‡]*

[1]Laboratory of Cell Therapies and Respiratory Medicine, Department of Medical and Surgical Sciences for Children and Adults University Hospital of Modena and Reggio Emilia, Modena, Italy, [2]University Hospital of Modena, Respiratory Diseases Unit, Department of Medical and Surgical Sciences, University of Modena Reggio Emilia, Modena, Italy, [3]Clinical and Experimental Medicine PhD Program, University of Modena Reggio Emilia, Modena, Italy, [4]University of Groningen, Departments of Pathology & Medical Biology and Pulmonology, GRIAC Research Institute, University Medical Center Groningen, Groningen, Netherlands, [5]IdISBa (Institut d'Investigacio Sanitaria Illes Balears), Palma de Mallorca, Spain, [6]Laboratory of Cellular Therapy, Program of Cell Therapy and Immuno-Oncology, Division of Oncology, Department of Medical and Surgical Sciences for Children & Adults, University Hospital of Modena and Reggio Emilia, Modena, Italy, [7]Department of Medicine, University of Vermont, Burlington, VT, United States, [8]Oncology Unit, University Hospital of Modena, University of Modena and Reggio Emilia, Modena, Italy

***Correspondence:**
Massimo Dominici
massimo.dominici@unimore.it

[†]These authors share first authorship

[‡]These authors share senior authorship

Idiopathic pulmonary fibrosis (IPF) is one of the most aggressive forms of idiopathic interstitial pneumonias, characterized by chronic and progressive fibrosis subverting the lung's architecture, pulmonary functional decline, progressive respiratory failure, and high mortality (median survival 3 years after diagnosis). Among the mechanisms associated with disease onset and progression, it has been hypothesized that IPF lungs might be affected either by a regenerative deficit of the alveolar epithelium or by a dysregulation of repair mechanisms in response to alveolar and vascular damage. This latter might be related to the progressive dysfunction and exhaustion of the resident stem cells together with a process of cellular and tissue senescence. The role of endogenous mesenchymal stromal/stem cells (MSCs) resident in the lung in the homeostasis of these mechanisms is still a matter of debate. Although endogenous MSCs may play a critical role in lung repair, they are also involved in cellular senescence and tissue ageing processes with loss of lung regenerative potential. In addition, MSCs have immunomodulatory properties and can secrete anti-fibrotic factors. Thus, MSCs obtained from other sources administered systemically or directly into the lung have been investigated for lung epithelial repair and have been explored as a potential therapy for the treatment of lung diseases including IPF. Given these multiple potential roles of MSCs, this review aims both at elucidating the role of resident lung MSCs in IPF pathogenesis and the role of administered MSCs from other sources for potential IPF therapies.

Keywords: cell based therapy, extracellular matrix, exosomes, idiopathic pulmonary fibrosis, mesenchymal stem cells

INTRODUCTION

Idiopathic pulmonary fibrosis (IPF) is a chronic progressive fibrosing lung disease of unknown cause that occurs primarily in older adults with a median survival of 3 years after diagnosis. It is diagnosed by clinicopathological criteria, including (Raghu et al., 2011) the radiographic and/or histological hallmark pattern of usual interstitial pneumonia (UIP). Prognosis remains extremely poor with most patients dying from progressive respiratory failure, often precipitated by acute events, namely disease exacerbations (Collard et al., 2016). As a therapeutic strategy, the two antifibrotic drugs Pirfenidone and nintedanib can slow down the respiratory functional decline of IPF patients, and according both the real-word data and randomized controlled trials, such as CAPACITY and ASCEND improve survival in patients (Guenther et al., 2018; Jo et al., 2017). Despite that, IPF still has a high mortality rate and that survival times are quite heterogenous (Noble et al., 2011; Glaspole et al., 2014; Sgalla et al., 2016; Richeldi et al., 2017; Lederer and Martinez, 2018; Cerri et al., 2019).

The pathogenesis of IPF is complex and far from being fully understood (Ley et al., 2011; Ryu et al., 2014). Current hypotheses center on alveolar epithelial and vascular endothelial injuries that lead to fibroblast activation, abnormal matrix collagen deposition (King et al., 2011; Bellaye and Kolb, 2015; Bitterman, 2018), aberrant repair mechanisms, inflammation, and a regenerative deficit of the alveolar tissue (Noble et al., 2011; Betensley et al., 2016). According to more recent studies, the onset and progression of IPF is due to the aberrant damage and activation of alveolar epithelial cells (AECs) that lead to the secretion of pro-fibrotic, coagulant, and inflammatory cytokines controlling the proliferation, activation and differentiation of fibroblasts into myofibroblasts and the consequent secretion and deposition of extracellular matrix (ECM) proteins (Selman and Pardo, 2020). These mechanisms translate into increased overall lung structural rigidity and thickening of the alveolar-capillary barrier with decline in alveolar gas exchange function. Since current evidence indicates epithelial cells as primers of disease and myofibroblasts as the key effectors in perpetrating fibrosis, recent investigations have focused on the cellular origin of the myofibroblasts including the potential role of resident mesenchymal progenitors as major source (Selman and Pardo, 2020). In particular, among myofibroblasts precursors, lung resident MSCs (LR-MSCs) have recently been gaining attention as to whether their aberrant behavior might be crucial in the fibrotic process (Agha et al., 2014; Enes et al., 2017; Cao et al., 2019). While research on resident lung MSCs as key protagonists in the pathogenesis of lung fibrosis is still emerging, there are many studies focusing on different roles of MSCs obtained from other sources outside of the lung namely their therapeutic potential given a range of immunomodulatory and anti-inflammatory properties (Uccelli et al., 2008; Mastrolia et al., 2019). To this purpose, a large number of pre-clinical investigations demonstrated efficacy of systemically or intratracheally administered MSCs obtained from bone marrow, adipose tissue, and other sources in a range of lung injury models. This has led to consideration and initial clinical investigations in IPF and other chronic lung diseases. (Weiss and Ortiz, 2013; Burgess and Irene, 2019). In parallel, a growing number of clinical investigations have been exploring systemic MSCs administration for the potential treatment of acute lung injury including the acute respiratory distress syndrome (ARDS) as well as most recently as potential treatment of COVID-19 respiratory failure (Golchin et al., 2020; Meng et al., 2020; Zumla et al., 2020). Although the mechanism of actions of MSCs in lung diseases have not yet been fully elucidated, and are likely to be different depending on the disease, the beneficial effects seem to be mainly dependent on paracrine mechanisms including release of bioactive molecules (soluble proteins, nucleic acids, lipids) and extracellular vesicles (EVs) (Kim et al., 2012; Chen et al., 2018; Cruz and Patricia, 2020; Harrell et al., 2019; Beer et al., 2017; Vizoso et al., 2017). In general, the EVs consists of exosomes, micro-vesicles (MVs), and apoptotic bodies that can be discriminated by their size and origin in the cells. Exosomes contain several molecules such as protein, lipids, mRNA, miRNA (Valadi et al., 2007), mitochondrial DNA (Guescini et al., 2010) and others non coding RNAs (Ferguson and Nguyen 2016). MSCs-derived exosomes have demonstrated immunoregulatory (Dabrowska et al., 2021), angiomodulatory (Lee et al., 2013; Alcayaga-miranda et al., 2016) and anti-apoptotic effects that control tissue repair and regeneration (Vishnubhatla et al., 2014; Lou et al., 2017) in both tissue culture and animal models. This includes a growing literature in which MSCs-derived EVs can be as effective as the MSCs themselves in pre-clinical models of lung injuries (Cruz and Patricia, 2020; Harrell et al., 2019; Beer et al., 2017; Vizoso et al., 2017).

In this dualistic scenario, the aim of this review is to explore the updated evidence on the molecular mechanisms of IPF from the alveolar epithelium damage to fibrotic changes, highlighting the role of resident lung MSCs as emerging key cellular determinant in IPF onset and progression and providing an overview of the potential role of MSCs from different sources and their secretome in cell-based therapies for lung fibrosis.

KEY MOLECULAR MECHANISMS OF IDIOPATHIC PULMONARY FIBROSIS AS AN EPITHELIUM DRIVEN DISEASE

Nowadays IPF is described as an epithelium-driven disease characterized by aberrant functional epithelium due to aging and exposure to alveolar injuries in combination with compromised lung tissue regeneration, leading to abnormal repair with an imbalance between profibrotic and antifibrotic factors. Notably, this aberrant reparative mechanism leads to an increased fibroblast proliferation and myofibroblast activity resulting in ECM deposition. It is known that the lung consists of quiescent tissue with little cell turnover at rest, compared for example to intestinal epithelial tissues. However, after injury it has the capability to efficiently regenerate the damage in both airway and alveolar niches (Beers and Morrisey, 2011). In normal lung, alveolar injuries are followed by depletion of type 1 alveolar epithelial cells (AECI) that are located at the interface with vascular endothelium and participate in alveolar gas exchange function. The lack of AECI is compensated by the alveolar epithelial cell 2 (AECII) that normally secrete the pulmonary surfactant to maintain the surface tension, but also have capacity to proliferate and differentiate into AECI, restoring the alveolar epithelium once injured (Fomby et al., 2010). The abnormal reparative response to injury of epithelial cells in IPF represents an initial and crucial mechanism of disease. The epithelial secretion of pro-fibrotic factors promotes fibroblast migration, proliferation, activation and differentiation into myofibroblasts with deposition of exaggerated ECM and subsequently distortion of the lung architecture. Several mechanisms and molecular pathways in lung IPF epithelium have been demonstrated to contribute to the development of the disease. Among these, abnormal AECII hyperplasia in response to injury results in the formation of mucus-filled microcystic structures that can evolve into macrocysts, compromising epithelial differentiation and alveolar epithelial cell function (Seibold et al., 2013; Vaughan et al., 2015). Indeed, in the damaged alveolar epithelium of IPF lungs the process named "bronchiolization" leads to migration of abnormal basal cells with accumulation of nuclear β-catenin (basal-cell hyperplasia) from adjacent bronchioles toward areas of alveolar injury colonizing them leading to aberrant re-epithelialization and contributing to disease progression. The integrity of the alveolar epithelium is severely disrupted in IPF lungs where abnormal epithelium covering the fibroblastic foci displayed a bronchiolar immunophenotype (Chilosi et al., 2003) Different works support the concept that bronchiolar abnormalities in IPF are due to changes in lung epithelial cell differentiation (Plantier et al., 2011). In particular, abnormal basal cells may differentiate into non-ciliated Club cells or ciliated FoxJ1 expressing bronchial cells, resulting in bronchiolization of damaged alveoli. Thus, bronchiolization of enlarged alveolar ducts, cysts and alveoli, results in the typical honeycombing that can be seen in the lung of IPF patients (Plantier et al., 2011).

Recently, it has been shown that the oncogene epithelial cell transforming sequence 2 (ECT2), a guanine nucleotide exchange factor (GEF) for Rho GTPases, is upregulated in hyperplastic AECII of IPF patients, and can contribute to the hyperplastic and proliferative lung epithelial cell phenotype (Ulke et al., 2019). In addition, pro-fibrotic mediators including transforming growth factor beta-1 (TGF-β1), platelet-derived growth factor (PDGF), tumor necrosis factor (TNF), endothelin-1, connective tissue growth factor (CTGF), osteopontin, and CXC chemokine ligand 12 (CXCL12) (Pardo et al., 2005; Selman and Pardo, 2020) are up-regulated in AECs and can contribute to the progression of fibrosis and aberrant extracellular matrix remodeling.

TGFβ SIGNALING AND CROSS-TALK WITH WNT AND SONIC HEDGEHOG PATHWAYS ACTIVATED IN EPITHELIAL CELLS OF IDIOPATHIC PULMONARY FIBROSIS PATIENTS

TGFβ can be considered a key regulator of fibrotic process favoring migration, proliferation, and activation of fibroblasts, differentiation into myofibroblasts, and deposition of ECM proteins (Meng et al., 2016; Horowitz and Thannickal, 2019). Indeed, TGFβ receptor complex activation leads to downstream canonical (SMAD2 & 3) (Massagué, 2014) and non-canonical signaling cascades (PI3K, MEK, mTOR, etc) (Hu et al., 2018), which orchestrate the transcription of profibrotic mediators, growth factors, microRNAs, and ECM proteins (Andrianifahanana et al., 2013). Furthermore, cross-talks exists with TGFβ1 signaling and pathways overexpressed by epithelial cells of IPF patients such as Wnt and Sonic hedgehog (Shh) (Bolaños et al., 2012; Cigna et al., 2012). Zhou et al. (2012) found that TGF-β1 and Wnt/β-catenin crosstalk played a role in IPF pathogenesis since TGF-β1 activate Wnt/β-catenin pathway and together with Wnt/β-catenin signaling induced epithelial-mesenchymal transition and myofibroblast activation (Zhou et al., 2012). Hasaneen et al.; found that TGF-β1 triggered the release of a glycosylated transmembrane protein named EMMPRIN (Extracellular Matrix metalloproteinase Inducer) that increases the expression of some matrix metalloproteinase (MMP) and activates β-catenin/canonical Wnt signaling pathway. Here, EMMPRIN overexpression led to an anti-apoptotic and pro-fibrotic phenotype in lung fibroblasts of IPF patients (Hasaneen et al., 2016). Indeed, ICG-001, an inhibitor of T-cell factor (TCF)/β-catenin transcription, has been shown to repress TGFβ1-induced EMT and reverse pulmonary fibrosis in mice (Henderson et al., 2010). More recently, it was demonstrated that chronic Wnt/β-catenin activity in the IPF lung increased AECII senescence, leading to further progenitor cells dysfunction and impaired lung repair (Lehmann et al., 2020). In contrast, previous studies have shown that a particular lineage of Wnt responsive alveolar epithelial progenitor cells within the AECII population acted as a central player in lung regeneration after acute injury, being able to self-renew (Zacharias et al., 2018). Bolanos et al. (2012) found that Shh pathway is activated in IPF lungs and might contribute to IPF pathogenesis by increasing fibroblast proliferation, migration and ECM production. They measured the expression of Shh, Patched-1, Smoothened, and transcription factors glioma-associated oncogene homolog GLI1 and GLI2 in IPF and normal lungs finding that most of them were overexpressed in IPF (Bolanos et al., 2012). Further, TGF-β1 modulates the expression of key components of the hedgehog pathway in lung fibroblasts, while the activity of the transcription factor GLI from the primary cilium is required to induce and maintain myofibroblast differentiation (Cigna et al., 2012).

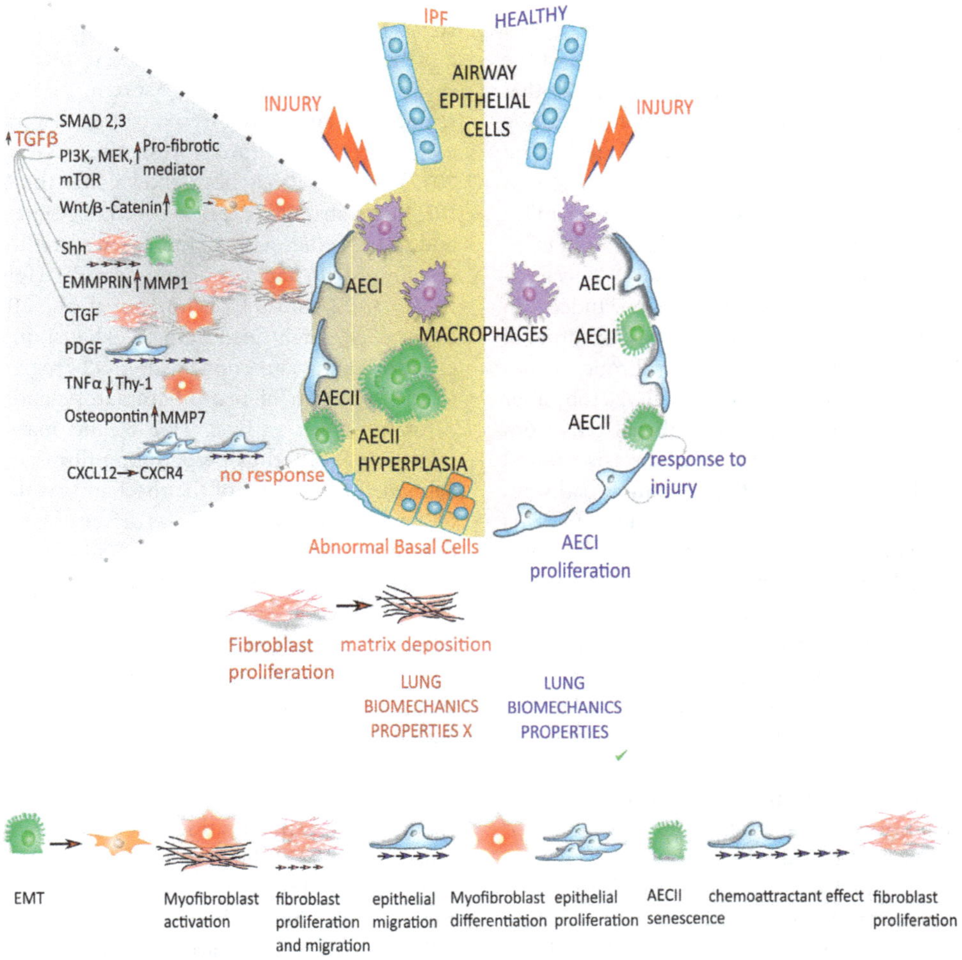

FIGURE 1 | Different response from the epithelium to lung injury in normal and IPF lung. In normal lung, the depletion of alveolar epithelial cells 1 (AECI) that play a pivotal role in gas exchange with the adjacent blood vessels after injuries, is compensated/replenished by/upon the differentiation of alveolar epithelial cells 2 (AECII) in AECI, restoring the alveolar epithelium. In lung epithelium of IPF patients, the regeneration of AECI by AECII progenitors is compromised, leading to impaired alveolar re-epithelialization. Together with the aberrant repair mechanisms the AECs start to secrete pro-fibrotic mediators that through different molecular pathway and down-stream effectors lead to fibroblast migration, proliferation, activation and differentiation into myofibroblasts with deposition of exaggerated ECM that drastically compromise the lung biomechanics properties.

Among other pathways involved, PDGF showed mitogenic and chemoattractant effects on fibroblasts while connective tissue growth factor (CTGF) was found to promote the progression of fibrosis either activating fibroblasts or through TGF-β pathway (Allen and Spiteri 2002).

TNF-α, OSTEOPONTIN, CXCL12, AND MATRIX METALLOPROTEASES INVOLVEMENT IN THE IDIOPATHIC PULMONARY FIBROSIS PATHOGENESIS

Tumor necrosis factor-alpha (TNF-α) was found to cause loss of fibroblast Thy-1 surface expression, thus contributing to myofibroblast differentiation (Kis et al., 2011). Selman and Pardo reported that osteopontin acted on both neighboring epithelial cells and fibroblast to trigger a migratory and proliferative phenotype (Selman and Pardo, 2020). Recently CXCL12 was reported to act on CXCR4, which is expressed in advanced form of interstitial lung diseases, particularly when cystic lesions are present (Jaffar et al., 2020). Furthermore, matrix metalloproteases (MMPs) showed to play a role in the progression of IPF. Particularly, MMP1 and MMP7 are strongly expressed in the IPF epithelial cells compared to the epithelium in normal tissue. MMP1 increases cell proliferation and protects epithelial cells from apoptosis (Herrera et al., 2013), while MMP7 is involved in the fibrotic response upon osteopontin (Pardo et al., 2005). **Figure 1** summarizes the different pathways involved in alveolar epithelial response to lung injury in normal and IPF lung.

HIPPO PATHWAY IN THE LUNG FIBROSIS PROGRESSION

It has been reported that Yes-associated protein (YAP) and the transcriptional coactivator with PDZ-binding motif (TAZ) that belong to the Hippo pathway are aberrantly activated in lung fibrosis. In particular, YAP/TAZ that act as sensors of mechanical forces in cell microenvironment, are activated in fibroblasts of fibrotic lung due to ECM stiffness thus subjected to mechanical stretch, leading to the secretion of profibrotic mediators and ECM proteins (Noguchi et al., 2018; Marchioni et al., 2020). This feed-forward loop enhances the lung fibrosis progression. Indeed, in epithelial cells, YAP/TAZ are also activated with the disruption of cell polarity and increased ECM stiffness in fibrotic tissues (Noguchi et al., 2018). To this purpose, (Xu et al., 2016b) after performing single-cell RNA sequencing of epithelial cells from IPF patients (Xu et al 2016), through Pathway analysis showed that the YAP/TAZ, TGF-β, Wnt, and PI3K signaling pathways were aberrantly activated in epithelial cells of IPF lung patients (Gokey et al., 2018). They suggested that YAP interacted with mTOR/PI3K/AKT signaling increasing the proliferation and migration of lung epithelial cells. Then, YAP/TAZ pathway contributes to the pathogenesis of IPF in lung fibroblasts and epithelial cells. Recently, Sun and collaborators have shown that Hippo/TAZ signaling also affects the regenerative capacity of AECII progenitors. TAZ also named WW Domain Containing Transcription Regulator 1(WWTR1) plays a crucial role in AECII to AECI differentiation and thus contribute to the maintenance of alveolar integrity after injury. Notably, conditional deletion of TAZ in AECII dramatically reduced AECI regeneration during recovery leading to exacerbated alveolar lesions and fibrosis in a bleomycin induced lung injury model. In addition, TAZ signaling can activate pro-fibrotic responses in fibroblasts (Sun et al., 2019).

Despite all these insights, the complete molecular mechanisms behind/underlying the differentiation of AECII in AECI after acute lung injury and how this is dysregulated in IPF are far from being fully understood.

CELLULAR SENESCENCE, GENETIC AND ENVIRONMENTAL RISKS IN THE PATHOGENESIS OF IDIOPATHIC PULMONARY FIBROSIS

As described above, epithelial damage and activation can drive myofibroblasts proliferation and the release of pro-fibrotic factors. What causes initial epithelial damage during the onset of IPF is not fully understood. To date, an integral model of IPF pathogenesis has been proposed where the presence of rare or common gene variants (genetic), cellular senescence and epigenetic reprogramming, converge to the initiation and progression of the disease (Michalski and Schwartz, 2020; Selman and Pardo, 2020). Indeed, aging-associated alterations as mitochondrial dysfunction and altered proteostasis could promote epithelial and fibroblast senescence in IPF lungs through the loss of proteome integrity and the shortening of telomeres (Mora et al., 2017; Lederer and Martinez, 2018). Cellular senescence leads to replicative arrest, apoptosis resistance, and the acquisition of a senescence-associated secretory phenotype (SASP), that involves the release of several inflammatory, growth-regulating and tissue-remodeling factors and could thus contribute to pro-fibrotic responses (Kirkland and Tchkonia, 2017). Hence, it has been shown that the epithelial cells from IPF lungs strongly expressed cellular senescence markers p16 and p21 together with an increased secretion of SASP factors as insulin growth factor binding proteins (Igfbp) 3, 4 and 7 and MMP 3, 12 and 14 (Lehmann et al., 2017). Then, cellular senescence, might lead both to exhaustion of stem/progenitor cell renewal (dysfunction) with loss of regenerative abilities and to the secretion of pro-inflammatory and matrix-remodeling cytokines, such as IL-6, TGF-β, and matrix metalloproteases related to SASP, thus perpetrating fibrosis (Pardo and Moisé s Selman, 2021). Some of the mechanisms that have been shown to induce AECII senescence as driver of IPF progression involve the overexpression of Wnt/β-catenin signaling, DNA damage and telomere shortening (Mora et al., 2017). Recently, it has been demonstrated that loss of PTEN (phosphatase and tension homolog deleted on chromosome ten) triggers senescence in AECs through the activation of the protein kinase B (Akt) signaling pathway leading to a reduction of the autophagy. In particular, in a murine model of bleomycin induced AECs senescence, repression of Akt2 with the pharmacological inhibition of the Akt pathway (LY294002 and MK2206), resulted in ameliorating fibrotic lesions. The cellular senescence in IPF lungs was then found to be modulated by Akt/PTEN pathway (Qiu et al., 2019). Recently, Yao and collaborators have shown the transcriptomic features of cellular senescence characterizing the AECII isolated from IPF lung tissue. In particular, they showed how the conditional loss of Sin3a in adult mouse brought to p53-dependent cellular senescence of AECII, cell depletion, and spontaneous and progressive pulmonary fibrosis. The authors suggested that progressive fibrosis might be caused by senescence rather than loss of AECII and that targeting of p53 could block fibrogenesis (Yao et al., 2020). To this purpose, with the advanced technology of single-cell RNA-seq, Adams and collaborators identified a new population of IPF lung epithelial cells that was transcriptionally distinct from any epithelial cell type previously described in the lung, named aberrant basaloid cells, characterized by senescence-related genes including CDKN1A, CDKN2A, CCND1, CCND2, MDM2, and GDF15 (Adams et al., 2019). Besides the direct role of senescence of epithelial cells in the progression of IPF, it has been demonstrated that senescence of lung fibroblasts might decrease the AECII proliferation and promote migration in wound healing, affecting the re-epithelialization process after injury in IPF lung (Blokland et al., 2020). It has been widely demonstrated that genetic susceptibility together with the environmental risks play a pivotal role in disease initiation and progression in both sporadic and familial IPF. In this context, the most validated and strongest genetic risk factor for both familial and sporadic IPF, is represented by the single nucleotide polymorphism rs35705950 in the promoter region of the mucin 5B (MUC5B) gene (Steele et al., 2011; Allen et al., 2017; Allen et al., 2020). Normally, together with mucin 5AC (MUC5AC), MUC5B plays a crucial role in the muco-ciliary clearance (MCC) that is essential for removing inhaled debris and pathogens in the normal lung homeostasis (Roy et al., 2013; Bonser and Erle 2017). *In vivo* studies have demonstrated that full-length murine MUC5B overexpression in AECII of two lines of C57BL/6 mice resulted in muco-ciliary clearance dysfunction thus worsening bleomycin-induced lung fibrosis (Hancock et al., 2018). Indeed, in genetically susceptible individuals bearing the rs35705950 SNP that cause MUC5B overexpression and impaired MCC, it might happen that exposure to inhaled pro-fibrotic particles could compromise the epithelial repair response to cell injury (Ley et al., 2017). Genome wide-association studies have revealed several common and rare variants associated with sporadic and familial IPF (Fingerlin et al., 2013; Allen et al., 2017; Allen et al., 2020; Dressen et al., 2018). To this purpose, the common genetic variants associated with IPF are represented by gene involved in the airway mucin production (MUC5B, MUC2), cell-cell adhesion (DSP, DPP9) playing a critical role in the maintenance of epithelial integrity, innate and adaptive immune response (Toll-Like receptor signaling, TOLLIP, TLR3), cytokine and growth factor signaling (IL1RN, IL8, IL4, TGFβ1), telomere maintenance (TERT, OBFC1) and cell cycle regulation (KIF15, MAD1L1, CDKN1A, TP53) (Michalski and Schwartz, 2020).

Rare variants of genes encoding proteins involved in telomere biology and maintenance have been identified in about 30% of patients with familial IPF whose AECII are characterized by short telomeres and proteins for surfactant production and secretion. These proteins include TERT, TERC (telomerase RNA component) TINF2 (TERF1 interacting nuclear factor 2), DKC1 (dyskerin), RTEL1, PARN (poly(A)-specific ribonuclease) and NAF1 (nuclear assembly factor 1 ribonucleoprotein) (Kropski et al., 2014; Kropski et al., 2015; Alder et al., 2015; Stuart et al., 2015; Stanley et al., 2016), SFPTA1, SFPTA2, SFPTC (surfactant protein A1, A2, C) and ABCA3 (ATP Binding Cassette Subfamily A Member 3) (Nureki et al., 2018; Doubková et al., 2019; Takezaki et al., 2019).

Finally, as mentioned above there are environmental risks such as cigarette smoke, inhalation of wood and metal dust, and other exposures that might contribute to the onset and progression of IPF, causing injury in the "genetically susceptible" patients (Barczyk et al., 2015; Phan et al., 2020; Shull et al., 2020). Indeed, the environmental risks might result in epigenomic modifications, with the alteration in key genes regulation contributing to the pathogenesis of IPF. To this purpose, exposure of cigarette smoke (CS) triggers DNA damage-related chromatin binding changes, and alterations in DNA methylation, influencing gene transcription and the downstream response of cells to injury (Vaz et al., 2017). Overall, however, the mechanisms and the correlation between environmental risk factors, genetic predisposition, aging and IPF pathogenesis need to be further elucidated.

THE EFFECT OF AGING ON MESENCHYMAL STROMAL/STEM CELLS

The cellular senescence of MSCs is a cellular mechanism that compromises their regenerative potential involving the oxidative state of the cell and mitochondrial dysfunction (Li Y et al., 2017). Despite lack of complete understanding of the molecular mechanisms and signaling pathways of senescence in MSCs, the senescence-associated phenotypes are characterized by an increase in the SA-β-gal activity, in the G1 cell cycle arrest, in the reactive oxygen species (ROS) production and expression of p53 and p21 (Jiang et al., 2008) and in a compromised autophagy process. One effect of MSCs aging can be seen in their decreased osteogenic activity. The molecular pathway behind the osteogenic activity is related to the expression of the transcription factor RUNX2/CBFA1 and the PI3K-AKT pathway that both decrease with age (Atashi et al., 2015). Additionally, it has been demonstrated that the adipogenic potential of MSCs tend to decline with aging and after different passages in *in vitro* culture mediated in part through the PPARγ modulation, an adipogenic-specific transcription and cross-talk with Wnt/β-catenin signaling pathway (Xu C et al., 2016).

Cellular senescence leads to replicative arrest, apoptosis resistance, and the acquisition of a senescence-associated secretory phenotype (SASP), that involves the release of several inflammatory, growth-regulating and tissue-remodeling factors and could thus contribute to pro-fibrotic responses (Kirkland and Tchkonia, 2017). Then, cellular senescence, might lead both to exhaustion of stem/progenitor cell renewal (dysfunction) with loss of regenerative abilities and to the secretion of pro-inflammatory and matrix-remodeling cytokines, such as IL-6, TGF-β, and matrix metalloproteases related to SASP, causing persistent fibrosis. (Pardo and Moisé s Selman, 2021). Indeed, a crucial mechanism that leads to MSCs senescence is the oxidative stress that leads to the production of free radicals/ROS (reactive oxygen species) the majority of which are produced by the mitochondrial respiratory chain (Liu et al., 2020). From a molecular point of view the p38/MAPK axis triggers MSCs senescence through ROS production and accumulation initiating the oxidative process that can lead to mitochondrial dysfunction, DNA damage and protein damage. In the endoplasmic reticulum (ER) take place correct folding and assembling of the proteins into their native conformation prior to be transported to intracellular organelles or cell surface. In general, during the ER stress the correct protein folding is impaired and the unfolded or misfolded proteins accumulate in the ER lumen compromising the ER homeostasis. Then, the accumulation of aberrant folded proteins activates as a cellular protective mechanism, the unfolded protein response (UPR) ameliorating cell hemostasis and survival during ER stress process. (Schröder and Kaufman, 2005; Cao and Kaufman, 2012). Indeed, it has been demonstrated that accumulation of misfolded, or unfolded, proteins into the lumen of ER might contribute to the progression of age-related diseases (Powers et al., 2009; López-Otín et al.,). Then, the oxidative stress, with compromised mechanism of UPR, might cause aging in MSCs affecting their cell functions and survival (Geissler et al., 2013; Wang et al., 2018). Recently, it has been demonstrated that a deficiency in the UPR lead to inactivation of ATF6, which can contribute to MSCs aging (Wang et al., 2018). In human MSCs, ATF6 is involved in cellular proteostasis, the process responsible for the preservation of a functional proteome and telomere shortening. The inactivation of ATF6 cause the accumulation of protein aggregates and compromise the integrity of various membrane organelles (Wang et al., 2018).

Indeed, these aging-associated alterations, including mitochondrial dysfunction and altered proteostasis, can also promote epithelial and fibroblast senescence in IPF lungs (Lederer and Martinez, 2018; Mora et al., 2017). Conceivable strategies to prevent aging in MSCs, for example genetic engineering through the knockdown of the tumor suppressor p16INK4a/CDKN2A (p16, cyclin-dependent kinase inhibitor 2A, CDKN2A) might lead to increase of proliferation rate and clonogenicity of MSCs (Gu et al., 2012). However, these might also increase the tumorigenesis risks. Finally, the use of growth factors such as exogenous FGF-2, PDGF and EGF have been demonstrated to reduce MSCs senescence and increase proliferation (Gharibi and Hughes, 2012). These might also be potential therapeutic interventions.

THE ROLE OF RESIDENT LUNG FIBROBLASTS AND BONE MARROW PROGENITOR CELLS IN PULMONARY FIBROSIS

Resident lung fibroblasts represent key effector cells in IPF pathogenesis since under the action of TGF-β can proliferate and differentiate into myofibroblasts promoting fibrogenesis and impairing normal alveolar epithelial repair in response to damage (David and Cory, 2017; Chanda et al., 2019). Here, the resident fibroblasts increase the synthesis of collagen and mesenchymal proteins, such as Vimentin and α-SMA with the activation of Wnt/β-catenin axis favoring the progression of IPF (Shi et al., 2017). Then, myofibroblasts, expressing α-SMA, trigger ECM accumulation and deposition with an increase in the structural rigidity, decrease in contractility of lung tissue, and impaired support of alveolar repair (Zhang et al., 1996; Wu and Tang, 2021). According to recent studies, it has been shown that there are several populations of resident lung fibroblasts including fibroblasts localized in the lung interstitium adjacent to alveolar epithelial cells and lipofibroblasts, mainly characterized by neutral lipids, located adjacent to AECII. Lipofibroblasts are implicated in alveolar maturation and surfactant production as well as FGF10 secretion, and have been shown to modulate the epithelial stem-cell niche in adult mouse lungs (Alam et al., 2015; Agha et al., 2017). These lipofibroblasts are characterized by specific markers such as Sca-1, CD248 (Bartis et al., 2016) and PDGFRα (Iwayama et al., 2015; Wang et al., 2017). Particularly, PDGFRα allows the discrimination between interstitial resident fibroblasts and lipofibroblasts from pericytes, mesenchymal cells closely related to vascular smooth muscle cells (VSMCs) that underlie and envelop capillaries, forming focal contacts with adjacent endothelial cells (Green et al., 2016). Recent studies of lineage tracing revealed that PDGFRα-expressing interstitial fibroblasts and/or lipofibroblasts can each differentiate into myofibroblasts after lung injury and that myofibroblast to lipofibroblast *trans*-differentiation is required for fibrosis attenuation in the mouse lung (El Agha et al., 2017).

As myofibroblasts represent key effector cells in lung fibrosis due to deposition of collagen and formation of scar tissue, their cellular origin and potential precursors have been extensively studied (Hinz et al., 2007; Fernandez and Oliver, 2012; Bochaton-Piallat et al., 2016; Horowitz and Thannickal, 2019). In this scenario, several population have been analyzed: 1) resident lung fibroblasts that under the influence of the profibrotic microenvironment directly differentiate into myofibroblasts (Phan 2002), 2) epithelial cells that lose their characteristic markers (such as E-cadherin and zona occludens-1) and acquire mesenchymal properties (such as fibroblast-specific protein-1 and α-SMA expression) in a process named epithelial-mesenchymal transition (EMT) (Willis et al., 2005; Kim et al., 2006) 3) bone marrow (BM)-derived cells as circulating fibrocytes (Phillips et al., 2004; Moore et al., 2005) and 4) pericytes (Scotton and Chambers, 2007; Wipff et al., 2007; Hinz, 2012; Hung et al., 2013). While more recent investigations have moved away from any significant roles of EMT or circulating fibrocytes as myofibroblast sources (Rock et al., 2011; Kleaveland et al., 2014; Barron et al., 2016; Chong et al., 2019), cell-lineage tracing experiments using reporter mouse models have focused attention on resident mesenchymal cell populations that can acquire myofibroblastic phenotype. These include:

- interstitial lung fibroblasts localized in the interstitium immediately adjacent to alveolar epithelial cells (Angeles, 2015; Barron et al., 2016),
- lipofibroblasts, that are lipid-droplet-containing interstitial fibroblasts located within close proximity to AECIIs (El Agha et al., 2017; Alam et al., 2015),
- pericytes localized within the capillary basement membrane connected to each other and with one or more endothelial cells (Marriott et al., 2014; Barron et al., 2016),
- mesothelial cells from pleural-mesothelium that line the visceral and parietal pleural surfaces (Karki et al., 2014), and
- resident lung mesenchymal progenitors (Xie et al., 2016), whose contribution in myofibroblast differentiating process seems prevalent.

Since the first isolation and characterization of LR-MSCs from human transplanted lungs, there has been increasing interest in their characterization with specific molecular markers for recognition, their exact location in the lung niche, their role in regulation of lung tissue homeostasis, and their role in the lung repair and regeneration after injury (Burgess and Irene, 2019; Sveiven and Nordgren, 2020). In particular, the expression of mesenchyme-specific t-box transcription factor (TBX4), that characterizes early mesenchyme progenitors during embryonic lung development, correlates with the activation and proliferation of myofibroblast accumulation in lung fibrosis. Then, in the adult lung the TBX4 positive lineage are fibroblasts, smooth muscle cells, pericytes, and endothelial cells (Xie et al., 2016). Indeed, it has been shown that the numbers of LR-MSCs decreases during experimentally induced fibrosis in mice. This cell population has also been shown to express ATP-binding cassette sub-family G member 2 (ABCG2) (Jun et al., 2011) and lineage tracing experiments revealed that ABCG2+ cells are located in perivascular regions and in proximity of AECI in the mouse lung. In a bleomycin mouse model ABCG2+ cells are amplified and significantly transform into myofibroblasts, contributing to the progression of lung fibrosis (Marriott et al., 2014). Moreover, another GLI1 (glioma-associated oncogene homolog 1) positive perivascular lung resident MSCs population has been shown to contribute to myofibroblast formation in the bleomycin pulmonary fibrosis mouse model (Kramann et al., 2015). Recently in a bleomycin mouse model, Cao et al. showed that Wnt10a had a pivotal role in pulmonary fibrosis as they found an increased expression level of Wnt10a secreted by LR-MSCs undergoing myofibroblastic differentiation. Indeed, after isolation of LR-MSCs with myofibroblast characteristics from fibrotic lungs they found an increase in Shh pathway activity in these cells. They demonstrated that the Shh/glioblastoma (Gli) pathway was a key regulator of LR-MSCs-to-myofibroblast transition in pulmonary fibrosis. Finally, they showed that the suppression of the Shh-Wnt signaling prevented myofibroblast differentiation from LR-MSCs ameliorating pulmonary fibrotic lesions (Cao et al., 2019).

Furthermore, the role of lipofibroblasts and their contribution to the myofibroblast cell population in IPF lungs have been studied in recent works. Among them, in the study from Kheirollhai and colleagues they demonstrated that the antidiabetic drug, metformin, inhibits collagen production in primary human lung fibroblasts and in *ex vivo* cultured human IPF model and triggers the myo-to lipofibroblast transdifferentiation leading to a recovery from fibrosis. They further demonstrated that treatment of bleomycin-injured mice with metformin resulted in a resolution of fibrosis altering the fate of myofibroblasts and enhanced their lipogenic differentiation (Kheirollahi et al., 2019). Finally, they showed that the antidiabetic drug metformin had potent antifibrotic effects in the lung, through the inhibition of TGFβ1 signaling and collagen formation together with PPARγ signaling activation and lipogenic differentiation.

In another study from Zysman and colleagues (Zysman et al., 2020); they investigated whether the cell-cycle inhibitor p16INK4a limits lung regeneration after newborn bronchopulmonary dysplasia (BPD), that lead to the arrest of alveolar development. They found that p16INK4a decrease leads to an increase of neutral lipid synthesis promoting lipofibroblast and AECII development within the lung stem-cell niche. Indeed, they found that treatment with a PPARγ (peroxisome proliferator-activated receptor γ) agonist increased lipofibroblast and AECII, restoring alveolar architecture after hyperoxia-exposure in mice (Zysman et al., 2020). Thus, the "plasticity" of myofibroblasts that are able under proper conditions and treatment to transdifferentiate back into lipofibroblasts, that contribute to the progression of IPF, provides the possibility to study novel drugs and compound to revert the fibrotic process in the lung niche.

To date, the emerging picture in the alveolar niche of IPF lung, indicates that there is a heterogenous myofibroblast population that may derive from different sources including interstitial lung fibroblasts, lipofibroblasts, pericytes, mesothelial cells and lung-resident MSCs rather than from EMT processes/epithelial or BM-derived cells (**Figure 2**).

THE ROLE OF LUNG RESIDENT MESENCHYMAL STROMAL/STEM CELLS IN LUNG HOMEOSTASIS, INJURY AND REPAIR

Adult resident stem cells are distributed in organ-specific niches which provide an appropriate microenvironment that regulates their development and functionality. Therefore, MSCs of all tissue origins have a common cellular signature even if there are also certain molecular features that seem to be organ-specific including the lung niche (Klein, 2020). In this regard, the characterization of human LR-MSCs meets the minimal suggested ISCT criteria for MSCs (Dominici et al., 2006) including expression of cell surface proteins as CD29, CD73, CD90, CD105 and CD146 (Kruk et al., 2021) besides being negative for hematopoietic markers. *In vitro* differentiation experiments have further demonstrated multilineage differentiation of LR-MSCs isolated from central and peripheral transbronchial biopsies, into adipocytes, osteoblasts and chondrocytes (Rolandsson et al., 2014). Nevertheless, it has been reported that LR-MSCs express higher level of FGFR2 as compared to BM-MSCs in mouse and rats. FGFR2 is bound by FGF10 leading to LR-MSCs activation and migration (Agha et al., 2014; Enes et al., 2017). To this purpose, Tong et al.; showed that in rats intratracheal administration of FGF-10 in lungs, led to LR-MSCs mobilization that allowed their collection through bronchoalveolar lavage. The collected LR-MSCs were cultured *in vitro* and then intratracheally delivered to rats after LPS-induced lung injury with more beneficial effects as compared to BM-MSCs used as positive control (Tong et al., 2016). Then, Sveiven and Nordgren in a recent review gave an update on both differences and similarities between BM-MSCs and LR-MSCs about the surface protein expression profile, the transcriptome, proteome and secretome (Sveiven and Nordgren, 2020). In particular, both the transcriptomic data and the pathway analysis of proteomic data showed that pathways involving Wnt, elasticity, motility, MET signaling, and integrins were more up-regulated in LR-MSCs as compared to BM-MSCs. Among the differences regarding the secretome, it has been shown that BM-MSCs secreted significantly less monocyte chemoattractant protein-1 (MCP-1, CCL2), crucial for macrophage recruitment, than LR-MSCs, while no significant differences in immunosuppressive effects on lymphocytes were observed between the two cell populations (Larsson et al., 2016). In another study comparing murine LR-MSCs and BM-MSCs in

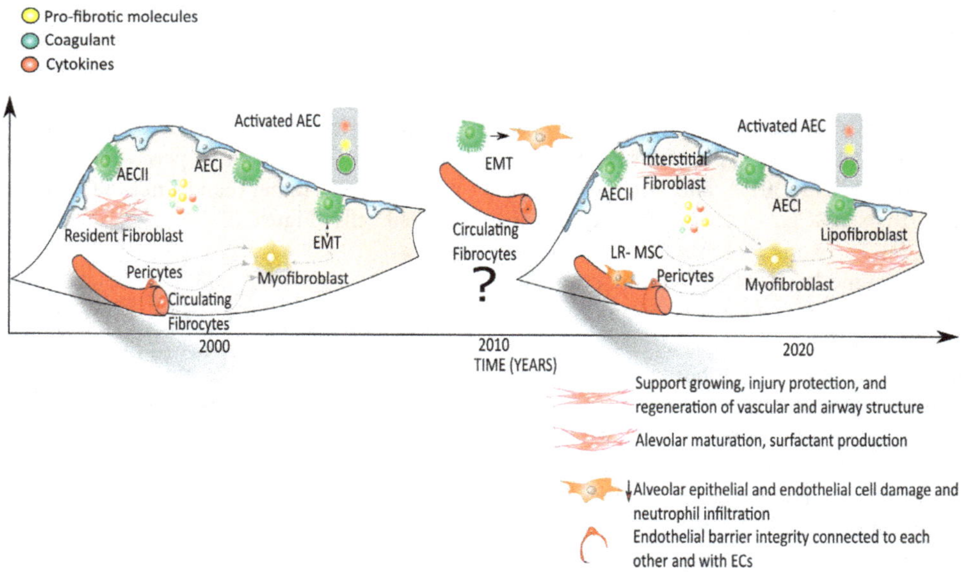

FIGURE 2 | Onset and progression of IPF: the myofibroblast in focus. According to the first hypothesis, the activation of alveolar epithelial cells (AECs) leads to the secretion of pro-fibrotic molecules, coagulant and cytokines that activate several cells from different sources: the resident fibroblast, the resident mesenchymal stromal/stem cells, the epithelial cells that undergo to the epithelial mesenchymal transition, the pericytes and the endothelial cells progenitors. These different cell types in IPF lungs may differentiate into myofibroblasts with the consequent secretion and deposition of extracellular matrix proteins followed by an overall lung structural rigidity and decline of alveolar function. According to the most recent publications (Etc 2019; Xie et al., 2016), interstitial lung fibroblasts, pericytes, lipofibroblasts, mesothelial cells and LR-MSCs, whose roles within the alveolar lung niche are list in the legend within the figure, give rise to the myofibroblast population representing the key cells for the onset and progression of fibrosis.

an elastase-injury mouse model it was suggested that LR-MSCs displayed prolonged retention in the lungs upon intravenous administration, which might be attributed to the specific expression of adhesion molecules (Hoffman et al., 2011). In a similar elastase model, effects of murine LR-MSCs, BM-MSCs and adipose derived (AD)-MSCs were compared. All sources reduced alveolar epithelial and endothelial cell damage and neutrophil infiltration and increased elastic fiber content (**Figure 2**). In contrast to intravenous delivery, intratracheal MSCs administration further reduced alveolar hyperinflation and collagen fiber content, while AD-MSCs and LR-MSCs showed a more significant reduction in fractional area of alveolar collapse compared to BM-MSCs (Antunes et al., 2014). In 2012 Ricciardi et al.; showed that LR-MSCs do not significantly differ from human BM-MSCs with regards to the immunophenotype, stemness gene profile and mesodermal differentiation potential. Indeed, *in vitro* co-culture of either LR-MSCs and BM-MSCs with activated T cells or NK cells showed the same inhibitory effect of T-cell and NK cells proliferation from the two different cell lines. They found that lung-MSCs expressed higher basal level of the nestin marker; moreover *in vitro* treatment with retinoic acid showed that the LR-MSCs led to higher epithelial cell differentiation and polarization compared to BM-MSCs (Ricciardi et al., 2012). The authors evaluated the effect of retinoic acid treatment *in vitro* on LR-MSCs and BM-MSCs after 4 weeks of RA culture and through phase-contrast microscopy. While, both LR-MSCs and BM-MSCs showed a round-cuboid shape as epithelial cells at the end of the culture, LR-MSCs cultured with RA displayed a stronger phenotype. Further, after analyzing LR-MSCs by trans epithelial electric resistance (TEER) assay after RA treatment to measure and quantify the formation of tight and adherence junctions it was found a higher polarization tendency in LR-MSCs compared to BM-MSCs (Ricciardi et al., 2012). Recently, LR-MSCs were isolated from allografts of human lung transplant recipients (Jarvinen et al., 2021). *In vitro* studies demonstrated that these LR-MSCs could suppress the proliferative capacity of T cells in response to a mitogenic or an allogeneic stimulus. The authors found that the immunosuppressive capacity of LR-MSCs was related to the secretion of PGE_2 since it was shown even in the absence of direct cell contact (Jarvinen et al., 2021).

Among studies aiming at characterizing the functional role of LR-MSCs, Kruk et al.: showed that human LR-MSCs can also be forced to differentiate *in vitro* toward adipocytes (Kruk et al., 2021), which closely resemble lipofibroblasts that support alveolar epithelial regeneration by secretion of FGF10 and assist in surfactant production. Thus, it might be speculated that such events, depending on cues from the microenvironment, may result in improved support of alveolar repair. *In vitro*, LR-MSCs secrete substantial levels of HFG as well as ECM molecules such as decorin, which is known to bind and inhibit TGF-β signaling (Kruk et al., 2021), acquiring of a role in alveolar repair. *In vitro* expanded LR-MSCs were also able to engraft decellularized lung tissue scaffolds and produce growth factors (Kruk et al., 2021). Concerning the role of LR-MSCs in lung pathologies and in particular in lung fibrosis several studies highlight a potential pathological role that is mediated by Wnt signaling. Cao et al. found that inhibition of the Shh-Wnt pathway in the bleomycin mouse model prevented LR-MSCs from differentiating into myofibroblasts and reduced lung fibrosis (Cao et al., 2018). Summers et al., further report in the same model that genetic

TABLE 1 | *In vitro* and *in vivo* studies involving LR-MSCs in lung homeostasis, injury and repair.

Study	Method	Source of MSCs	Outcome
Tong et al. (2016)	Intratracheal administration to rat	LR-MSCs/BM-MSCs	↓ inflammation after LPS-induced lung injury
Antunes et al. (2014)	Elastase murine model/intratracheal administration	LR/AD/BM-MSCs	↓ alveolar hyperinflation ↓Collagen fibers ↓Alveolar area collapse
Ricciardi et al. (2012)	*In vitro* co-culture and RA treatment	LR-MSCs/BM-MSCs	↓ T-cells/NK cells proliferation ↑LR-MSCs polarization after RA treatment
Jarvinen et al. (2021)	*In vitro* studies	LR-MSCs/allograft of human lung transplant	↓ T-cells proliferation ↑immunosuppressive capacity-PGE_2 secretion
Kruk et al. (2021)1	*In vitro* studies-differentiation	LR-MSCs	↑ HGF,↑ ECM proteins (decorin), ↑ engraftment of decellularized lung tissue scaffold
Cao et al. (2019)	Inhibition of Shh/WNT sigmalling.in bleomycin model	Analysis on murine LR-MSCs	↓ myofibroblast differentiation of LR-MSCs ↓lung fibrosis
Summers et al. (2020)	Knock out mouse model for MVPC	Murine MVPC-ABCG2$^+$cells	↑ microvascular dysfunction ↑lung fibrosis
Jun et al. (2011)	Intravenous injection of LR-MSCs	LR-MSCs	↓ bleomycin-induced fibrosis ↓ arterial hypertension (PAH)
Marriott et al. (2014)	*In vitro* functional study/*in vivo* study bleomycin mouse model	Human LR-MSCs/ ABCG2$^+$MSC	↓ LR-MSCs cell number in IPF patients ↑pro-fibrotic reprogramming
Martin et al. (2020)	*In vitro* studies	LR-MSCs from donor and IPF patients	↓ decreased genetic profile in the ox-phospho. Pathway in LR_MSCs from IPF ↓*in vitro* repair potential (lung epithelial wound)

activation of Wnt in linage labeled ABCG2 positive pulmonary mesenchymal vascular progenitor cells (MVPC) drive microvascular dysfunction and exacerbated fibrosis (Summers et al., 2021). In 2011 Jun and collaborators demonstrated that treatment of mice with bleomycin led to the decrease of endogenous LR-MSCs population identified as H33342^{low}CD45^{neg} by flow cytometry and *in vivo* by immunostaining to detect the multidrug resistance transporter ATP binding cassette (ABCG2.) Indeed, they hypothesized that decrease in the LR-MSCs population favored the progression of fibrosis measured with Aschroft score inflammation, and pulmonary arterial hypertension (PAH). The replacement of lung resident stem cells by intravenous injection of exogenous LR-MSCs immediately after the intratracheal administration of bleomycin reduced both the bleomycin-associated fibrosis and the PAH (Jun et al., 2011). The study from Marriott et al.; described the functional role of LR-MSCs in IPF. They found that LR-MSCs were located in the distal lung and expresses ABCG2 contributing to the myofibroblast population and lung tissue remodeling in IPF. They found that in patients with IPF or ILD ABCG2^{pos} cell numbers were decreased relative to control, possibly because most of them differentiated into myofibroblasts contributing to the lung remodeling during IPF (Marriott et al., 2014). In another functional study, Martin et al. compared LR-MSCs from donor and IPF patients and found that IPF derived LR-MSCs presented a decreased genetic profile in the oxidative phosphorylation pathway and had reduced potential to induce the repair of a lung epithelial wound in an *in vitro* indirect co-culture system (Martin et al., 2020). Thus, abnormalities in endogenous LR-MSCs may contribute to aberrant alveolar repair responses in IPF. For their use in autologous cell-based therapies, more insight into LR-MSCs function and potential abnormalities in IPF is crucial and may guide pre-conditioning strategies of LR-MSCs.

Finally, in addition to their molecular and functional properties, understanding the spatial location of LR-MSCs within the lung is crucial in order to elucidate their physiological role in maintaining lung homeostasis. Although the exact location of LR-MSCs remains under debate, recent studies found that human LR-MSCs express the so called "HOX code" characteristic of vascular wall MSCs (VW-MSCs derived from the vascular wall of adult human blood vessels) therefore pointing at a vascular nature. According to this picture, LR-MSCs would be located within two areas: 1. a vascular niche situated at the perivascular space between the vessels and the surrounding tissue, and 2. an alveolar niche in close contact with the capillary endothelial cells and the alveolar epithelial cells (Steens et al., 2021).

To date, given the poor functional characterization of LR-MSCs related to the bone marrow counterpart, their role in the lung homeostasis and pathologies should be inferred both from the studies published on LR-MSCs (Steens et al., 2021), and essentially from studies based on the comparison of those to BM-MSCs. Indeed, a deeper characterization of LR-MSCs, with more *in vitro* and *in vivo* studies that will recapitulate both the spatial location and the functional effects of these cells in the lung would clarify their role within lung tissue microenvironment to enrich the knowledge in the LR-MSCs biology in order to perform new and effective LR-MSCs-based therapy. (**Table 1**).

THE ROLE OF EXOGENOUSLY ADMINISTERED MESENCHYMAL STROMAL/STEM CELLS IN LUNG REPAIR AFTER INJURY

MSCs are able to regulate the adaptive and innate immune systems by either their paracrine effect via soluble factors or

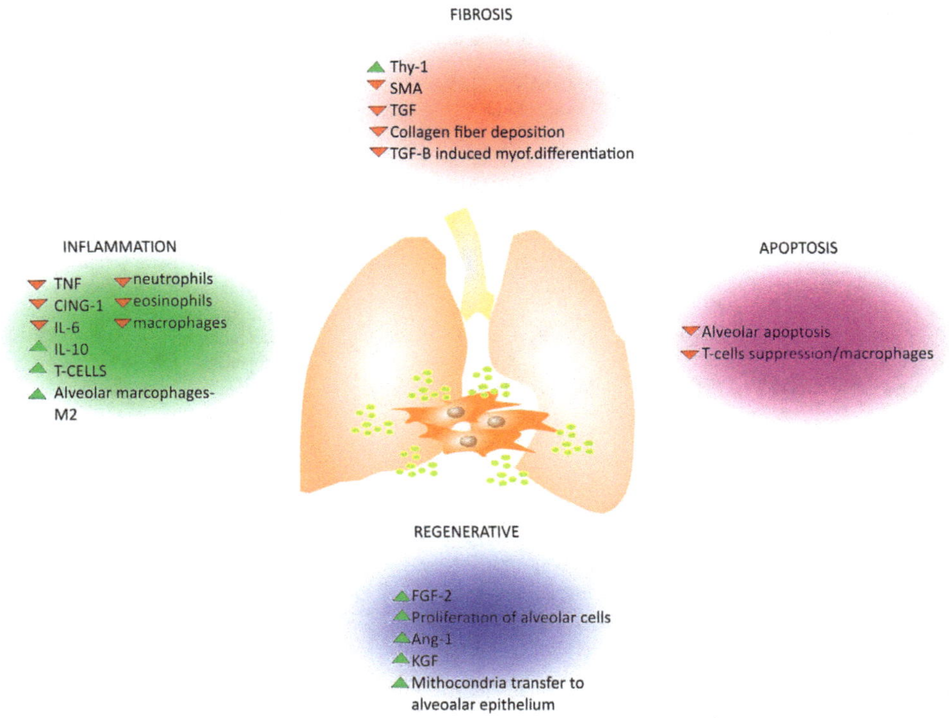

FIGURE 3 | Paracrine effects of MSCs in lung disease. Since the MSCs derived EVs play pivotal roles in different pathways that are common in lung disease, several works describe the effect of their administration for lung diseases treatment. In general, the MSCs derived EVs display antifibrotic, antiapoptotic, anti-inflammatory effects and counteract fibrosis with different mechanisms where they can either enhance (green head-arrow) or down-regulate (red head-arrow) growth factors and cytokines secretion as well as functional activity in lungs (e.g., collagen deposition, mitochondria transfer, etc) as summarized in the cartoon.

by cell–cell contact mechanisms with inhibition of T-lymphocyte proliferation, modulation of regulatory T-cells (Tregs) function, maturation of dendritic cells, reduction of B-cell activation and proliferation, inhibition of proliferation and cytotoxicity of NK cells, and stimulation of regulatory T cells (Gharibi and Hughes, 2012; Gao et al., 2016). The paracrine effect of different sources of MSCs is expressed through the secretion of soluble anti-inflammatory factors including but not limited to TGF-β, hepatocyte growth factor (HGF), interleukin (IL)-10, IL-1 receptor antagonist (IL-1Ra) prostaglandin E2 (PGE2) microRNAs (Vishnubhatla et al., 2014; Gazdic et al., 2015; Maguire, 2013), and factors that drive endothelial and epithelial repair and regeneration such as angiopoetin 1 (ANGPT1), FGFs (FGF2, FGF10) keratinocyte growth factor (KGF)/FGF7, hepatocyte growth factor (HGF), epidermal growth factor (EGF) and vascular endothelial growth factor alpha (VEGFA). In addition, MSCs can modulate repair responses by the deposition and remodeling of extracellular matrix (Kruk et al., 2021) providing cues to instruct cellular behavior such as survival, migration and proliferation (**Figure 3**).There have been a wide range of MSCs anti-inflammatory and immunomodulatory properties demonstrated in preclinical models of lung injuries including pulmonary fibrosis (Behnke et al., 2020). Although BM-derived MSCs are the most extensively investigated (Zhang et al., 2019), MSCs from other sources such as umbilical cord, placenta and adipose tissue have been studied (Aguilar et al., 2009; Yamada et al., 2004) (**Table 2**). As one example, in a bleomycin-induced lung injury model in mice, Moodley et al.; demonstrated that umbilical cord derived MSCs (uMSCs) can reduce lung inflammation and prevent fibrosis by up-regulating anti-inflammatory modulators and downregulating both cytokine production and pro-fibrotic factor release as measured through quantitative real-time PCR from whole lung suspensions from mice at 14 days post-bleomycin (Moodley et al., 2009). Indeed, in another study using the bleomycin mouse model of lung fibrosis, placenta-derived MSCs suppressed the infiltration of neutrophils, mitigated the inflammatory response and promoted lung tissue regeneration (Cargnoni et al., 2009; Antoniou et al., 2018). However, as shown in **Table 2**, in most of the preclinical studies, MSCs were administered after a few hours or days following the induction of lung damage and prevented the development of fibrotic changes (Jenkins et al., 2017). In contrast, when MSCs were administered at weeks 8, 10, 12, and 14 after-BLM induction (Moeller et al., 2008), no effect on lung collagen content was found while only improvement in Ashcroft score and lung TGF-β levels was reported. These studies mirror findings in one of the original studies on MSCs effects in the bleomycin lung model in which MSCs administration immediately after bleomycin significantly reduces inflammation, collagen deposition, and MMPs activation preventing development of fibrosis whereas delayed application decreased the inflammation but failed to reduce lung fibrosis (Ortiz et al., 2003). In another pre-clinical study Yu et al.;

TABLE 2 | Pre-clinical applications of MSCs in lung diseases. DAB = days after bleomycin administration.

Study	Lung disease model	Type of MSCs	Source of MSCs	Effect	Timing of administration
Li et al. (2017a)	Pulmonary fibrosis	Human fpMSCs	Placenta	↓ collagen deposition, ↑ pro-fibrotic cytokines	1 × 10^{5}cells-tail vein-3DAB
Cargnoni et al. (2009)	Pulmonary fibrosis	Murine/human MSCs	Placenta	↓ neutrophil infiltration	1–4X10^{5}cells - intraper.intrajug.intratrach.-15mAB
Moodley et al. (2009)	ARDS	Human MSCs	Umbilical cord	↓ TIMP expression, ↓ lung cytokine, ↑ MMP expression	1 × 10^{6}cells-tail vein-1DAB
Jun et al. (2011)	Pulmonary fibrosis	Murine MSCs	Lung	↓ lymphocyte and granulocyte infiltration, ↓ PAH	1.5–2.5 × 10^6-tail vein-14DAB
Moodley et al. (2013)	COPD- pulmonary fibrosis	Murine/human MSCs	Bone marrow, amnion	↓ TGF-β, ↑ MMP-9,↑ GM-CSF, ↑ IL-1RA	1 × 10^{6}cells-tail vein-3DAB
Huleihel et al. (2017)	Pulmonary fibrosis	Human MSCs	Bone marrow	↓ collagen deposition and CD45-positive cells	5 × 10^{5}cells-tail vein-7DAB
Ortiz et al. (2003)	IPF	Murine MSCs	Bone marrow	↓ collagen deposition, ↓ inflammation	5 × 10^{5}cells-intrajug. 0-7DAB
Ortiz et al. (2007)	ILD	Murine MSCs	Bone marrow	↓ IL-1 and TNF-α	5 × 10^{5}cells-intrajug-0DAB
Huang et al. (2015)	Pulmonary fibrosis	Rat MSCs	Bone marrow	↓ oxidative stress and collagen deposition	2,5 × 10^{6}cells-tail vein -0-7DAB
Lee et al. (2014)	ALI	Murine MSCs	Bone marrow	↓ TGF-β, ↓ IL-1β, ↓ VEGF, ↓ TNF-α, ↓ IL-6, ↓ NOS	1 × 10^7-tail vein-4DAB
Ono et al. (2015)	IPF	Human MSCs	Bone marrow	↓ endoplasmic reticulum stress, ↓ oxidative stress, ↓ TGF-β1	5 × 10^{5}cells-tail vein-0-1DAB
Lan et al. (2015)	IPF	Murine MSCs	Bone marrow	↓ inflammation, ↑ lung function	5 × 10^{5}cells-intratrach-0-3DAB
Cahill et al. (2016)	IPF	Murine MSCs	Bone marrow	↓ IL-1β, ↓ apoptosis, ↑ HGF	5 × 10^{4}cells-tail vein-6h-9DAB
Kotani T et al. (2017)	IP	Murine ADSCs	Adipose tissue	↓ inflammation, ↓ fibrosis	2,5 × 10^{4}cells-tail vein-0-7DAB
Lee et al. (2014)	IPF	Human ADSCs	Adipose tissue	↓ fibrosis, ↓ apoptosis, ↓ TGF-β, ↓ epithelial cell hyperplasia	3 × 10^{5}cells-intraper. 0-DAB
Tashiro et al. (2015)	IPF	Murine ADSCs	Adipose tissue	↓ oxidative stress, ↓ fibrosis, ↓ apoptosis, ↓ TGF-β, ↓ MMP-2	5 × 10^{5}cells-tail vein-1DAB
Yu et al. (2015)	IPF	Murine MSCs	Bone marrow	↑ lung injury repair↓ fibrosis, ↓ INFγ↓ MMP-1 ↓ TGF-β, ↓ MMP-9	2.5 × 10^{6}cells-tail vein-1,3,6DAB
Rubio et al. (2017)	IPF	Murine MSCs	Adipose tissue	↓lung and skin fibrosis, ↓ miR-199–3p↑CAV-1	5 × 10^{5}cells-tail vein-1DAB

further investigated the mechanism and timing of MSCs administration in bleomycin-induced pulmonary fibrosis. They demonstrated that BM-MSCs administration at day 3 and day 6 decreased lung fibrosis and inflammation down-regulating MMP9, TIMP-1, INF-γ and TGF-β to the same extent as after day 1 of bleomycin treatment. Thus, they stated that delayed BM-MSCs administration for up to 6 days after bleomycin treatment might be effective but did not look at longer intervals (Yu et al., 2015). Ni et al. demonstrated that in a humanized mouse model of BLM-induced lung fibrosis, human BM-MSCs administered at day 2 after bleomycin injection could prevent the progression of pulmonary fibrosis suppressing bleomycin-induced human T-cell infiltration and pro-inflammatory cytokine production targeting the PD-1/programmed death-ligand 1 pathway. However, BM-MSCs administration at day 7 after BLM injection did not improve lung function nor reverse established fibrosis. The authors concluded that human BM-MSCs administration displayed anti-fibrotic effects only in the early phase of BLM induced lung damage, namely the inflammatory phase (Ni et al., 2018). Taken together, these studies demonstrate that while MSCs are effective in mitigating acute lung inflammation and preventing development of lung fibrosis, they do not reverse established fibrosis. As IPF is usually diagnosed only after extensive fibrotic changes are present, this raises questions as to whether MSCs administration will be beneficial in IPF. However, in a recent study from Zakaria et al. in albino rats BM-MSCs systemically administered 28 days after bleomycin-induction of lung damage; resulted in reversion of established fibrosis, restored lung architecture, and improved lung functions (Zakaria et al., 2021). The mechanisms by which these effects occurred need further study and may open up better understanding that will support use of systemically administered MSCs in IPF.

To date, the immunomodulatory effects of systemic or intratracheal administration of allogeneic and also xenogeneic MSCs on both the innate and adaptive immune response have been intensively explored (Masterson et al., 2019). In contrast, less is known about the interaction of lung resident MSCs with the immune system and role of LR-MSCs in pathogenesis or repair from lung injuries.

Finally, along with the beneficial role of exogenous MSCs administration, there are studies using gene therapy to improve the MSCs potency for the resolution of lung injury in different animal models. To this purpose, overexpressing of MSCs with

HGF (HGF-MSCs) which is a growth factor with anti-inflammatory, antiapoptotic, and reparative properties, have also been tested in acute lung injury models. To this purpose, MSC-based hepatocyte growth factor (HGF) has been used as gene therapy for RILI (radiation-induced lung injury). Mice receiving single dose radiation with 20 Gy of γ rays locally to the lung and-HGF-modified MSCs (MSCs-HGF) revealed improved histopathological and biochemical markers of lung injury. MSCs-HGF reduced secretion and expression of proinflammatory cytokines, such as TNF-α, interferon-γ, interleukin (IL)-6, and intercellular adhesion molecule-1, increasing the expression level of anti-inflammatory cytokine IL-10 and decreasing the expression levels of profibrotic factors TGF-β, Col1a1 and Col3a1 culminating in the reduction of lung fibrosis progression (Wang et al., 2013) In another study from Chen and collaborators, rat bone marrow-derived MSCs transfected to express HGF increased MSCs viability, and inhibit the proinflammatory phenotype of MSCs in the inflammatory condition. In the rat model of ischemia/reperfusion I/R-induced lung injury, MSCs-HGF administration enhanced PaO_2 level and ameliorate lung pathological injury, compared with MSCs treatment (Chen et al., 2017).

PRE-CLINICAL STUDIES INVOLVING EXTRACELLULAR VESICLES DERIVED MESENCHYMAL STROMAL/STEM CELLS IN LUNG FIBROSIS

Given their ability to reduce inflammation and their action on myofibroblast activity, MSC-derived secretome and EVs have been increasingly investigated for development of new therapeutic strategies for lung fibrosis (Worthington and Hagood, 2020). In bleomycin-induced fibrosis in immunocompetent CD1 mice, lung spheroid cell-secretome (LSC-Sec) and exosomes (LSC-Exo) derived from human LSCs generated from whole lung samples were administered by inhalation to treat fibrosis progression. Starting at day 10 mice received daily nebulized inhalations for seven consecutive days with a dose of 10 mg of secretome protein per kg of body weight or 10×10^9 exosomes particles per kg of body weight or an equal volume of PBS (Dinh et al., 2020). The results demonstrated that both LSC-Sec and LSC-Exo treatments could attenuate and resolve bleomycin-induced lung fibrosis, restoring normal alveolar structure and decreasing both collagen accumulation and myofibroblast proliferation. Indeed, they showed that LSC-Exo reproduced part of the regenerative potency of the full secretome, while LSC-Exo overcame MSC-Exo in resolving pulmonary fibrosis and healthy lung function (Dinh et al., 2020).

Shentu and co-workers demonstrated in *in vitro* studies that MSC-derived EVs can play an antifibrotic role demonstrating down-regulation of TGF-β induced differentiation of isolated lung fibroblasts into myofibroblast, interaction with resident myofibroblasts through Thy 1, and delivery of miRNAs targeting profibrotic genes. To this purpose, MSC-EVs bearing miR-630, a powerful suppressor of pro-fibrotic genes in lung fibroblasts, was used to reduce α-SMA expression in lung fibroblasts (Shentu et al., 2017; Fujita et al., 2018). Mansouri and collaborators demonstrated that human BM-MSCs-derived exosomes prevented and reverted experimental pulmonary fibrosis along with the modulation of monocyte phenotypes in bleomycin mice model (Mansouri et al., 2019). In particular, they initially evaluated the preventive effect of a single dose of human BM-derived MSCs (Mex) administered concurrently with endotracheal administration of bleomycin in 14-week-old mice on day 0. The results demonstrated that at day 7, Mex administration significantly reduced the bleomycin-induced pulmonary fibrosis and restored collagen content to levels similar to their bleomycin untreated-counterparts. In parallel studies, Mex administration at either day 7 or on day 21 decreased collagen content compared to control animals, although the administration after 21 days was not able to decrease the Aschroft score (Mansouri et al., 2019). Since it is known that in lung diseases LR-MSCs can migrate from their tissue niche toward the alveolar space and can be recovered from the BAL fluid, LR-MSCs EVs have been isolated from BAL fluid (Sinclair et al., 2016; Shah et al., 2019). To this purpose, Martin-Medina et al.; isolated EVs from BALF collected from mice 14 days after intratracheal bleomycin, IPF patients, non IPF ILD patients, non ILD patients where BALF was performed for diagnostic evaluation (unclear cough) and ILD was excluded, and healthy volunteers as controls. The EVs were then characterized by transmission electron microscopy, nanoparticle tracking analysis, and Western blotting which demonstrated increased number of exosomes, according to their size distribution, in BALF from experimental lung fibrosis (bleomycin mouse model) and from patients with IPF compared to patients with non- ILD/non-IPF ILD. Notably, EVs from IPF BALF stimulated Wnt5A-mediated proliferation of primary human lung fibroblasts in *in vitro* studies (Martin-Medina et al., 2018).

CLINICAL STUDIES INVOLVING MESENCHYMAL STROMAL/STEM CELLS IN LUNG FIBROSIS

Clinical studies of MSCs administration in IPF patients to date have mainly consisted of small phase I safety investigations. MSCs are known to express major histocompatibility complex I (MHC I) and lack MHC II expression, a mechanism that allows them to escape immune host reaction. However, when MSCs are systemically infused, the high level of procoagulant tissue factor (TF) expressed might trigger the instant blood-mediated inflammatory reaction (IBMIR) with potential lethal consequences for patients. Thus, it has become crucial to find strategies aiming at modulating MSCs hemocompatibility in order to increase safety and efficacy of intravascular MSCs therapies (Moll et al., 2019). Focusing on IPF, the first phase I trial performed by Tzouvelekis et al.; showed safety of MSCs application. This was a phase Ib, non-randomized, open label clinical trial to study the safety of three endobronchial infusions of autologous adipose derived stromal cells (ADSCs)-stromal vascular fraction (SVF) in patients with IPF (n = 14) of mild to moderate disease severity. They showed an acceptable safety profile with attributable serious short and long-term adverse events in all patients. However, there was no apparent suggestion of efficacy and the study was not designed to detect efficacy (Tzouvelekis et al., 2013). Another phase I safety clinical trial (AETHER) utilized a single intravenous infusion of allogeneic BM-MSCs in nine patients with mild to moderate IPF. No serious adverse events as death, pulmonary embolism, stroke and hospitalization for worsening dyspnea were observed through 60 weeks although two deaths occurred because of progression of IPF. Secondary exploratory end points demonstrated a decline in % predicted FVC and DLCO below the defined thresholds for IPF disease progression, however, this non-controlled trial was not designed to evaluate changes in lung function (Glassberg et al., 2017). However, as the pre-clinical data, to date, more strongly suggests a potential beneficial role of MSCs administration in reducing inflammation and preventing development of fibrosis rather than reversing established fibrosis, it would be informative to explore the effect of MSCs administration in an acute exacerbation of IPF for instance following a respiratory virus infection. However, to the best of our knowledge there are not as yet pre-clinical studies based on the induction of experimental respiratory virus infection in mice with bleomycin-induced fibrosis treated with administered MSCs.

CONCLUSION AND FUTURE PERSPECTIVE

There are multiple potential roles of MSCs in lung fibrosis. On one hand, given the lessons learned from preclinical studies, further strategies can be developed in which exogenously administered MSCs might contribute to prevent disease progression or might even revert established lung fibrosis, suppressing inflammation and supporting alveolar repair. This will involve further clarification on the route and timing of MSCs administration, source and age of MSCs administered and other factors that have thus far given rise to the heterogeneous results of available preclinical data. On the other hand, lung resident MSCs might contribute to IPF pathogenesis and progression as they might differentiate into myofibroblast following lung damage. Moreover, whereas the role of LR-MSCs in lung fibrosis pathology is still being elucidated, it remains presently unknown whether healthy LR-MSCs could potentially restore/rescue this function. Since the microenvironment to which MSCs are exposed seems to regulate function and to affect further cellular development, it is arguable that healthy LR-MSCs might have a therapeutical effect in terms of lung regeneration. Thus, further work on characterizing MSCs from different sources, including LR-MSCs, in terms of function, phenotype and secretome will contribute to a greater understanding of the mechanism of disease in the aim of developing specialized and targeted approaches to treat lung fibrosis. Furthermore, besides the characterization of different MSCs sources, the gene therapy based on a deeper knowledge of molecular scenario of MSCs after their administration, would improve their potency and potentiate their effect to treat specific disease.

AUTHOR CONTRIBUTIONS

AS and RT equally contributed to the conception, design, writing, and editing of the manuscript and they should be considered both first author. IH and AM (4th author) wrote and critically edited the manuscript. AM (5th author), GB, IC, DA and FG reviewed the literature, designed the review, wrote the manuscript, and produced figures. LM, AM (11th author), SC, RF, LT, CN and IM wrote the manuscript and produced figures. DW, MD and EC critically reviewed and edited the manuscript. All the authors read and approved the final version of the manuscript.

ACKNOWLEDGMENTS

We thank FIMARP (Federazione Italiana MAlattie Rare del Polmone), Modena Golf Country Club, and AMMI (Associazione Mogli di Medici Italiani) for their support to our research.

REFERENCES

Adams, T. S., Schupp, J. C., Poli, S., Ayaub, E. A., Neumark, N., Ahangari, F., et al. (2019). *Single Cell RNA-Seq Reveals Ectopic and Aberrant Lung Resident Cell Populations in Idiopathic Pulmonary Fibrosis*. bioRxiv. doi:10.1101/759902

Agha, E. E., Herold, S., Alam, D. A. L., Quantius, J., Mackenzie, B., Carraro, G., et al. (2014). *Fgf10 -positive Cells Represent a Progenitor Cell Population during Lung Development and Postnatally*, 296–306. doi:10.1242/dev.099747

Agha, E. E. L., Moiseenko, A., Kheirollahi, V., De Langhe, S., Crnkovic, S., Kwapiszewska, G., et al. (2017). Two-Way Conversion between Lipogenic and Myogenic Fibroblastic Phenotypes Marks the Progression and Resolution of Lung Fibrosis. *Cell Stem Cell* 20 (2), 261–273.e3. doi:10.1016/j.stem.2016.10.004

Aguilar, S., Chris, J. S., Katrina, M., Emma, N., Gordon, S., Geoff, L., et al. (2009). Bone Marrow Stem Cells Expressing Keratinocyte Growth Factor via an Inducible Lentivirus Protects against Bleomycin-Induced Pulmonary Fibrosis. *PLoS ONE* 4 (11), e8013. doi:10.1371/journal.pone.0008013

Alam, D. A. L., El Agha, E., Sakurai, R., Kheirollahi, V., Moiseenko, A., Danopoulos, S., et al. (2015). Evidence for the Involvement of Fibroblast Growth Factor 10 in Lipofibroblast Formation during Embryonic Lung Development. *NIH* 142, 4139–4150. doi:10.1242/dev.109173

Alcayaga-miranda, F., González, P. L., Lopez-verrilli, A., Aguila-díaz, C., Contreras, L., and Maroun Khoury., S. D. (2016). Prostate Tumor-Induced Angiogenesis Is Blocked by Exosomes Derived from Menstrual Stem Cells through the Inhibition of Reactive Oxygen. *species* 7 (28), 44462–44477. doi:10.18632/oncotarget.9852

Alder, J. K., Stanley, S. E., Wagner, C. L., and Hamilton, M. (2015). Exome Sequencing Identifies Mutant TINF2 in a Family with Pulmonary Fibrosis. *CHEST* 147 (5), 1361–1368. doi:10.1378/chest.14-1947

Allen, J. T., and Spiteri, M. A. (2002). Growth Factors in Idiopathic Pulmonary Fibrosis: Relative Roles. *Respir. Res.* 3 (1), 13. doi:10.1186/rr162

Allen, R. J., Guillen-Guio, B., Oldham, J. M., Ma, S. F., Amy, D., Paynton, M. L., et al. (2020). Genome-wide Association Study of Susceptibility to Idiopathic Pulmonary Fibrosis. *Am. J. Respir. Crit. Care Med.* 201 (5), 564–574. doi:10.1164/rccm.201905-1017OC

Allen, R. J., Porte, J., Braybrooke, R., Flores, C., Fingerlin, T. E., Oldham, J. M., et al. (2017). Genetic Variants Associated with Susceptibility to Idiopathic Pulmonary Fibrosis in People of European Ancestry: a Genome-wide Association Study. *Lancet Respir. Med.* 5 (11), 869–880. doi:10.1016/S2213-2600(17)30387-9

Andrianifahanana, M., Wilkes, M. C., Gupta, S. K., Rahimi, R. A., Repellin, C. E., Edens, M., et al. (2013). Profibrotic TGFβ Responses Require the Cooperative Action of PDGF and ErbB Receptor Tyrosine Kinases. *FASEB J.* 27 (11), 4444–4454. doi:10.1096/fj.12-224907

Angeles, L. (2015). TISSUE -SPECIFIC STEM CELLS Progenitors of Secondary Crest Myofibroblasts Are Developmentally Committed in Early Lung. *Stem Cells* 33 (3), 999–1012. doi:10.1002/stem.1911

Antoniou, K. M., Karagiannis, K., Tsitoura, E., Bibaki, E., Lasithiotaki, I., Proklou, A., et al. (2018). Clinical Applications of Mesenchymal Stem Cells in Chronic Lung Diseases (Review). *Biomed. Rep.* 8 (4), 314–318. doi:10.3892/br.2018.1067

Antunes, M. A., Laffey, J. G., Pelosi, P., and Patricia, R. M. (2014). Mesenchymal Stem Cells Trials for Pulmonary Disease. *J. Cel Biochem* 115 (6), 1023–1032. doi:10.1002/jcb.24783

Atashi, F., Modarressi, A., and Pepper, M. S. (2015). The Role of Reactive Oxygen Species in Mesenchymal Stem Cell Adipogenic and Osteogenic Differentiation: a Review. *Stem Cell Dev* 24 (10), 1150–1163. doi:10.1089/scd.2014.0484

Barczyk, M., Matthias, S., and Sabrina, M. (2015). Stem Cell-Based Therapy in Idiopathic Pulmonary Fibrosis. *Stem Cel Rev. Rep.* 11 (4), 598–620. doi:10.1007/s12015-015-9587-7

Barron, L., Gharib, S. A., and Duffield, J. S. (2016). Lung Pericytes and Resident Fibroblasts: Busy Multitaskers. *Am. J. Pathol.* 186 (10), 2519–2531. doi:10.1016/j.ajpath.2016.07.004

Bartis, D., Louise, E. C., Vijay, K. D., Lee, B., Fisher, A. J., Croft, A. P., et al. (2016). Role of CD248 as a Potential Severity Marker in Idiopathic Pulmonary Fibrosis. *BMC Pulm. Med.* 16 (1), 1–10. doi:10.1186/s12890-016-0211-7

Beer, L., Mildner, M., and Jan Ankersmit, H. (2017). Cell Secretome Based Drug Substances in Regenerative Medicine: when Regulatory Affairs Meet Basic Science. *Ann. Transl Med.* 5 (7), 5–7. doi:10.21037/atm.2017.03.50

Beers, M. F., and Morrisey, E. E. (2011). Science in Medicine the Three R 's of Lung Health and Disease: Repair, Remodeling, and Regeneration. *J. Clin. Invest.* 121 (6), 2065–2073. doi:10.1172/JCI45961.respiratory

Behnke, J., Kremer, S., Shahzad, T., Chao, C., Böttcher-Friebertshäuser, E., Morty, R. E., et al. (2020). MSC Based Therapies—New Perspectives for the Injured Lung. *J. Clin. Med.* 9 (3), 682. doi:10.3390/jcm9030682

Bellaye, P. S., and Kolb, M. (2015). Why Do Patients Get Idiopathic Pulmonary Fibrosis? Current Concepts in the Pathogenesis of Pulmonary Fibrosis. *BMC Med.* 13 (1), 1–3. doi:10.1186/s12916-015-0412-6

Betensley, A., Sharif, R., and Karamichos, D. (2016). A Systematic Review of the Role of Dysfunctional Wound Healing in the Pathogenesis and Treatment of Idiopathic Pulmonary Fibrosis. *J. Clin. Med.* 6 (1), 2. doi:10.3390/jcm6010002

Bitterman, P. (2018). Fibroblast–Matrix Cross-Talk in Idiopathic Pulmonary Fibrosis: Cross-Links at the Crossroads. *Am. J. Respir. Cel Mol. Biol.* 58 (5), 547–548. doi:10.1165/rcmb.2017-0402ED

Blokland, K. E. C., Waters, D. W., Schuliga, M., Read, J., Pouwels, S. D., Grainge, C. L., et al. (2020). Senescence of Ipf Lung Fibroblasts Disrupt Alveolar Epithelial Cell Proliferation and Promote Migration in Wound Healing. *Pharmaceutics* 12 (4). doi:10.3390/pharmaceutics12040389

Bochaton-Piallat, L., Gabbiani, G., and Hinz, B. (2016). The Myofibroblast in Wound Healing and Fibrosis: Answered and Unanswered Questions. *F1000Research* 5 (0), 1–8. doi:10.12688/f1000research.8190.1

Bolanos, A. L., Mendoza Milla, C., Lira, J. C., Ramírez, R., Checa, M., Barrera, L., et al. (2012). Role of Sonic Hedgehog in Idiopathic Pulmonary Fibrosis. *Am. J. Physiol. - Lung Cell Mol. Physiol.* 303 (11), 978–990. doi:10.1152/ajplung.00184.2012

Bonser, L., and Erle, D. (2017). Airway Mucus and Asthma: The Role of MUC5AC and MUC5B. *J. Clin. Med.* 6 (12), 112. doi:10.3390/jcm6120112

Burgess, J. K., and Irene, H. H. (2019). *Stem Cell-Based Therapy for Lung Disease.* Springer. doi:10.1007/978-3-030-29403-8

Cahill, E. F., Kennelly, H., Carty, F., Mahon, B. P., and English, K. (2016). Hepatocyte Growth Factor Is Required for Mesenchymal Stromal Cell Protection against Bleomycin-Induced Pulmonary Fibrosis. *Stem Cell Transl Med* 5 (10), 1307–1318. doi:10.5966/sctm.2015-0337

Cao, H., Chen, X., Hou, J., Wang, C., Zou, X., Shen, Y., et al. (2019). The Shh/Gli Signaling cascade Regulates Myofibroblastic Activation of Lung-Resident Mesenchymal Stem Cells via the Modulation of Wnt10a Expression during Pulmonary Fibrogenesis. *Lab. Invest.* 100 (3), 363–377. doi:10.1038/s41374-019-0316-8

Cao, H., Wang, C., Chen, X., Hou, J., Zou, X., Shen, Y., et al. (2018). Inhibition of Wnt/β-Catenin Signaling Suppresses Myofibroblast Differentiation of Lung Resident Mesenchymal Stem Cells and Pulmonary Fibrosis. *Scientific Rep.* 8 (1), 1–14. doi:10.1038/s41598-018-28968-9

Cao, S. S., and Kaufman, R. J. (2012). Unfolded Protein Response. *Curr. Biol.* 22 (16), R622–R626. PMID: 22917505. doi:10.1016/j.cub.2012.07.004

Cargnoni, A., Gibelli, L., Tosini, A., Signoroni, P. B., Nassuato, C., Arienti, D., et al. (2009). Transplantation of Allogeneic and Xenogeneic Placenta-Derived Cells Reduces Bleomycin-Induced Lung Fibrosis. *Cel Transplant.* 18 (4), 405–422. doi:10.3727/096368909788809857

Cerri, S., Monari, M., Guerrieri, A., Donatelli, P., Bassi, I., Garuti, M., et al. (2019). Real-life Comparison of Pirfenidone and Nintedanib in Patients with Idiopathic Pulmonary Fibrosis: A 24-month Assessment. *Respir. Med.* 159 (10), 105803. doi:10.1016/j.rmed.2019.105803

Chanda, D., Otoupalova, E., Smith, S. R., Volckaert, T., Stijn, P. D., and Victor, J. T. (2019). Developmental Pathways in the Pathogenesis of Lung Fibrosis. *Mol. Aspects Med.* 65 (7), 56–69. doi:10.1016/j.mam.2018.08.004

Chen, S., Chen, X., Wu, X., Wei, S., Han, W., Lin, J., et al. (2017). Hepatocyte Growth Factor-Modified Mesenchymal Stem Cells Improve Ischemia/reperfusion-Induced Acute Lung Injury in Rats. *Gene Ther.* 24 (1), 3–11. Epub 2016 Aug 24: PMID: 27556817. doi:10.1038/gt.2016.64

Chen, X., Shi, C., Cao, H., Chen, L., Hou, J., Zou, X., et al. (2018). The Hedgehog and Wnt/β-Catenin System Machinery Mediate Myofibroblast Differentiation of LR-MSCs in Pulmonary. *Cel Death Dis.* 9 (6), 639. doi:10.1038/s41419-018-0692-9

Chilosi, M., Poletti, V., Zamò, A., Lestani, M., Montagna, L., Piccoli, P., et al. (2003). Aberrant Wnt/beta-Catenin Pathway Activation in Idiopathic Pulmonary Fibrosis. *Am. J. Pathol.* 162 (5), 1495–1502. PMID: 12707032; PMCID: PMC1851206. doi:10.1016/s0002-9440(10)64282-4

Chong, S., Sato, S., Kolb, M., and Gauldie, J. (2019). Fibrocytes and Fibroblasts—Where Are We Now. *Int. J. Biochem. Cel Biol.* 116 (August), 105595. doi:10.1016/j.biocel.2019.105595

Cigna, N., Elika, F. M., Brayer, S., Marchal-Somme, J., Wémeau-Stervinou, L., Fabre, A., et al. (2012). The Hedgehog System Machinery Controls Transforming Growth Factor-β-dependent Myofibroblastic Differentiation in Humans: Involvement in Idiopathic Pulmonary Fibrosis. *Am. J. Pathol.* 181 (6), 2126–2137. doi:10.1016/j.ajpath.2012.08.019

Collard, H. R., Ryerson, C. J., Corte, T. J., Jenkins, G., Kondoh, Y., Lederer, D. J., et al. (2016). Acute Exacerbation of Idiopathic Pulmonary Fibrosis an International Working Group Report. *Am. J. Respir. Crit. Care Med.* 194 (3), 265–275. doi:10.1164/rccm.201604-0801CI

Cruz, F. F., and Patricia, R. M. R. (2020). The Potential of Mesenchymal Stem Cell Therapy for Chronic Lung Disease. *Expert Rev. Respir. Med.* 14 (1), 31–39. doi:10.1080/17476348.2020.1679628

Dabrowska, S., Anna, A., and Janowski, M. (2021). Immunomodulatory and Regenerative Effects of Mesenchymal Stem Cells and Extracellular Vesicles: Therapeutic Outlook for in Fl Ammatory and Degenerative Diseases. *Front. Immunol.* 11 (2), 591065. doi:10.3389/fimmu.2020.591065

David, M. H., and Cory, M. H. (2017). Heterogeneity of Fibroblasts and Myofibroblasts in Pulmonary Fibrosis. *Physiol. Behav.* 176 (3), 139–148. doi:10.1007/s40139-017-0134-x

Dinh, P., Uyen, C. D., Paudel, D., Brochu, H., Kristen, D. P., Gracieux, M. C., et al. (2020). Inhalation of Lung Spheroid Cell Secretome and Exosomes Promotes Lung Repair in Pulmonary Fibrosis. *Nat. Commun.* 11 (1). doi:10.1038/s41467-020-14344-7

Dominici, M., Le Blanc, K., Mueller, I., Slaper-Cortenbach, I., Marini, F. C., Krause, D. S., et al. (2006). Minimal Criteria for Defining Multipotent Mesenchymal Stromal Cells. The International Society for Cellular Therapy Position Statement. *Cytotherapy* 8 (4), 315–317. doi:10.1080/14653240600855905

Doubková, M., Radová, L., Michaela, P., Trizuljak, J., Karol, P., Svobodová, K., et al. (2019). *A Novel Germline Mutation of the SFTPA1 Gene in Familial Interstitial Pneumonia*, 4–9. doi:10.1038/s41439-019-0044-z

Dressen, A., Abbas, A. R., Cabanski, C., Reeder, J., Ramalingam, T. R., Neighbors, M., et al. (2018). Analysis of Protein-Altering Variants in Telomerase Genes and Their Association with MUC5B Common Variant Status in Patients with Idiopathic Pulmonary Fibrosis: a Candidate Gene Sequencing Study. *Lancet Respir. Med.* 6 (8), 603–614. doi:10.1016/S2213-2600(18)30135-8

El Agha, E., Moiseenko, A., Kheirollahi, V., De Langhe, S., Crnkovic, S., and Kwapiszewska, G. (2017). Two-Way Conversion Between Lipogenic and Myogenic Fibroblastic Phenotypes Marks the Progression and Resolution of Lung Fibrosis. *Cell Stem Cell* 20 (4), 571. doi:10.1016/j.stem.2017.03.011. Erratum for: Cell Stem Cell. 2017 Feb 2;20(2):261-273.e3. PMID: 28388434

Enes, R. S., Ahrman, E., Palani, A., Hallgren, O., Bjermer, L., Malmström, A., et al. (2017). *Quantitative Proteomic Characterization of Lung-MSC and Bone Marrow-MSC Using DIA-Mass Spectrometry.* Springer, 1–12. doi:10.1038/s41598-017-09127-y

Ferguson, S. W., and Nguyen, J. (2016). Exosomes as Therapeutics: The Implications of Molecular Composition and Exosomal Heterogeneity. *J. Controlled Release* 228, 179–190. doi:10.1016/j.jconrel.2016.02.037

Fernandez, I. E., and Oliver, E. (2012). New Cellular and Molecular Mechanisms of Lung Injury and Fi Brosis in Idiopathic Pulmonary Fi Brosis. *The Lancet* 380 (9842), 680–688. doi:10.1016/S0140-6736(12)61144-1

Fingerlin, T. E., Murphy, E., Zhang, W., Peljto, A. L., Brown, K. K., Steele, M. P., et al. (2013). Genome-wide Association Study Identifies Multiple Susceptibility Loci for Pulmonary Fibrosis. *Nat. Genet.* 45 (6), 613–620. doi:10.1038/ng.2609

Fomby, P., Cherlin, A. J., Hadjizadeh, A., Doillon, C. J., Sueblinvong, V., Weiss, D. J., et al. (2010). Stem Cells and Cell Therapies in Lung Biology and Diseases: Conference Report. *Ann. Am. Thorac. Soc.* 12 (3), 181–204. doi:10.1002/term

Fujita, Y., Kadota, T., Araya, J., Ochiya, T., and Kuwano, K. (2018). Clinical Application of Mesenchymal Stem Cell-Derived Extracellular Vesicle-Based Therapeutics for Inflammatory Lung Diseases. *J. Clin. Med.* 7 (10), 355. doi:10.3390/jcm7100355

Gao, F., Chiu, S. M., Motan, D. A. L., Zhang, Z., Chen, L., Ji, H. L., et al. (2016). Mesenchymal Stem Cells and Immunomodulation: Current Status and Future Prospects. *Cel Death Dis.* 7 (1). doi:10.1038/cddis.2015.327

Gazdic, M., Volarevic, V., Arsenijevic, N., and Stojkovic, M. (2015). Mesenchymal Stem Cells: A Friend or Foe in Immune-Mediated Diseases. *Stem Cel Rev. Rep.* 11 (2), 280–287. doi:10.1007/s12015-014-9583-3

Geissler, S., Textor, M., Schmidt-Bleek, K., Klein, O., Thiele, M., Ellinghaus, A., et al. (2013). In Serum Veritas-In Serum Sanitas? Cell Non-autonomous Aging Compromises Differentiation and Survival of Mesenchymal Stromal Cells via the Oxidative Stress Pathway. *Cell Death Dis* 4 (12), e970, 2013. PMID: 24357801; PMCID: PMC3877568. doi:10.1038/cddis.2013.501

Gharibi, B., and Hughes, F. J. (2012). Effects of Medium Supplements on Proliferation, Differentiation Potential, and *In Vitro* Expansion of Mesenchymal Stem Cells. *Stem Cell Transl Med* 1 (11), 771–782. Epub 2012 Oct 23. PMID: 23197689; PMCID: PMC3659663. doi:10.5966/sctm.2010-0031

Glaspole, I., Glassberg, M. K., Gorina, E., Hopkins, P. M., David, K., Teherani, A., et al. (2014). A Phase 3 Trial of Pirfenidone in Patients with Idiopathic Pulmonary Fibrosis. *N. Engl. J. Med.* 2014, 2083–2092. doi:10.1056/NEJMoa1402582

Glassberg, M. K., Julia, M., Rebecca, L. T., Emmanuelle, S. S., Gustavo, A. R., Darcy, D., et al. (2017). Allogeneic Human Mesenchymal Stem Cells in Patients with Idiopathic Pulmonary Fibrosis via Intravenous Delivery (AETHER): A Phase I Safety Clinical Trial. *Chest* 151 (5), 971–981. doi:10.1016/j.chest.2016.10.061

Gokey, J. J., Sridharan, A., Xu, Y., Green, J., Carraro, G., Stripp, B. R., et al. (2018). Active Epithelial Hippo Signaling in Idiopathic Pulmonary Fibrosis. *JCI insight* 3 (6), e98738. doi:10.1172/jci.insight.98738

Golchin, A., Seyedjafari, E., and Ardeshirylajimi, E. (2020). Mesenchymal Stem Cell Therapy for COVID-19: Present or Future. *Stem Cel Rev. Rep.* 16 (3), 427–433. doi:10.1007/s12015-020-09973-w

Green, J., Endale, M., Auer, H., and Anne Karina, T. P. (2016). Diversity of Interstitial Lung Fibroblasts Is Regulated by Platelet-Derived Growth Factor Receptor a Kinase Activity. *Am. J. Respir. Cel Mol. Biol.* 54 (4), 532–545. doi:10.1165/rcmb.2015-0095OC

Gu, Z., Cao, X., Jiang, J., Li, L., Da, Z., Liu, H., et al. (2012). Upregulation of p16INK4A Promotes Cellular Senescence of Bone Marrow-Derived Mesenchymal Stem Cells from Systemic Lupus Erythematosus Patients. *Cell Signal* 24 (12), 2307–2314. Epub 2012 Jul 20. PMID: 22820504. doi:10.1016/j.cellsig.2012.07.012

Guenther, A., Krauss, E., Tello, S., Wagner, J., Paul, B., Kuhn, S., et al. (2018). The European IPF Registry (eurIPFreg): Baseline Characteristics and Survival of Patients With Idiopathic Pulmonary Fibrosis. *Respir Res.* 28 (1), 141. doi:10.1186/s12931-018-0845-5

Guescini, M., Genedani, S., Stocchi, V., and Agnati, L. F. (2010). Astrocytes and Glioblastoma Cells Release Exosomes Carrying mtDNA. *J. Neural Transm.* 117 (1), 1–4. doi:10.1007/s00702-009-0288-8

Hancock, L. A., Hennessy, C. E., Solomon, G. M., Dobrinskikh, E., Estrella, A., Hara, N., et al. (2018). Muc5b Overexpression Causes Mucociliary Dysfunction and Enhances Lung Fibrosis in Mice. *Nat. Commun.* 9 (1), 1–10. doi:10.1038/s41467-018-07768-9

Harrell, C., Fellabaum, C., Jovicic, N., Djonov, V., Arsenijevic, N., and Volarevic, V. (2019). Molecular Mechanisms Responsible for Therapeutic Potential of Mesenchymal Stem Cell-Derived Secretome. *Cells* 8 (5), 467. doi:10.3390/cells8050467

Hasaneen, N. A., Cao, J., Pulkoski-gross, A., Zucker, S., and Hussein, D. F. (2016). Extracellular Matrix Metalloproteinase Inducer (EMMPRIN) Promotes Lung Fibroblast Proliferation, Survival and Differentiation to Myofibroblasts. *Respir. Res.* 17, 1–14. doi:10.1186/s12931-016-0334-7

Henderson, W., Chi, E. Y., Ye, X., Nguyen, C., Tien, Y. T., Zhou, B., et al. (2010). *Inhibition of Wnt/β -catenin/CREB Binding Protein (CBP) Signaling Reverses Pulmonary Fi Brosis*, 14309–14314. doi:10.1073/pnas.1001520107

Herrera, I., Cisneros, J., Maldonado, M., Ramírez, R., Ortiz-Quintero, B., Elena, A., et al. (2013). Matrix Metalloproteinase (MMP)-1 Induces Lung Alveolar Epithelial Cell Migration and Proliferation, Protects from Apoptosis, and Represses Mitochondrial Oxygen Consumption. *J. Biol. Chem.* 288 (36), 25964–25975. doi:10.1074/jbc.M113.459784

Hinz, B. (2012). Mechanical Aspects of Lung Fibrosis: A Spotlight on the Myofibroblast. *Proc. Am. Thorac. Soc.* 9 (3), 137–147. doi:10.1513/pats.201202-017AW

Hinz, B., Phan, S. H., Thannickal, V. J., and Galli, A. (2007). Marie Luce Bochaton-Piallat, Giulio Gabbiani. 2007. The Myofibroblast: One Function, Multiple Origins. *Am. J. Pathol.* 170 (6), 1807–1816. doi:10.2353/ajpath.2007.070112

Hoffman, A. M., Paxson, J. A., Mazan, M. R., Davis, A. M., Tyagi, S., Murthy, S., et al. (2011). Lung-derived Mesenchymal Stromal Cell post-transplantation Survival, Persistence, Paracrine Expression, and Repair of Elastase-Injured Lung. *Stem Cell Dev* 20 (10), 1779–1792. Epub 2011 Jul 6. PMID: 21585237; PMCID: PMC3182034. doi:10.1089/scd.2011.0105

Horowitz, J. C., and Thannickal, V. J. (2019). Mechanisms for the Resolution of Organ Fibrosis. *Physiology* 34 (1), 43–55. doi:10.1152/physiol.00033.2018

Hu, H. H., Chen, D. Q., Wang, Y. N., Feng, Y. L., Cao, G., Vaziri, N. D., et al. (2018). New Insights into TGF-β/Smad Signaling in Tissue Fibrosis. *Chem. Biol. Interact* 292, 76–83. Epub 2018 Jul 11. PMID: 30017632. doi:10.1016/j.cbi.2018.07.008

Huang, K., Kang, X., Wang, X., Wu, S., Xiao, J., Li, Z., et al. (2015). Conversion of Bone Marrow Mesenchymal Stem Cells into Type II Alveolar Epithelial Cells Reduces Pulmonary Fibrosis by Decreasing Oxidative Stress in Rats. *Mol. Med. Rep.* 11, 1685–1692. doi:10.3892/mmr.2014.2981

Huleihel, L., Sellares, J., Cardenes, N., Álvarez, D., Faner, R., Sakamoto, K., et al. (2017). Modified Mesenchymal Stem Cells Using miRNA Transduction Alter Lung Injury in a Bleomycin Model. *Am. J. Physiol. - Lung Cel. Mol. Physiol.* 313, L92–L103. doi:10.1152/ajplung.00323.2016

Hung, C., Linn, G., Chow, Y., Kobayashi, A., Mittelsteadt, K., Altemeier, W. A., et al. (2013). Role of Lung Pericytes and Resident Fibroblasts in the Pathogenesis of Pulmonary Fibrosis. *Am. J. Respir. Crit. Care Med.* 188 (7), 820–830. PMID: 23924232; PMCID: PMC3826269. doi:10.1164/rccm.201212-2297OC

Iwayama, T., Steele, C., Yao, L., Dozmorov, M. G., Karamichos, D., Wren, J. D., et al. (2015). PDGFRα Signaling Drives Adipose Tissue Fibrosis by Targeting Progenitor Cell Plasticity. *Genes Dev.* 29 (11), 1106–1119. doi:10.1101/gad.260554.115

Jaffar, J., Griffiths, K., Oveissi, S., Duan, M., Foley, M., Glaspole, I., et al. (2020). CXCR4+cells Are Increased in Lung Tissue of Patients with Idiopathic Pulmonary Fibrosis. *Respir. Res.* 21 (1), 1–16. doi:10.1186/s12931-020-01467-0

Jarvinen, L., Badri, L., Scott, W., Standiford, T. J., Toews, G. B., David, J., et al. (2021). Lung Resident Mesenchymal Stem Cells Isolated from Human Lung Allografts Inhibit T Cell Proliferation via a Soluble Mediator. *J. Immunol.* 181 (6), 4389–4396. doi:10.4049/jimmunol.181.6.4389

Jenkins, R. G., Moore, B. B., Chambers, R. C., Oliver, E., Konigshoff, M., Kolb, M., et al. (2017). An Official American Thoracic Society Workshop Report: Use of Animal Models for the Preclinical Assessment of Potential Therapies for Pulmonary Fibrosis. *Am. J. Respir. Cel Mol. Biol.* 56 (5), 667–679. doi:10.1165/rcmb.2017-0096ST

Jessica Germaine, S., Teresa Pay, M., Lara Compte, C., Olid, M., Bermudo, G., Portillo, K., et al. (2020). Mapping IPF Helps Identify Geographic Regions at Higher Risk for Disease Development and Potential Triggers. *Respirology* 26, 1–8. doi:10.1111/resp.13973

Jiang, Y., Mishima, H., Sakai, S., Liu, Y. K., Ohyabu, Y., and Uemura, T. (2008). Gene Expression Analysis of Major Lineage-Defining Factors in Human Bone Marrow Cells: Effect of Aging, Gender, and Age-Related Disorders. *J. Orthop. Res.* 26 (7), 910–917. PMID: 18302252. doi:10.1002/jor.20623

Jun, D., Garat, C., West, J., Thorn, N., Chow, K., Cleaver, T., et al. (2011). The Pathology of Bleomycin-Induced Fibrosis Is Associated with Loss of Resident Lung Mesenchymal Stem Cells that Regulate Effector T-Cell Proliferation. *Stem Cells* 29 (4), 725–735. doi:10.1002/stem.604

Jo, H. E., Glaspole, I., Grainge, C., Goh, N., Hopkins, P. M., Moodley, Y., Reynolds, P. N., et al. (2017). Baseline Characteristics of Idiopathic Pulmonary Fibrosis: Analysis From the Australian Idiopathic Pulmonary Fibrosis Registry. *Eur. Respir J.* 49 (2), 1601592. doi:10.1183/13993003.01592-2016. Erratum in: Eur Respir J. 2017 Mar 29;49(3): PMID: 28232409

Karki, S., Surolia, R., David Hock, T., Guroji, P., Zolak, J. S., Ryan, D., et al. (2014). Wilms' Tumor 1 (Wt1) Regulates Pleural Mesothelial Cell Plasticity and Transition into Myofibroblasts in Idiopathic Pulmonary Fibrosis. *FASEB J.* 28 (3), 1122–1131. doi:10.1096/fj.13-236828

Kheirollahi, V., Wasnick, R. M., Biasin, V., Vazquez-Armendariz, A. I., Chu, X., Moiseenko, A., et al. (2019). Metformin Induces Lipogenic Differentiation in Myofibroblasts to Reverse Lung Fibrosis. *Nat. Commun.* 10 (1), 2987, 2019. PMID: 31278260; PMCID: PMC6611870. doi:10.1038/s41467-019-10839-0

Kim, K. K., Kugler, M. C., Paul, J., Robillard, L., Galvez, M. G., Alexis, M., et al. (2006). Alveolar Epithelial Cell Mesenchymal Transition Develops *In Vivo* during Pulmonary Fibrosis and Is Regulated by the Extracellular Matrix. *Proc. Natl. Acad. Sci. United States America* 103 (35), 13180–13185. doi:10.1073/pnas.0605669103

Kim, S. Y., Lee, J. H., Kim, H. J., Park, M. K., Huh, J. W., Ro, J. Y., et al. (2012). Mesenchymal Stem Cell-Conditioned media Recovers Lung Fibroblasts from Cigarette Smoke-Induced Damage. *Am. J. Physiol. - Lung Cell Mol. Physiol.* 302 (9), L891–L908. doi:10.1152/ajplung.00288.2011

King, T. E., Pardo, A., and Selman, M. (2011). Idiopathic Pulmonary Fibrosis. *The Lancet* 378 (9807), 1949–1961. doi:10.1016/S0140-6736(11)60052-4

Kirkland, J. L., and Tchkonia, T. (2017). Cellular Senescence: A Translational Perspective. *EBioMedicine* 21, 21–28. doi:10.1016/j.ebiom.2017.04.013

Kis, K., Liu, X., James, S., and Hagood, S. (2011). Myofibroblast Differentiation and Survival in Fibrotic Disease. *Expert Rev. Mol. Med.* 13 (2), e27. doi:10.1017/S1462399411001967

Kleaveland, K. R., Miranda, V., Yang, J., Agarwal, M., Rippe, R. A., Bethany, B., et al. (2014). Fibrocytes Are Not an Essential Source of Type I Collagen during Lung Fibrosis. *J. Immunol.* 193 (10), 5229–5239. doi:10.4049/jimmunol.1400753

Klein, D. (2020). Lung Multipotent Stem Cells of Mesenchymal Nature : Cellular Basis. *Clin. relevance implications Stem Cel. Ther.* 5, 1–38. doi:10.1089/ars.2020.8190

Kotani, T., Masutani, R., Suzuka, T., Oda, K., Makino, S., and Li, M. (2017). Anti-Inflammatory and Anti-Fibrotic Effects of Intravenous Adipose-Derived Stem Cell Transplantation in a Mouse Model of Bleomycin-Induced Interstitial Pneumonia. *Sci. Rep.* 7 (1), 14608, 2017. Erratum in: Sci Rep. 2018 Jan 8;8(1):454. Erratum in: Sci Rep. 2018 Mar 6;8(1):4222. PMID: 29097816.

Kramann, R., Schneider, R. K., Dirocco, D. P., Machado, F., Fleig, S., Bondzie, P. A., et al. (2015). Perivascular Gli1+ Progenitors Are Key Contributors to Injury-Induced Organ Fibrosis. *Cell Stem Cell* 16 (1), 51–66. doi:10.1016/j.stem.2014.11.004

Kropski, J. A., Daphne, B. M., Cheryl, M., Vasiliy, V. P., Choi, L., Joyce, E. J., et al. (2014). A Novel Dyskerin (DKC1) Mutation Is Associated with Familial Interstitial Pneumonia. *CHEST* 146 (1), e1–7. doi:10.1378/chest.13-2224

Kropski, J. A., Jason, M. P., Donald, F. Z., Peter, F. C., Markin, C., Garnett, E. T., et al. (2015). Extensive Phenotyping of Individuals at Risk for Familial Interstitial Pneumonia Reveals Clues to the Pathogenesis of Interstitial Lung Disease. *Am. J. Respir. Crit. Care Med.* 191 (4), 417–426. doi:10.1164/rccm.201406-1162OC

Kruk, D. M. L. W., Wisman, M., de Bruin, H. G., Lodewijk, M. E., Danique, J., Borghuis, T., et al. (2021). Abnormalities in Reparative Function of Lung-Derived Mesenchymal Stromal Cells in Emphysema. *Am. J. Physiology-Lung Cell Mol. Physiol. marzo* 320. doi:10.1152/ajplung.00147.2020

Lan, Y. W., Choo, K. B., Chen, C. M., Hung, T. H., Chen, Y. Bin., Hsieh, C. H., et al. (2015). Hypoxia-preconditioned Mesenchymal Stem Cells Attenuate Bleomycin-Induced Pulmonary Fibrosis. *Stem Cel Res. Ther.* 6, 1–17. doi:10.1186/s13287-015-0081-6

Larsson, H., Le Blanc, K., Eriksson, L., Bjermer, L., and Scheding, S. (2016). *MSC from Fetal and Adult Lungs Possess Lung-specific Properties Compared to Bone Marrow-Derived.* Nature Publishing Group, 1–10. doi:10.1038/srep29160

Lederer, D. J., and Martinez, F. J. (2018). Idiopathic Pulmonary Fibrosis. *New Engl. J. Med.* 378 (19), 1811–1823. doi:10.1056/NEJMra1705751

Lee, J. K., Park, S., Jung, B., Jeon, Y., Lee, Y., Kim, K., et al. (2013). Exosomes Derived from Mesenchymal Stem Cells Suppress Angiogenesis by Down-Regulating VEGF Expression in Breast Cancer. *Cells* 8 (12). doi:10.1371/journal.pone.0084256

Lee, S., Lee, E., Lee, S., Kim, J., Shim, J., Shin, C., et al. (2014). The Effect of Adipose Stem Cell Therapy on Pulmonary Fibrosis Induced by Repetitive Intratracheal Bleomycin in Mice. *Exp. Lung Res.* 40 (3), 117–125. doi:10.3109/01902148.2014.881930

Lehmann, M., Hu, Q., Hu, Y., Hafner, K., Costa, R., van den Berg, A., et al. (2020). Chronic Wnt/β-Catenin Signaling Induces Cellular Senescence in Lung Epithelial Cells. *Cell Signal.* 70 (October), 109588. doi:10.1016/j.cellsig.2020.109588

Lehmann, M., Korfei, M., Mutze, K., Klee, S., Skronska-wasek, W., Alsafadi, H. N., et al. (2017). Senolytic Drugs Target Alveolar Epithelial Cell Function and Attenuate Experimental. *Eur. Respir. J.* 50 (2), 1602367. doi:10.1183/13993003.02367-2016

Ley, B., Collard, H. R., and King, T. E. (2011). Clinical Course and Prediction of Survival in Idiopathic Pulmonary Fibrosis. *Am. J. Respir. Crit. Care Med.* 183 (4), 431–440. doi:10.1164/rccm.201006-0894CI

Ley, B., Newton, C. A., Arnould, I., Elicker, B. M., Henry, T. S., Vittinghoff, E., et al. (2017). The MUC5B Promoter Polymorphism and Telomere Length in Patients with Chronic Hypersensitivity Pneumonitis: an Observational Cohort-Control Study. *Lancet Respir. Med.* 5 (8), 639–647. doi:10.1016/S2213-2600(17)30216-3

Li, F., Han, F., Li, H., Zhang, J., Qiao, X., Shi, J., et al. (2017a). Human Placental Mesenchymal Stem Cells of Fetal Origins-Alleviated Inflammation and Fibrosis by Attenuating MyD88 Signaling in Bleomycin-Induced Pulmonary Fibrosis Mice. *Mol. Immunol.* 90, 11–21. doi:10.1016/j.molimm.2017.06.032

Li, Y., Wu, Q., Wang, Y., Li, L., Bu, H., and Bao, J. (2017b). Senescence of Mesenchymal Stem Cells (Review). *Int. J. Mol. Med.* 39 (4), 775–782. Epub 2017 Mar 9. PMID: 28290609. doi:10.3892/ijmm.2017.2912

Liu, J., Ding, Y., Liu, Z., and Liang, X. (2020). Senescence in Mesenchymal Stem Cells: Functional Alterations, Molecular Mechanisms, and Rejuvenation Strategies. *Front Cel Dev Biol* 8, 258, 2020 . PMID: 3. doi:10.3389/fcell.2020.00258

López-Otín, C., Blasco, M. A., Partridge, L., Serrano, M., and Kroemer, G. (2013). The Hallmarks of Aging. *Cell.* 153 (6), 1194–1217. PMID: 23746838; PMCID: PMC3836174. doi:10.1016/j.cell.2013.05.039

Lou, G., Chen, Z., Zheng, M., and Liu, E. Y. (2017). Mesenchymal Stem Cell-Derived Exosomes as a New Therapeutic Strategy for Liver Diseases. *Exp. Mol. Med.* 49 (6), e346. doi:10.1038/emm.2017.63

Maguire, Greg. (2013). Stem Cell Therapy without Cells. *Communicative Integr. Biol.* 6 (6), e2663. doi:10.4161/cib.26631

Mansouri, N., Willis, G. R., Fernandez-Gonzalez, A., Reis, M., Nassiri, S., Alex Mitsialis, S., et al. (2019). Mesenchymal Stromal Cell Exosomes Prevent and Revert Experimental Pulmonary Fibrosis through Modulation of Monocyte Phenotypes. *JCI Insight* 4 (21), 1–17. doi:10.1172/jci.insight.128060

Marchioni, A., Tonelli, R., Rossi, G., Spagnolo, P., Luppi, F., Cerri, S., et al. (2020). Ventilatory Support and Mechanical Properties of the Fibrotic Lung Acting as a "squishy ball". *Ann. Intensive Care* 10 (1), 13, 2020 . PMID: 32020548; PMCID: PMC7000609. doi:10.1186/s13613-020-0632-6

Marriott, S., Baskir, R. S., Gaskill, C., Menon, S., Carrier, E. J., Williams, J., et al. (2014). ABCG2pos Lung Mesenchymal Stem Cells Are a Novel Pericyte Subpopulation that Contributes to Fibrotic Remodeling. *Am. J. Physiol. - Cel Physiol.* 307 (8), C684–C698. doi:10.1152/ajpcell.00114.2014

Martin, A., Jahn, A., Rio, C., Iglesias, A., Mercader, J., Montes, A., et al. (2020). Characterizing Lung Resident Mesenchymal Stem Cells in Idiopathic Pulmonary Fibrosis. *Eur. Respir. J.* 56 (Suppl. 64). doi:10.1183/13993003.congress-2020.457

Martin-Medina, A., Lehmann, M., Olivier, B., Hermann, S., Baarsma, H. A., Wagner, D. E., et al. (2018). Increased Extracellular Vesicles Mediate Wnt5A Signaling in Idiopathic Pulmonary Fibrosis. *Am. J. Respir. Crit. Care Med.* 198 (12), 1527–1538. doi:10.1164/rccm.201708-1580OC

Massagué, J. (2014). TGFbeta Signalling in Context. *Nat. Rev. Mol. Cel Biol* 13 (10), 616–630. doi:10.1038/nrm3434.TGF

Masterson, C. H., Curley, G. F., and Laffey, J. G. (2019). Modulating the Distribution and Fate of Exogenously Delivered. *MSCs enhance Ther. potential: knowns unknowns* 7 (Suppl. 1), 1–21. doi:10.1186/s40635-019-0235-4

Mastrolia, I., Foppiani, E. M., Alba, M., Candini, O., Samarelli, A. V., Grisendi, G., et al. (2019). Challenges in Clinical Development of Mesenchymal Stromal/Stem Cells: Concise Review. *Stem Cell Translational Med.* 8 (11), 1135–1148. doi:10.1002/sctm.19-0044

Meng, F., Xu, R., Wang, S., Xu, Z., Zhang, C., Li, Y., et al. (2020). Human Umbilical Cord-Derived Mesenchymal Stem Cell Therapy in Patients with COVID-19: a Phase 1 Clinical Trial. *Signal. Transduction Targeted Ther.* 5 (1). doi:10.1038/s41392-020-00286-5

Meng, X. M., Nikolic-Paterson, D. J., and Lan, H. Y. (2016). TGF-β: The Master Regulator of Fibrosis. *Nat. Rev. Nephrol.* 12 (6), 325–338. doi:10.1038/nrneph.2016.48

Michalski, J. E., and Schwartz, D. A. (2020). Genetic Risk Factors for Idiopathic Pulmonary Fibrosis: Insights into Immunopathogenesis. *J. Inflamm. Res.* 13, 1305–1318. doi:10.2147/JIR.S280958

Moeller, A., Kjetil, A., Warburton, D., Gauldie, J., and Kolb, M. (2008). The Bleomycin Animal Model: A Useful Tool to Investigate Treatment Options for Idiopathic Pulmonary Fibrosis? *Int. J. Biochem. Cel Biol.* 40 (3), 362–382. doi:10.1016/j.biocel.2007.08.011

Moll, G., James, A. A., Julian, K-M., Karen, B., Olle, R., Hans, D. V., et al. (2019). Intravascular Mesenchymal Stromal/Stem Cell Therapy Product Diversification: Time for New Clinical Guidelines. *Trends Mol. Med.* 25 (2), 149–163. doi:10.1016/j.molmed.2018.12.006

Moodley, Y., Atienza, D., Manuelpillai, U., Samuel, C. S., Tchongue, J., Ilancheran, S., et al. (2009). Human Umbilical Cord Mesenchymal Stem Cells Reduce Fibrosis of Bleomycin-Induced Lung Injury. *Am. J. Pathol.* 175 (1), 303–313. doi:10.2353/ajpath.2009.080629

Moodley, Y., Vaghjiani, V., Chan, J., Baltic, S., Ryan, M., Tchongue, J., et al. (2013). Anti-Inflammatory Effects of Adult Stem Cells in Sustained Lung Injury: A Comparative Study. *PLoS One* 8, e69299. doi:10.1371/journal.pone.0069299

Moore, B. B., Jill, E. K., Victor, J. T., Cooke, K., Moore, T. A., Hogaboam, C., et al. (2005). CCR2-mediated Recruitment of Fibrocytes to the Alveolar Space after Fibrotic Injury. *Am. J. Pathol.* 166 (3), 675–684. doi:10.1016/S0002-9440(10)62289-4

Mora, A. L., Rojas, M., Pardo, A., and Selman, M. (2017). Emerging Therapies for Idiopathic Pulmonary Fibrosis, a Progressive Age-Related Disease. *Nat. Rev. Drug Discov.* 16 (11), 755–772. doi:10.1038/nrd.2017.170

Ni, K., Liu, M., Zheng, J., Wen, L., Chen, Q., Zheng, X., et al. (2018). PD-1/PD-L1 Pathway Mediates the Alleviation of Pulmonary Fibrosis by Human Mesenchymal Stem Cells in Humanized Mice. *Am. J. Respir. Cel Mol. Biol.* 58 (6), 684–695. doi:10.1165/rcmb.2017-0326OC

Noble, P. W., Albera, C., Williamson, Z. B., Ulrich, C., Glassberg, M. K., Kardatzke, D., et al. (2011). Pirfenidone in Patients with Idiopathic Pulmonary Fi Brosis (CAPACITY): Two Randomised Trials. *The Lancet* 377 (9779), 1760–1769. doi:10.1016/S0140-6736(11)60405-4

Noguchi, S., Saito, A., and Nagase, T. (2018). YAP/TAZ Signaling as a Molecular Link between Fibrosis and Cancer. *Int. J. Mol. Sci.* 19 (11). doi:10.3390/ijms19113674

Nureki, S. I., Tomer, Y., Venosa, A., Katzen, J., Russo, A. J., Jamil, S., et al. (2018). Expression of Mutant Sftpc in Murine Alveolar Epithelia Drives Spontaneous Lung Fibrosis. *J. Clin. Invest.* 128 (9), 4008–4024. doi:10.1172/JCI99287

Ono, M., Ohkouchi, S., Kanehira, M., Tode, N., Kobayashi, M., Ebina, M., et al. (2015). Mesenchymal Stem Cells Correct Inappropriate Epithelial-Mesenchyme Relation in Pulmonary Fibrosis Using Stanniocalcin-1. *Mol. Ther.* 23, 549–560. doi:10.1038/mt.2014.217

Ortiz, L. A., Gambelli, F., McBride, C., Gaupp, D., Baddoo, M., Kaminski, N., et al. (2003). Mesenchymal Stem Cell Engraftment in Lung Is Enhanced in Response to Bleomycin Exposure and Ameliorates its Fibrotic Effects. *Proc. Natl. Acad. Sci. United States America* 100 (14), 8407–8411. doi:10.1073/pnas.1432929100

Ortiz, L. A., DuTreil, M., Fattman, C., Pandey, A. C., Torres, G., Go, K., et al. (2007). Interleukin 1 Receptor Antagonist Mediates the Antiinflammatory and Antifibrotic Effect of Mesenchymal Stem Cells during Lung Injury. *Proc. Natl. Acad. Sci. U. S. A.* 104, 11002–11007. doi:10.1073/pnas.0704421104

Pardo, A., Gibson, K., Cisneros, J., Richards, T. J., Yang, Y., Becerril, C., et al. (2005). Up-regulation and Profibrotic Role of Osteopontin in Human Idiopathic Pulmonary Fibrosis. *PLoS Med.* 2 (9), 0891–0903. doi:10.1371/journal.pmed.0020251

Pardo, A., and Moisés Selman, E. (2021). The Interplay of the Genetic Architecture, Aging, and Environmental Factors in the Pathogenesis of Idiopathic Pulmonary Fibrosis. *Am. J. Respir. Cel Mol. Biol.* 64 (2), 163–172. doi:10.1165/rcmb.2020-0373ps

Phan, Sem. H. (2002). The Myofibroblast in Pulmonary Fibrosis. *Chest* 122 (6 Suppl. L), 286S–289S. doi:10.1378/chest.122.6_suppl.286S

Phan, T., Paliogiannis, P., Nasrallah, G. K., Giordo, R., Hussein Eid, A., Giuseppe Fois, A., et al. (2020). Emerging Cellular and Molecular Determinants of Idiopathic Pulmonary Fibrosis. *Cell Mol. Life Sci.* 78, 2031–2057. doi:10.1007/s00018-020-03693-7

Phillips, R. J., Burdick, M. D., Hong, K., Lutz, M. A., Murray, L. A., Ying Xue, Y., et al. (2004). Circulating Fibrocytes Traffic to the Lungs in Response to CXCL12 and Mediate Fibrosis. *J. Clin. Invest.* 114 (3), 438–446. doi:10.1172/JCI200420997

Plantier, L., Crestani, B., Wert, S. E., Dehoux, M., Zweytick, B., Guenther, A., et al. (2011). Ectopic Respiratory Epithelial Cell Differentiation in Bronchiolised Distal Airspaces in Idiopathic Pulmonary Fibrosis. *Thorax* 66 (8), 651–657. Epub 2011 Mar 21: PMID: 21422041. doi:10.1136/thx.2010.151555

Powers, E. T., Morimoto, R. I., Dillin, A., Kelly, J. W., and Balch, W. E. (2009). Biological and Chemical Approaches to Diseases of Proteostasis Deficiency. *Annu. Rev. Biochem.* 78, 959–991. PMID: 19298183. doi:10.1146/annurev.biochem.052308.114844

Qiu, T., Tian, Y., Gao, Y., Ma, M., Li, H., Liu, X., et al. (2019). PTEN Loss Regulates Alveolar Epithelial Cell Senescence in Pulmonary Fibrosis Depending. *Akt activation* 11 (18), 7492–7509. doi:10.18632/aging.102262 on

Raghu, G., Harold, C., Egan, J. J., Martinez, F. J., Behr, J., Brown, K. K., et al. (2011). An Official ATS/ERS/JRS/ALAT Statement: Idiopathic Pulmonary Fibrosis: Evidence-Based Guidelines for Diagnosis and Management. *Am. J. Respir. Crit. Care Med.* 183 (6), 788–824. doi:10.1164/rccm.2009-040GL.Ricciardi

Ricciardi, M., Giorgio, M., Francesco, B., Giulio, B., Luciano, P., and Nwabo, K. A. H. (2012). Comparison of Epithelial Differentiation and Immune Regulatory Properties of Mesenchymal Stromal Cells Derived from Human Lung and Bone Marrow. *PLoS One* 7 (5), 1–10. doi:10.1371/journal.pone.0035639

Richeldi, L., Collard, H. R., and Jones, M. G. (2017). Idiopathic Pulmonary Fibrosis. *The Lancet* 389 (10082), 1941–1952. doi:10.1016/S0140-6736(17)30866-8

Rock, J. R., Christina, E., Michael, J., Xue, Y., Harris, J. R., Liang, J., et al. (2011). "Multiple Stromal Populations Contribute to Pulmonary Fibrosis without Evidence for Epithelial to Mesenchymal Transition," in *Proceedings of the National Academy of Sciences of the United States of America* (US: NIH). doi:10.1073/pnas.1117988108

Rolandsson, S., Andersson Sjöland, S., Brune, J. C., Li, H., Kassem, M., Mertens, F., et al. (2014). Primary Mesenchymal Stem Cells in Human Transplanted Lungs Are CD90/CD105 Perivascularly Located Tissue-Resident Cells. *BMJ Open Respir. Res.* 1 (1), 1–12. doi:10.1136/bmjresp-2014-000027

Roy, M. G., Livraghi-butrico, S., Fletcher, A. A., Mcelwee, M. M., Scott, E. E., Ryan, M. B., et al. (2013). Muc5b Is Required for Airway Defence. *Nature* 505 (7483), 412–416. doi:10.1038/nature12807

Rubio, G. A., Elliot, S. J., Wikramanayake, T., Xia, X., Pereira-simon, S., Seth, R., et al. (2017). Mesenchymal Stromal Cells Prevent Bleomycin-Induced Lung and Skin Fibrosis in Aged Mice and Restore Wound Healing †. *J. Cel Physiol* 233 (8), 5503–5512. doi:10.1002/jcp.26418

Ryu, J. H., Teng, M., Daniels, C. E., Hartman, T. E., Yi, E. S., Utz, J. P., et al. (2014). Idiopathic Pulmonary Fibrosis: Evolving Concepts. *Mayo Clinic Proc.* 89 (8), 1130–1142. doi:10.1016/j.mayocp.2014.03.016

Schröder, M., and Kaufman, R. J. (2005). The Mammalian Unfolded Protein Response. *Annu. Rev. Biochem.* 74, 739–789. PMID: 15952902. doi:10.1146/annurev.biochem.73.011303.074134

Scotton, C. J., and Chambers, R. C. (2007). Molecular Targets in Pulmonary Fibrosis: The Myofibroblast in Focus. *Chest* 132 (4), 1311–1321. doi:10.1378/chest.06-2568

Seibold, M. A., Smith, R. W., Urbanek, C., Steve, D. G., Cosgrove, G. P., Brown, K. K., et al. (2013). The Idiopathic Pulmonary Fibrosis Honeycomb Cyst Contains A Mucocilary Pseudostratified Epithelium. *PLoS ONE* 8 (3). doi:10.1371/journal.pone.0058658

Selman, M., and Pardo, A. (2020). The Leading Role of Epithelial Cells in the Pathogenesis of Idiopathic Pulmonary Fibrosis. *Cell Signal.* 66 (November 2019), 109482. doi:10.1016/j.cellsig.2019.109482

Sgalla, G., Cocconcelli, E., Tonelli, R., and Richeldi, L. (2016). Novel Drug Targets for Idiopathic Pulmonary Fibrosis. *Expert Rev. Respir. Med.* 10 (4), 393–405. doi:10.1586/17476348.2016.1152186

Shah, T. G., Predescu, D., and Predescu, S. (2019). Mesenchymal Stem Cells-derived Extracellular Vesicles in Acute Respiratory Distress Syndrome: a Review of Current Literature and Potential Future Treatment Options. *Clin. Translational Med.* 8 (1), 4–9. doi:10.1186/s40169-019-0242-9

Shentu, T. P., Huang, T. S., Cernelc-Kohan, M., Chan, J., Wong, S. S., Espinoza, C. R., et al. (2017). Thy-1 Dependent Uptake of Mesenchymal Stem Cell-Derived Extracellular Vesicles Blocks Myofibroblastic Differentiation. *Scientific Rep.* 7 (1), 1–11. doi:10.1038/s41598-017-18288-9

Shi, J., Li, F., Luo, M., Wei, J., and Liu, X. (2017). Distinct Roles of Wnt/β-Catenin Signaling in the Pathogenesis of Chronic Obstructive Pulmonary Disease and Idiopathic Pulmonary Fibrosis. *Mediators Inflamm.* 2017, 3520581. doi:10.1155/2017/3520581

Sinclair, K. A., Yerkovich, S. T., Chen, T., McQualter, J. L., Hopkins, P. M. A., Wells, C. A., et al. (2016). Mesenchymal Stromal Cells Are Readily Recoverable from Lung Tissue, but Not the Alveolar Space, in Healthy Humans. *Stem Cells* 34 (10), 2548–2558. doi:10.1002/stem.2419

Stanley, S. E., Gable, D. L., Wagner, C. L., Carlile, T. M., Vidya Sagar, H., Joshua, D. P., et al. (2016). Loss-of-function Mutations in the RNA Biogenesis Factor NAF1 Predispose to Pulmonary Fibrosis – Emphysema. *Sci. Transl Med.* 8 (351), 1–10. doi:10.1126/scitranslmed.aaf7837

Steele, M. P., Brown, K. K., James, E. L., Tasha E Fingerlin, D., Zhang, W., Adler, K. B., et al. (2011). A Common. *N. Engl. J. Med.* 364 (16), 1503–1512.

Steens, J., Klar, L., Hansel, C., Alexis, S., Hager, T., Jendrossek, V., et al. (2021). The Vascular Nature of Lung-Resident Mesenchymal Stem Cells. *Stem Cell Translational Med.* 10 (1), 128–143. doi:10.1002/sctm.20-0191

Stuart, B. D., Choi, J., Zaidi, S., Xing, C., Holohan, B., Chen, R., et al. (2015). Exome Sequencing Links Mutations in PARN and RTEL1 with Familial Pulmonary Fibrosis and Telomere Shortening. *Nat. Genet.* 47 (5), 512–517. doi:10.1038/ng.3278

Summers, M. E., Richmond, B. W., Kropski, J. A., Majka, S. A., Bastarache, J. A., Hatzopoulos, A. K., et al. (2021). Balanced Wnt/Dickkopf-1 Signaling by Mesenchymal Vascular Progenitor Cells in the Microvascular Niche Maintains Distal Lung Structure and Function. *Am. J. Physiol. Cel Physiol* 320 (1), C119–C131. Epub 2020 Oct 21. PMID: 33085496; PMCID: PMC7846975. doi:10.1152/ajpcell.00277.2020

Sveiven, S. N., and Nordgren, T. M. (2020). Lung-resident Mesenchymal Stromal Cells Are Tissue-specific Regulators of Lung Homeostasis. *Am. J. Physiol. - Lung Cell Mol. Physiol.* 319 (2), L197–L210. doi:10.1152/AJPLUNG.00049.2020

Sun, T., Huang, Z., Zhang, H., Posner, C., Posner, G., and Ramalingam, T. R. (2019). TAZ is Required for Lung Alveolar Epithelial Cell Differentiation After Injury. *JCI Insight* 5, e128674. doi:10.1172/jci.insight.128674

Takezaki, A., Tsukumo, S., Setoguchi, Y., Ledford, J. G., Goto, H., Hosomichi, K., et al. (2019). A Homozygous SFTPA1 Mutation Drives Necroptosis of Type II Alveolar Epithelial Cells in Patients with Idiopathic Pulmonary Fibrosis. *J. Exp. Med.* 216 (12), 2724–2735. doi:10.1084/jem.20182351

Tashiro, J., Elliot, S. J., Gerth, D. J., Xia, X., Pereira-Simon, S., Choi, R., et al. (2015). Therapeutic Benefits of Young, but Not Old, Adipose-Derived Mesenchymal Stem Cells in a Chronic Mouse Model of Bleomycin-Induced Pulmonary Fibrosis. *Transl. Res.* 166, 554–567. doi:10.1016/j.trsl.2015.09.004

Tong, L., Zhou, J., Rong, L., Seeley, E. J., Pan, J., Zhu, X., et al. (2016). Fibroblast Growth Factor-10 (FGF-10) Mobilizes Lung-Resident Mesenchymal Stem Cells and Protects against Acute Lung Injury. *Scientific Rep.* 6 (September), 1–12. doi:10.1038/srep21642

Tzouvelekis, A., Paspaliaris, V., George, K., Ntolios, P., Bouros, E., Oikonomou, A., et al. (2013). A Prospective, Non-randomized, No Placebo-Controlled, Phase Ib Clinical Trial to Study the Safety of the Adipose Derived Stromal Cells-Stromal Vascular Fraction in Idiopathic Pulmonary Fibrosis. *J. Transl Med.* 11, 171. doi:10.1186/1479-5876-11-171

Uccelli, A., Moretta, L., and Pistoia, V. (2008). Mesenchymal Stem Cells in Health and Disease. *Nat. Rev. Immunol.* 8 (9), 726–736. doi:10.1038/nri2395

Ulke, H. M., Mutze, K., Lehmann, M., Wagner, D. E., Heinzelmann, K., Günther, A., et al. (2019). The Oncogene ECT2 Contributes to a Hyperplastic, Proliferative Lung Epithelial Cell Phenotype in Idiopathic Pulmonary Fibrosis. *Am. J. Respir. Cel Mol. Biol.* 61 (6), 713–726. doi:10.1165/rcmb.2019-0047OC

Valadi, H., Ekström, K., Bossios, A., Sjöstrand, M., James, J., and Lee, O. (2007). Exosome-mediated Transfer of mRNAs and microRNAs Is a Novel Mechanism of Genetic Exchange between Cells. *Nat. Cel Biol.* 9 (6), 654–659. doi:10.1038/ncb1596

Vaughan, A. E., Brumwell, A. N., Xi, Y., Gotts, J. E., Brownfield, D. G., Treutlein, B., et al. (2015). Lineage-negative Progenitors Mobilize to Regenerate Lung Epithelium after Major Injury. *Nature* 517 (7536), 621–625. doi:10.1038/nature14112

Vaz, M., Hwang, S. Y., Kagiampakis, I., Phallen, J., Patil, A., O'Hagan, H. M., et al. (2017). Chronic Cigarette Smoke-Induced Epigenomic Changes Precede Sensitization of Bronchial Epithelial Cells to Single-step Transformation by KRAS Mutations. *Cancer Cell* 32 (3), 360–376.e6. doi:10.1016/j.ccell.2017.08.006

Vishnubhatla, I., Randolph, C., Stevanato, L., Hicks, C., and Sinden, J. (2014). The Development of Stem Cell-Derived Exosomes as a Cell-free Regenerative Medicine. *J. Circulating Biomarkers* 3, 1–14. doi:10.5772/58597

Vizoso, F. J., Eiro, N., Cid, S., Schneider, J., and Perez-Fernandez, R. (2017). Mesenchymal Stem Cell Secretome: Toward Cell-free Therapeutic Strategies in Regenerative Medicine. *Int. J. Mol. Sci.* 18 (9), 1852. doi:10.3390/ijms18091852

Wang, H., Yang, Y. F., Zhao, L., Xiao, F. J., Zhang, Q. W., Wen, M. L., et al. (2013). Hepatocyte Growth Factor Gene-Modified Mesenchymal Stem Cells Reduce Radiation-Induced Lung Injury. *Hum. Gene Ther.* 24 (3), 343–353. Epub 2013 Mar 4. PMID: 23458413. doi:10.1089/hum.2012.177

Wang, L., Yuan, Y., Yang, X., Fan, T., Mei, B., Hou, J., et al. (2017). Platelet Derived Growth Factor Alpha (PDGFRα) Induces the Activation of Cardiac Fibroblasts by Activating C-Kit. *Med. Sci. Monitor* 23, 3808–3816. doi:10.12659/MSM.906038

Wang, S., Hu, B., Ding, Z., Dang, Y., Wu, J., Li, D., et al. (2018). ATF6 Safeguards Organelle Homeostasis and Cellular Aging in Human Mesenchymal Stem Cells.

Cell Discov 4, 2, 2018. PMID: 29423270; PMCID: PMC5798892. doi:10.1038/s41421-017-0003-0

Weiss, D. J., and Ortiz, L. A. (2013). Cell Therapy Trials for Lung Diseases: Progress and Cautions. *Am. J. Respir. Crit. Care Med.* 188 (2), 123–125. doi:10.1164/rccm.201302-0351ED

Willis, B. C., Liebler, J. M., Luby-Phelps, K., Nicholson, A. G., Crandall, E. D., Roland, M., et al. (2005). Induction of Epithelial-Mesenchymal Transition in Alveolar Epithelial Cells by Transforming Growth Factor-B1: Potential Role in Idiopathic Pulmonary Fibrosis. *Am. J. Pathol.* 166 (5), 1321–1332. doi:10.1016/S0002-9440(10)62351-6

Wipff, P. J., Rifkin, D. B., Jean, J. M., and Hinz, B. (2007). Myofibroblast Contraction Activates Latent TGF-B1 from the Extracellular Matrix. *J. Cel Biol.* 179 (6), 1311–1323. doi:10.1083/jcb.200704042

Worthington, E. N., and Hagood, J. S. (2020). Therapeutic Use of Extracellular Vesicles for Acute and Chronic Lung Disease. *Int. J. Mol. Sci.* 21 (7). doi:10.3390/ijms21072318

Wu, H., and Tang, N. (2021). Stem Cells in Pulmonary Alveolar Regeneration. *Development* 148 (2), dev193458. doi:10.1242/dev.193458

Xie, T., Liang, J., Liu, N., Huan, C., Zhang, Y., Liu, W., et al. (2016). Transcription Factor TBX4 Regulates Myofibroblast Accumulation and Lung Fibrosis. *J. Clin. Invest.* 126 (8), 3063–3079. doi:10.1172/JCI85328

Xu, C., Wang, J., Zhu, T., Shen, Y., Tang, X., Fang, L., et al. (2016a). Cross-Talking between PPAR and WNT Signaling and its Regulation in Mesenchymal Stem Cell Differentiation. *Curr. Stem Cel Res Ther* 11 (3), 247–254. PMID: 26201865. doi:10.2174/1574888x10666150723145707

Xu, Y., Mizuno, T., Sridharan, A., Du, Y., Guo, M., Tang, J., et al. (2016b). Single-cell RNA Sequencing Identifies Diverse Roles of Epithelial Cells in Idiopathic Pulmonary Fibrosis. *JCI Insight* 1 (20), e90558. doi:10.1172/jci.insight.90558

Yamada, M., Kubo, H., Kobayashi, S., Ishizawa, K., Numasaki, M., Ueda, S., et al. (2004). Bone Marrow-Derived Progenitor Cells Are Important for Lung Repair after Lipopolysaccharide-Induced Lung Injury. *J. Immunol.* 172 (2), 1266–1272. doi:10.4049/jimmunol.172.2.1266

Yao, C., Guan, X., Carraro, G., Parimon, T., Liu, X., Huang, G., et al. (2020). Senescence of Alveolar Type 2 Cells Drives Progressive Pulmonary Fibrosis. *Am. J. Respir. Crit. Care Med.* 203 (6), 707–717. doi:10.1164/rccm.202004-1274oc

Yu, S., Liu, L-J., Lv, B., Che, C-li., Fan, D-P., Wang, L-F., et al. (2015). Inhibition of Bleomycin-Induced Pulmonary Fi Brosis by Bone Marrow- Derived Mesenchymal Stem Cells Might Be Mediated by Decreasing. *Cell Biochem Funct* 33 (6), 356–366. July. doi:10.1002/cbf.3118

Zacharias, W. J., Frank, D. B., Zepp, J. A., Morley, M. P., Alkhaleel, F., Kong, J., et al. (2018). *HHS Public Access* 555 (7695), 251–255. doi:10.1038/nature25786.Regeneration

Zakaria, D. M., Noha, M. Z., Samia, A. A. A., Radwa, A. M., and Rehab, A. M. (2021). Histological and Physiological Studies of the Effect of Bone Marrow-Derived Mesenchymal Stem Cells on Bleomycin Induced Lung Fibrosis in Adult Albino Rats. *Tissue Eng. Regenerative Med.* 18 (1), 127–141. doi:10.1007/s13770-020-00294-0

Zhang, E., Yang, Y. E., Zhang, J., Ding, G., Chen, S., Cheng, P., et al. (2019). Efficacy of Bone Marrow Mesenchymal Stem Cell Transplantation in Animal Models of Pulmonary Fibrosis after Exposure to Bleomycin : A Meta - Analysis. *Exp. Ther. Med.* 17 (3), 2247–2255. doi:10.3892/etm.2019.7205

Zhang, H. Y., Gharaee-Kermani, M., Zhang, K., Karmiol, S., and Sem, H. (1996). Lung Fibroblast α-smooth Muscle Actin Expression and Contractile Phenotype in Bleomycin-Induced Pulmonary Fibrosis. *Am. J. Pathol.* 148 (2), 527–537.

Zhou, B., Liu, Y., Kahn, M., David, K. A., Han, A., Wang, H., et al. (2012). Interactions between -Catenin and Transforming Growth Factor- Signaling Pathways Mediate Epithelial- Mesenchymal Transition and Are Dependent on the Element-Binding Protein (CREB) -binding Protein (CBP). *J. Biol. Chem.* 287 (10), 7026–7038. doi:10.1074/jbc.M111.276311

Zumla, A., Fu, S. W., Chang, C., Giuseppe, I., Petrosillo, N., Agrati, C., et al. (2020). Reducing Mortality and Morbidity in Patients with Severe COVID-19 Disease by Advancing Ongoing Trials of Mesenchymal Stromal (Stem) Cell (MSC) Therapy — Achieving Global Consensus and Visibility for Cellular Host-Directed Therapies. *Int. J. Infect. Dis.* 96, 431–439. doi:10.1016/j.ijid.2020.05.040

Zysman, M., Baptista, B. R., Essari, L. A., Taghizadeh, S., Thibault de Ménonville, C., Giffard, C., et al. (2020). Targeting p16INK4a Promotes Lipofibroblasts and Alveolar Regeneration after Early-Life Injury. *Am. J. Respir. Crit. Care Med.* 202 (8), 1088–1104. PMID: 32628504. doi:10.1164/rccm.201908-1573OC

GLOSSARY

IPF idiopathic pulmonary fibrosis
IIPs idiopathic interstitial pneumonias
MSCs mesenchymal stem cells
ECT2 epithelial cell transforming sequence 2
AECI alveolar epithelial cells 1
AECII alveolar epithelial cell 2
AEP alveolar epithelial progenitor
TGF-β1 transforming growth factor beta 1
PDGF platelet-derived growth factor
VEGF vascular endothelial growth factor
FGF fibroblast growth factor
IL-1 interleukin 1
TNF-α tumor necrosis factor-alpha
ERS endoplasmic reticulum stress
EMMPRIN extracellular matrix metalloproteinase inducer
CXCL12 C-X-C motif chemokine 12
CCL2 chemokine C-C motif ligand 2
EMT epithelial mesenchymal transition
α-SMA alpha smooth-muscle actin
Shh sonic hedgehog
PTEN phosphatase and tensin homologuephosphatase and TENsin homolog
INFγ interferon γ
PDGFRα platelet-derived growth factor receptor A
ABCA3 ATP binding cassette subfamily A member 3
DKC1 dyskerin pseudouridine synthase 1
TP53 tumor protein P53
TOLIP toll interacting protein
MUC5B mucin 5B
ECM extracellular matrix
BM bone marrow
hMSCs human mesenchymal stem cells
KGF keratinocyte growth factor
ARDS acute respiratory distress syndrome
Thy-1 or CD90 cluster of differentiation 90
BAL bronchoalveolar Lavage
SASP senescence associated secretory phenotype
uMSCs umbilical cord derived Mesenchymal Stem Cells
DLCO diffuse lung coefficient for carbon dioxide
Igfb insulin growth factor binding protein
FVC forced vital capacity
CT computed tomography
ADMSCs adipose tissue-derived mesenchymal stem cells
GEF guanine nucleotide exchange factor
CTGF connective tissue growth factor
EV extracellular vesicles
PI3K phosphatidylInositol 3-Kinase
TCF T cell factor
miRNA micro RNA
MVs micro vesicles
MHC I major histocompatibility complex I
HGF hepathocyte growth factor
IDO-1 indolamine 2,3-dioxygenase-1
IL-1Ra IL-1 receptor antagonist
PGE2 prostaglandin E2
PTEN phosphatase and tensin homologuephosphatase and TENsin homolog
NK natural killer cells
YAP yes-associated protein
TAZ transcriptome coactivator with PDZ-binding motif
ECs endothelial cells
GLI1 transcription factors glioma-associated homologue
MHC-1 major histocompatibility complex I
BLM bleomycin
CS cigarette smoke
SFPTA1 surfactant protein 1
CDKN1A cyclin dependent kinase inhibitor 1A
TERT telomerase reverse transcriptase
MCC mucociliary clearance
MCP1 CCL2 monocyte chemotacticprotein 1
SDF1 stromal cell-derived factor 1
TIMP tissue inhibitors of metalloproteinase
BDNF brain-derived neurotrophic factor
NGF nerve growth factor
CINC-1 cytokine-induced neutrophil chemoattractant 1
AT-MSCs adipose tissue-derived mesenchymal stem cells
COPD chronic obstructive pulmonary disease
LSC-Sec lung spheroid cell-secretome
LSC-Exo lung spheroid cell exosomes
lncRNAs long non coding RNA

17

The Influenza A Virus H3N2 Triggers the Hypersusceptibility of Airway Inflammatory Response *via* Activating the lncRNA TUG1/ miR-145-5p/NF-κB Pathway in COPD

You-Hui Tu[†1,2], *Yan Guo*[†1,2], *Shuang Ji*[1,2], *Ji-Long Shen*[3] *and Guang-He Fei*[1,2*]

[1]Department of Respiratory and Critical Care Medicine, The First Affiliated Hospital of Anhui Medical University, Hefei, China, [2]Key Laboratory of Respiratory Disease Research and Medical Transformation of Anhui Province, The First Affiliated Hospital of Anhui Medical University, Hefei, China, [3]Department of Pathogen Biology and Provincial Laboratories of Pathogen Biology and Zoonoses, Anhui Medical University, Hefei, China

***Correspondence:**
Guang-He Fei
guanghefei@126.com

[†]These authors have contributed equally to this work

Background: Patients with chronic obstructive pulmonary disease (COPD) are more susceptible to influenza A virus (IAV) with more severe symptoms, yet the underlying molecular mechanisms of the hypersusceptibility of airway inflammatory response remain unclear.

Methods: The primary human bronchial epithelial cells (pHBECs) were isolated from normal and COPD bronchial tissues (NHBE and DHBE) and cultured with/without IAV infection *in vitro*. DHBE cells were exposed to IAV for 24 h after knockdown of lncRNA TUG1 with short hairpin RNA (shRNA). Gain-of-function assays were performed with the miR-145-5p inhibitor and NF-κBp65 transfection. The expressions of lncRNA TUG1, miR-145-5p, phospho-NF-κBp65, NF-κBp65, TNF-α, and (Interleukin) IL-1β were examined with qRT-PCR, Western blotting, and ELISA. The interactions of lncRNA TUG1, miR-145-5p, and NF-κB were verified with luciferase reporter assay.

Results: The expressions of lncRNA TUG1, phospho-NF-κBp65, TNF-α, and IL-1β were increased significantly in pHBECs after being infected with IAV for 24 h (all $p < 0.05$). The detailed time analysis revealed that the NF-κBp65 in DHBE was activated earlier than that in NHBE by Western blotting and immunofluorescence. Knockdown of lncRNA TUG1 and miR-145-5p mimic attenuated the expressions of NF-κBp65, TNF-α, and IL-1β significantly. The miR-145-5p inhibitor and NF-κBp65 transfection reversed the attenuated expressions of NF-κBp65, TNF-α, and IL-1β.

Conclusion: The IAV causes the hypersusceptibility of airway inflammatory response, which may be closely associated with more severe symptoms in AECOPD patients. The lncRNA TUG1 inhibitor may be a promising therapeutic strategy for AECOPD caused by IAV.

Keywords: COPD, influenza A virus, airway inflammatory hypersusceptibility, lncRNA TUG1, miR-145-5p, NF-κB

INTRODUCTION

Chronic obstructive pulmonary disease (COPD) is a chronic airway inflammatory disease characterized by progressive airway inflammation and impaired lung function. Exacerbation of COPD (AECOPD) is the main source of hospitalization and mortality in COPD patients (Vogelmeier et al., 2017). The majority of exacerbation is related to respiratory viral infection (Wedzicha et al., 2014; Zwaans et al., 2014); accumulative evidence shows that influenza virus is one of the most frequently detected pathogens that induce AECOPD in Asian countries (Dai et al., 2015; Koul et al., 2017). Exacerbations triggered by viral infections are usually associated with hypersusceptibility of greater airway inflammatory response, more severe symptoms, and delayed recovery compared to those without viral infections (Almansa et al., 2012; Dickson et al., 2013). However, the underlying molecular mechanisms of the hypersusceptibility of airway inflammatory response induced by influenza A virus (IAV) in COPD patients remain unclear.

Long noncoding RNAs (lncRNAs) are defined as noncoding RNAs that have a length greater than 200 nucleotides, which may participate in the gene expressions of many inflammatory diseases, including COPD (Shi et al., 2013; Tang et al., 2016). The lncRNA taurine-upregulated gene 1 (TUG1) is a highly conserved lncRNA, originally identified in taurine-treated retinal cells. Previous studies have revealed the critical roles of lncRNA TUG1 played in the progression of various diseases (Li et al., 2016; Wang et al., 2019a; Su et al., 2020). Gu and colleagues found a higher expression of lncRNA TUG1 in the sputum and lung tissues of COPD patients as compared with nonsmokers (Gu et al., 2019), and lncRNA TUG1 can regulate the cigarette smoke induced airway remodeling by sponging miR-145-5p in COPD patients. Active nuclear factor kappa B (NF-κB) pathway is vital for the progression of the inflammatory response, and the protection of NF-κB inhibitor from inflammatory injury may be correlated with the lncRNA TUG1 (Cao et al., 2020). However, the biological role that lncRNA TUG1 plays in the hypersusceptibility of airway inflammatory response induced by respiratory viruses in COPD is barely reported.

The aim of this study is to investigate the underlying molecular mechanisms that the lncRNA TUG1/miR-145-5p/NF-κB pathway mediates in the hypersusceptibility of airway inflammatory response induced by H3N2 in COPD, thus exploring the underlying mechanisms why AECOPD patients induced by IAV have more severe symptoms and the possible therapeutic strategy.

MATERIALS AND METHODS

Study Approval

The study was approved by the ethics committee of the First Affiliated Hospital of Anhui Medical University (Quick-PJ2019-15-22); all participants provided their written consent and were informed the purpose of this study. All experiments that involved working with the IAV H3N2 were performed according to the biosafety level two requirements and personal protection equipment was provided for all the researchers. The characteristics of all subjects were shown in **Supplementary Table S1**.

Cell Isolation and Culture

pHBECs were isolated from the bronchial tissues of patients with lung carcinoma *in situ* comorbidity with and without COPD (DBHE and NHBE) according to the method modified from previous studies (Fulcher et al., 2005; Yamaya et al., 2011). The definition of COPD was based on the signs and symptoms and spirometry according to the 2017 GOLD guidelines (Vogelmeier et al., 2017). The bronchial tissues were cut at the site more than 2 cm distant from the edge of lung carcinoma. The isolated bronchial tissues were cut into pieces and incubated in solution comprised of 100 μg/ml pronase and 1 μg/ml deoxyribonuclease (both from Sigma-Aldrich) at 4°C overnight, then the supernatant was removed, and the tissue was resuspended and digested in another solution comprising of Ethylenediaminetetraacetic Acid (EDTA 2 nm), $CaCl_2$ (0.75 mg/ml), $MgCl_2$ (1 mg/ml), DL-Dithiothreitol (0.05 mg/ml), collagenase (0.25 mg/ml), and deoxyribonuclease (10 μg/ml) (all from Sigma-Aldrich) for 1 h. The pHBECs were finally isolated from the mixture with a centrifugation of 500 g 5 min and carefully rinsed with phosphate buffer solution (PBS) and plated on collagen-coated culture dishes (10 $\mu g/cm^2$ rat type I collagen; Sigma) in bronchial epithelial growth medium (BEGM) (Lonza, NJ, United States), comprising bronchial epithelial basal medium (BEBM) supplemented with bovine pituitary extract (52 μg/ml), hydrocortisone (0.5 μg/ml), human recombinant epidermal growth factor (25 ng/ml), epinephrine (0.5 μg/ml), transferrin (10 μg/ml), insulin (5 μg/ml), retinoic acid (50 nm), triiodothyronine (6.5 ng/ml), gentamycin (40 μg/ml), amphotericin B (50 ng/ml), and bovine serum albumin (BSA) (1.5 μg/ml). The pHBECs were observed in the cultured dishes after 3–5 days, and the medium was replaced once every one or two days. After trypsinization (passage one), cells were cultured accordingly for different experiments, and all the experiments performed in this study with pHBECs were done on monolayer cultures. The identity of the monolayer as bronchial epithelial cells was confirmed as previously described (Ji et al., 2020).

IAV Infection

pHBECs were seeded at a density of $1*10^6$ cells/well in 6-well plates coated with type I rat-tail collagen and cultured for 24 h to allow monolayer formation. Then cells were infected with IAV H3N2 (Multiplicity of Infection (MOI) = 2) for 24 h. The supernatants were collected and stored at −80°C for further examination; then the cells were rinsed with PBS three times and the protein or RNA was further extracted.

Quantitative Reverse Transcriptase Polymerase Chain Reaction

RNA was extracted using TRIzol reagent kit (Invitrogen) and transcribed to cDNA using the high capacity cDNA reverse transcription. Quantitative reverse transcriptase polymerase chain reaction (qRT-PCR) was performed using the SYBR Premix Ex Taq II (Tli RNaseH Plus) (Takara Biotechnology,

Dalian, China). The relative expression levels were calculated by the relative quantification ($2^{-\triangle\triangle Ct}$) method, and data were normalized to β-actin as endogenous control. The following primer sequences were as follows:

TUG1 (human) forward: 5′-TGAGCAAGCACTACCACC AG-3′, reverse: 5′-ACTCAGCAATCAGGAGGCAC-3′; miR-145-5p (human) forward: 5′-CAGTCTTGTCCAGTTTTCCCA G-3′, reverse: 5′-TATGCTTGTTCTCGTCTCTGTGTC-3′; NF-κBp65(human) forward: 5′-TGTGAAGAAGCGGGACCT GGAG-3′, reverse: 5′-AAGCAGAGCCGCACAGCATTC-3′; IL-1β (human) forward: 5′-CTCCACCTCCAGGGACAG GATATG-3′, reverse:5′-TCATCTTTCAACACGCAGGACAGG-3′; TNF-α(human) forward:5′-TGGCGTGGAGCTGAGAGATAACC-3′, reverse: 5′-CGA TGCGGCTGATGGTGTGG-3′ ; U6 (human) forward:5′-TGGAACGCTTCACGAATTTGCG-3′, reverse: 5′-AGACTGCCG CCTGGTAGTTGT-3′

Plasmid Construction, Lentivirus Production, and Cell Transduction

miR-145-5p mimic and its negative control mimic (miR-NC) and miR-145-5p inhibitor and its negative control inhibitor were purchased from Hanbio Biotechnology Co., Ltd. (Shanghai, China). The sequences were as follows:

miR-145-5p mimic:5′-GUCCAGUUUUCCCAGGAAUCCCU-3′ and 5′-AGGGAUUCCUGGGAAAACUGGAC-3′; negative control:5′-UCACAACCUCCUAGAAAGAGUAGA-3′ and 5′-UCUACUCUUUCUAGGAGGUUGUGA-3′; miR-145-5p inhibitor: 5′-AGGGAUUCCUGGGAAAACUGGAC-3′; scrambled control: 5′-UCUACUCUUUCUAGGAGGUUGUGA-3′.

The coding region of the NF-κBp65 mRNA was cloned into the pcDNA3.1 vector. The lentiviral vector expressing short hairpin RNA (shRNA) targeting TUG1 was designed and constructed by Hanbio Biotechnology Co., Ltd. (Shanghai, China). All cell transfection procedures were performed with Lipofectamine 3000 (Invitrogen, CA, United States) according to the manufacturer's instructions.

Western Blotting Analysis

Total protein extracts were prepared by using RIPA lysis buffer (ShangHai Biocolor BioScience Technology Company, Shanghai, China) with phosphatase and protease inhibitors. Nuclear proteins were extracted with the nuclear and cytoplasmic extraction kit (ShangHai Beyotime Biotechnology Company, Shanghai, China), and the efficacy of the fractionation was evaluated by the expression of nuclear protein Histone H3 and cytoplasmic protein β-actin in nuclear protein with Western blotting. The protein concentration was determined by BCA assay (Thermo Scientific, Rockford, IL, United states). Equal amounts of protein extracts were separated by SDS-PAGE (Bio-Rad, Hercules, CA, United States) and electrophoretically transferred to a PVDF membrane (Millipore, Bedford, NY, United States). After blockade with BSA for 2 h at room temperature, membrane was incubated with human primary antibodies specific to phospho-NF-κBp65(Ser536) (1:1,000, Cell Signaling Technology, MA, United States), NF-κBp65 (1:1,000, Cell Signaling Technology, MA, United States), Histone H3 (1: 1,000, Cell Signaling Technology, MA, United States), and β-actin (1:1,000, Cell Signaling Technology, MA, United States) at 4°C overnight. And subsequent incubation was done with a secondary horseradish peroxidase- (HRP-) conjugated antibody (KPL, Gaithersburg, MD, United States) at 1:5,000 dilution for 2 h at room temperature. The specific bands were visualized using the ECL detection kit (Thermo Fisher ScientificTM, Cleveland, OH, United States). Protein bands intensities were analyzed by Quantity One software (Bio-Rad Laboratories, Hercules, CA, United States).

Cell Immunofluorescence

pHBECs were grown on 15 mm Glass Bottom Cell Culture Dish (NEST, China) and then infected with IAV H3N2 (MOI = 2); cells were fixed at different time points (0, 2, 4, and 8 h post infection (hpi)) for 10 min with 4% phosphate-buffered paraformaldehyde at room temperature. Then the fixing solution was aspirated off and cells were rinsed with PBS and permeabilized with 0.5% Trixton-100 for 10 min. The cells were then rinsed with PBS and blocked with 5% BSA (FractionV, Beyotime, China) for 1 h. After incubation with the primary antibody of NF-κBp65 (1:200, Cell Signaling Technology, Beverly, MA, United States) at 4°C overnight, cells were rinsed for three times with PBS and incubated with the secondary antibody conjugated with FITC at a 1:500 dilution for 1 h at room temperature; the cells were followed by three rinsing steps for 5 min with PBS. Cells nuclei were stained using 4, 6-diamidino-2-pheylindole (DAPI, Sigma) and analyzed using a confocal laser scanning microscope (Leica SP8).

ELISA

Cell culture supernatants were collected and frozen at −80°C. The protein expression of proinflammatory cytokines (TNF-α and IL-1β) was quantified by ELISA kits purchased from Dakewe Biological Technology Co., Ltd. (Beijing, China), according to the manufacturer's instructions.

Luciferase Reporter Assay

Plasmid pmirGLO-TUG1 wildtype (wt) or pmirGLO-TUG1 mutant (mut) (relevant binding sites in miR-145-5p) was cotransfected with miR-145-5p mimics or miR-NC into HEK293T cells using a Lipofectamine 3000-mediated gene transfer. NF-κBp65-wt/mut 3UTR was constructed and transfected into HEK293T cells along with miR-145-5p mimic/miR-NC. Luciferase activity was detected using the Dual-Luciferase Reporter Assay System (Promega, Madison, WI, United States) according to the manufacturer's instructions.

Statistical Analysis

Data were expressed as the mean ± SD. Statistical analysis was performed using Prism software (version 6, GraphPad Software, La Jolla, CA, United States); differences between groups were analyzed by one-way analysis of variance (ANOVA), followed by

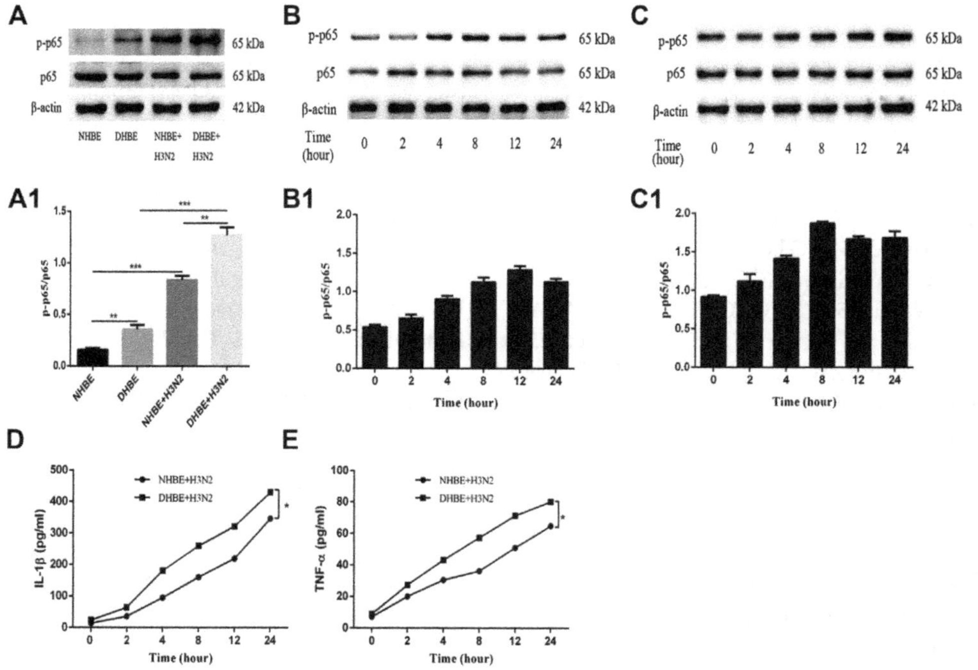

FIGURE 1 | IAV activated the NF-κB pathway in pHBECs. **(A,A1)** The protein expression and relative intensity of NF-κBp65 and phospho-p65 in pHBECs after infection with or without IAV for 24 h. **(B,B1)** The time-dependent protein expression and relative intensity of NF-κBp65 and phospho-p65 in NHBE after infection with IAV. **(C,C1)** The time-dependent protein expression and relative intensity of NF-κBp65 and phospho-p65 in DHBE after infection with IAV. **(D,E)** ELISA analyses of IL-1β and TNF-α in pHBECs after infection with IAV (*$p < 0.05$). Each dataset comprises three independent experiments.

the Student-Newman-Keuls test. Statistically significant differences were accepted at $p < 0.05$.

RESULTS

IAV Activates the NF-κB Pathway in pHBECs

The activity of NF-κB pathway was measured through the levels of NF-κBp65 and phospho-NF-κBp65. The expression of phospho-NF-κBp65 in DHBE was significantly higher than that in NHBE ($p < 0.01$); after infection with IAV for 24 h, the expression of phospho-NF-κBp65 increased significantly in pHBECs ($p < 0.001$) (shown in **Figures 1A, A1**). The detailed time analysis revealed that the expression of phospho-NF-κBp65 in pHBECs changed in a time-dependent manner (shown in **Figures 1B, B1, C, C1**); moreover, the intensity analysis showed the peak expression of phospho-NF-κBp65 in DHBE was observed at 8 hpi, earlier than that at 12 hpi in NHBE. Meanwhile, the IAV induced NF-κBp65 nuclear translocation was measured by immunofluorescence; as shown in **Figure 2A**, the IAV induced NF-κBp65 nuclear translocation in DHBE was obviously detected at two hpi and sustained up to four hpi, while in NHBE, the NF-κBp65 nuclear translocation was barely detected at two hpi and apparently increased at four hpi. The corresponding expressions of NF-κBp65 in the nucleus were also detected by Western blotting, as shown in **Figure 2B**. The efficacy of nuclear fractionation in nuclear protein was evaluated by Western blotting, as shown in **Supplementary Figure S1**. All these results may indicate that the NF-κB pathway in DHBE was activated earlier than NHBE after infection with IAV.

The downstream proinflammatory cytokines (IL-1β and TNF-α) of NF-κB pathway were quantified by ELISA. As shown in **Figures 1D, E**, IAV infection increased the expressions of IL-1β and TNF-α significantly in a time-dependent manner ($p < 0.05$). Moreover, the expressions of IL-1β and TNF-α measured in the culture supernatants of DHBE were significantly higher than those of NHBE at different time points.

The Differential Expressions of lncRNA TUG1 and miR-145-5p in COPD

The relative expressions of lncRNA TUG1 and miR-145-5p in pHBECs were examined with qRT-PCR. As shown in **Figure 3A**, the expression of lncRNA TUG1 measured in DHBE was significantly higher than that in NHBE ($p < 0.05$), but opposite in the expression of miR-145-5p (**Figure 3B**, $p < 0.05$). After infection with the IAV for 24 h, the expression of lncRNA TUG1 in pHBECs increased significantly, whereas the expression of miR-145-5p decreased significantly.

Knockdown of lncRNA TUG1 Reduced Airway Inflammation Induced by IAV in DHBE

To investigate whether the IAV induced airway inflammation was regulated by the lncRNA TUG1, we pretreated the DHBE

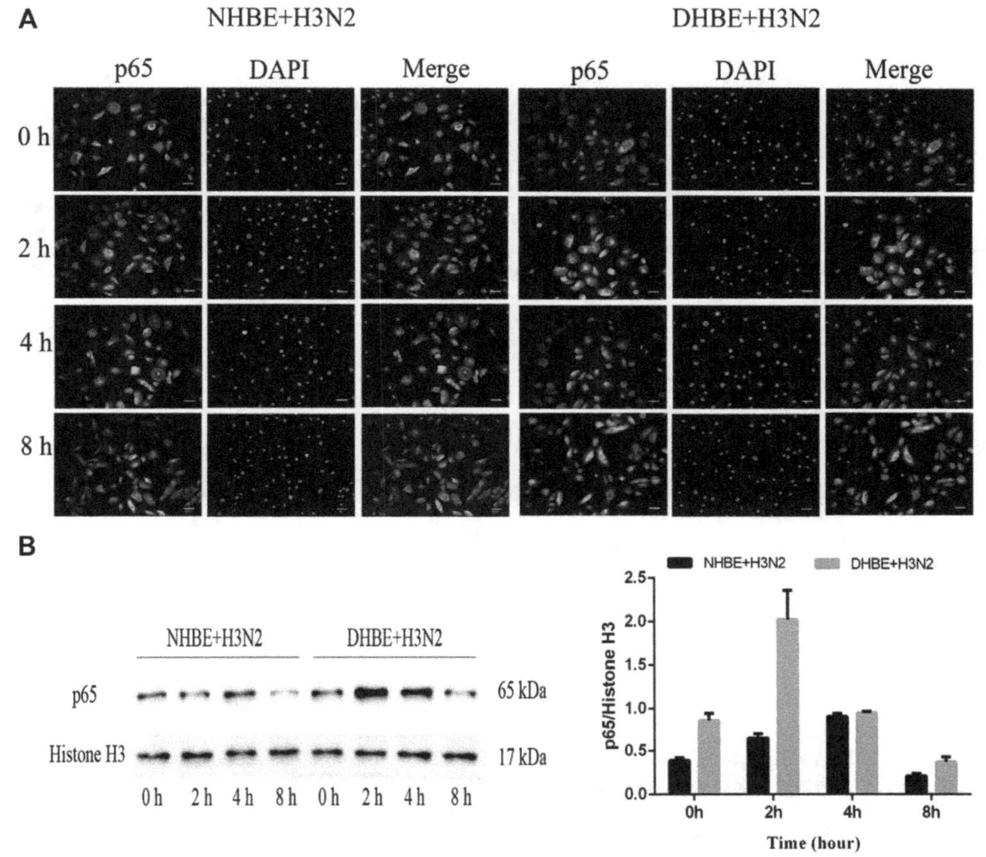

FIGURE 2 | IAV activated the NF-κB pathway earlier in DHBE. **(A)** Cell immunofluorescence of IAV induced NF-κBp65 nuclear translocation in pHBECs measured at different times. The IAV induced NF-κBp65 nuclear translocation was obviously detected at four hpi in NHBE **(left)** and two hpi in DHBE **(right)**, scale bar = 50 μm. Note: hpi: hours post infection, **(B)** NF-κB/p65 expression and relative intensity in the nucleus of pHBECs after infection with IAV for different times.

with shRNA specific to lncRNA TUG1 (sh-TUG1). As shown in **Figure 3C**, the expression of lncRNA TUG1 in DHBE attenuated significantly after treatment with sh-TUG1. Although the mRNA levels of NF-κBp65, IL-1β, and TNF-α in DHBE were increased significantly after infection with IAV, this effect was reduced significantly by sh-TUG1 (**Supplementary Figure S2**); consistent with this result, the protein expressions of phospho-NF-κBp65, IL-1β, and TNF-α were also reduced significantly by sh-TUG1 (shown in **Figures 3E–H**). These results indicated that knockdown of lncRNA TUG1 reduced airway inflammation induced by the IAV in DHBE.

lncRNA TUG1 Positively Regulated the IAV Induced Airway Inflammation by Sponging miR-145-5p in DHBE

To investigate the mechanisms by which the lncRNA TUG1 regulates the IAV induced airway inflammation, we predicted the miRNA target sites with bioinformatic database analysis and identified the miR-145-5p as the lncRNA with relevant binding site in the *TUG1* mRNA. We then constructed luciferase reporter vectors that contained the wildtype (wt) or mutated (mut) binding sequences for miR-145-5p in TUG1, and luciferase reporter assay results displayed that luciferase activity was suppressed in TUG1-wt cells but was not in TUG1-mut cells (**Figures 4A, B**), which suggested that miR-145-5p is a TUG1-targeting miRNA. Moreover, we demonstrated that miR-145-5p expression was significantly upregulated by lncRNA TUG1 knockdown in DHBE (**Figure 3D**). Bioinformatic database analysis revealed that miR-145-5p interacted with the 3UTR of NF-κBp65 mRNA. Dual-luciferase reporter assay revealed that the luciferase activity was significantly suppressed when cotransfected with NF-κBp65-wt and miR-145-5p mimic, whereas cotransfection with NF-κBp65-mut and miR-145-5p mimic failed to affect the luciferase activity (**Figures 4C, D**). The pretransfection of miR-145-5p mimic in DHBE partially inhibited the activation of NF-κB pathway induced by IAV infection, as well as the expressions of IL-1β and TNF-α (shown in **Figures 4E–H** and **Supplementary Figure S3**).

In addition, the lncRNA TUG1 knockdown attenuated the expressions of phospho-NF-κBp65, IL-1β and TNF-α significantly in DHBE after infection with IAV, and this effect

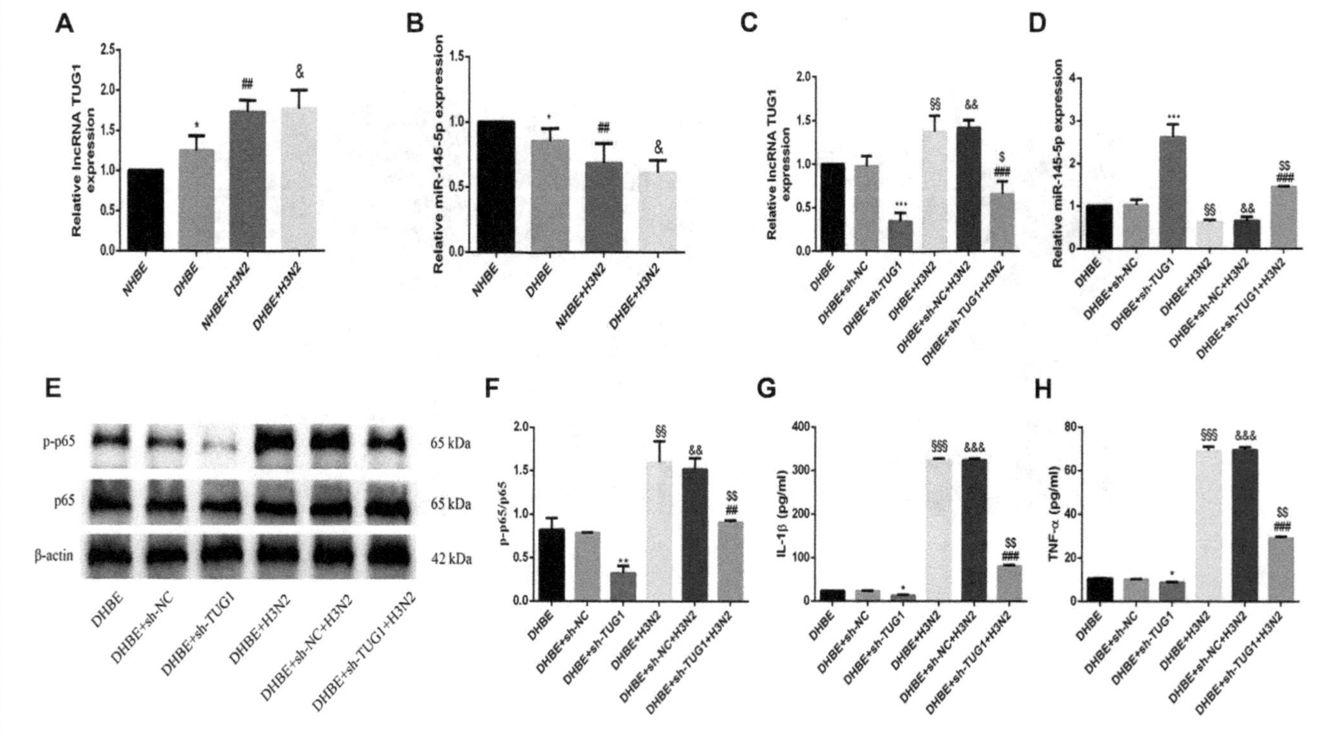

FIGURE 3 | Knockdown of lncRNA TUG1 reduced the IAV induced airway inflammation in DHBE. **(A,B)** The expression of lncRNA TUG1 and miR-145-5p was analyzed in pHBECs with or without IAV infection for 24 h (note: $^{*}p < 0.05$ as compared to NHBE, $^{\#\#}p < 0.01$ as compared to NHBE, $^{\&}p < 0.05$ as compared to DHBE). **(C,D)** The mRNA levels of lncRNA TUG1 and miR-145-5p were analyzed in DHBE pretreated with or without sh-TUG1. **(E,F)** The protein expressions of NF-κBp65 and phospho-NF-κBp65 were analyzed in DHBE pretreated with or without sh-TUG1 by Western blotting. **(G,H)** The protein expressions of IL-1β and TNF-α were analyzed in DHBE pretreated with or without sh-TUG1 by ELISA. ($^{*}p < 0.05$, $^{**}p < 0.01$, $^{***}p < 0.001$ as compared to DHBE + sh-NC group, $^{\#\#}p < 0.01$, $^{\#\#\#}p < 0.001$ as compared to DHBE + H3N2 group, $^{\S\S}p < 0.01$, $^{\S\S\S}p < 0.001$ as compared to DHBE group, $^{\&\&}p < 0.01$, $^{\&\&\&}p < 0.001$ as compared to DHBE + sh-NC group, $^{\$}p < 0.05$, $^{\$\$}p < 0.01$ as compared to DHBE + sh-NC + H3N2 group). Each dataset comprises three independent experiments.

was reversed by miR-145-5p inhibition, as shown in **Figures 4I–L** and **Supplementary Figure S4**. These results suggested that the lncRNA TUG1 positively regulated the IAV induced airway inflammation by sponging miR-145-5p in DHBE.

Overexpression of NF-κBp65 Reversed the Effects of lncRNA TUG1 Knockdown in DHBE After Infection With IAV

To further investigate the interaction of lncRNA TUG1 and NF-κB pathway, we performed gain-of-function assays by introducing the NF-κBp65 overexpression plasmid into DHBE with lncRNA TUG1 knockdown. As shown in **Figures 5A, B** and **Supplementary Figure S5A**, lncRNA TUG1 knockdown attenuated phospho-NF-κBp65 expression in IAV infected DHBE, whereas NF-κBp65 overexpression reversed this effect. Furthermore, NF-κBp65 overexpression attenuated the suppressive effect of lncRNA TUG1 knockdown on the expressions of IL-1β and TNF-α in IAV infected DHBE (shown in **Figures 5C, D** and **Supplementary Figures S5B, C**). These results revealed that lncRNA TUG1 knockdown might have a protective effect on the airway inflammatory response by repressing the activation of NF-κB pathway. We provide a schematic diagram to better illustrate the interactions among lncRNA TUG1/miR-145-5p/NF-κB pathway, as shown in **Figure 6**.

DISCUSSION

COPD patients are more susceptible to influenza virus infection, but the underlying molecular mechanism of its higher susceptibility is unknown. Respiratory epithelial cells are the first physical barrier to defense against respiratory viruses; they rapidly recognize the virus antigen with a variety of pattern recognition receptors, trigger the inflammatory responses by releasing cytokines, and regulate potentially harmful inflammation (Sajjan, 2013). In the present study, we demonstrated an earlier activation of NF-κB pathway in DHBE after IAV infection, accompanied with increased lncRNA TUG1 and decreased miR-145-5p. Knockdown of lncRNA TUG1 significantly attenuated the airway inflammation by inhibiting the NF-κB pathway and its downstream proinflammatory cytokines IL-1β and TNF-α. Meanwhile, mechanistic analysis revealed that the lncRNA TUG1 positively regulates the NF-κB pathway by sponging miR-145-5p.

NF-κB pathway is a key mediator in inflammatory injury and has been proven to participate in various cellular signaling transduction, including the influenza virus infection. Nimmerjahn and colleagues (Nimmerjahn et al., 2004) showed that an active NF-κB pathway was a prerequisite for influenza virus infection. Although previous research has studied the IAV

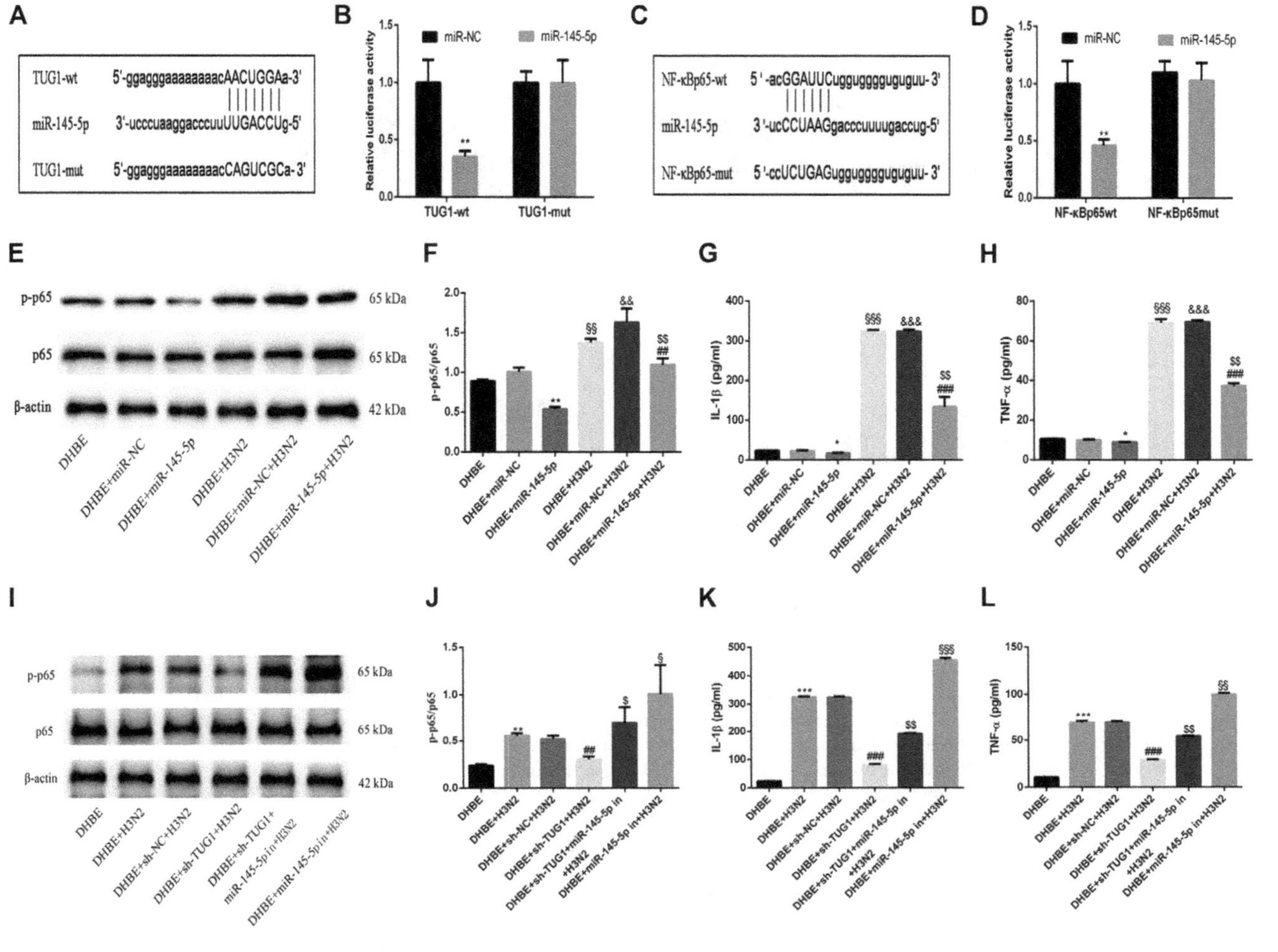

FIGURE 4 | lncRNA TUG1 positively regulated the IAV induced airway inflammation by sponging miR-145-5p in DHBE. **(A)** The putative miR-145-5p binding sequence of TUG1 mRNA. **(B)** Luciferase activity was measured between miR-145-5p (wt and mut) and TUG1 (wt and mut). **(C)** The putative miR-145-5p binding sequence of the 3′UTR of NF-κBp65. **(D)** Luciferase activity was measured between miR-145-5p (wt and mut) and NF-κBp65 (wt and mut). **(E,F)** The protein expressions of NF-κBp65 and phospho-NF-κBp65 were analyzed in DHBE pretreated with or without miR-145-5p mimic by Western blotting. **(G,H)** The protein expressions of proinflammatory cytokines IL-1β and TNF-α were analyzed in DHBE pretreated with or without miR-145-5p mimic by ELISA ($^{*}p < 0.05$, $^{**}p < 0.01$ as compared to DHBE + miR-NC group, $^{\#\#}p < 0.01$, $^{\#\#\#}p < 0.001$ as compared to DHBE + H3N2 group, $^{\S\S}p < 0.01$, $^{\S\S\S}p < 0.001$ as compared to DHBE group, $^{\&\&}p < 0.01$, $^{\&\&\&}p < 0.001$ as compared to DHBE+ miR-NC group, $^{\$\$}p < 0.01$ as compared to DHBE+ miR-NC +H3N2 group). Each dataset comprises three independent experiments. **(I,J)** The protein expressions of NF-κBp65 and phospho-NF-κBp65 were analyzed in DHBE pretreated with or without sh-TUG1/miR-145-5p inhibitor by Western blotting. **(K,L)** The protein expressions of proinflammatory cytokines IL-1β and TNF-α were analyzed in DHBE pretreated with or without sh-TUG1/miR-145-5p inhibitor by ELISA ($^{**}p < 0.01$, $^{***}p < 0.001$ as compared to DHBE group, $^{\#\#}p < 0.01$, $^{\#\#\#}p < 0.001$ as compared to DHBE + sh-NC + H3N2 group, $^{\$}p < 0.05$, $^{\$\$}p < 0.01$ as compared to DHBE+ sh-TUG1+H3N2 group, $^{\S}p < 0.05$, $^{\S\S}p < 0.01$, $^{\S\S\S}p < 0.001$ as compared to DHBE+ sh-TUG1+miR-145-5p in+H3N2 group). Each dataset comprises three independent experiments.

induced inflammatory response in pHBECs (Hsu et al., 2017; Huo et al., 2018), little have investigated the difference of the hypersusceptibility of airway inflammatory response caused by IAV between normal and COPD patients. Here we not only confirmed the activated NF-κB pathway in pHBECs after IAV infection, but also compared the differences in activation of NF-κB pathway between NHBE and DHBE at different time points. We found that the peak expression of phospho-NF-κBp65 observed in DHBE was 4 h earlier than NHBE with Western blotting, and the IAV induced NF-κBp65 nuclear translocation in DHBE was 2 h earlier than NHBE with cell immunofluorescence. The individual variation in susceptibility to virus directly affects the inflammatory responses of people with different immune status. An active NF-κB pathway may directly induce the exaggerated "cytokine storm" in the early stage after IAV infection (Nimmerjahn et al., 2004), and the inflammatory cytokines release may be quicker and stronger in COPD patients. Our results may partially explain the reason why COPD patients are more susceptible to IAV and have earlier and more severe symptoms than normal people, as well as the higher morbidity and mortality of emerging infectious diseases like Severe Acute Respiratory Syndrome (SARS) (Xu et al., 2020). All these indicate that we need to pay more attention and

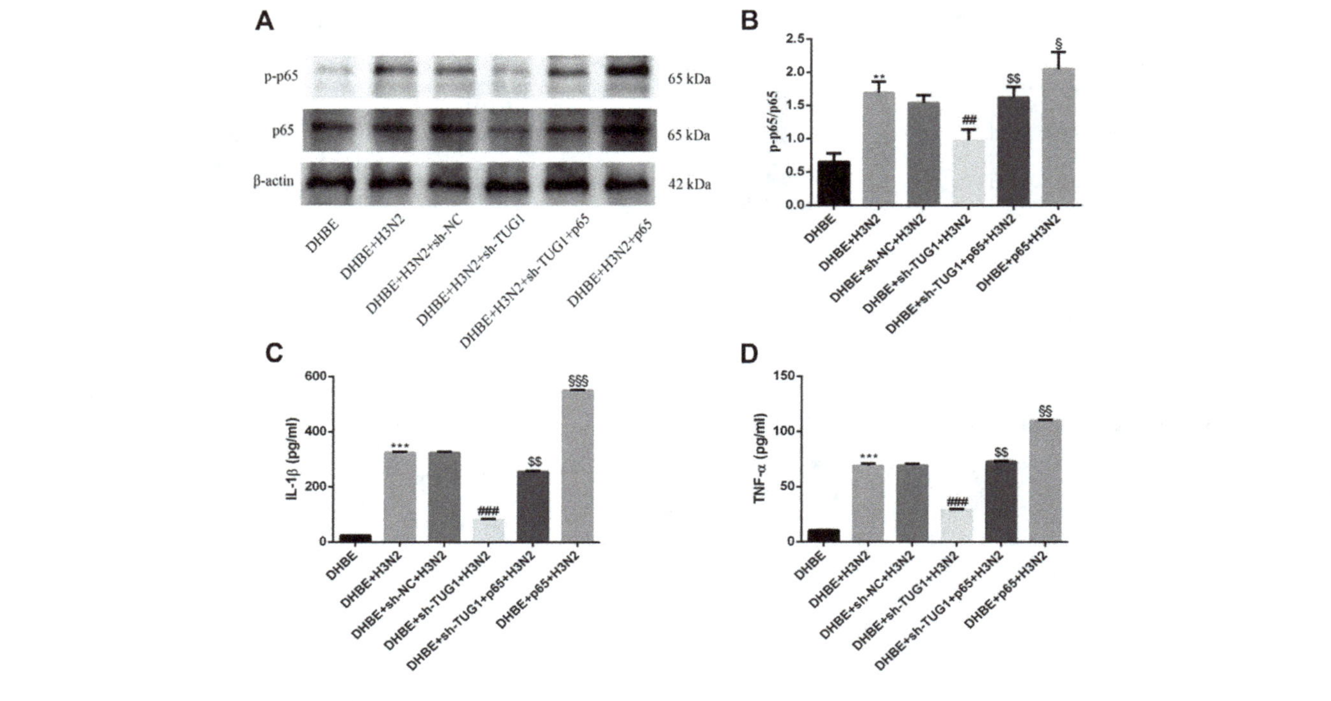

FIGURE 5 | Overexpression of NF-κBp65 reversed the effects of lncRNA TUG1 knockdown in DHBE after infection with IAV. **(A,B)** The protein expressions of NF-κBp65 and phospho-NF-κBp65 were analyzed in DHBE pretreated with or without sh-TUG1 and NF-κBp65 plasmid by Western blotting. **(C,D)** The protein expressions of proinflammatory cytokines IL-1β and TNF-α were analyzed in DHBE pretreated with or without sh-TUG1 and NF-κBp65 plasmid by ELISA ($^{**}p < 0.01$, $^{***}p < 0.001$ as compared to DHBE group, $^{\#\#}p < 0.01$, $^{\#\#\#}p < 0.001$ as compared to DHBE + sh-NC + H3N2 group, $^{\$\$}p < 0.01$ as compared to DHBE + sh-TUG1+H3N2 group, $^{\S}p < 0.05$, $^{\S\S}p < 0.01$, $^{\S\S\S}p < 0.001$ as compared to DHBE + sh-TUG1+p65 + H3N2 group). Each dataset comprises three independent experiments.

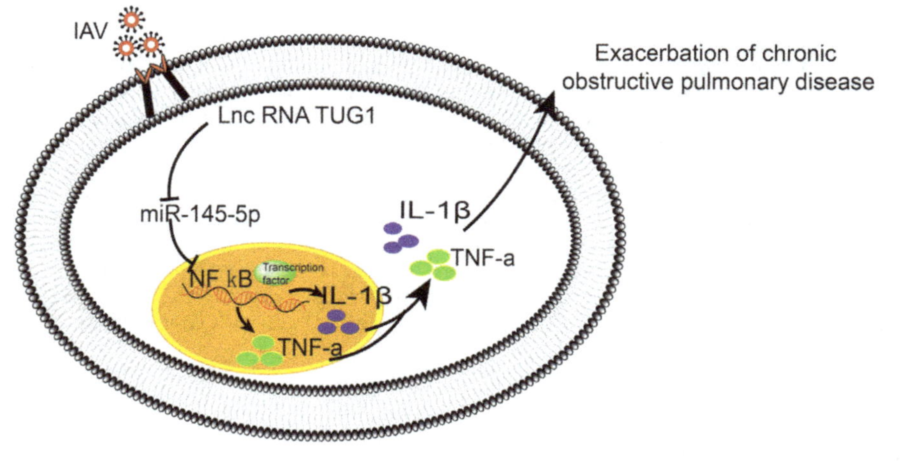

FIGURE 6 | Schematic diagram to illustrate the interactions of lncRNA TUG1/miR-145-5p/NF-κB pathway.

implement effective strategies to prevent the inflammatory injuries in the early stage of diseases.

lncRNA regulates the gene expression at the various levels, including transcriptional and posttranscriptional ones. Aberrant lncRNA may lead to dysfunction and contribute to the pathogenesis of various diseases (Chen, 2016). It interacts with a specific protein and regulates its functions or activities; moreover, lncRNA may interfere with the transcription by regulating the encoding sequences of protein genes (Shi et al., 2013). Furthermore, lncRNA can modulate a variety of biological activities or functions by acting as a competing endogenous RNA or miRNA sponge (Gu et al., 2019). In this study, we predicted the miR-145-5p as the binding target of lncRNA TUG1 with bioinformatic database analysis. We found that the DHBE had a significantly higher lncRNA TUG1 expression and lower miR-145-5p expression than NHBE, and the lncRNA TUG1 could regulate the airway inflammatory response by sponging miR-145-5p, which was consistent with Gu's study (Gu et al., 2019). Zhang et al. (Zhang et al., 2020) analyzed the expression profiles of lncRNAs and mRNAs in H3N2 infection by RNA sequencing. Different from our study, they did not report the expression of lncRNA TUG1 or miR-145-5p; we speculate this difference may be explained by the different research object we studied, and the pHBECs we studied may be more similar to the result *in vivo*. Previous studies have shown that the miR-145-5p attenuated significantly after being exposed to cigarette smoke extract and negatively regulated the proinflammatory cytokines expressions of airway smooth muscle cells in COPD patients (Pal et al., 2013; O'Leary et al., 2016). Here we found that the miR-145-5p expression in the pHBECs decreased significantly after IAV infection, accompanied with increased lncRNA TUG1 expression, activated NF-κB pathway, and increased IL-1β and TNF-α. Furthermore, this effect was significantly reversed by downregulation of lncRNA TUG1 or miR-145-5p mimic, which was quite consistent with Wang's study (Wang et al., 2019b) that the overexpression of miR-145-5p can inhibit the secretion of proinflammatory cytokines by suppressing NF-κB pathway in high glucose-induced retinal endothelial cells. It is reasonable to speculate that the NF-κB pathway was regulated positively by lncRNA TUG1 and negatively by miR-145-5p.

CONCLUSION

In conclusion, the present study demonstrated that the IAV can induce an exaggerated hypersusceptibility of airway inflammatory response in COPD by activating the lncRNA TUG1/miR-145-5p/NF-κB pathway *in vitro*, which may associate with the more severe symptoms induced by IAV in COPD. We speculate that the lncRNA TUG1 inhibitor may be a promising therapeutic strategy for AECOPD caused by IAV.

AUTHOR CONTRIBUTIONS

Conception and design of the study were done by YT and GF. Research was performed by YT and SJ. Drafting the article was done by YT. YG analyzed the data . Language edit was done by JS and GF. Manuscript revision was done by YT and GF. All authors gave their consent for publication.

ACKNOWLEDGMENTS

The authors would like to sincerely thank the professor Yan Liu in the Laboratory of Pathogenic Microorganism, Anhui Medical University, for providing the influenza virus H3N2 and the assistance with the related guidance and support of experimental techniques.

REFERENCES

Almansa, R., Socias, L., Andaluz-Ojeda, D., Martín-Loeches, I., Bobillo, F., Blanco, J., et al. (2012). Viral infection is associated with an increased proinflammatory response in chronic obstructive pulmonary disease. *Viral Immunol.* 25 (4), 249. doi:10.1089/vim.2011.0095

Cao, H. Y., Li, D., Wang, Y. P., Lu, H. X., Sun, J., and Li, H. B. (2020). The protection of NF-κB inhibition on kidney injury of systemic lupus erythematosus mice may be correlated with lncRNA TUG1. *Kaohsiung J. Med. Sci.* 36 (5), 354–362. doi:10.1002/kjm2.12183

Chen, L. L. (2016). Ling-ling Chen: linking long noncoding RNA processing and function to RNA biology. *Trends Biochem. Sci.* 41 (9), 733–734. doi:10.1016/j.tibs.2016.07.006

Dai, M. Y., Qiao, J. P., Xu, Y. H., and Fei, G. H. (2015). Respiratory infectious phenotypes in acute exacerbation of COPD: an aid to length of stay and COPD Assessment Test. *.Int. J. Chron. Obstruct Pulmon. Dis.* 10 (1), 2257–2263. doi:10.2147/COPD.S92160

Dickson, R. P., Huang, Y. J., Martinez, F. J., and Huffnagle, G. B. (2013). The lung microbiome and viral-induced exacerbations of chronic obstructive pulmonary disease: new observations, novel approaches. *Am. J. Respir. Crit. Care Med.* 188 (10), 1185–1186. doi:10.1164/rccm.201309-1573ed

Fulcher, M. L., Gabriel, S., Burns, K. A., Yankaskas, J. R., and Randell, S. H. (2005). Well-differentiated human airway epithelial cell cultures. *Methods Mol. Med.* 107, 183–206. doi:10.1385/1-59259-861-7:183

Gu, W., Yuan, Y., Wang, L., Yang, H., Li, S., Tang, Z., et al. (2019). Long non-coding RNA TUG1 promotes airway remodelling by suppressing the miR-145-5p/DUSP6 axis in cigarette smoke-induced COPD. *J. Cell Mol. Med.* 23 (11), 7200–7209. doi:10.1111/jcmm.14389

Hsu, A. C., Dua, K., Starkey, M. R., Haw, T. J., Nair, P. M., Nichol, K., et al. (2017). MicroRNA-125a and -b inhibit A20 and MAVS to promote inflammation and impair antiviral response in COPD. *Jci Insight* 2 (7), e90443. doi:10.1172/jci.insight.90443

Huo, C., Jin, Y., Zou, S., Qi, P., Xiao, J., Tian, H., et al. (2018). Lethal influenza A virus preferentially activates TLR3 and triggers a severe inflammatory response. *Virus Res.* 257, 102–112. doi:10.1016/j.virusres.2018.09.012

Ji, S., Bai, Q., Wu, X., Zhang, D.-W., Wang, S., Shen, J.-L., et al. (2020). Unique synergistic antiviral effects of Shufeng Jiedu Capsule and oseltamivir in influenza A viral-induced acute exacerbation of chronic obstructive pulmonary disease. *Biomed. Pharmacother.* 121, 109652. doi:10.1016/j.biopha.2019.109652

Koul, P. A., Mir, H., Akram, S., Potdar, V., and Chadha, M. S. (2017). Respiratory viruses in acute exacerbations of chronic obstructive pulmonary disease. *Lung India* 34 (1), 29–33. doi:10.4103/0970-2113.197099

Li, Z., Shen, J., Chan, M. T., and Wu, W. K. (2016). TUG1: a pivotal oncogenic long non-coding RNA of human cancers. *Cell Prolif.* 49 (4), 471–475. doi:10.1111/cpr.12269

Nimmerjahn, F., Dudziak, D., Dirmeier, U., Hobom, G., Riedel, A., Schlee, M., et al. (2004). Active NF-kappaB signalling is a prerequisite for influenza virus infection. *J. Gen. Virol.* 85 (8), 2347–2356. doi:10.1099/vir.0.79958-0

O'Leary, L., Sevinç, K., Papazoglou, I. M., Tildy, B., Detillieux, K., Halayko, A. J., et al. (2016). Airway smooth muscle inflammation is regulated by microRNA-145 in COPD. *FEBS Lett.* 590 (9), 1324–1334. doi:10.1002/1873-3468.12168

Pal, A., Melling, G., Hinsley, E. E., Kabir, T. D., Colley, H. E., Murdoch, C., et al. (2013). Cigarette smoke condensate promotes pro-tumourigenic stromal-epithelial interactions by suppressing miR-145. *J. Oral Pathol. Med.* 42 (4), 309–314. doi:10.1111/jop.12017

Sajjan, U. S. (2013). Susceptibility to viral infections in chronic obstructive pulmonary disease: role of epithelial cells. *Curr. Opin. Pulm. Med.* 19 (2), 125–132. doi:10.1097/MCP.0b013e32835cef10

Shi, X., Sun, M., Liu, H., Yao, Y., and Song, Y. (2013). Long non-coding RNAs: a new Frontier in the study of human diseases. *Cancer Lett.* 339 (2), 159–166. doi:10.1016/j.canlet.2013.06.013

Su, Q., Liu, Y., Lv, X.-W., Dai, R.-X., Yang, X.-H., and Kong, B.-H. (2020). LncRNA TUG1 mediates ischemic myocardial injury by targeting miR-132-3p/HDAC3 axis. *Am. J. Physiol. Heart Circ. Physiol.* 318 (2), H332–H344. doi:10.1152/ajpheart.00444.2019

Tang, W., Shen, Z., Guo, J., and Sun, S. (2016). Screening of long non-coding RNA and TUG1 inhibits proliferation with TGF-β induction in patients with COPD. *Int. J. Chron. Obstruct Pulmon. Dis.* 11, 2951–2964. doi:10.2147/COPD.S109570

Vogelmeier, C. F., Criner, G. J., Martinez, F. J., Anzueto, A., Barnes, P. J., Bourbeau, J., et al. (2017). Global strategy for the diagnosis, management, and prevention of chronic obstructive lung disease 2017 report. GOLD executive summary. *Am. J. Respir. Crit. Care Med.* 195 (5), 557. doi:10.1164/rccm.201701-0218PP

Wang, S., Cao, W., Gao, S., Nie, X., Zheng, X., Xing, Y., et al. (2019a). TUG1 regulates pulmonary arterial smooth muscle cell proliferation in pulmonary arterial hypertension. *Can. J. Cardiol.* 35 (11), 1534–1545. doi:10.1016/j.cjca.2019.07.630

Wang, H., Liao, S., Li, H., Chen, Y., and Yu, J. (2019b). Long non-coding RNA TUG1 sponges mir-145a-5p to regulate microglial polarization after oxygen-glucose deprivation. *Front. Mol. Neurosci.* 12, 215. doi:10.3389/fnmol.2019.00215

Wedzicha, J. A., Singh, R., and Mackay, A. J. (2014). Acute COPD exacerbations. *Clin. Chest Med.* 35 (1), 157–163. doi:10.1016/j.ccm.2013.11.001

Xu, G., Yang, Y., Du, Y., Peng, F., Hu, P., Wang, R., et al. (2020). Clinical pathway for early diagnosis of COVID-19: updates from experience to evidence-based practice. *Clin. Rev. Allergy Immunol.* 59 (1), 89–100. doi:10.1007/s12016-020-08792-8

Yamaya, M., Nishimura, H., Hatachi, Y., Yoshida, M., Fujiwara, H., Asada, M., et al. (2011). Procaterol inhibits rhinovirus infection in primary cultures of human tracheal epithelial cells. *Eur. J. Pharmacol.* 650 (1), 431–444. doi:10.1016/j.ejphar.2010.09.056

Zhang, Y., Yu, T., Ding, Y., Li, Y., Lei, J., Hu, B., et al. (2020). Analysis of expression profiles of long noncoding RNAs and mRNAs in A549 cells infected with H3N2 swine influenza virus by RNA sequencing. *Virol. Sin.* 35 (2), 171–180. doi:10.1007/s12250-019-00170-9

Zwaans, W. A., Mallia, P., van Winden, M. E., and Rohde, G. G. (2014). The relevance of respiratory viral infections in the exacerbations of chronic obstructive pulmonary disease—a systematic review. *J. Clin. Virol.* 61 (2), 181–188. doi:10.1016/j.jcv.2014.06.025

18

Gene Therapy: A Possible Alternative to CFTR Modulators?

J. Mercier[1], *M. Ruffin*[1], *H. Corvol*[1,2] *and L. Guillot*[1]*

[1]Sorbonne Université, Inserm, Centre de Recherche, Saint Antoine, F-75012, Paris, France, [2]Pneumologie Pédiatrique, APHP, Hôpital Trousseau, Paris, France

***Correspondence:**
L. Guillot
loic.guillot@inserm.fr

Cystic fibrosis (CF) is a rare genetic disease that affects several organs, but lung disease is the major cause of morbidity and mortality. The gene responsible for CF, the *CFTR* (Cystic Fibrosis Transmembrane Conductance Regulator) gene, has been discovered in 1989. Since then, gene therapy i.e., defective gene replacement by a functional one, remained the ultimate goal but unfortunately, it has not yet been achieved. However, patients care and symptomatic treatments considerably increased CF patients' life expectancy ranging from 5 years old in the 1960s to 40 today. In the last decade, research works on CFTR protein structure and activity led to the development of new drugs which, by readdressing CFTR to the plasma membrane (correctors) or by enhancing its transport activity (potentiators), allow, alone or in combination, an improvement of CF patients' lung function and quality of life. While expected, it is not yet known whether taking these drugs from an early age and for years will improve the quality of life of CF patients in the long term and further increase their life expectancy. Besides, these molecules are not available (specific variants of *CFTR*) or accessible (national health policies) for all patients and there is still no curative treatment. Another alternative that could benefit from new technologies, such as gene therapy, is therefore still attractive, although it is not yet offered to patients. Faced with the development of new CFTR correctors and potentiators, the question arises as to whether there is still a place for gene therapy and this is discussed in this perspective.

Keywords: cystic fibrosis, gene therapy, ivacaftor, lumacaftor, tezacaftor, personalized medicine

INTRODUCTION

Cystic fibrosis (CF) is a rare genetic disease caused by pathogenic variants in the *CFTR* (Cystic Fibrosis Transmembrane Conductance Regulator) gene, which encodes for a chloride channel expressed ubiquitously within epithelia. As a result, ionic and hydric imbalances across epithelia are observed in several organs, affecting their function. Specifically, manifestations can occur in the pancreas, liver, kidneys, and intestine, but lung disease is the main cause of morbidity and mortality of CF patients.

Since the *CFTR* gene discovery in 1989, more than 2000 variants of the *CFTR* gene have been identified. They were classified into six classes depending on their consequences on the CFTR protein. CF patients' life expectancy increased considerably between the 1960s and the beginning of the 21st century mainly due to symptomatic treatment development and to patient management standardization. However, even if new promising drugs (called "CFTR modulators") directly targeting the CFTR protein are already available for some CF patients, there is still no curative treatment. Gene therapy, as defined by the delivery of a wild-type *CFTR* gene in cells, might be this curative treatment but is not yet available.

TABLE 1 | CFTR modulators available for the treatment of CF patients. ppFEV1: percent-predicted Forced Expiratory Volume in 1 s; m.o.: months old; y.o.: years old. *only initial Phase III studies are cited. [detailed in (Lopes-Pacheco, 2019)].

Molecules	First approval date	Eligibility age	Indication*	Absolute change in ppFEV1
Ivacaftor	2012	≥6 m.o.	G551D/other Ramsey et al. (2011)	10.6%
			Class III variants/Other Davies et al. (2013)	12.5%
Lumacaftor/ivacaftor	2015	≥2 y.o.	F508del/F508del Wainwright et al. (2015)	2.8%
Tezacaftor/ivacaftor	2018	≥6 y.o.	F508del/F508del Taylor-Cousar et al. (2017)	4%
			F508del/residual function variant in *trans* Rowe et al. (2017)	6.8%
Elexacaftor/tezacaftor/ivacaftor	2019	≥12 y.o.	F508del/minimal function variant in *trans* Middleton et al. (2019)	13.8%
			F508del/F508del Heijerman et al. (2019)	10.4%

This perspective briefly describes the latest development of CFTR modulators and *CFTR* gene delivery strategies and discusses whether gene therapy is a still relevant alternative to be considered with respect to these promising molecules.

CFTR Modulators

In the last decade, new drugs called "CFTR modulators" addressing the direct consequences of *CFTR* variants on the CFTR protein have been identified thanks to high-throughput screening (extensively reviewed in (Lopes-Pacheco, 2019)). The two major types of CFTR modulators are correctors and potentiators. Correctors are intended to improve CFTR trafficking to the plasma membrane, while potentiators are designed to increase CFTR channel conductance. Thus, correctors and potentiators can only be effective on certain classes of *CFTR* variants i.e., those affecting CFTR protein trafficking (class II) and conductance (class III and IV). *CFTR* class I variants, that result in the absence of protein synthesis, and *CFTR* class V and VI variants, that lead to decreased CFTR protein quantity production, are excluded from modulator therapies. CFTR modulators approval represents a breakthrough in CF care because a significant improvement in patient's lung function (evaluated by measurements of FEV1 (forced expiratory volume in 1 s)) has been observed (**Table 1**).

Ivacaftor, the first potentiator designed to target the G551D gating variant (the most prevalent *CFTR* class III gating variant), showed in phase 3 clinical trial that patients gain more than 10% of FEV1 (Ramsey et al., 2011). Ivacaftor was then validated for other *CFTR* class III gating variants. A few years after, modulators targeting the most common *CFTR* variant called F508del (a class II variant) emerged. The combination of the corrector lumacaftor with the potentiator ivacaftor was approved for patient homozygotes for the F508del variant but showed limited FEV1 improvement. New correctors and combinations emerged further, which have more interesting effects on FEV1, allowing to address patients carrying only one F508del variant (**Table 1**). The latest combination (elexacaftor/tezacaftor/ivacaftor) showed indeed impressive results with a 14% increase in FEV1 (Heijerman et al., 2019; Middleton et al., 2019). Even if the level of increased lung function remains the principal measurement of treatment efficiency, these modulators have also been shown to be beneficial for other clinical parameters including increased body-mass index, improved life quality, and decreased exacerbations frequency.

Altogether, based on their age and genotype, around 80% of the patients reported in the Cystic Fibrosis Foundation Patient Registry are eligible for CFTR modulators (https://www.cff.org/Research/Researcher-Resources/Patient-Registry/). According to this registry, 10% of the patients are still too young to be eligible for CFTR modulators; and the remaining 10% carry *CFTR* variants not currently known to be responsive to modulators or have unknown or incomplete genotypes. Among these patients, it has been estimated that 7% may require genetic-based therapy.

In this new promising era, some other concerns remain. For example, it should be noted that the hindsight on these treatments is limited, which makes it difficult to assess their long-term efficacy and tolerance. According to national health policies, the cost of these treatments might also be an obstacle to their access for all CF patients. Finally, as shown in a recent retrospective study, among 845 CF patients who initiated lumacaftor/ivacaftor, 22.8% fully or temporarily discontinued their treatment mostly because of respiratory adverse events (Burgel et al., 2020). This could result in limiting the total number of patients who can benefit from these treatments.

The latest generation of modulator, the triple therapy, elexacaftor/tezacaftor/ivacaftor, showed impressive results leading us to question in this perspective whether gene therapy is still attractive.

GENE THERAPY: WHAT'S UP?

Gene therapy consists of introducing a functional gene into host cells to replace a defective gene. Theoretically, this could be a perfect match for the needs of a monogenic disease as CF and could lead to a universal treatment for CF patients. Especially since Johnson and colleagues stated in 1992 that 6–10% of CFTR-corrected cells are sufficient to observe a therapeutic effect *in vitro* (Johnson et al., 1992), we can speculate that correction of all CF airway cells may not be mandatory to observe the same effect *in vivo*. However, the race for CF gene therapy turned out to be more challenging than expected so far.

Lungs: Barriers to Delivery

The lung represents an organ of choice for the delivery of organ-specific treatments due to its ease of access. Therefore, aerosol administration has been widely used in previous clinical trials of pulmonary gene therapy as reviewed by Resnier et al. (Resnier et al., 2016). However, the major difficulty encountered in these

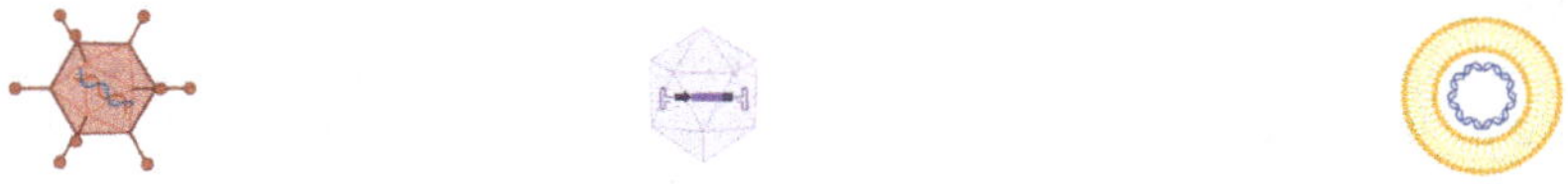

	Adenovirus[1-4]	Adeno-associated virus [5-11]	Liposome[12-21]
Administration	-Nasal ([1] Zabner et al., 1993; [2] Crystal et al., 1994; [3] Knowles et al., 1995; [4] Zabner et al., 1996) -Bronchial ([3] Knowles et al., 1995)	-Nasal ([5] Flotte et al., 2003) -Bronchial ([7] Aitken et al., 2001; [9] Flotte et al., 2003; [10] Moss et al., 2004; [11] Moss et al., 2007) -Maxillary sinus ([5] Wagner et al., 1998; [6] Wagner et al., 1999; [8] Wagner et al., 2002)	-Nasal ([12] Caplen et al., 1995; [13] Gill et al., 1997; [14] Porteous et al., 1997; [15] Zabner et al., 1997; [17] Noone et al., 2000; [18] Konstan et al., 2004) -Lung ([16] Alton et al., 1999; [19] Alton et al., 2015a; [20] Alton et al., 2015b; [21] Alton et al., 2016)
Transfection efficiency	Low	-Low ([8] Wagner et al., 2002; [9] Flotte et al., 2003; [10] Moss et al., 2004) -Good ([5] Wagner et al., 1998; [6] Wagner et al., 1999) -High ([7] Aitken et al., 2001) -Not measured ([11] Moss et al., 2007)	Good
Safety profile	Yes	Yes	Yes
Adverse events	Some immune responses No long-term adverse events	Little or no inflammatory response	Little or no inflammatory response
Functional effect	Cl^- transport defect partially restored or not	Cl^- transport defect partially restored or not	Transient Cl^- transport correction No change or modest improvement of FEV_1 (increase of 3.7%)

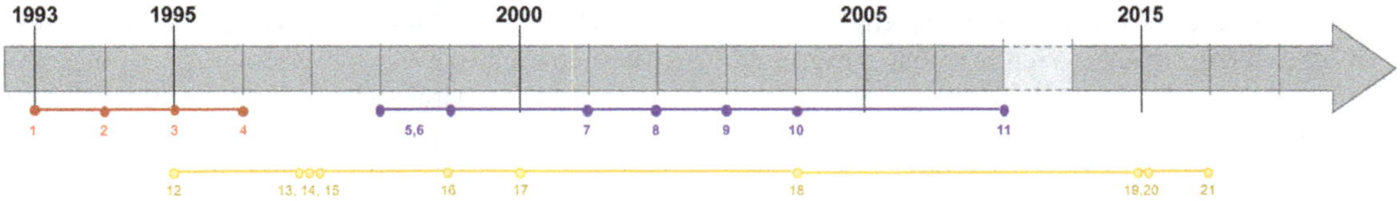

FIGURE 1 | Summary of CF gene therapy clinical trials. Colors represent vector agent used (red: Ad, purple: AAV, yellow: liposome). Vectors agent made with biorender: https://biorender.com.

trials is the delivery of the gene into airway epithelial cells. Indeed, mucus, mucociliary clearance, and lung immune responses complicate the entry of the gene transfer agent into target cells, and the few that succeed encounters a new obstacle: the nuclear membrane (Yonemitsu et al., 2000; Stern et al., 2003; Schuster et al., 2014; Xia et al., 2014). Moreover, since the airway epithelium renews itself gradually, another challenge is to target progenitor cells to obtain a permanent treatment and avoid repeated required deliveries (Gill and Hyde, 2014).

CFTR Gene Delivery Methods: Advantages and Limitations

Only 1 year after the *CFTR* gene discovery in 1989 (Kerem et al., 1989; Riordan et al., 1989; Rommens et al., 1989), two groups independently showed that it was possible to produce a functional CFTR protein by using a viral vector to introduce the full-length *CFTR* gene *in vitro* (Drumm et al., 1990; Rich et al., 1990). This proof of concept paved the way for the beginning of CF gene therapy clinical trials (**Figure 1**). To efficiently introduce a normal *CFTR* gene into cells, various delivery strategies have been developed for three decades, including viral and non-viral vector systems, and are briefly presented after (recently reviewed in detail by (Cooney et al., 2018; Schneider-Futschik, 2019; Yan et al., 2019)).

Viral Vectors

Viruses have a high natural capacity to infect host cells and were modified by scientists to decrease their pathogenicity. Thus, recombinant vectors expressing a foreign antigenic protein or a functional protein were created and used for vaccines or gene therapy, respectively.

Recombinant Adenovirus Vector

Recombinant Adenovirus-based vectors (rAd-vector) were the first viral vectors used in CF gene therapy clinical trials. They are non-enveloped viruses with a linear and double-stranded DNA genome. Commonly, two serotypes are observed beyond Ad - type 2 (Ad2) or type 5 (Ad5) which allow host-cell binding. *In vivo* studies showed that Ad-vectors were transduced in all airway epithelial cell types (Mastrangeli et al., 1993) and also in submucosal glands (Pilewski et al., 1995). The first use of Ad-vectors with *CFTR* gene in CF gene therapy clinical trial showed that their delivery was safe, with little or no immune response and a partial correction of Cl^- transport defect (Zabner et al., 1993; Zabner et al., 1996). Crystal et al. showed that rAd-CFTR protein was expressed in the airway epithelium 4 days after intra-bronchial administration. They tested doses up to 2×10^9 pfu, which led to short-term adverse events such as transient systemic inflammation (Crystal et al., 1994). No other adverse event was reported after a 6-months follow-up. Another trial showed no evidence of CFTR functional defect correction, probably due to inflammatory responses (Knowles et al., 1995). Thus, rAd-vectors are capable of transducing and occasionally correcting Cl^- transport defect in CF human airway epithelial cells. Yet, some inflammatory responses were observed. Besides, rAd-vector DNA does not integrate the host cell genome but rather persists within the cells as episomal DNA (Athanasopoulos et al., 2017). Finally, rAd-vector DNA is not replicated upon cell divisions, requiring multiple deliveries for patients.

Recombinant Adeno-Associated Virus Vector

Recombinant adeno-associated virus vectors (rAAV) are characterized by their ability to transduce both dividing and quiescent cells and by their high transduction efficiency in primary human airway (Yan et al., 2013). Those vectors are less immunogenic than Ad-vectors and were the most used vectors in CF gene therapy clinical trials, showing a strong safety profile record but failed in improving the lung function (Wagner et al., 1999; Wagner et al., 1998; Aitken et al., 2001; Wagner et al., 2002; Flotte et al., 2003; Moss et al., 2007) (**Figure 1**).

A limitation of rAAV vector is its packaging capacity limited to 4.8 kb (Blacklow et al., 1988; Wu et al., 2010). The small size of this vector may give it an advantage to enter cells more easily but considering that the size of the *CFTR* gene is 4.6 kb, there is almost no space left for regulatory sequences allowing *CFTR* gene expression enhancement. As reviewed by Cooney and coll., the shortening of the *CFTR* gene and other cassette sequences led to a generation of modified AAV vectors that expressed functional CFTR.

Moreover, rAAVs vectors genome integrates into the human genome (Kotin et al., 1991; Samulski et al., 1991; Kotin et al., 1992; Rivadeneira et al., 1998; Ding et al., 2003; Janovitz et al., 2014) and can also persist as episomal DNA in post-mitotic tissues when the replication protein rep is absent (Athanasopoulos et al, 2017). Besides, rAAV-mediated transduction has been proved to induce a long-lasting gene expression up to several months in pigs (Steines et al., 2016) and better rAAV vectors allowing an increased packaging capacity and higher tropism for airway epithelial cells are developed (Yan et al., 2019).

Helper-Dependent Adenovirus Vector

Helper-dependent adenovirus (Hd-Ad) vectors, which have had all viral genes deleted, were developed to circumvent inflammatory properties of rAd-vectors (Parks et al., 1996). With a 36 kb packaging capacity (Cots et al., 2013), they circumvent little packaging capacities of rAAV-vectors. Multiple serotypes of Hd-Ad vectors have been tested but serotype 5 showed effective transduction *in vivo* in airways basal cells in mouse and pig models and, *in vitro*, in primary human airway epithelial cell cultures (Cao et al., 2018; Palmer et al., 2020).

Lentivirus

Finally, the last type of viral vector used for CF gene therapy studies is lentiviral vector, which could allow a genomic integration and provide a long-term expression (Naldini et al., 1996) without repeated administrations. Even if LV vectors seem less likely to be destroyed by immune system than rAAVs, because of no-prexisting immunity (neutralizing antibodies), they activate the immune system as the other viral vectors (Nayak and Herzog, 2010). LV-mediated transgene integration site into the host genome can be multiple, extremely variable and potentially leading to proto-oncogenes activation. This property led to the interruption of a clinical trial in severe combined immunodeficiency patients (Hacein-Bey-Abina et al., 2003a; Hacein-Bey-Abina et al., 2003b; Fischer et al., 2004; Fischer and Cavazzana-Calvo, 2005; Hacein-Bey-Abina et al., 2008). In order to circumvent this, LV vectors design was then improved with self-inactivating (SIN) of long terminal repeats (LTRs), reducing the genotoxic risk of these strong enhancer-promoter sequences (Modlich and Baum, 2009; Milone and O'Doherty, 2018). Thus, lentiviruses still seem to be interesting vectors for CF gene therapy as some lentiviral vector pseudotypes demonstrated high vector production and apical tropism to airway epithelium *in vitro* and *in vivo* (Sinn et al., 2005; McKay et al., 2006). Plus, repeated administration was possible without blocking antibody immune responses (Sinn et al., 2008; Griesenbach et al., 2012) and LV efficiency was demonstrated in several animal models including mice, ferret and pigs (Oakland et al., 2013; Yan et al., 2015; Cooney et al., 2016). Recently, a study with a promising lentiviral vector developed by the United Kingdom Cystic Fibrosis Gene Therapy consortium showed a 14% airway cells transduction efficiency *in vitro*, low toxicity and an integration site profile supporting a future first-in-man trial (Alton et al., 2017).

Nevertheless, viral vectors use can be limited by several factors. Firstly, neutralizing antibodies to Ad or AAV, due to the immune response to previous natural infection, are frequently found in patients, rendering them ineligible for this kind of treatments (Erles et al., 1999). Secondly, viral vectors internalization into host cells requires receptors such as α_V integrins (Wickham et al., 1993), Coxsackie-Adenovirus Receptor (Bergelson et al., 1997), heparan sulfate glycosaminoglycans (Dechecchi et al., 2001) or fibroblast growth factor receptors (Duan et al., 1998) that are expressed on the basolateral membrane of bronchial epithelial cells, thus explaining the lack of transduction efficiency (Duan et al., 1998; Pickles et al., 1998; Marquez Loza et al., 2019). Pseudotyping viral vectors with proteins able to interact with apical membrane receptors of airway epithelial cells is thus required to enhance delivery efficiency.

Non-Viral Vectors

Non-viral vectors allow genomic material delivery into cells by direct administration as naked DNA or associated with different compounds. Those vectors have theoretically no size restrictions and have mainly three possible configurations: lipid-based, peptide-based or polymer-based delivery. They can carry plasmid or linear DNA as well as RNA molecules. A non-viral strategy for *CFTR* delivery was considered as an alternative to viral vectors. Indeed, several studies showed that cationic lipids were safe delivery vehicles for gene transfer (Kollen et al., 1996; Fasbender et al., 1998; McDonald et al., 1998), their main issue remaining the limited transgene delivery into the nucleus (Brisson et al., 1999). However, as recently reviewed (Cooney et al., 2018), several clinical trials using cationic lipids showed transient expression of vector related-*CFTR* for few days and partial restoration of nasal potential differences in CF patients without significant clinical effect on lung function (Caplen et al., 1995; Gill et al., 1997; Porteous et al., 1997; Zabner et al., 1997; Alton et al., 1999; Noone et al., 2000; Ruiz et al., 2001; Konstan et al., 2004). In 2015, Alton and colleagues reported an increase in FEV1 of 3.7% (0.07–7.25%) after using pGM169/GL67A cationic lipid (Alton et al., 2015b) in patients who received nebulized vector at 28 days intervals for 12 months (Alton et al., 2015a). However, as FEV1 improvements observed were only comparable to those obtained with some CFTR modulators, trial did not result in the current clinical application for CF patients. Alton et al. now focused on alternative lentiviral vectors candidates, such as the lentiviral vector based on simian immunodeficiency virus (SIV) pseudotyped with Sendaï virus envelope proteins Fusion (F) and Hemagglutinin-Neuraminidase (HN) (rSIV.F/HN), which retains 90–100% transduction efficiency and leads to a functional CFTR expression in preclinical models (Alton et al., 2016; Alton et al., 2017).

GENE THERAPY STILL TO CONSIDER?

To date, CF gene therapy clinical trials have not been conclusive, with a weak effect observed on CF patients' lung function, associated with important immune responses, which may render the treatment ineffective. Moreover, as mentioned previously, the recent developments of effective drugs such as the triple combination elexacaftor/tezacaftor/ivacaftor, which greatly improves patients' lung function and quality of life, has given rise to the idea that "cystic fibrosis is almost cured". Thus, it is therefore legitimate to wonder to what extent gene therapy still has a place in the treatment of CF. However, it should be remembered that the drugs currently on the market still leave aside at least 10% of CF patients without curative treatment, as highlighted by the Cystic Fibrosis Foundation patient registry. In addition, current CFTR modulators are not well tolerated by all eligible patients and real-life studies show that numerous patients stop their treatment. Besides, we do not have enough hindsight to predict effectiveness of these promising drugs in the long term.

Over the last 20 years, gene therapy has shown successful transient or permanent results for several diseases such as X-linked severe combined immune deficiency (Cavazzana-Calvo et al., 2000), adenosine deaminase deficiency (Cicalese et al., 2016), Leber congenital amaurosis (Cideciyan et al., 2013), hemophilia (Nathwani et al., 2011), severe beta-Thalassemia (Cavazzana-Calvo et al., 2010; Persons, 2010), but also Parkinson's disease (Palfi et al., 2014) or leukemia, with 27 children who experienced complete remission after treatment (Maude et al., 2014). In 2012, the first viral gene-therapy treatment was approved in Europe for treatment of lipoprotein lipase deficiency (Yla-Herttuala, 2012) and showed good results even years later (Gaudet et al., 2016). Recently, gene therapy also showed promising results for Leber hereditary optic neuropathy by improving bilateral vision in patients over 96 weeks of follow-up after a unilateral intravitreal injection (Yu-Wai-Man et al., 2020). These successful trials were carried out on easily accessible hematopoietic stem cells or by direct vectors injections into specific tissues, which may explain previous trials failure in CF compared to other diseases.

In addition to wild-type *CFTR* gene delivery strategy, *CFTR* gene editing with CRISPR/Cas9 technology emerged as a promising therapeutic option for CF patients (Hodges and Conlon, 2019). New strategies are also currently tested in on-going trials, such as RESTORE-CF phase I/II clinical trial (http://ClinicalTrials.gov Identifier: NCT03375047), which evaluates safety and tolerability of MRT5005, an RNA-based therapy. RNA-based therapy has the advantage of not disturbing the genome, however would require repeated doses. Another promising strategy is to combine gene therapy with pluripotent stem cells (iPSCs). As a proof of concept, Hawkins et al. succeeded to derive airway basal cells from human iPSCs, to perform an engraftment and to allow epithelial regeneration *in vivo* using a tracheal xenograft model in immune-compromized mice, with similar structure and composition than *in vivo* airways (Hawkins et al., 2020). The long-term goal is to obtain a *de novo* generation of the full diversity of lung lineages and transplantable 3D lung tissues, that could be corrected by gene therapy and transferred into CF patients (Kotton, 2012).

In conclusion, CF gene therapy still has a bright future ahead. The main current challenge is to circumvent technical problems of transduction encountered in the lung. If this happens one day, not only will CF be truly cured, but the gene therapy might also be applied to other lung genetic diseases.

AUTHOR CONTRIBUTIONS

JM, MR, HC, and LG wrote the manuscript.

ACKNOWLEDGMENTS

MR received a postdoctoral fellowship from the French cystic fibrosis non-profit organization Vaincre la mucoviscidose (RF20190502451).

REFERENCES

Aitken, M. L., Moss, R. B., Waltz, D. A., Dovey, M. E., Tonelli, M. R., McNamara, S. C., et al. (2001). A phase I study of aerosolized administration of tgAAVCF to cystic fibrosis subjects with mild lung disease. *Hum. Gene Ther.* 12 (15), 1907–1916. doi:10.1089/104303401753153956

Alton, E., Armstrong, D. K., Ashby, D., Bayfield, K. J., Bilton, D., Bloomfield, E. V., et al. (2016). *A randomised, double-blind, placebo-controlled trial of repeated nebulisation of non-viral cystic fibrosis transmembrane conductance regulator (CFTR) gene therapy in patients with cystic fibrosis* (Southampton (UK):NIHR Journals Library. doi:10.3310/eme03050

Alton, E., Stern, M., Farley, R., Jaffe, A., Chadwick, S., Phillips, J., et al. (1999). Cationic lipid-mediated CFTR gene transfer to the lungs and nose of patients with cystic fibrosis: a double-blind placebo-controlled trial. *The Lancet* 353 (9157), 947–954. doi:10.1016/s0140-6736(98)06532-5

Alton, E. W. F. W., Armstrong, D. K., Ashby, D., Bayfield, K. J., Bilton, D., Bloomfield, E. V., et al. (2015a). Repeated nebulisation of non-viral CFTR gene therapy in patients with cystic fibrosis: a randomised, double-blind, placebo-controlled, phase 2b trial. *Lancet Respir. Med.* 3 (9), 684–691. doi:10.1016/S2213-2600(15)00245-3

Alton, E. W. F. W., Beekman, J. M., Boyd, A. C., Brand, J., Carlon, M. S., Connolly, M. M., et al. (2017). Preparation for a first-in-man lentivirus trial in patients with cystic fibrosis. *Thorax* 72 (2), 137–147. doi:10.1136/thoraxjnl-2016-208406

Alton, E. W. F. W., Boyd, A. C., Porteous, D. J., Davies, G., Davies, J. C., Griesenbach, U., et al. (2015b). A phase I/IIa safety and efficacy study of nebulized liposome-mediated gene therapy for cystic fibrosis supports a multidose trial. *Am. J. Respir. Crit. Care Med.* 192 (11), 1389–1392. doi:10.1164/rccm.201506-1193LE

Athanasopoulos, T., Munye, M. M., and Yáñez-Muñoz, R. J. (2017). Nonintegrating gene therapy vectors. *Hematology/Oncology Clin. North America* 31 (5), 753–770. doi:10.1016/j.hoc.2017.06.007

Bergelson, J. M., Cunningham, J. A., Droguett, G., Kurt-Jones, E. A., Krithivas, A., Hong, J. S., et al. (1997). Isolation of a common receptor for Coxsackie B viruses and adenoviruses 2 and 5. *Science* 275 (5304), 1320–1323. doi:10.1126/science.275.5304.1320

Blacklow, S. C., Raines, R. T., Lim, W. A., Zamore, P. D., and Knowles, J. R. (1988). Triosephosphate isomerase catalysis is diffusion controlled. *Biochemistry* 27 (4), 1158–1165. doi:10.1021/bi00404a013

Brisson, M., Tseng, W.-C., Almonte, C., Watkins, S., and Huang, L. (1999). Subcellular trafficking of the cytoplasmic expression system. *Hum. Gene Ther.* 10 (16), 2601–2613. doi:10.1089/10430349950016645

Burgel, P. R., Munck, A., Durieu, I., Chiron, R., Mely, L., Prevotat, A., et al. (2020). Real-life safety and effectiveness of lumacaftor-ivacaftor in patients with cystic fibrosis. *Am. J. Respir. Crit. Care Med.* 201 (2), 188–197. doi:10.1164/rccm.201906-1227OC

Cao, H., Ouyang, H., Grasemann, H., Bartlett, C., Du, K., Duan, R., et al. (2018). Transducing airway basal cells with a helper-dependent adenoviral vector for lung gene therapy. *Hum. Gene Ther.* 29 (6), 643–652. doi:10.1089/hum.2017.201

Caplen, N. J., Alton, E. W. F. W., Mddleton, P. G., Dorin, J. R., Stevenson, B. J., Gao, X., et al. (1995). Liposome-mediated CFTR gene transfer to the nasal epithelium of patients with cystic fibrosis. *Nat. Med.* 1 (1), 39–46. doi:10.1038/nm0195-39

Cavazzana-Calvo, M., Hacein-Bey, S., de Saint Basile, G., Gross, F., Yvon, E., Nusbaum, P., et al. (2000). Gene therapy of human severe combined immunodeficiency (SCID)-X1 disease. *Science* 288 (5466), 669–672. doi:10.1126/science.288.5466.669

Cavazzana-Calvo, M., Payen, E., Negre, O., Wang, G., Hehir, K., Fusil, F., et al. (2010). Transfusion independence and HMGA2 activation after gene therapy of human β-thalassaemia. *Nature* 467 (7313), 318–322. doi:10.1038/nature09328

Cicalese, M. P., Ferrua, F., Castagnaro, L., Pajno, R., Barzaghi, F., Giannelli, S., et al. (2016). Update on the safety and efficacy of retroviral gene therapy for immunodeficiency due to adenosine deaminase deficiency. *Blood* 128 (1), 45–54. doi:10.1182/blood-2016-01-688226

Cideciyan, A. V., Jacobson, S. G., Beltran, W. A., Sumaroka, A., Swider, M., Iwabe, S., et al. (2013). Human retinal gene therapy for Leber congenital amaurosis shows advancing retinal degeneration despite enduring visual improvement. *Proc. Natl. Acad. Sci. U. S. A.* 110 (6), E517–E525. doi:10.1073/pnas.1218933110

Cooney, A. L., Abou Alaiwa, M. H., Shah, V. S., Bouzek, D. C., Stroik, M. R., Powers, L. S., et al. (2016). Lentiviral-mediated phenotypic correction of cystic fibrosis pigs. *JCI Insight* 1 (14), e88730. doi:10.1172/jci.insight.88730

Cooney, A., McCray, P., Jr., and Sinn, P. (2018). Cystic fibrosis gene therapy: looking back, looking forward. *Genes* 9 (11), 538. doi:10.3390/genes9110538

Cots, D., Bosch, A., and Chillón, M. (2013). Helper dependent adenovirus vectors: progress and future prospects. *Cgt* 13 (5), 370–381. doi:10.2174/1566523211305131212125338

Crystal, R. G., McElvaney, N. G., Rosenfeld, M. A., Chu, C.-S., Mastrangeli, A., Hay, J. G., et al. (1994). Administration of an adenovirus containing the human CFTR cDNA to the respiratory tract of individuals with cystic fibrosis. *Nat. Genet.* 8 (1), 42–51. doi:10.1038/ng0994-42

Davies, J. C., Wainwright, C. E., Canny, G. J., Chilvers, M. A., Howenstine, M. S., Munck, A., et al. (2013). Efficacy and safety of ivacaftor in patients aged 6 to 11 years with cystic fibrosis with aG551D Mutation. *Am. J. Respir. Crit. Care Med.* 187 (11), 1219–1225. doi:10.1164/rccm.201301-0153OC

Dechecchi, M. C., Melotti, P., Bonizzato, A., Santacatterina, M., Chilosi, M., and Cabrini, G. (2001). Heparan sulfate glycosaminoglycans are receptors sufficient to mediate the initial binding of adenovirus types 2 and 5. *J. Virol.* 75 (18), 8772–8780. doi:10.1128/jvi.75.18.8772-8780.2001

Ding, W., Yan, Z., Zak, R., Saavedra, M., Rodman, D. M., and Engelhardt, J. F. (2003). Second-strand genome conversion of adeno-associated virus type 2 (AAV-2) and AAV-5 is not rate limiting following apical infection of polarized human airway epithelia. *J Virol.* 77 (13), 7361–7366. doi:10.1128/jvi.77.13.7361-7366.2003

Drumm, M. L., Pope, H. A., Cliff, W. H., Rommens, J. M., Marvin, S. A., Tsui, L.-C., et al. (1990). Correction of the cystic fibrosis defect *in vitro* by retrovirus-mediated gene transfer. *Cell* 62 (6), 1227–1233. doi:10.1016/0092-8674(90)90398-x

Duan, D., Yue, Y., Yan, Z., McCray, P. B., Jr., and Engelhardt, J. F. (1998). Polarity influences the efficiency of recombinant adenoassociated virus infection in differentiated airway epithelia. *Hum. Gene Ther.* 9 (18), 2761–2776. doi:10.1089/hum.1998.9.18-2761

Erles, K., Sebokova, P., and Schlehofer, J. R. (1999). Update on the prevalence of serum antibodies (IgG and IgM) to adeno-associated virus (AAV). *J. Med. Virol.* 59 (3), 406–411. doi:10.1002/(sici)1096-9071(199911)59:3<406::aid-jmv22>3.0.co;2-n

Fasbender, A., Lee, J. H., Walters, R. W., Moninger, T. O., Zabner, J., and Welsh, M. J. (1998). Incorporation of adenovirus in calcium phosphate precipitates enhances gene transfer to airway epithelia *in vitro* and *in vivo*. *J. Clin. Invest.* 102 (1), 184–193. doi:10.1172/JCI2732

Fischer, A., and Cavazzana-Calvo, M. (2005). Integration of retroviruses: a fine balance between efficiency and danger. *Plos Med.* 2 (1), e10. doi:10.1371/journal.pmed.0020010

Fischer, A., Abina, S. H., Thrasher, A., von Kalle, C., and Cavazzana-Calvo, M. (2004). LMO2 and gene therapy for severe combined immunodeficiency. *N. Engl. J. Med.* 350 (24), 2526–2527. doi:10.1056/NEJM200406103502422

Flotte, T. R., Zeitlin, P. L., Reynolds, T. C., Heald, A. E., Pedersen, P., Beck, S., et al. (2003). Phase I trial of intranasal and endobronchial administration of a recombinant adeno-associated virus serotype 2 (rAAV2)-CFTR vector in adult cystic fibrosis patients: a two-part clinical study. *Hum. Gene Ther.* 14 (11), 1079–1088. doi:10.1089/104303403322124792

Gaudet, D., Stroes, E. S., Méthot, J., Brisson, D., Tremblay, K., Bernelot Moens, S. J., et al. (2016). Long-term retrospective analysis of gene therapy with alipogene tiparvovec and its effect on lipoprotein lipase deficiency-induced pancreatitis. *Hum. Gene Ther.* 27 (11), 916–925. doi:10.1089/hum.2015.158

Gill, D. R., and Hyde, S. C. (2014). Delivery of genes into the CF airway. *Thorax* 69 (10), 962–964. doi:10.1136/thoraxjnl-2014-205835

Gill, D., Southern, K., Mofford, K., Seddon, T., Huang, L., Sorgi, F., et al. (1997). A placebo-controlled study of liposome-mediated gene transfer to the nasal epithelium of patients with cystic fibrosis. *Gene Ther.* 4 (3), 199–209. doi:10.1038/sj.gt.3300391

Griesenbach, U., Inoue, M., Meng, C., Farley, R., Chan, M., Newman, N. K., et al. (2012). Assessment of F/HN-pseudotyped lentivirus as a clinically relevant vector for lung gene therapy. *Am. J. Respir. Crit. Care Med.* 186 (9), 846–856. doi:10.1164/rccm.201206-1056OC

Hacein-Bey-Abina, S., Garrigue, A., Wang, G. P., Soulier, J., Lim, A., Morillon, E., et al. (2008). Insertional oncogenesis in 4 patients after retrovirus-mediated gene therapy of SCID-X1. *J. Clin. Invest.* 118 (9), 3132–3142. doi:10.1172/JCI35700

Hacein-Bey-Abina, S., von Kalle, C., Schmidt, M., Le Deist, F., Wulffraat, N., McIntyre, E., et al. (2003a). A serious adverse event after successful gene therapy for X-linked severe combined immunodeficiency. *N. Engl. J. Med.* 348 (3), 255–256. doi:10.1056/NEJM200301163480314

Hacein-Bey-Abina, S., Von Kalle, C., Schmidt, M., McCormack, M. P., Wulffraat, N., Leboulch, P., et al. (2003b). LMO2-associated clonal T cell proliferation in two patients after gene therapy for SCID-X1. *Science* 302 (5644), 415–419. doi:10.1126/science.1088547

Hawkins, F. J., Suzuki, S., Beermann, M. L., Barillà, C., Wang, R., Villacorta-Martin, C., et al. (2021). Derivation of airway basal stem cells from human pluripotent stem cells. *Cell Stem Cell* 28, 79. doi:10.1016/j.stem.2020.09.017

Heijerman, H. G. M., McKone, E. F., Downey, D. G., Van Braeckel, E., Rowe, S. M., Tullis, E., et al. (2019). Efficacy and safety of the elexacaftor plus tezacaftor plus ivacaftor combination regimen in people with cystic fibrosis homozygous for the F508del mutation: a double-blind, randomised, phase 3 trial. *The Lancet* 394 (10212), 1940–1948. doi:10.1016/S0140-6736(19)32597-8

Hodges, C. A., and Conlon, R. A. (2019). Delivering on the promise of gene editing for cystic fibrosis. *Genes Dis.* 6 (2), 97–108. doi:10.1016/j.gendis.2018.11.005

Janovitz, T., Oliveira, T., Sadelain, M., Falck-Pedersen, E., and Imperiale, M. J. (2014). Highly divergent integration profile of adeno-associated virus serotype 5 revealed by high-throughput sequencing. *J. Virol.* 88 (5), 2481–2488. doi:10.1128/JVI.03419-13

Johnson, L. G., Olsen, J. C., Sarkadi, B., Moore, K. L., Swanstrom, R., and Boucher, R. C. (1992). Efficiency of gene transfer for restoration of normal airway epithelial function in cystic fibrosis. *Nat. Genet.* 2 (1), 21–25. doi:10.1038/ng0992-21

Kerem, B., Rommens, J., Buchanan, J., Markiewicz, D., Cox, T., Chakravarti, A., et al. (1989). Identification of the cystic fibrosis gene: genetic analysis. *Science* 245 (4922), 1073–1080. doi:10.1126/science.2570460

Knowles, M. R., Hohneker, K. W., Zhou, Z., Olsen, J. C., Noah, T. L., Hu, P.-C., et al. (1995). A controlled study of adenoviral-vector-mediated gene transfer in the nasal epithelium of patients with cystic fibrosis. *N. Engl. J. Med.* 333 (13), 823–831. doi:10.1056/NEJM199509283331302

Kollen, W. J. W., Midoux, P., Erbacher, P., Yip, A., Roche, A. C., Monsigny, M., et al. (1996). Gluconoylated and glycosylated polylysines as vectors for gene transfer into cystic fibrosis airway epithelial cells. *Hum. Gene Ther.* 7 (13), 1577–1586. doi:10.1089/hum.1996.7.13-1577

Konstan, M. W., Davis, P. B., Wagener, J. S., Hilliard, K. A., Stern, R. C., Milgram, L. J. H., et al. (2004). Compacted DNA nanoparticles administered to the nasal mucosa of cystic fibrosis subjects are safe and demonstrate partial to complete cystic fibrosis transmembrane regulator reconstitution. *Hum. Gene Ther.* 15 (12), 1255–1269. doi:10.1089/hum.2004.15.1255

Kotin, R. M., Linden, R. M., and Berns, K. I. (1992). Characterization of a preferred site on human chromosome 19q for integration of adeno-associated virus DNA by non-homologous recombination. *EMBO J.* 11 (13), 5071–5078. doi:10.1002/j.1460-2075.1992.tb05614.x

Kotin, R. M., Menninger, J. C., Ward, D. C., and Berns, K. I. (1991). Mapping and direct visualization of a region-specific viral DNA integration site on chromosome 19q13-qter. *Genomics* 10 (3), 831–834. doi:10.1016/0888-7543(91)90470-y

Kotton, D. N. (2012). Next-generation regeneration: the hope and hype of lung stem cell research. *Am. J. Res. Crit. Care Med.* 185, 1255–1260. doi:10.1164/rccm.201202-0228PP

Lopes-Pacheco, M. (2019). CFTR modulators: the changing face of cystic fibrosis in the era of precision medicine. *Front. Pharmacol.* 10, 1662. doi:10.3389/fphar.2019.01662

Marquez Loza, L., Yuen, E., and McCray, P., Jr. (2019). Lentiviral vectors for the treatment and prevention of cystic fibrosis lung disease. *Genes* 10 (3), 218. doi:10.3390/genes10030218

Mastrangeli, A., Danel, C., Rosenfeld, M. A., Stratford-Perricaudet, L., Perricaudet, M., Pavirani, A., et al. (1993). Diversity of airway epithelial cell targets for *in vivo* recombinant adenovirus-mediated gene transfer. *J. Clin. Invest.* 91 (1), 225–234. doi:10.1172/JCI116175

Maude, S. L., Frey, N., Shaw, P. A., Aplenc, R., Barrett, D. M., Bunin, N. J., et al. (2014). Chimeric antigen receptor T cells for sustained remissions in leukemia. *N. Engl. J. Med.* 371 (16), 1507–1517. doi:10.1056/NEJMoa1407222

McDonald, R. J., Liggitt, H. D., Roche, L., Nguyen, H. T., Pearlman, R., Raabe, O. G., et al. (1998). Aerosol delivery of lipid:DNA complexes to lungs of rhesus monkeys. *Pharm. Res.* 15 (5), 671–679. doi:10.1023/a:1011902532163

McKay, T., Patel, M., Pickles, R. J., Johnson, L. G., and Olsen, J. C. (2006). Influenza M2 envelope protein augments avian influenza hemagglutinin pseudotyping of lentiviral vectors. *Gene Ther.* 13 (8), 715–724. doi:10.1038/sj.gt.3302715

Middleton, P. G., Mall, M. A., Dřevínek, P., Lands, L. C., McKone, E. F., Polineni, D., et al. (2019). Elexacaftor-Tezacaftor-Ivacaftor for Cystic Fibrosis with a Single Phe508del Allele. *N. Engl. J. Med.* 381 (19), 1809–1819. doi:10.1056/NEJMoa1908639

Milone, M. C., and O'Doherty, U. (2018). Clinical use of lentiviral vectors. *Leukemia* 32 (7), 1529–1541. doi:10.1038/s41375-018-0106-0

Modlich, U., and Baum, C. (2009). Preventing and exploiting the oncogenic potential of integrating gene vectors. *J. Clin. Invest.* 119 (4), 755–758. doi:10.1172/jci38831

Moss, R. B., Milla, C., Colombo, J., Accurso, F., Zeitlin, P. L., Clancy, J. P., et al. (2007). Repeated aerosolized AAV-CFTR for treatment of cystic fibrosis: a randomized placebo-controlled phase 2B trial. *Hum. Gene Ther.* 18 (8), 726–732. doi:10.1089/hum.2007.022

Moss, R. B., Rodman, D., Spencer, L. T., Aitken, M. L., Zeitlin, P. L., Waltz, D., et al. (2004). Repeated adeno-associated virus serotype 2 aerosol-mediated cystic fibrosis transmembrane regulator gene transfer to the lungs of patients with cystic fibrosis. *Chest* 125 (2), 509–521. doi:10.1378/chest.125.2.509

Naldini, L., Blomer, U., Gallay, P., Ory, D., Mulligan, R., Gage, F. H., et al. (1996). *In vivo* gene delivery and stable transduction of nondividing cells by a lentiviral vector. *Science* 272 (5259), 263–267. doi:10.1126/science.272.5259.263

Nathwani, A. C., Tuddenham, E. G. D., Rangarajan, S., Rosales, C., McIntosh, J., Linch, D. C., et al. (2011). Adenovirus-associated virus vector-mediated gene transfer in hemophilia B. *N. Engl. J. Med.* 365 (25), 2357–2365. doi:10.1056/NEJMoa1108046

Nayak, S., and Herzog, R. W. (2010). Progress and prospects: immune responses to viral vectors. *Gene Ther.* 17 (3), 295–304. doi:10.1038/gt.2009.148

Noone, P. G., Hohneker, K. W., Zhou, Z., Johnson, L. G., Foy, C., Gipson, C., et al. (2000). Safety and biological efficacy of a lipid-CFTR complex for gene transfer in the nasal epithelium of adult patients with cystic fibrosis. *Mol. Ther.* 1 (1), 105–114. doi:10.1006/mthe.1999.0009

Oakland, M., Maury, W., McCray, P. B., Jr., and Sinn, P. L. (2013). Intrapulmonary versus nasal transduction of murine airways with GP64-pseudotyped viral vectors. *Mol. Ther. Nucleic Acids* 2, e69. doi:10.1038/mtna.2012.60

Palfi, S., Gurruchaga, J. M., Ralph, G. S., Lepetit, H., Lavisse, S., Buttery, P. C., et al. (2014). Long-term safety and tolerability of ProSavin, a lentiviral vector-based gene therapy for Parkinson's disease: a dose escalation, open-label, phase 1/2 trial. *The Lancet* 383 (9923), 1138–1146. doi:10.1016/S0140-6736(13)61939-X

Palmer, D. J., Turner, D. L., and Ng, P. (2020). A single "All-in-One" helper-dependent adenovirus to deliver donor DNA and CRISPR/Cas9 for efficient homology-directed repair. *Mol. Ther. Methods Clin. Dev.* 17, 441–447. doi:10.1016/j.omtm.2020.01.014

Parks, R. J., Chen, L., Anton, M., Sankar, U., Rudnicki, M. A., and Graham, F. L. (1996). A helper-dependent adenovirus vector system: removal of helper virus by Cre-mediated excision of the viral packaging signal. *Proc. Natl. Acad. Sci.* 93 (24), 13565–13570. doi:10.1073/pnas.93.24.13565

Persons, D. A. (2010). Targeting β-thalassaemia. *Nature* 467 (7313), 277–278. doi:10.1038/467277a

Pickles, R. J., McCarty, D., Matsui, H., Hart, P. J., Randell, S. H., and Boucher, R. C. (1998). Limited entry of adenovirus vectors into well-differentiated airway epithelium is responsible for inefficient gene transfer. *J. Virol.* 72 (7), 6014–6023. doi:10.1128/JVI.72.7.6014-6023.1998

Pilewski, J. M., Engelhardt, J. F., Bavaria, J. E., Kaiser, L. R., Wilson, J. M., and Albelda, S. M. (1995). Adenovirus-mediated gene transfer to human bronchial submucosal glands using xenografts. *Am. J. Physiol.-Lung Cell. Mol. Physiol.* 268 (4 Pt 1), L657–L665. doi:10.1152/ajplung.1995.268.4.L657

Porteous, D., Dorin, J., McLachlan, G., Davidson-Smith, H., Davidson, H., Stevenson, B., et al. (1997). Evidence for safety and efficacy of DOTAP cationic liposome mediated CFTR gene transfer to the nasal epithelium of patients with cystic fibrosis. *Gene Ther.* 4 (3), 210–218. doi:10.1038/sj.gt.3300390

Ramsey, B. W., Davies, J., McElvaney, N. G., Tullis, E., Bell, S. C., Dřevínek, P., et al. (2011). A CFTR potentiator in patients with cystic fibrosis and theG551DMutation. *N. Engl. J. Med.* 365 (18), 1663–1672. doi:10.1056/NEJMoa1105185

Resnier, P., Mottais, A., Sibiril, Y., Le Gall, T., and Montier, T. (2016). Challenges and successes using nanomedicines for aerosol delivery to the airways. *Cgt* 16 (1), 34–46. doi:10.2174/1566523216666160104142013

Rich, D. P., Anderson, M. P., Gregory, R. J., Cheng, S. H., Paul, S., Jefferson, D. M., et al. (1990). Expression of cystic fibrosis transmembrane conductance regulator corrects defective chloride channel regulation in cystic fibrosis airway epithelial cells. *Nature* 347 (6291), 358–363. doi:10.1038/347358a0

Riordan, J. R., Rommens, J., Kerem, B., Alon, N., Rozmahel, R., Grzelczak, Z., et al. (1989). Identification of the cystic fibrosis gene: cloning and characterization of complementary DNA. *Science* 245 (4922), 1066–1073. doi:10.1126/science.2475911

Rivadeneira, E. D., Popescu, N. C., Zimonjic, D. B., Cheng, G. S., Nelson, P. J., Ross, M. D., et al. (1998). Sites of recombinant adeno-associated virus integration. *Int. J. Oncol.* 12 (4), 805–810. doi:10.3892/ijo.12.4.805

Rommens, J., Iannuzzi, M., Kerem, B., Drumm, M., Melmer, G., Dean, M., et al. (1989). Identification of the cystic fibrosis gene: chromosome walking and jumping. *Science* 245 (4922), 1059–1065. doi:10.1126/science.2772657

Rowe, S. M., Daines, C., Ringshausen, F. C., Kerem, E., Wilson, J., Tullis, E., et al. (2017). Tezacaftor-ivacaftor in residual-function heterozygotes with cystic fibrosis. *N. Engl. J. Med.* 377 (21), 2024–2035. doi:10.1056/NEJMoa1709847

Ruiz, F. E., Clancy, J. P., Perricone, M. A., Bebok, Z., Hong, J. S., Cheng, S. H., et al. (2001). A clinical inflammatory syndrome attributable to aerosolized lipid-DNA administration in cystic fibrosis. *Hum. Gene Ther.* 12 (7), 751–761. doi:10.1089/104303401750148667

Samulski, R. J., Zhu, X., Xiao, X., Brook, J. D., Housman, D. E., Epstein, N., et al. (1991). Targeted integration of adeno-associated virus (AAV) into human chromosome 19. *EMBO J.* 10 (12), 3941–3950. doi:10.1002/j.1460-2075.1991.tb04964.x

Schneider-Futschik, E. K. (2019). Beyond cystic fibrosis transmembrane conductance regulator therapy: a perspective on gene therapy and small molecule treatment for cystic fibrosis. *Gene Ther.* 26 (9), 354–362. doi:10.1038/s41434-019-0092-5

Schuster, B. S., Kim, A. J., Kays, J. C., Kanzawa, M. M., Guggino, W. B., Boyle, M. P., et al. (2014). Overcoming the cystic fibrosis sputum barrier to leading adeno-associated virus gene therapy vectors. *Mol. Ther.* 22 (8), 1484–1493. doi:10.1038/mt.2014.89

Sinn, P. L., Arias, A. C., Brogden, K. A., and McCray, P. B., Jr. (2008). Lentivirus vector can be readministered to nasal epithelia without blocking immune responses. *Jvi* 82 (21), 10684–10692. doi:10.1128/JVI.00227-08

Sinn, P. L., Penisten, A. K., Burnight, E. R., Hickey, M. A., Williams, G., McCoy, D. M., et al. (2005). Gene transfer to respiratory epithelia with lentivirus pseudotyped with Jaagsiekte sheep retrovirus envelope glycoprotein. *Hum. Gene Ther.* 16 (4), 479–488. doi:10.1089/hum.2005.16.479

Steines, B., Dickey, D. D., Bergen, J., Excoffon, K. J. D. A., Weinstein, J. R., Li, X., et al. (2016). CFTR gene transfer with AAV improves early cystic fibrosis pig phenotypes. *JCI Insight* 1 (14), e88728. doi:10.1172/jci.insight.88728

Stern, M., Ulrich, K., Geddes, D. M., and Alton, E. W. F. W. (2003). Poly (D, L-lactide-co-glycolide)/DNA microspheres to facilitate prolonged transgene expression in airway epithelium *in vitro*, *ex vivo* and *in vivo*. *Gene Ther.* 10 (16), 1282–1288. doi:10.1038/sj.gt.3301994

Taylor-Cousar, J. L., Munck, A., McKone, E. F., van der Ent, C. K., Moeller, A., Simard, C., et al. (2017). Tezacaftor-ivacaftor in patients with cystic fibrosis homozygous for Phe508del. *N. Engl. J. Med.* 377 (21), 2013–2023. doi:10.1056/NEJMoa1709846

Wagner, J. A., Messner, A. H., Moran, M. L., Daifuku, R., Kouyama, K., Desch, J. K., et al. (1999). Safety and biological efficacy of an adeno-associated virus vector-cystic fibrosis transmembrane regulator (AAV-CFTR) in the cystic fibrosis maxillary sinus. *Laryngoscope* 109 (2 Pt 1), 266–274. doi:10.1097/00005537-199902000-00017

Wagner, J. A., Moran, M. L., Messner, A. H., Daifuku, R., Conrad, C. K., Reynolds, T., et al. (1998). A phase I/II study of tgAAV-CF for the treatment of chronic sinusitis in patients with cystic fibrosis. Stanford University, Stanford, California. *Hum. Gene Ther.* 9 (6), 889–909. doi:10.1089/hum.1998.9.6-889

Wagner, J. A., Nepomuceno, I. B., Messner, A. H., Moran, M. L., Batson, E. P., Dimiceli, S., et al. (2002). A phase II, double-blind, randomized, placebo-controlled clinical trial of tgAAVCF using maxillary sinus delivery in patients with cystic fibrosis with antrostomies. *Hum. Gene Ther.* 13 (11), 1349–1359. doi:10.1089/104303402760128577

Wainwright, C. E., Elborn, J. S., Ramsey, B. W., Marigowda, G., Huang, X., Cipolli, M., et al. (2015). Lumacaftor-Ivacaftor in patients with cystic fibrosis homozygous for Phe508del CFTR. *N. Engl. J. Med.* 373 (3), 220–231. doi:10.1056/NEJMoa1409547

Wickham, T. J., Mathias, P., Cheresh, D. A., and Nemerow, G. R. (1993). Integrins αvβ3 and αvβ5 promote adenovirus internalization but not virus attachment. *Cell* 73 (2), 309–319. doi:10.1016/0092-8674(93)90231-e

Wu, Z., Yang, H., and Colosi, P. (2010). Effect of genome size on AAV vector packaging. *Mol. Ther.* 18 (1), 80–86. doi:10.1038/mt.2009.255

Xia, E., Munegowda, M. A., Cao, H., and Hu, J. (2014). Lung gene therapy-How to capture illumination from the light already present in the tunnel. *Genes Dis.* 1 (1), 40–52. doi:10.1016/j.gendis.2014.06.001

Yan, Z., Lei-Butters, D. C. M., Keiser, N. W., and Engelhardt, J. F. (2013). Distinct transduction difference between adeno-associated virus type 1 and type 6 vectors in human polarized airway epithelia. *Gene Ther.* 20 (3), 328–337. doi:10.1038/gt.2012.46

Yan, Z., McCray Jr, P. B., Jr., and Engelhardt, J. F. (2019). Advances in gene therapy for cystic fibrosis lung disease. *Hum. Mol. Genet.* 28 (R1), R88–R94. doi:10.1093/hmg/ddz139

Yan, Z., Stewart, Z. A., Sinn, P. L., Olsen, J. C., Hu, J., McCray, P. B., Jr., et al. (2015). Ferret and pig models of cystic fibrosis: prospects and promise for gene therapy. *Hum. Gene Ther. Clin. Dev.* 26 (1), 38–49. doi:10.1089/humc.2014.154

Ylä-Herttuala, S. (2012). Endgame: glybera finally recommended for approval as the first gene therapy drug in the European Union. *Mol. Ther.* 20 (10), 1831–1832. doi:10.1038/mt.2012.194

Yonemitsu, Y., Kitson, C., Ferrari, S., Farley, R., Griesenbach, U., Judd, D., et al. (2000). Efficient gene transfer to airway epithelium using recombinant Sendai virus. *Nat. Biotechnol.* 18 (9), 970–973. doi:10.1038/79463

Yu-Wai-Man, P., Newman, N. J., Carelli, V., Moster, M. L., Biousse, V., Sadun, A. A., et al. (2020). Bilateral visual improvement with unilateral gene therapy injection for Leber hereditary optic neuropathy. *Sci. Transl. Med.* 12 (573), eaaz7423. doi:10.1126/scitranslmed.aaz7423

Zabner, J., Cheng, S. H., Meeker, D., Launspach, J., Balfour, R., Perricone, M. A., et al. (1997). Comparison of DNA-lipid complexes and DNA alone for gene transfer to cystic fibrosis airway epithelia *in vivo*. *J. Clin. Invest.* 100 (6), 1529–1537. doi:10.1172/JCI119676

Zabner, J., Couture, L. A., Gregory, R. J., Graham, S. M., Smith, A. E., and Welsh, M. J. (1993). Adenovirus-mediated gene transfer transiently corrects the chloride transport defect in nasal epithelia of patients with cystic fibrosis. *Cell* 75 (2), 207–216. doi:10.1016/0092-8674(93)80063-k

Zabner, J., Ramsey, B. W., Meeker, D. P., Aitken, M. L., Balfour, R. P., Gibson, R. L., et al. (1996). Repeat administration of an adenovirus vector encoding cystic fibrosis transmembrane conductance regulator to the nasal epithelium of patients with cystic fibrosis. *J. Clin. Invest.* 97 (6), 1504–1511. doi:10.1172/JCI118573

19

Circulating Plasma miRNA and Clinical/ Hemodynamic Characteristics Provide Additional Predictive Information about Acute Pulmonary Thromboembolism, Chronic Thromboembolic Pulmonary Hypertension and Idiopathic Pulmonary Hypertension

Alexandre Todorovic Fabro[1,2†], Juliana Machado-Rugolo[1,3†], Camila Machado Baldavira[1†], Tabatha Gutierrez Prieto[1†], Cecília Farhat[1‡], Flavia Regina Rotea ManGone[4‡], Sabrina Setembre Batah[2‡], Heloísa Resende Cruvinel[2‡], Maiara Almeida Aldá[2‡], Jhonatas Sirino Monteiro[5‡], Adriana Inacio Pádua[6‡], Sirlei Siani Morais[2‡], Rogério Antônio de Oliveira[7‡], Marcel Koenigkam Santos[6‡], José Antônio Baddini-Martinez[6‡], João Carlos Setubal[5‡], Claudia Aparecida Rainho[8‡], Hugo Hyung Bok Yoo[9‡], Pedro Leme Silva[10,11,$], Maria Aparecida Nagai[4,12,$] and Vera Luiza Capelozzi[1,$]*

[1]Department of Pathology, Laboratory of Histomorphometry and Lung Genomics, Faculty of Medicine, University of São Paulo, São Paulo, Brazil, [2]Department of Pathology and Legal Medicine, Respiratory Medicine Laboratory, Ribeirão Preto Medical School, University of São Paulo (USP), São Paulo, Brazil, [3]Health Technology Assessment Center (NATS), Clinical Hospital (HCFMB), Medical School of São Paulo State University (UNESP), Botucatu, Brazil, [4]Laboratory of Molecular Genetics, Center for Translational Research in Oncology, Cancer Institute of São Paulo (ICESP), São Paulo, Brazil, [5]Bioinformatic Laboratory, Institute of Chemistry, University of São Paulo (USP), São Paulo, Brazil, [6]Pulmonary Hypertension Care Center, Department of Internal Medicine, Ribeirão Preto Medical School, University of São Paulo (USP), São Paulo, Brazil, [7]Department of Biostatistics, Plant Biology, Parasitology and Zoology, Institute of Biosciences, São Paulo State University (UNESP), Botucatu, Brazil, [8]Department of Chemical and Biological Sciences, Institute of Biosciences, São Paulo State University (UNESP), Botucatu, Brazil, [9]Pulmonary Hypertension Care Center, Department of Internal Medicine, Botucatu Medical School, São Paulo State University (UNESP), São Paulo, Brazil, [10]Laboratory of Pulmonary Investigation, Carlos Chagas Filho Biophysics Institute, Federal University of Rio de Janeiro, Centro de Ciências da Saúde, Rio de Janeiro, Brazil, [11]National Institute of Science and Technology for Regenerative Medicine, Rio de Janeiro, Brazil, [12]Department of Radiology and Oncology, Medical School of São Paulo State University (UNESP), São Paulo, Brazil

***Correspondence:**
Alexandre Todorovic Fabro
fabro@fmrp.usp.br

†These authors have contributed equally to this work and share first authorship
‡These authors have contributed equally to this work
$These authors share senior authorship

Idiopathic pulmonary artery hypertension (IPAH), chronic thromboembolic pulmonary hypertension (CTEPH), and acute pulmonary embolism (APTE) are life-threatening cardiopulmonary diseases without specific surgical or medical treatment. Although APTE, CTEPH and IPAH are different pulmonary vascular diseases in terms of clinical presentation, prevalence, pathophysiology and prognosis, the identification of their circulating microRNA (miRNAs) might help in recognizing differences in their outcome evolution and clinical forms. The aim of this study was to describe the APTE, CTEPH, and IPAH-associated miRNAs and to predict their target genes. The target genes of the key differentially expressed miRNAs were analyzed, and functional enrichment analyses were carried out. The miRNAs were detected using RT-PCR. Finally, we incorporated plasma circulating miRNAs in baseline and clinical characteristics of the patients to detect differences between APTE and CTEPH in time of evolution, and differences between CTEPH and IPAH in diseases form. We found five top circulating plasma miRNAs in common with APTE, CTEPH and IPAH assembled in one conglomerate. Among them, miR-let-7i-5p expression was upregulated in APTE and IPAH, while miRNA-320a was upregulated in CTEP and IPAH. The network construction for target genes showed 11 genes regulated by let-7i-5p and 20 genes regulated by miR-320a, all of them regulators of pulmonary arterial adventitial fibroblasts, pulmonary artery endothelial cell, and pulmonary artery smooth muscle cells. AR (androgen receptor), a target gene of hsa-let-7i-5p and has-miR-320a, was enriched in pathways in cancer, whereas PRKCA (Protein Kinase C Alpha), also a target gene of hsa-let-7i-5p and has-miR-320a, was enriched in KEGG pathways, such as pathways in cancer, glioma, and PI3K-Akt signaling pathway. We inferred that CTEPH might be the consequence of abnormal remodeling in APTE, while unbalance between the hyperproliferative and apoptosis-resistant phenotype of pulmonary arterial adventitial fibroblasts, pulmonary artery endothelial cell and pulmonary artery smooth muscle cells in pulmonary artery confer differences in IPAH and CTEPH diseases form. We concluded that the incorporation of plasma circulating let-7i-5p and miRNA-320a in baseline and clinical characteristics of the patients reinforces differences between APTE and CTEPH in outcome evolution, as well as differences between CTEPH and IPAH in diseases form.

Keywords: microRNA, RNA-sequencing, blood plasma, pulmonary hypertension, thromboemboilc disease

INTRODUCTION

Acute pulmonary thromboembolism (APTE), chronic thromboembolic pulmonary hypertension (CTEPH) and idiopathic pulmonary artery hypertension (IPAH) are pulmonary vascular diseases, that can reveal a pathophysiological continuum. On the other hand, they are rather different pulmonary vascular diseases in terms of clinical presentation, prevalence, pathophysiology, and prognosis. Acute pulmonary thromboembolism is characterized by acute obstruction of the pulmonary artery usually leading to pulmonary artery hypertension (PH), being the third most common cause of acute cardiovascular death (Douma et al., 2010; Goldhaber et al., 2012; Konstantinides et al., 2014). However, due to the non-specific clinical symptoms and signs, the diagnosis of APTE is often missed or delayed (Kostadima and Zakynthinos, 2007). CTEPH, a complication of APTE and the fourth types of PH, is characterized by the remodeling of the pulmonary arteries by fibro-organized tissue Connell et al., 2015 (Simonneau et al., 2018). The incidence of CTEPH in APTE survivors is about 3–9%, and 2 years survival in untreated patients with a mean pulmonary artery pressure greater than 50 mmHg was as low as 10% (Simonneau et al., 2018). However, the early recognition of CTEPH progression is difficult due to the gradual beginning and absence of effective biomarker (Guo et al., 2014; Miao et al., 2017). IPAH is a rare but life-threatening cardiopulmonary disease of unknown etiology, with progressive loss of quality of life, showing a 5 years overall survival rate of 50% (Berger et al., 2011; Simonneau et al., 2018; Koudstaal et al., 2020). IPAH characterizes by progressively increased pulmonary artery pressure and pulmonary vascular resistance, and up to now, there is no specific treatment (Santos-Ferreira et al., 2020; Zhang et al., 2020). Thus, comprehensive analyses of potential mechanisms with possible implications in time of evolution and disease form in APTE, CTEPH and IPAH are urgently needed. Interestingly, they share common pathophysiology changes, including fibrinolysis, pulmonary artery endothelial cell (PAEC) proliferation; pulmonary artery smooth muscle cell (PASMC) proliferation, migration, and contraction; inflammation; and pulmonary arterial adventitial fibroblasts (PAAF) proliferation, activation, and migration. Therefore, there should be some differences between these three pulmonary vascular diseases at molecular level, especially microRNAs (miRNAs).

MicroRNAs (miRNAs) are small, non-coding endogenous RNA molecules consisting of approximately 20 nucleotides that suppress gene expression post-transcriptionally by binding to the "seed sequences" in 39 untranslated regions (UTRs) mRNAs (Chen et al., 2008; Kosaka et al., 2010). Identified as stable cell-free miRNAs in serum or plasma, circulating miRNAs are discharged passively and selectively to blood by various cells, and may play as receiver or messenger in cell communication (Kosaka et al., 2010). Through illness, miRNAs in the sick cells are released into the circulation, and the circulating miRNA profile is adopted with the disease characteristics (Chen et al., 2008).

Therefore, circulating miRNAs have been widely explored as potential blood-based biomarkers for individual cardiovascular diseases diagnosis. Furthermore, it is also reasonable to assume that identification of molecular pathways and axon guidance enriched by differentially expressed miRNAs target genes and interactions between them provide a molecular basis for the unbalance between hyperproliferative and apoptosis-resistant phenotype particularly in the three principal pulmonary artery cell involved including PAEC, PASMC, and PAAF (Graham et al., 2010; Chen and Jiang, 2018; Yuan, 2019; Santos-Ferreira et al., 2020). Thus, we hypothesize that analyzing different circulating plasma miRNAs in APTE, CTEPH and IPAH, we can describe the early APTE evolution to CTEPH, as well as irreversible fibro-cellular narrowing of pulmonary arteries in diseases form, including CTEPH and IPAH.

This study aimed to describe the APTE, CTEPH, and IPAH-associated miRNAs. miRNAs differentially expressed in APTE, CTEPH, and IPAH samples, compared with healthy samples were identified, and the target genes were predicted. The target genes of the key differentially expressed miRNAs were analyzed, and functional enrichment analyses were carried out. The miRNAs were detected using RT-PCR. Finally, we incorporated plasma circulating miRNAs in baseline and clinical characteristics of the patients to detect differences between APTE and CTEPH in time of evolution, as well as differences between CTEPH and IPAH in diseases form.

METHODS

Diagnosis and Clinical Characterization of Patients and Healthy Subjects

The Research Ethics Committee of Botucatu Medical School, Botucatu, Brazil (CAAE: 27704714.4.0000.5411) approved this study, and all participants provided their written informed consent for study participation under the Declaration of Helsinki. This study is reported in accordance with the Strengthening the Reporting of Observational Studies in Epidemiology (STROBE) reporting guideline.

The New Generation Sequencing (NGS) cohort was composed of 19 APTE, 14 CTEPH, 14 IPAH patients and 13 healthy subjects (CTR). For RT-PCR confirmation, 5 APTE, 6 CTEPH, 6 IPAH patients and 4 healthy subjects were included. The patients were recruited over approximately 3 years (from 2015 to 2018) from the Pulmonary Hypertension Center and the Emergency Room of University Hospital of Botucatu Medical School (FMB-UNESP, Botucatu, Brazil). To participate of the study, healthy subjects should present normal tricuspid annular plane systolic pressure (TAPSE) by echocardiogram. In patients with APTE, the study was performed with less than 48 h in relation to the acute episode. Only CTEPH patients with distal thrombotic lesions participated in the study. Reported characteristics of patients were assessed at diagnosis moment. Hemodynamic and clinical classification of idiopathic pulmonary hypertension was done according to the 2018 World Symposium on Pulmonary Hypertension (Simonneau et al., 2019). Patients with CTEPH were inoperable and managed with targeted IPAH therapy according to the 2018 guideline (Simonneau et al., 2019).

Table 1 summarizes the baseline and clinical characteristics of our NGS cohort and healthy subjects.

Blood Plasma Collection and RNA Isolation

Blood samples (6 ml each) were collected into EDTA anticoagulant tubes and mixed by upside-down rotation ten times. After a two-step centrifugation process (1,100 g at 4°C for 10 min, followed by 1,300 g at 4°C for 20 min), the plasma was transferred into rnase/DNase-free tubes and stored at −80°C until further analysis. We obtained RNA plasma using the miRNeasy Serum/Plasma kit (QIAGEN, Hilden, Germany) according to the manufacturer's instructions. The RNA quantity and integrity were determined by Qubit® 3.0 Fluorometer (Invitrogen, Life Technologies, CA, United States) and the Agilent 2100 Bioanalyzer (Agilent Technologies, Santa Clara, CA, United States), respectively.

Library Preparation and High-Throughput Sequencing

Small RNA library was built with TruSeq Small RNA Library Prep kit (Illumina Inc, San Diego, CA, United States) following the manufacturer's recommendations. We transcribed the RNA to cDNA and amplified it using a common primer and a primer containing the barcode index sequences. This cDNA was separated by PAGE 6%. Libraries was recovered via purification and quality checked on Bioanalyzer 2100 (Agilent Technologies). Library concentration was confirmed (>2 nmol/L) by qPCR using the KAPA Library Quantification kit (KAPA Biosystems). Indexed small RNA libraries were multiplexed in equimolar amounts, denatured, and loaded on flow-cell lanes for sequencing. All samples were sequenced at the Institute of Biotechnology (IBTEC-UNESP, Botucatu, Brazil) using the Illumina NextSeq 500 according to the manufacturer's instructions consisting of 36bp single-end reads in 50 cycles.

Bioinformatic Analysis

Screening of Differentially Expressed miRNAs

Small RNA sequencing raw data was translated into a raw FASTQ sequence one. Then, we filtered the FASTQ format reads to remove rows with low quality via adaptor sequences and sequences inclusion with a quality score <20, using Fastx-Toolkit (http://hannonlab.cshl.edu/fastxtoolkit/). We aligned the filtered reads against the reference human genome, version hg19, using Bowtie v2.0.6. Then, the reads from each individual were merged to identify mature miRNAs using miRDeep2.0.0.8. In detail, the reads were mapped and quantified using the miRDeep2 mapper. pl module and quantifier. pl module, respectively, with standard parameters. Mature miRNAs were downloaded from mirbase v21 (http://www.mirbase.org). The differentially expressed miRNAs (DEmiRNAs) between the samples were normalized and identified by the Bioconductor/R DESeq2 package using ten counts per miRNA as a detection threshold. The criteria for microRNA expression level measuring was CPM (counts per million) value, and we adjusted p values to control the false discovery rate (FDR). We identified significant DEmiRNAs using log2 (fold change) >1 and adjusted FDR.

TABLE1 | Baseline and clinical characteristics of the NGS cohort and healthy subjects.

Characteristic	CTR *N* = 13	APTE *N* = 19	CTEPH *N* = 14	IPAH *N* = 14	*P*-value[a]
Age (yr. Median and interval quartile)	42 (32–52)	55 (39–71)	53 (42–68)	45 (25–65)	0.85
Gender (female/%)	11/84%	17/89%	10/71%	11/78%	0.07
Race category					0.90
White	11/84%	13/68%	7/50%	10/71%	
Black	2/16%	6/32$^{\&}$	7/50%	4/29%	
Smoking	0	3/16%	4/28%	1/7%	0.20
DVT (positive/total)	0	1/5%	3/21%	2/14%	0.13
mPAP (mmHg), mean ± SD	–	–	25.2 ± 13.4	43.3 ± 12.3$^{\&}$	**0.02**
sPAP (mmHg), mean ± SD	–	–	75.4 ± 9.4	89.2 ± 8.6$^{\#}$	**0.01**
PVR (dyn s cm^{-5})	–	–	336 ± 2.48	586 ± 5.38$^{\&\&}$	**0.009**
Oxygen saturation, mean ± SD	–	95.42 ± 2.4	90.92 ± 8.07	89.42 ± 6.22$^{\#\#}$	**0.001**
Respiratory rate, mean ± SD	–	20.89 ± 5.34	18.64 ± 3.02	19.14 ± 3.48	0.05
Heart rate, mean ± SD	–	92.05 ± 18.38†	81.71 ± 15.19	78.78 ± 11.53	**0.001**
CI (L min^{-1} m^{-2})					0.05
>4	–	–	12/85%	5/36%	
WHO functional class					**0.002**
>2	–	–	9/14†	5/14	
TAPSE (mm)	16.9 ± 0.4	17.6 ± 0.6	15.1 ± 1.3	14.2 ± 1.5$^{\#\#\#}$	**0.001**
NTproBNP (pg/ml)*1	–	74.6 ± 4.2	182 ± 7.7$^{\&\&\&}$	47 ± 5.3$^{\#\#\#\#}$	**0.001**
CRP (mg/L)*l	–	17.33 ± 2.35††	6.14 ± 1.34	4.2 ± 1.2	**0.009**
D-dimer (μg/L)	–	8,161.86 ± 1729.89†††	217.78 ± 92.12	–	**0.001**

Abbreviations: CTR, controls; APTE, acute pulmonary thromboembolism; CTEPH, chronic pulmonary thromboembolism with pulmonary hypertension; PAH, idiopathic pulmonary arterial hypertension; DVT, deep venous thrombosis; mPAP, mean pulmonary arterial pression; sPAP, systolic pulmonary arterial pressure; PVR, pulmonary vascular resistance; CI, cardiac index; TAPSE, tricuspid annular plane systolic excursion; NTproBNP, N-terminal pro-brain natriuretic peptide; CRP, C-reactive protein.

[a]The Mann–Whitney U test, two-sample Kolmogorov–Smirnov test were used to examine differences between two groups.

Chi-square test were used to examine differences between categorical variables. Multiple comparison was done by non-parametric Kruskall–Wallis test. & = mPAP different between CPTEH and PAH; # = sPAP different between PAH and CPTEH; && = PRV different between CPTEH and PAH; ## = oxygen saturation different between CTR and PAH; † = Heart rate different from CTR; † = WHO Functional Class different between CPTEH and PAH; ### TAPSE different from PAH to CPTEH and APTE; &&& = NTproBNP different from CTR, CPTEH and PAH; †† = CRP different from CTR, CPTEH and PAH; ††† = D-dimer different between APTE and CPTEH.

Bolded values are statically significant.

Functional Enrichment Analysis for Differentially Expressed miRNAs

Gene Ontology (GO) and Kyoto Encyclopedia of Genes and Genomes (KEGG) were used to assess the functional annotation of the DEmiRNAs and their enrichment in different biological pathways, respectively. Functional annotation and miRNAs pathways were performed using the DIANA-miRPath v3.0 database according to the published instructions (Vlachos et al., 2015). The Gene Ontology (GO) and Kyoto Encyclopedia of Genes and Genomes (KEGG) were used to assess the functional annotation of the DEmiRNAs and their enrichment in different biological pathways, respectively. The functional annotation and miRNAs pathways were performed using the DIANA-miRPath v3.0 database according to the published instructions (Vlachos et al., 2015).

Construction of the Differentially Expressed miRNAs-Gene Regulatory Network

In order to predict the DEmiRNA target genes (Hamberg et al., 2016), we used the miRTargetLink (www.ccb.uni-saarland.de/mirtargetlink) to predict the DEmiRNA target genes (Hamberg et al., 2016). Then, we calculated and visualized the mirtarbase and miRanda interaction network information (Enright et al., 2003; Chou et al., 2016). Thus, we only considered the validated targets with strong evidence. The Venn diagram indicating the intersected targets genes was generated by a Draw Venn Diagram online tool (http://bioinformatics.psb.ugent.be/webtools/Venn/).

Quantitative Reverse-Transcription PCR Confirmation

For quantitative real-time reverse transcription PCR (qRT-PCR) confirmation, we selected the miRNAs with the highest significant differences in expression revealed by next-generation sequencing experiment. Then, we performed the quantification of miRNA expression using miScript miRNA PCR primer assays and miScript SdYBRGreen PCR kit (Qiagen, Valencia, CA, United States) on a StepOnePlus™ Real-Time PCR System (Applied Biosystems, Foster, United States) following the manufacturer's instructions. Finally, we calculated each miRNA levels using the comparative cycle threshold method (ddCT method) relative to the mean of *miR-16* and *miR-483*. All samples were performed in triplicate.

Statistical Analysis

The chi-square or Fisher's exact test were performed to assess differences in clinical variables. In addition, General Linear Model was applied to evaluate the associations between miRNAs and clinically related parameters. The statistical software program IBM SPSS (version 22; Armonk, NY, United States of America) performed all analyses. p value < 0.05 was considered as statistically significant.

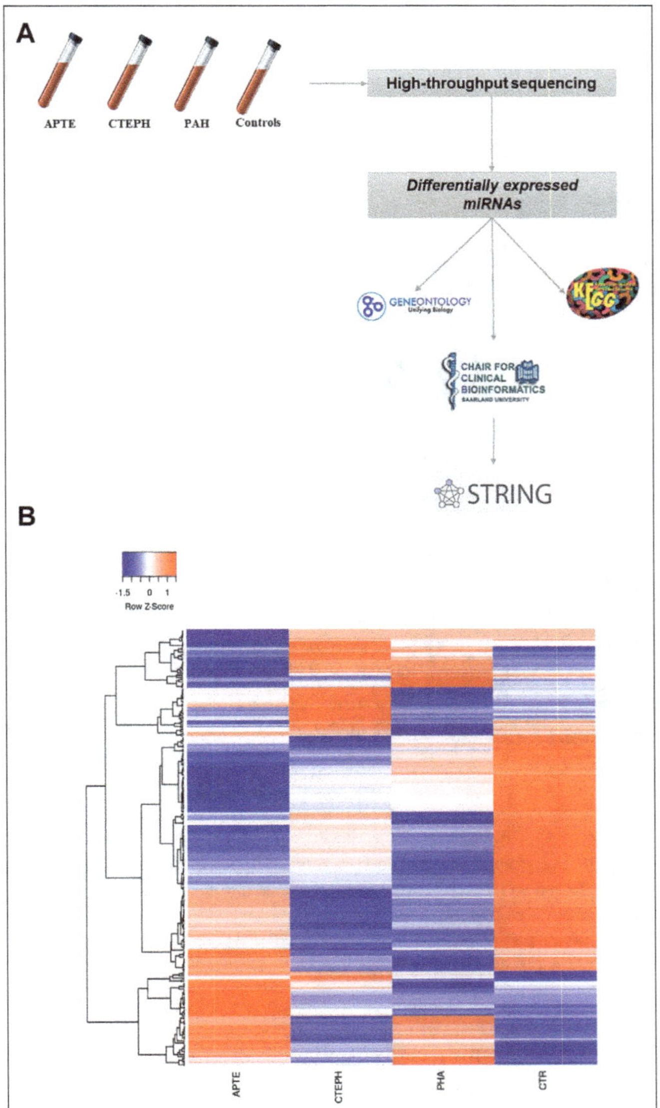

FIGURE 1 | (A) Flowchart showing the strategy for detection of differentially expressed miRNAs through next-generation technology. **(B)** Hierarchical clustering of the four experimental groups based on their miRNA expression patterns (*p* adj <0.05, |log 2 (foldchange)| > 1) filtering of next-generation sequencing results. 299 miRNAs were subjected to hierarchical clustering by average linkage method calculating with Pearson distance. Green and red colors represent increased and decreased expression levels (transformed into *z*-scores), respectively, when compared with the average level of each miRNA. Columns and lines represent samples and miRNA, respectively. APTE, acute pulmonary thromboembolism; CTEPH, thromboembolic pulmonary hypertension; PAH, idiopathic pulmonary hypertension; and CTR, Controls.

RESULTS

Screening of Differentially Expressed miRNA

Overall, 299 known mature miRNAs were identified in our NGS cohort according to the QC inclusion criteria (**Supplementary Table S2; Figures 1A,B**). Among these, a total of 21 differentially expressed miRNAs were obtained according to the cut-off criteria (*p* adj <0.05, |log 2 (foldchange)| >1) (**Supplementary Table S2**). The heat map of these differentially expressed miRNAs is shown in **Figure 2**.

Target Gene of Differentially Expressed miRNA Prediction Analysis

The top five results for the number of target genes regulated by differentially expressed miRNAs are shown in **Figure 3**. Of the 21 miRNAs, let-7i-5p, miR-320a miR-320b-1, miR-320b-2, and miR-1291 regulated the most target genes. The heatmap represents all of them (**Figure 3**). The five miRNAs-let-7i-5p, miR-320a, miR-320b-1, miR-320b-2, and miR-1291 were up-regulated in APTE and, with exception of miR-320b-1, down-regulated in CTEPH (**Table 2** and **Figure 3**). In IPAH, we found miRNA-320a and miR-1291 down-regulated and up-regulation of let-7i-5p and miR-320b-1 (**Table 2** and **Figure 3**).

Functional Enrichment Analysis for Differentially Expressed miRNAs

As shown in **Supplementary Tables S1–S3** and **Figure 4**, the upregulated miRNAs in APTE (let-7i-5p, miR-320a, miR-320b-1, miR-320b-2, and miR-1291) and CTEPH (miR-320b-1) were significantly enriched in pathways of cancer, glioma, and PI3K-Akt signaling pathway, whereas the downregulated miRNAs in CTEPH (let-7i-5p, miR-320a, miR-320b-2, and miR-1291) and IPAH (miR-320a and miR-1291) were mainly enriched in pathways of cancer and apelin signaling pathway. Among them, let-7i-5p and miR-320a were significantly enriched in pathways of cancer and axon guidance.

The Network Construction for Target Genes Regulated by Differentially Expressed miRNAs

We constructed the miRNA-Target network for the differentially expressed miRNAs. MiRTargetLink found 126 genes targeted by two or more of the selected microRNAs (**Figure 5A**). We performed the Venn diagram to indicate the possibly targeted intersected genes upregulated in APTE, down-regulated in CTEPH and IPAH (**Figure 5B**). Finally, we evaluated the potential targets for each miRNA. The *let-7i-5p* presented 11 possible targets: *IL13, EIF2C1, TLR4, COPS8, NEUROG1, BMP4, ASCL1, COPS6, IGF1, GPS1,* and *SOCS1* (**Figure 5C**). The *miR-320a* showed 20 targets: *MAPK1, TAC1, RAC1, GNAI1, HSPB6, BMI1, AQP4, NPR1, ITGB3, ARF1, AQP1, NRP1, MCL1, TRPC5, IGF1R, POLR3D, NFATC3, TFRC, PTEN,* and *BANP* (**Figure 5D**). There were no strongly evident targets for *miR-320b-1/b-2* (**Figure 5E**). Lastly, *miR-1291* possibly targeted the *SLC2A1, ERN1,* and *ABCC1* genes (**Figure 5F**).

Functional Enrichment Analysis of the Target Genes of the Key miRNAs

The target genes regulated by upregulated differentially expressed miRNAs in APTE (let-7i-5p, miR-320a, miR-320b-1, miR-320b-

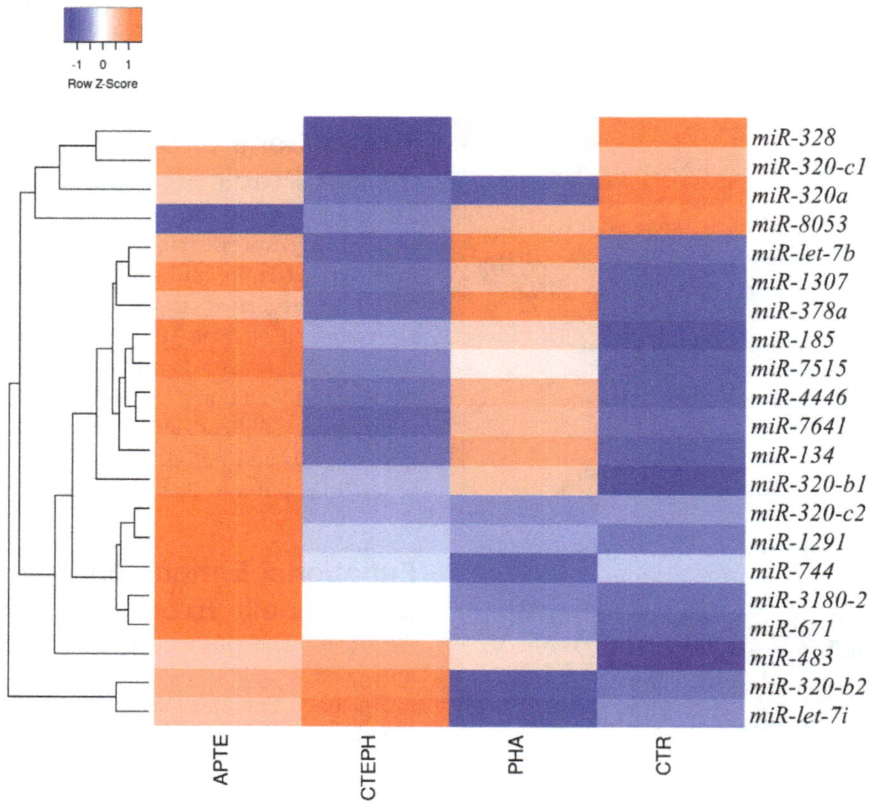

FIGURE 2 | Circulating miRNAs signature in APTE, CTEPH, PAH patients, and healthy controls. Hierarchical clustering and heatmap diagram of the optimum circulating miRNAs from APTE (n = 7), CTEPH (n = 8), PAH (n = 5), and healthy controls (n = 2). Green and red colors represent increased and decreased expression levels (transformed into z-scores), respectively, when compared with the average level of each miRNA. Columns and lines represent samples and miRNA, respectively. APTE, Acute Pulmonary Thromboembolism; CTEPH, Chronic Thromboembolic Pulmonary Hypertension; PAH, Pulmonary artery Hypertension; and CTR, Controls.

2, and miR-1291) and CTEPH (miR-320b-1) were mainly enriched in 11 GO terms (**Supplementary Table 1S**) and 5 KEGG pathways (**Supplementary Table 3S**), and the target genes regulated by downregulated differentially expressed miRNAs in CTEPH (let-7i-5p, miR-320a, miR-320b-2, and miR-1291) and IPAH (miR-320a and miR-1291) were mainly enriched in 40 GO terms and calcium signaling pathway. Androgen receptor (AR), a target gene of hsa-let-7i-5p and has-miR-320a, was enriched in pathways in cancer. Protein kinase C Alpha (PRKCA), also a target gene of hsa-let-7i-5p and has-miR-320a, was enriched in 14 of 18 KEGG pathways, such as pathways in cancer, glioma, and PI3K-Akt signaling pathway.

Detection of miRNAs Using RT-PCR

The expression of let-7i-5p and miRNA-320a in APTE samples was significantly higher than that of the control samples (p = 0.01 and p = 0.02, respectively; **Figures 6A,B**). In contrast, the expression of let-7i-5p and miRNA-320a was significantly lower in CTEPH compared to the control samples (p = 0.02 and p = 0.01, respectively; **Figures 6C,D**). IPAH samples presented significant higher expression of let-7i-5p than control samples ($p < 0.01$; **Figure 6E**) and significant lower expression of miRNA-320a compared to the control samples (p = 0.02; **Figure 6F**).

Baseline and Clinical Characteristics of Patients and Healthy Subjects

Table 1 summarizes the baseline and clinical characteristics of patients and healthy subjects. Patients and healthy subjects presented a similar distribution of age, gender, race, and tobacco history. Deep venous thrombosis was detected in six out of 47 (13%) patients. In patients who underwent right cardiac catheterization, the level of mean pulmonary artery pressure (mPAP) in IPAH was significantly higher than CTEPH. Equally significant was the increased systolic pulmonary artery pressure (sPAP) in IPAH compared to CTEPH. Furthermore, pulmonary vascular resistance (PVR) was significantly increased in IPAH compared to patients with CTEPH. Oxygen saturation and heart rate were lower in IPAH patients than CTEPH groups. The WHO functional class major than two was significantly associated with CTEPH patients. Tricuspid annular plane systolic excursion (TAPSE) done by echocardiography, was reduced in patients with IPAH when compared to APTE. Brain natriuretic peptide (BNP) or its stable inactive pro-

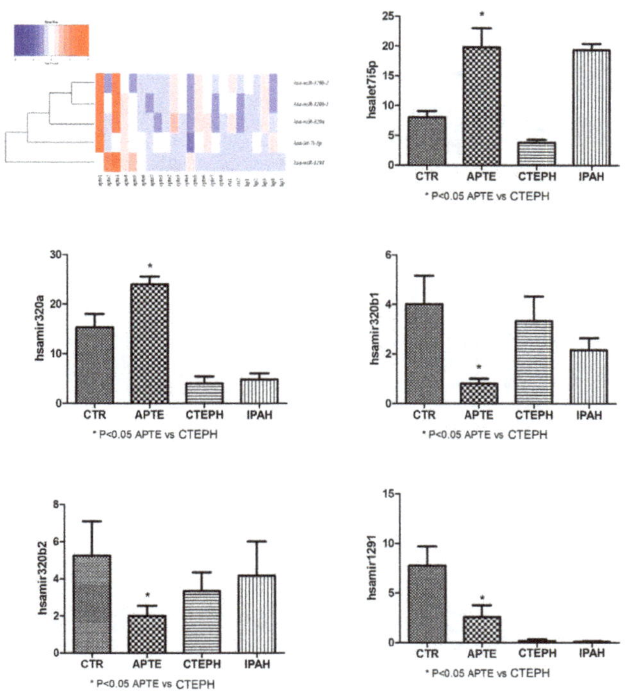

FIGURE 3 | Heatmap and box plots graphs representing the five miRNAs—*let-7i-5p*, *miR-320a*, *miR-320b-1*, *miR-320b-2*, and *miR-1291* significantly associated with the APTE group compared to the CTEPH group after testing adjustment by FDR (Benjamini–Hochberg). Red and blue colors represent increased and decreased expression levels (transformed into *z*-scores), respectively, when compared with the average level of each miRNA. APTE, acute pulmonary thromboembolism; CTEPH, thromboembolic pulmonary hypertension; PAH, idiopathic pulmonary hypertension; and CTR, Controls.

hormone (NT-proBNP) was higher in CTEPH than IPAH patients. Patients with APTE presented a significantly increased level of CRP and D-dimer compared to CTEPH and PAH.

Association Between Circulating Plasma miRNA Expression, Clinical and Baseline Characteristics of the Patients

Differentially expressed miRNAs were associated with baseline and clinical characteristics of the patients, as shown in **Table 3**. Expression of let-7i-5p > 2.30 and miRNA-320a >2.58 was associated with APTE, high level of C-reactive protein and D-dymer. In contrast, miRNA-320a expression ≤2.58 was associated with CTEPH (p = 0.04) and IPAH (p = 0.03).

DISCUSSION

Rationale of the Study

We described five highly expressed circulating plasma miRNAs present in APTE, CTEPH and IPAH assembled in one conglomerate. APTE, CTEPH and IPAH are rather different pulmonary vascular diseases in terms of clinical presentation, prevalence, pathophysiology, and prognosis, making it difficult to extrapolate the results among them. However, incorporating miRNA panel into baseline and clinical characteristics of the patients, we provide additional information about outcome evolution (APTE and CTEPH) and the disease form (CTEPH and IPAH), which may have implications in life-threatening cardiopulmonary disease, and specific surgical or medical treatment. To our knowledge it is an innovative study suggesting a differential spectrum of evolution and form of the disease among APTE, CTEPH and IPAH.

Among the miRNA 5-signature, let-7i-5p and miR-320a were the most expressed and functionally enriched by cancer, glioma, and PI3K-Akt signaling pathways. The network construction for target genes showed 11 genes regulated by let-7i-5p and 20 genes regulated by miR-320a. These genes regulated by let-7i-5p and miR-320a are modulators of PAAF, PAEC, and PASMC, respectively involved in proliferation, vasoconstriction, inflammation, and DNA damage. These target genes regulated by differentially expressed miRNAs were mainly enriched in GO terms and KEGG pathways. AR (androgen receptor), a target gene of hsa-let-7i-5p and has-miR-320a, was enriched in pathways in cancer, whereas PRKCA (Protein kinase C Alpha), also a target gene of hsa-let-7i-5p and has-miR-320a, was enriched in KEGG pathways, such as pathways in cancer, glioma, and PI3K-Akt signaling pathway.

Taken together, the interaction between genes and their miRNA may play important roles in the time of evolution and disease form in pulmonary hypertensive and thromboembolic diseases, as discussed below.

Outcome Evolution in Pulmonary Thromboembolism (APTE and CTEPH)

Our results demonstrated that miR-let-7i-5p expression was upregulated in APTE and downregulated in CTEPH. Furthermore, these upregulated miRNAs in APTE were significantly enriched in cancer, glioma, and PI3K-Akt signaling pathways, whereas the downregulated miRNAs observed in CTEPH were mainly enriched in cancer and apelin signaling pathways.

Yang's group showed that 24 miRNAs were upregulated, and 22 miRNAs were downregulated (including miR-let-7i-5p) in CTEPH compared with APTE (Miao et al., 2017). Likewise, Guo

TABLE 2 | miRNAs with ID starting with "ENSG" are known miRNAs.

Id	logFC	PValue	FDR
ENSG00000199179	3.16	0.00023	0.02525
2_dna:REF_16,302	4.53	0.00024	0.2525
ENSG00000211543	4.26	0.00025	0.2525
ENSG00000208037	4.50	0.00028	0.2525
ENSG00000281842	5.21	0.00071	0.04868
ENSG00000221406	4.29	0.00082	0.04868

The only one with a different ID "2_dna: REF_16,302" is a likely new miRNA. LogFC represents how many times the miRNA is expressed in the APTE group in relation to CTEPH. FDR is a statistical method for correcting the p-value for multiple tests.

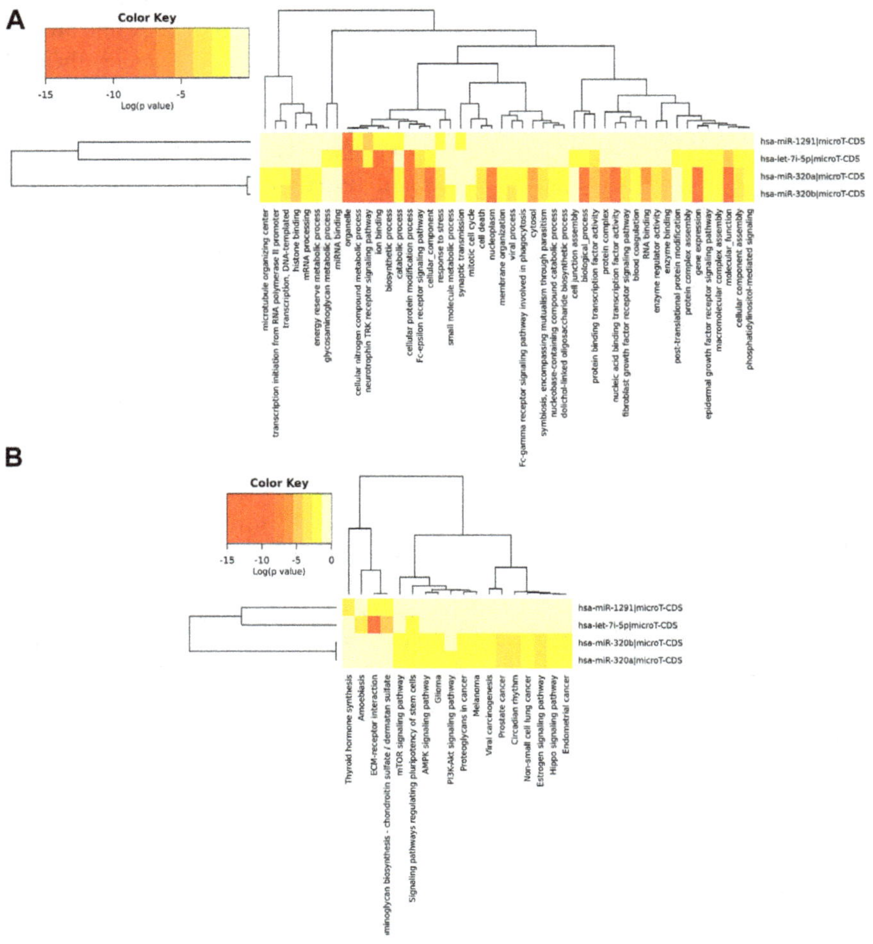

FIGURE 4 | Hierarchical clustering based on predicted target genes of upregulated miRNAs in APTE samples. **(A)** Ontology-based hierarchical clustering of genes identified as predicted targets of upregulated miRNAs in APTE. Using mirPath from DIANA tools, the upregulated miRNAs APTE samples were used to prepare a heatmap based on the gene ontology of predicted target genes. **(B)** Pathways based hierarchical clustering of predicted target genes as part of upregulated miRNAs in APTE samples. Kyoto Encyclopedia of Genes and Genomes (KEGG) based mapping of putative target genes in various pathways as part of the upregulated miRNAs and their canonical target genes.

et al. also found that miR-let-7i-5p was downregulated in CTEPH patients when compared to healthy controls, as well as miR-140-3p, miR-93, miR-22, miR-106b; and that miR-1260, miR-602, miR-129-5p, miR-1908 and miR-483-5p were upregulated (Guo et al., 2014). As a tumor suppressor or tumor promoter, miR-let-7b has been found to halt cell proliferation, adhesion, and invasion by targeting Protein Code Gene (*PKA1*), Diaphanous Related Formin 2 (*DIAPH2*), Radixin (*RDX*), *RAS, MYC,* and High Mobility Group A2 (*HMGA2*) genes and their respective proteins. *Let-7b* expression is also differently regulated in breast cancer and the data reveal its possible role in DNA repair capacity during breast carcinogenesis (Hu et al., 2013). Similarly, miR-let-7b was shown to be significantly downregulated in osteosarcoma tissues and cell lines and the functional studies revealed that the antitumor effect of miR-let-7b was probably due to targeting and suppressing Insulin Like Growth Factor 1 Receptor (*IGF1R*) expression (Zhang et al., 2019). Wang et al. demonstrated that miR-let-7b binds the 3′-UTR of Angiopoietin (*ANGPT2*) to induce migration and tube formation of Human Umbelical Vein Endothelial Cells (HUVECs), and Human Cardiac Progenitor Cells (*hCPFs*)-exosome transport to endothelial cells expressing relatively low amounts of miR-let-7b, promoting angiogenesis through upregulation of Angiopoietin 2 (*ANGPT2*) (Wang et al., 2015).

MiR-let-7i-5p has been reported as pivotal in regulating cell proliferation and migration. In fact, investigations have demonstrated that PASMCs excessively proliferate and migrate to the intima layer of pulmonary artery after APTE, remodeling the pulmonary vasculature and increasing pulmonary vascular resistance (Douma et al., 2010; Goldhaber et al., 2012; Konstantinides et al., 2014). Thus, we hypothesize that upregulation of miR-let-7i-5p may be intimately associated with excessive proliferation and migration of PASMCs following APTE which may evolve to CTEPH. Ham et al. showed that the levels of miR-let-7i-5p were upregulated in APTE compared with CTEPH, thus suppressing apoptosis via caspase in HUVECs (Ham et al., 2015).

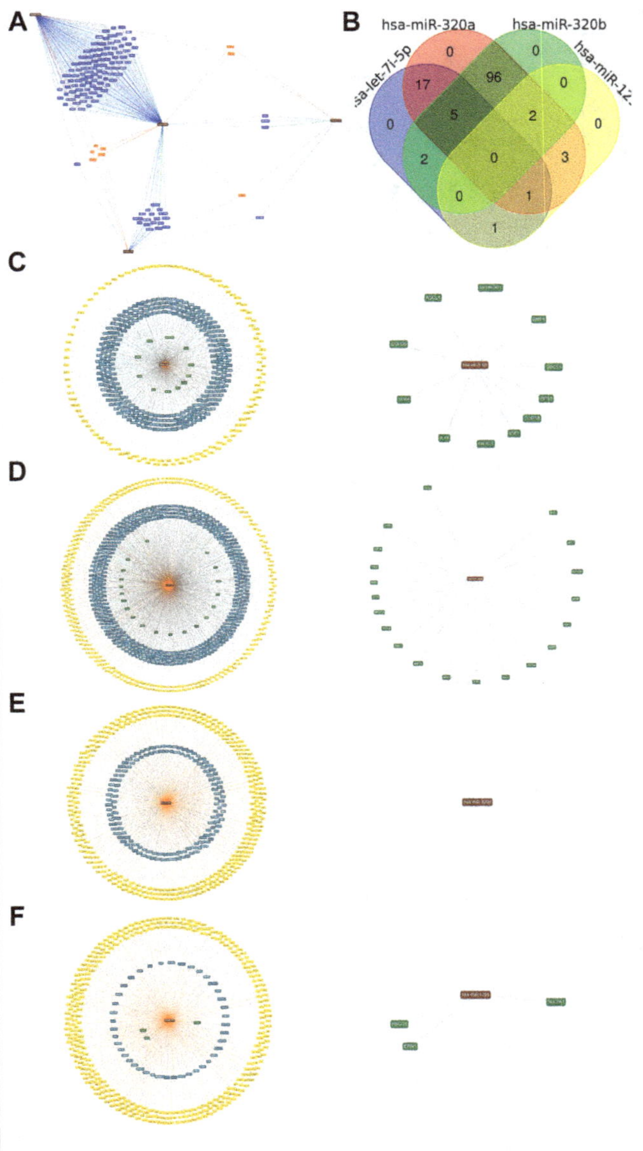

FIGURE 5 | The target and predicted genes of the upregulated miRNAs in APTE samples **(A)** The bioinformatics tool miRTargetLink Human executed the network. **(B)** The Draw Venn Diagram online tool generated the Venn diagram. **(C)** The central node represents the *hsa-let-7i-5p*. **(D)** the *hsa-mir-320a*. **(E)** the *hsa-mir-320b*; and **(F)** the *hsa-mir-1291* surrounded by the validated target with predicted targets in yellow, weak (blue), and strong (green) evidence, which was highlighted in circles.

In this way, we have also shown that 11 genes were a direct target of miR-let-7i-5p, which upregulation modulates the proliferation of human PASMCs. Among them, Interleukin13 (*IL13*) upregulation induces PASMCs in the pulmonary artery through signal transducer and activator of transcription STAT6 or through phosphatidylinositol 3-kinase (PI3K), STAT3 and mitogen activated protein kinase (MAPK) pathways (Yuan, 2019). Oxidant, arginase 2 (*ARG2*) and hypoxia-inducible factor 1α (*HIF1*) are also involved in the proliferation of PASMCs (Yuan, 2019). The experimental Schistosomiasis-associated PAH potentially depends on upregulation of *IL-13*, which can activate TGF-β1 via phospho-STAT6 signaling, or via increased matrix metalloproteinase-inducing muscular hypertrophy and periadventitial fibrosis in pulmonary arteries (Graham et al., 2010). The human eukaryotic initiation factor *EIF2C1* gene downregulates protein synthesis in response to amino acid starvation, hypoxia, and viral infection but up-regulated specific stress response proteins. *EIF2C1* expression is increased in smooth muscle cells in the vessel wall and interstitial tissue (Chen and Jiang, 2018). Toll-Like Receptor four Signaling (*TLR4*) has a prominent functional impact on platelet activity, hemostasis, and thrombosis (Vallance et al., 2017). Bone morphogenetic protein-4 (*BMP4*) acts downstream of *HIF-1* and mediates hypoxia-induced up-regulation of transient receptor potential canonical (*TRPC*), leading to increased basal [Ca2+]i in pulmonary arterial smooth muscle cells (PASMCs), promoting chronic hypoxia-induced pulmonary hypertension pathogenesis (Wang et al., 2015).

The up-regulation in miR-let-7i-5p observed only in APTE and the downregulation of miR-let-7i-5p observed only in CTEPH reinforces the abnormal remodeling between APTE and CTEPH. These differences may be associated with time of evolution, since differences were observed in cardiac index, C-reactive protein and D-dimer.

Disease Form in Pulmonary Artery Hypertension (CTEPH and IPAH)

IPAH is an isolated small-vessel disease comprising vasoconstriction, remodeling, and thrombosis of distal vessels. On the other hand, CTEPH is characterized by large-vessel occlusion with a concomitant small-vessel disease following thromboembolism event. The pulmonary microvascular disease as a common denominator of IPAH and CTEPH probably plays a major role in pathophysiology (Berger et al., 2011; Koudstaal et al., 2020).

In the current study, we carried out NGS analysis and detection of miRNAs to understand the key miRNAs associated with disease form in CTEPH and IPAH. We found that let-7i-5p and miR-320a were down-regulated in CTEPH, while let-7i-5p was up-regulated in IPAH. Furthermore, 20 target genes were coregulated by miR-320a and other miRNAs. Androgen receptor (*AR*), a target gene of hsa-miR-320a, was enriched in cancer pathways. Protein kinase C Alpha (*PRKCA*), also a target gene of hsa-let-7i-5p and has-miR-320a, was enriched in 14 of 18 KEGG pathways, such as in cancer, glioma, and PI3K-Akt signaling pathway.

Recent studies have shown that miRNA dysregulation plays an important role in the hyperproliferative and apoptosis-resistant phenotype of pulmonary vascular cells in PH, including PAAF, PAEC, and PASMC respectively involved in proliferation, vasoconstriction, inflammation, and DNA damage (Santos-Ferreira et al., 2020). Previous studies have also uncovered that dysregulation of miRNAs such as miR-204 and miR-21 was associated with the pathobiology of IPAH (Courboulin et al., 2011; Rhodes et al., 2013; Bienertova-Vasku et al., 2015), suggesting that miRNAs may configure novel therapeutic targets.

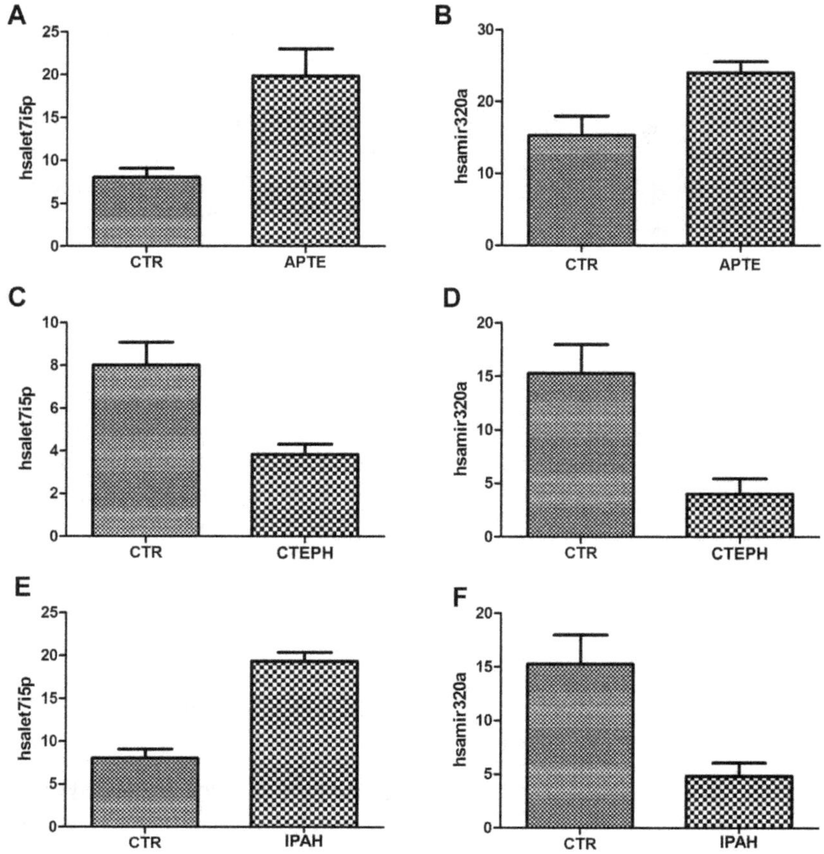

FIGURE 6 | (A)–(F) Plot graphs of the expression of miRNAs in APTE, CTEPH and IPAH samples compared with that in control samples by qRT-PCR. $^*p < 0.05$ (Independent-Samples Mann–Whitney test). APTE group $n = 5$; CTEPH ($N = 6$), IPAH ($N = 6$) and CTR ($N = 4$). APTE, acute pulmonary thromboembolism; CTEPH, chronic thromboembolism pulmonary hypertension; iPAH, idiopathic pulmonary hypertension; CTR, healthy subjects; qRT-PCR, Quantitative Reverse-Transcription.

In this line, the downregulation of miR-let-7i-5p has also been observed elsewhere (Wang et al., 2013). While miR-let-7i-5p was downregulated in CTEPH, it was upregulated in IPAH and this inverse association may be crucial to differentiate both disease forms. As a tumor promoter, miR-let-7b has been found to enhance cell proliferation, adhesion, and invasion by targeting the genes of *PKA1*, *DIAPH2*, *RDX*, *RAS*, *MYC*, and *HMGA2* and respective proteins, creating an unbalance between hyperproliferative and apoptosis-resistant phenotype of PAAF, PAEC and PASMC in IPAH.

Moreover, in the present study, we demonstrated that 20 genes were a direct target of miR-320a. It has been reported these miRNA regulates cell proliferation, differentiation, and invasion in human colon cancer (Sun et al., 2012), and erythroid differentiation (Mittal et al., 2013) as well as bladder carcinoma (Shang et al., 2014) and when upregulated, miRNA-320a act toward proliferation of human PASMCs. Among the 20 target genes, a family of water-selective membrane channels promoting endothelial cell migration and angiogenesis (aquaporin—*AQP*) was found to be overexpressed in PAH patients, indicating its potential role in the treatment of PH (Saadoun et al., 2005; Schuoler et al., 2017; Gräf et al., 2018).

Considering the above evidence, we inferred that unbalance between the hyperproliferative and apoptosis-resistant phenotype of PAAF, PAEC and PASMC in pulmonary artery confer differences in IPAH and CTEPH about the diseases form. The incorporation of miRNA-320a and the unbalance of miR-let-7i-5p in baseline added by clinical characteristics signatures reinforce differences between CTEPH and IPAH.

CONCLUSION

We concluded that circulating plasma miRNA and clinical/hemodynamic characteristics provide additional predictive information about the evolution outcome and the form of pulmonary thromboembolic and hypertensive diseases.

TABLE 3 | Association between baseline and clinical characteristics of the patients and miRNA microarray signature.

	Dependent variables									
Clinical features	***let-7i-5p* Mean ΔCt ±SE 2.30 ± 0.74**		***miR-320a* Mean ΔCt ±SE 2.58 ± 1.41**		***miR-320b-1* mean ΔCt ±SE 2.07 ± 1.61**		***miR-320b-2* mean ΔCt ±SE 2.34 ± 1.44**		***miR-1291* mean ΔCt ±SE 2.43 ± 1.62**	
	β	*p*	*B*	*p*	*β*	*p*	*β*	*p*	*B*	*p*
Age yr (median, 51)	−0.35	**0.0001**	0.48	**0.0001**	−0.41	**0.0001**	−0.44	**0.0001**	0.11	0.11
Gender		4.49								
Female (49/60)	−6.93	**0.0001**	−8.65	**0.0001**	−7.89	**0.0001**	−4.93	**0.0001**	4.30	**0.02**
Etiology[a]										
APTE	3.16	**0.00023**	4.50	**0.00028**	4.26	**0.00025**	4.29	**0.00082**	5.21	**0.00071**
CPTEH	1.86	0.60	−2.09	**0.04**	0.81	0.74	1.16	0.57	2.78	0.47
IPAH	3.85	0.39	−3.76	**0.03**	4.01	0.33	4.21	0.33	5.40	0.05
mPAH (mmHg) (mean, 45.9)	2.96	0.19	0.19	**0.0001**	3.12	0.49	3.99	0.41	4.97	0.40
sPAH (mmHg) (mean, 75.9)	−0.03	0.07	0.17	**0.0001**	2.91	0.12	3.21	0.21	4.49	0.06
PVR (dyn s cm^{-5}) (mean, 349.94)	−0.001	0.16	−0.001	0.06	−0.002	0.15	0.002	0.15	−0.000026	1.00
TAPSE (mmHg) (mean, 14.50)	−0.07	0.09	−0.35	**0.0001**	−0.004	1.00	2.12	**0.0001**	3.39	**0.26**
CI (L min^{-1} m^{-2})										
1–2	−1.90	**0.009**	8.35	**0.0001**	2.13	0.67	1.98	0.83	−0.24	1.00
3–4	−0.64	**0.009**	10.17	**0.0001**	8.88	**0.0001**	6.58	**0.0001**	−0.006	1.00
WHO functional class[a]										
I vs. II	4.30	0.35	4.73	0.29	5.14	0.28	5.32	0.28	8.21	0.05
III vs. IV	3.48	0.22	3.09	0.24	3.03	1.98	2.22	0.20	4.12	0.07
CRP (mg/L) (mean, 7.63)	5.21	**0.0001**	−0.20	**0.0001**	−0.18	**0.0001**	−0.18	**0.0001**	0.07	**0.04**
D-dymer (μg/L)	4.39	**0.0001**	−0.19	**0.0001**	−0.16	**0.0001**	−0.17	**0.0001**	0.09	**0.03**

Abbreviations: APTE, acute pulmonary thromboembolism; CPTEH, chronic pulmonary thromboembolism with pulmonary hypertension; IPAH, idiopathic pulmonary hypertension; mean pulmonary arterial pression sPAH, systolic pulmonary arterial pressure; PVR, pulmonary vascular resistance; TAPSE, tricuspid annular plane systolic pressure; CI, cardiac index; CRP, C-reactive protein. General Linear Model was carried out to analyze the effect of several dependent variables on clinical features of the subjects. β = β coefficient. P = P value.
[a]FDR statistical test (statistical method for correcting the p value for multiple tests) was carried out to compare independent variables between two groups.
Bolded values are statically significant.

AUTHOR CONTRIBUTIONS

ATF, JMR and SSB have contributed equally to this work and share first authorship. CMB, TGP, CF, FRRM, HRC, MAA, JSM, AIP, SSM, RAO, MKS, JABM have contributed equally to this work. JCS, CAR, HHBY, PLS, MAN, VLC share senior authorship.

ACKNOWLEDGMENTS

This work was supported by São Paulo Research Foundation (FAPESP) [2018/20403-6 to V.L.C; 2015/06708-0 and 2015/06387-0 to A.T.F]; the National Council for Scientific and Technological Development (CNPq) [483005/2012-6 to V.L.C]; and Coordenação de Aperfeiçoamento de Pessoal de Nível Superior - Brasil (CAPES) [Finance Code 001 to C.M.B].

REFERENCES

Berger, G., Azzam, Zs., Hardak, E., Tavor, Y., and Yigla, M. (2011). Idiopathic Pulmonary Arterial Hypertension or Chronic Thromboembolic Pulmonary Hypertension: Can We Be Certain? *Isr. Med. Assoc. J.* 13, 106–110. doi:10.15420/ecr.2006.0.2.1r

Bienertova-Vasku, J., Novak, J., and Vasku, A. (2015). MicroRNAs in Pulmonary Arterial Hypertension: Pathogenesis, Diagnosis and Treatment. *J. Am. Soc. Hypertens.* 9, 221–234. doi:10.1016/j.jash.2014.12.011

Chen, Lt., and Jiang, Cy. (2018). MicroRNA Expression Profiles Identify Biomarker for Differentiating the Embolic Stroke from Thrombotic Stroke. *Biomed. Res. Int.* 2018, 4514178. doi:10.1155/2018/4514178

Chen, X., Ba, Y., Ma, L., Cai, X., Yin, Y., Wang, K., et al. (2008). Characterization of microRNAs in Serum: a Novel Class of Biomarkers for Diagnosis of Cancer and Other Diseases. *Cell Res.* 18, 997–1006. doi:10.1038/cr.2008.282

Chou, C.-H., Chang, N.-W., Shrestha, S., Hsu, S.-D., Lin, Y.-L., Lee, W.-H., et al. (2016). miRTarBase 2016: Updates to the Experimentally Validated miRNA-Target Interactions Database. *Nucleic Acids Res.* 44, D239–D247. doi:10.1093/nar/gkv1258

Courboulin, A., Paulin, R., giguère, N. J., Saksouk, N., Perreault, T., Meloche, J., et al. (2011). Role for miR-204 in Human Pulmonary Arterial Hypertension. *J. Exp. Med.* 208, 535–548. doi:10.1084/jem.20101812

Douma, R. A., Kamphuisen, P. W., and büller, H. R. (2010). Acute Pulmonary Embolism. Part 1: Epidemiology and Diagnosis. *Nat. Rev. Cardiol.* 7, 585–596. doi:10.1038/nrcardio.2010.106

Enright, A. J., John, B., Gaul, U., Tuschl, T., Sander, C., and Marks, D. S. (2003). MicroRNA Targets in Drosophila. *Genome Biol.* 5, R1. doi:10.1186/gb-2003-5-1-r1

Goldhaber, S. Z. (2012). Venous Thromboembolism: Epidemiology and Magnitude of the Problem. *Best Pract. Res. Clin. Haematol.* 25, 235–242. doi:10.1016/j.beha.2012.06.007

Gräf, S., Haimel, M., Bleda, M., Hadinnapola, C., Southgate, L., Li, W., et al. (2018). Identification of Rare Sequence Variation Underlying Heritable Pulmonary Arterial Hypertension. *Nat. Commun.* 9, 1416. doi:10.1038/s41467-018-03672-4

Graham, B. B., Mentink-Kane, M. M., El-Haddad, H., Purnell, S., Zhang, L., Zaiman, A., et al. (2010). Schistosomiasis-Induced Experimental Pulmonary Hypertension. *Am. J. Pathol.* 177, 1549–1561. doi:10.2353/ajpath.2010.100063

Guo, L., Yang, Y., Liu, J., Wang, L., Li, J., Wang, Y., et al. (2014). Differentially Expressed Plasma microRNAs and the Potential Regulatory Function of Let-7b in Chronic Thromboembolic Pulmonary Hypertension. *PLoS One* 9, e101055. doi:10.1371/journal.pone.0101055

Ham, O., Lee, S. Y., Lee, C. Y., Park, J. H., Lee, J., Seo, H. H., et al. (2015). let-7b Suppresses Apoptosis and Autophagy of Human Mesenchymal Stem Cells

Transplanted into Ischemia/reperfusion Injured Heart 7by Targeting Caspase-3. *Stem Cel Res Ther* 6, 147. doi:10.1186/s13287-015-0134-x

Hamberg, M., Backes, C., Fehlmann, T., Hart, M., Meder, B., Meese, E., et al. (2016). miRTargetLink-miRNAs, Genes and Interaction Networks. *Ijms* 17, 564. doi:10.3390/ijms17040564

Hu, X., Guo, J., Zheng, L., Li, C., Zheng, T. M., Tanyi, J. L., et al. (2013). The Heterochronic microRNA Let-7 Inhibits Cell Motility by Regulating the Genes in the Actin Cytoskeleton Pathway in Breast Cancer. *Mol. Cancer Res.* 11, 240–250. doi:10.1158/1541-7786.mcr-12-0432

Konstantinides, S. V., Torbicki, A., Agnelli, G., Danchin, N., Fitzmaurice, D., Galie, N., et al. (2014). 2014 ESC Guidelines on the Diagnosis and Management of Acute Pulmonary Embolism. *Eur. Heart J.* 35 (3033-69), 3069a–3069k. doi:10.1093/eurheartj/ehu243

Kosaka, N., Iguchi, H., Yoshioka, Y., Takeshita, F., Matsuki, Y., and Ochiya, T. (2010). Secretory Mechanisms and Intercellular Transfer of microRNAs in Living Cells. *J. Biol. Chem.* 285, 17442–17452. doi:10.1074/jbc.m110.107821

Kostadima, E., and Zakynthinos, E. (2007). Pulmonary Embolism: Pathophysiology, Diagnosis, Treatment. *Hellenic J. Cardiol.* 48, 94–107.

Koudstaal, T., Boomars, K. A., and Kool, M. (2020). Pulmonary Arterial Hypertension and Chronic Thromboembolic Pulmonary Hypertension: An Immunological Perspective. *Jcm* 9, 561. doi:10.3390/jcm9020561

Miao, R., Wang, Y., Wan, J., Leng, D., Gong, J., Li, J., et al. (2017). Microarray Analysis and Detection of MicroRNAs Associated with Chronic Thromboembolic Pulmonary Hypertension. *Biomed. Res. Int.* 2017, 8529796. doi:10.1155/2017/8529796

Mittal, S. P. K., Mathai, J., Kulkarni, A. P., Pal, J. K., and Chattopadhyay, S. (2013). miR-320a Regulates Erythroid Differentiation through MAR Binding Protein SMAR1. *Int. J. Biochem. Cel Biol.* 45, 2519–2529. doi:10.1016/j.biocel.2013.07.006

O'connell, C., Montani, D., Savale, L., Sitbon, O., Parent, F., Seferian, A., et al. (2015). Chronic Thromboembolic Pulmonary Hypertension. *Presse Med.* 44, e409–16. doi:10.1016/j.lpm.2015.10.010

Rhodes, C. J., Wharton, J., Boon, R. A., Roexe, T., Tsang, H., Wojciak-Stothard, B., et al. (2013). Reduced microRNA-150 Is Associated with Poor Survival in Pulmonary Arterial Hypertension. *Am. J. Respir. Crit. Care Med.* 187, 294–302. doi:10.1164/rccm.201205-0839oc

Saadoun, S., Papadopoulos, M. C., Hara-Chikuma, M., and Verkman, A. S. (2005). Impairment of Angiogenesis and Cell Migration by Targeted Aquaporin-1 Gene Disruption. *Nature* 434, 786–792. doi:10.1038/nature03460

Santos-Ferreira, C. A., Abreu, M. T., Marques, C. I., Gonçalves, L. M., Baptista, R., and Girão, H. M. (2020). Micro-RNA Analysis in Pulmonary Arterial Hypertension. *JACC: Basic Translational Sci.* 5, 1149–1162. doi:10.1016/j.jacbts.2020.07.008

Schuoler, C., Haider, T. J., Leuenberger, C., Vogel, J., Ostergaard, L., Kwapiszewska, G., et al. (2017). Aquaporin 1 Controls the Functional Phenotype of Pulmonary Smooth Muscle Cells in Hypoxia-Induced Pulmonary Hypertension. *Basic Res. Cardiol.* 112, 30. doi:10.1007/s00395-017-0620-7

Shang, C., Zhang, H., Guo, Y., Hong, Y., Liu, Y., and Xue, Y. (2014). MiR-320a Down-Regulation Mediates Bladder Carcinoma Invasion by Targeting ITGB3. *Mol. Biol. Rep.* 41, 2521–2527. doi:10.1007/s11033-014-3110-0

Simonneau, G., Montani, D., Celermajer, D. S., Denton, C. P., Gatzoulis, M. A., Krowka, M., et al. (2019). Haemodynamic Definitions and Updated Clinical Classification of Pulmonary Hypertension. *Eur. Respir. J.* 53, 1801913. doi:10.1183/13993003.01913-2018

Sun, J.-Y., Huang, Y., Li, J.-P., Zhang, X., Wang, L., Meng, Y.-L., et al. (2012). MicroRNA-320a Suppresses Human colon Cancer Cell Proliferation by Directly Targeting β-catenin. *Biochem. Biophysical Res. Commun.* 420, 787–792. doi:10.1016/j.bbrc.2012.03.075

Vallance, T. M., Zeuner, M. T., Williams, H. F., Widera, D., and Vaiyapuri, S. (2017). Toll-Like Receptor 4 Signalling and its Impact on Platelet Function, Thrombosis, and Haemostasis. *Mediators Inflamm.* 2017, 9605894. doi:10.1155/2017/9605894

Vlachos, I. S., Zagganas, K., Paraskevopoulou, M. D., Georgakilas, G., Karagkouni, D., Vergoulis, T., et al. (2015). DIANA-miRPath v3.0: Deciphering microRNA Function with Experimental Support. *Nucleic Acids Res.* 43, W460–W466. doi:10.1093/nar/gkv403

Wang, L., Guo, L.-J., Liu, J., Wang, W., Yuan, J. X.-J., Zhao, L., et al. (2013). MicroRNA Expression Profile of Pulmonary Artery Smooth Muscle Cells and the Effect of Let-7d in Chronic Thromboembolic Pulmonary Hypertension. *Pulm. Circ.* 3, 654–664. doi:10.1086/674310

Wang, X., Wang, H.-X., Li, Y.-L., Zhang, C.-C., Zhou, C.-Y., Wang, L., et al. (2015). MicroRNA Let-7i Negatively Regulates Cardiac Inflammation and Fibrosis. *Hypertension* 66, 776–785. doi:10.1161/hypertensionaha.115.05548

Yuan, S.-M. (2019). Interleukin-13 in the Pathogenesis of Pulmonary Artery Hypertension. *J. Lab. Med.* 43, 5–11. doi:10.1515/labmed-2018-0323

Zhang, K., Wang, W., Liu, Y., Guo, A., and Yang, D. (2019). Let-7b Acts as a Tumor Suppressor in Osteosarcoma via Targeting IGF1R. *Oncol. Lett.* 17, 1646–1654. doi:10.3892/ol.2018.9793

Zhang, R., Wang, L., Zhao, Q. H., Jiang, R., Gong, S. G., Jiang, X., et al. (2020). Alteration of Extracellular Superoxide Dismutase in Idiopathic Pulmonary Arterial Hypertension. *Front Med (Lausanne).* 7, 509. doi:10.3389/fmed.2020.00509

20

Bacterial Signatures of Paediatric Respiratory Disease: An Individual Participant Data Meta-Analysis

*David T. J. Broderick[1], David W. Waite[1], Robyn L. Marsh[2], Carlos A. Camargo Jr.[3,4,5], Paul Cardenas[6], Anne B. Chang[2,7,8], William O. C. Cookson[9,10], Leah Cuthbertson[10], Wenkui Dai[11], Mark L. Everard[12], Alain Gervaix[13], J. Kirk Harris[14], Kohei Hasegawa[3,4,5], Lucas R. Hoffman[15,16], Soo-Jong Hong[17], Laurence Josset[18], Matthew S. Kelly[19], Bong-Soo Kim[20], Yong Kong[21], Shuai C. Li[22,23], Jonathan M. Mansbach[5,24], Asuncion Mejias[25], George A. O'Toole[26], Laura Paalanen[27], Marcos Pérez-Losada[28,29], Melinda M. Pettigrew[30], Maxime Pichon[31,32], Octavio Ramilo[25], Lasse Ruokolainen[33], Olga Sakwinska[34], Patrick C. Seed[35], Christopher J. van der Gast[36], Brandie D. Wagner[37], Hana Yi[38], Edith T. Zemanick[14], Yuejie Zheng[39], Naveen Pillarisetti[40] and Michael W. Taylor[1]**

[1] School of Biological Sciences, University of Auckland, Auckland, New Zealand, [2] Child Health Division, Menzies School of Health Research, Charles Darwin University, Darwin, NT, Australia, [3] Department of Emergency Medicine, Massachusetts General Hospital, Boston, MA, United States, [4] Department of Epidemiology, Harvard T.H. Chan School of Public Health, Boston, MA, United States, [5] Harvard Medical School, Boston, MA, United States, [6] Colegio de Ciencias Biológicas y Ambientales, Instituto de Microbiología, Universidad San Francisco de Quito, Quito, Ecuador, [7] Department of Respiratory and Sleep Medicine, Queensland Children's Hospital, Brisbane, QLD, Australia, [8] Australian Centre for Health Services Innovation, Queensland University of Technology, Brisbane, QLD, Australia, [9] National Heart and Lung Institute, Imperial College London, London, United Kingdom, [10] Royal Brompton and Harefield NHS Foundation Trust, London, United Kingdom, [11] Department of Obstetrics and Gynecology, Peking University Shenzhen Hospital, Shenzhen, China, [12] School of Medicine, University of Western Australia, Perth, WA, Australia, [13] Department of Pediatrics, Gynecology and Obstetrics, Faculty of Medicine, University Hospitals of Geneva, Geneva, Switzerland, [14] Department of Pediatrics, University of Colorado School of Medicine, Aurora, CO, United States, [15] Seattle Children's Hospital, Seattle, WA, United States, [16] Department of Pediatrics and Microbiology, University of Washington, Seattle, WA, United States, [17] Department of Pediatrics, Childhood Asthma Atopy Center, Humidifier Disinfectant Health Center, Asan Medical Center, University of Ulsan College of Medicine, Seoul, South Korea, [18] Hospices Civils de Lyon, Lyon, France, [19] Division of Pediatric Infectious Diseases, Duke University, Durham, NC, United States, [20] Department of Life Science, Multidisciplinary Genome Institute, Hallym University, Chuncheon, South Korea, [21] Department of Biostatistics, Yale School of Public Health, Yale University, New Haven, CT, United States, [22] Department of Computer Science, City University of Hong Kong, Kowloon, Hong Kong SAR, China, [23] Department of Biomedical Engineering, City University of Hong Kong, Kowloon, Hong Kong SAR, China, [24] Department of Pediatrics, Boston Children's Hospital, Boston, MA, United States, [25] Division of Pediatric Infectious Diseases, Department of Pediatrics, Center for Vaccines and Immunity, Abigail Wexner Research Institute at Nationwide Children's Hospital, The Ohio State University College of Medicine, Columbus, OH, United States, [26] Department of Microbiology and Immunology, Geisel School of Medicine at Dartmouth, Hanover, NH, United States, [27] Finnish Institute for Health and Welfare (THL), Helsinki, Finland, [28] Department of Biostatistics and Bioinformatics, Computational Biology Institute, Milken Institute School of Public Health, George Washington University, Washington, DC, United States, [29] CIBIO-InBIO, Centro de Investigação em Biodiversidade e Recursos Genéticos, Universidade do Porto, Campus Agrário de Vairão, Vairão, Portugal, [30] Department of Epidemiology of Microbial Diseases, Yale School of Public Health, New Haven, CT, United States, [31] CHU Poitiers, Infectious Agents Department, Poitiers, France, [32] University of Poitiers, INSERM U1070, Poitiers, France, [33] Department of Biosciences, University of Helsinki, Helsinki, Finland, [34] Nestlé Research, Lausanne, Switzerland, [35] Department of Pediatrics, Feinberg School of Medicine, Northwestern University, Chicago, IL, United States, [36] Department of Life Sciences, Manchester Metropolitan University, Manchester, United Kingdom, [37] Department of Biostatistics and Informatics, Colorado School of Public Health, University of Colorado, Aurora, Aurora, CO, United States, [38] School of Biosystem and Biomedical Science, Korea University, Seoul, South Korea, [39] Shenzhen Children's Hospital, Shenzhen, China, [40] Starship Children's Hospital, Auckland, New Zealand

***Correspondence:**
Michael W. Taylor
mw.taylor@auckland.ac.nz

Introduction: The airway microbiota has been linked to specific paediatric respiratory diseases, but studies are often small. It remains unclear whether particular bacteria are associated with a given disease, or if a more general, non-specific microbiota association with disease exists, as suggested for the gut. We investigated overarching patterns of bacterial association with acute and chronic paediatric respiratory disease in an individual participant data (IPD) meta-analysis of 16S rRNA gene sequences from published respiratory microbiota studies.

Methods: We obtained raw microbiota data from public repositories or *via* communication with corresponding authors. Cross-sectional analyses of the paediatric (<18 years) microbiota in acute and chronic respiratory conditions, with >10 case subjects were included. Sequence data were processed using a uniform bioinformatics pipeline, removing a potentially substantial source of variation. Microbiota differences across diagnoses were assessed using alpha- and beta-diversity approaches, machine learning, and biomarker analyses.

Results: We ultimately included 20 studies containing individual data from 2624 children. Disease was associated with lower bacterial diversity in nasal and lower airway samples and higher relative abundances of specific nasal taxa including *Streptococcus* and *Haemophilus*. Machine learning success in assigning samples to diagnostic groupings varied with anatomical site, with positive predictive value and sensitivity ranging from 43 to 100 and 8 to 99%, respectively.

Conclusion: IPD meta-analysis of the respiratory microbiota across multiple diseases allowed identification of a non-specific disease association which cannot be recognised by studying a single disease. Whilst imperfect, machine learning offers promise as a potential additional tool to aid clinical diagnosis.

Keywords: microbiota (16S), respiratory tract, respiratory infection, paediatrics, meta-analysis, individual participant data (IPD) meta-analysis

INTRODUCTION

The human respiratory tract has long been of interest to clinicians and microbiologists, with a traditional focus on single, putatively pathogenic microorganisms (Huang and Lynch, 2011). More recent research, enabled by advances in DNA sequencing, has revealed the existence of complex bacterial communities (microbiota) throughout the airways of even healthy individuals (Charlson et al., 2011; Man et al., 2017; Cox et al., 2019). While a protective function of the respiratory microbiota has been proposed (Man et al., 2017), it is increasingly apparent that a microbiota imbalance, or dysbiosis, is frequently associated with disease. Understanding how, or even if, patterns within the microbiota correspond to different respiratory diagnoses is a key challenge.

Respiratory disease in children is a known risk factor for chronic disease in adulthood (Grimwood and Chang, 2015; Bui et al., 2018; Zhang, 2020). As such, any reduction in childhood disease burden could also improve the outlook for adult respiratory health. In particular, respiratory infections in children are associated with future impaired lung function as adults (Zhang, 2020). While connections between paediatric and adult respiratory disease remain enigmatic, it is likely that the airway microbiota plays a role. Indeed, atypical development of the infant upper airway microbiota has been linked to unfavourable respiratory outcomes in older children (Biesbroek et al., 2014; Teo et al., 2015), a pattern which may continue into adulthood. These findings, together with the role of microbes in early life immune education and evidence for a shared core microbiota across different respiratory diseases in children but not adults (van der Gast et al., 2014), suggest a potential therapeutic window aiming at a beneficial microbiota (e.g., *via* probiotics or targetted antibiotics). Although the microbiota of the upper airway may not contribute directly to pathogenesis of lower airway disease, it nonetheless demands consideration both as a reservoir for lower airway microorganisms as well as being a more clinically accessible site.

Studying the respiratory microbiota in children brings challenges including logistical and ethical considerations with sampling the paediatric lower airway and inherent difficulties with low-microbial-biomass samples (Marsh et al., 2018). Consequently, understanding of the paediatric respiratory microbiota is not as developed as for other organs with more accessible specimens, such as the bowel. However, with an ever-increasing body of studies, and a field that is already starting to look beyond the typical sequencing of amplified bacterial 16S rRNA genes, it is both feasible and timely to examine what these data as a whole reveal about the microbiota and paediatric respiratory illness. Indeed, rigorous examination of existing data should serve to guide future application of approaches based on microbial function, such as metagenomics and metatranscriptomics (Ritchie and Singanayagam, 2020).

Variation within the human microbiota is considerable, with differences among individuals sometimes swamping signals from clinical factors such as disease (Biswas et al., 2015). Further challenges arise due to a lack of standardisation among studies, such as anatomical site sampled, collection technique, DNA extraction method, 16S rRNA gene region sequenced, and bioinformatics approach. This signals the need for large sample numbers which are not always feasible in paediatric respiratory studies. By combining individual participant data (IPD) from multiple studies, IPD meta-analyses help identify biologically and/or clinically relevant patterns that may not otherwise be detected in small, unstratified studies. Standardised bioinformatics pipelines for re-processing microbiota data from multiple studies have been successfully applied to the human gut (Duvallet et al., 2017), sinus (Wagner Mackenzie et al., 2017), and cystic fibrosis (CF) lung microbiotas (Li et al., 2016).

The value of contextualising results across multiple diseases was eloquently demonstrated by Duvallet et al. (2017) in a recent IPD meta-analysis of the gut microbiota. As this approach has never been done for respiratory microbiota across a range of acute and chronic childhood diseases, we collated and re-analysed published 16S rRNA gene-based microbiota data from 20 studies encompassing such diagnoses. We aimed to test several hypotheses, namely that: (a) the airway microbiota differs between health and disease; (b) there is a consistent microbiota signature in children with lower airway disease, irrespective of specific diagnosis; and (c) airway microbiota profiles can be used to detect lower airway disease.

MATERIALS AND METHODS

Study Selection Strategy

To identify publications with 16S rRNA gene sequence data from cross-sectional analyses containing paediatric respiratory samples, Scopus and PubMed databases were searched on January 2, 2018 using 25 search terms (**Supplementary File A**). To be included in the analysis studies could only have a single timepoint per individual within that publication and investigate one of the following illnesses: bronchiolitis, bronchiectasis, CF, asthma, wheeze, acute respiratory infections, chronic suppurative lung disease, and protracted or persistent bacterial bronchitis. Studies which focused on lung transplants, individuals undergoing mechanical ventilation, contained 10 or fewer disease samples, or where age, sex, or diagnosis were unclear, were excluded. We also contributed new, at the time unpublished, data of our own (Pillarisetti et al., 2019). Overall, we obtained data from 4884 samples across 21 studies. Separate ethics approvals had been obtained for each original study and the University of Auckland Human Participants Ethics Committee deemed that re-use of these published data did not require additional approval.

Sequence Data Processing

We used a uniform bioinformatics pipeline to analyze all of the included studies (code is supplied in **Supplementary Material**). The analysis pipeline utilised USEARCH (v.11.0667) (Edgar, 2010) for quality filtering and, where applicable, merging of paired-end reads, after which reference gene alignment and chimaera removal (chimera.uchime) (Edgar et al., 2011) were performed using mothur (v1.38.1) (Schloss et al., 2009). Taxonomic classification (classify.otu) was performed in mothur using the SILVA SSU database (v132) as reference (Quast et al., 2012). Sequences assigned to non-bacterial lineages or that could not be identified to genus level were removed. Reprocessing of the data led to removal of 557 samples not containing any reads which could be identified at genus level through our uniform pipeline. The wide range of sequenced 16S rRNA regions (**Supplementary File A** and **Supplementary Figure E1**) necessitated a genus-level phylotype approach (Waite and Taylor, 2014; Callahan et al., 2017). Following data reprocessing, our uniformly applied bioinformatics approach was able to successfully recapitulate most testable claims identified in the original papers, across multiple normalisation approaches and rarefaction depths (**Supplementary File C**). Removal of samples with <1000 sequences (348 total) resulted in removal of a single study (Langevin et al., 2017), as retention of only 8% of their samples meant this study could not be fairly represented. Hence, only 20 studies were ultimately included. Following normalisation, pseudoreplication bias (i.e., over-representation of a particular bacterial community) was avoided by splitting data into four broad anatomical sites with distinct physicochemical features [nasal, oral, sputum, lower airways (bronchoalveolar lavage or bronchial brushings)] (Marsh et al., 2016; Man et al., 2017; Ronchetti et al., 2018), and avoiding cross-site comparisons. Ultimately, 2789 samples (from 2624 individuals) were retained.

Defining Diagnostic Groupings

Given variations in how clinical diagnoses are reported across studies, we grouped reported diagnoses into separate groups on two levels. The first, broad level grouped diagnoses into (a) controls, comprising individuals deemed healthy or suitable to use as disease controls in the original study; and (b) disease, comprising individuals with diagnosed respiratory disease. For the second, more nuanced level we defined seven mutually exclusive diagnostic groupings: acute infections, asthma, CF, disease control, healthy, suppurative lung diseases (e.g., bronchiectasis, protracted bacterial bronchitis), and wheezing illness.

Data Analysis

Statistical analyses were performed in R (v3.6.2) (R Core Team, 2019), using vegan (Jari et al., 2015) for diversity calculations, and ggplot2 (Wickham, 2016) for generating plots. Genus-level phylotypes differing significantly between diagnostic groupings were identified using linear discriminant analysis effect size (LEfSe) (Segata et al., 2011). We identified the core microbiota for specific anatomical sites and diagnostic groupings by applying a prevalence threshold of ≥75% in the relevant samples, and an abundance filter whereby a genus must represent ≥10% in at least one sample.

Sensitivity Analyses

In addition to anatomical site and clinical condition, we attempted to account for other factors affecting the respiratory microbiota. In sensitivity analyses we examined effect of participant age, data normalisation approach and influence of two specific studies on our overall findings. While results shown here are based on rarefaction to 1000 sequence reads/sample, we also considered a size factor-based normalisation approach (GMPR) (Chen et al., 2018). This allowed for an accounting of the flaws in each method, namely data compositionality in rarefaction and bias caused by differing sequencing depths in GMPR. The data from one study (Wang et al., 2016) formed a distinctly separate cluster in ordination (principle coordinates analysis, multidimensional scaling) analyses (**Supplementary Figure E6**). The second study (Luna et al., 2018) represented such a large proportion of the overall dataset that we had concerns our findings could simply reflect that study's original findings. To test for any such effects, we: (a) eliminated all samples from a particular category (e.g., a specific age group/study) then repeated the analyses; and (b) retained only samples pertaining to the single category in question and re-analysed these independently. Both approaches aimed to determine whether our initial overall findings could be recapitulated.

Machine Learning

To determine whether diagnostic groups could be identified based only on microbiota composition, machine learning trials were performed on rarefied data in python (Pedregosa et al., 2011). For this, 60% of samples from a given anatomical site were selected at random to use as training data, with the remaining 40% used for validation. Of five different initial approaches [random forest; neural network; support vector machine (SVM): linear; SVM: radial bias function; SVM: polynomial], random forest was most successful across the

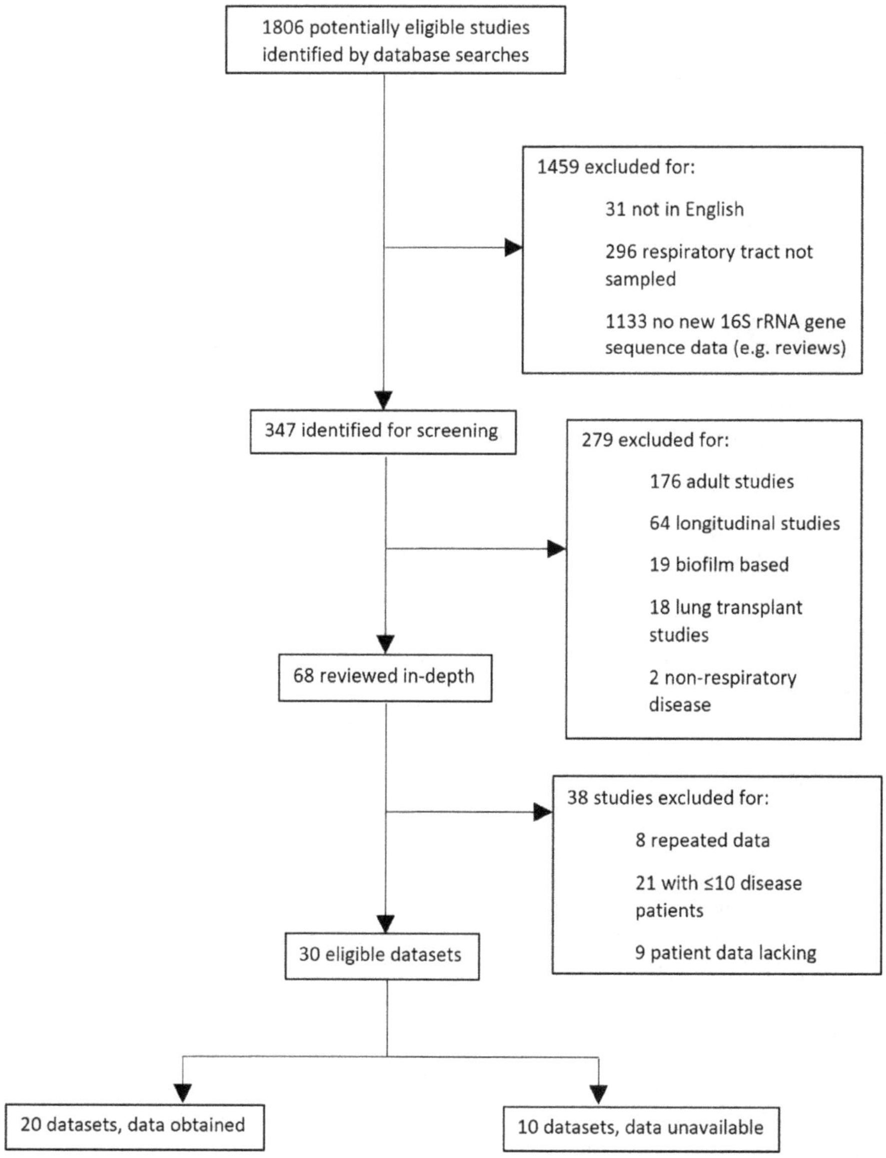

FIGURE 1 | Schematic showing protocol for selecting meta-analysis studies.

majority of trials. Success in this context was determined by the accuracy value (the fraction of correct calls over all calls) (Sokolova et al., 2006). The random forest approach was then applied independently to both the rarefied and GMPR-normalised datasets using the training and validation strategy outlined above. In addition, for both normalisation methods we generated a sample dataset in which the contribution of different diagnostic groupings was set as equivalent to account for differences in sample numbers. These final machine learning approaches were assessed for both their positive predictive value (defined as the fraction of calls of a diagnostic grouping which are correct) and sensitivity (defined as the fraction of samples within a diagnostic grouping which are correctly identified) for all specific diagnostic groupings.

For more details see **Supplementary File A**.

RESULTS

In total, 1806 potentially eligible studies were identified by literature database searches, of which 347 required screening and evaluation against specific criteria (**Supplementary File A**). Thirty eligible datasets were ultimately interrogated, and we were able to access 16S rRNA gene sequences and essential metadata for 20 of these, in addition to our own new data (Pillarisetti et al., 2019; **Figure 1**). After removal of one study (Langevin et al., 2017) due to low sample retention, ultimately 20 datasets were included.

Bioinformatic processing using a uniform analysis pipeline resulted in a final dataset comprising 2789 samples, from 2624 individuals. Following sequence data reprocessing, the assembled dataset encompassed 20 unique studies (**Table 1**) spanning chronic and acute diagnoses, multiple anatomical sites, and 11 countries. Technical, clinical, and demographic heterogeneity were considerable (**Table 2**). While use of a uniform bioinformatics pipeline is expected to reduce some underlying data variation, other technical factors such as sequencing technology used, 16S rRNA gene region sequenced, and DNA extraction method could not be readily controlled. This was evident in that the variables "Study," "Extraction method," "16S rRNA gene region," and "sequencing platform" accounted for 12.4, 6.75, 4.76, and 0.438% of underlying data variation, respectively, according to PERMANOVA analysis (**Table 3**). The most substantial of these technical factors was DNA extraction method, as accounting for this factor could reduce the explanatory power

TABLE 1 | Summary of studies which contributed to the final dataset; for more detailed summaries see **Supplementary File A (Supplementary Tables E2–E5)**.

Studys	Age (years)	Sample site(s)	Disease	N disease	Control individuals	N control
Cardenas et al., 2012	0.5–1.083	OP	Early onset wheeze	21	Healthy	23
Cuthbertson et al., 2017	0.8–15.4	Bronchial brushings	PBB	23	Healthy	19
de Steenhuijsen Piters et al., 2016	0.025–1.83	NP	RSV infections	105	Healthy	26
Hampton et al., 2014	9.86–17.58	IS	Cystic fibrosis	13		
Kelly et al., 2017	0.083–1.99	NP	Pneumonia	374	Control	90
			URI symptoms	82		
Kim et al., 2017	6–14	NP	Asthma	26	Healthy	21
			Asthma remission	17		
Lu et al., 2017	0.1–12.7	NP, OP	Pneumonia	120	Healthy	113
Luna et al., 2018	0.027–1	NP	Bronchiolitis	814		
Marsh et al., 2016*	0.4–10.1	BAL, NP, OP	Bronchiectasis	46	Disease control	9
			CSLD	6		
			PBB	21		
Perez-Losada et al., 2016	6–17	NP	Asthma	29		
Pettigrew et al., 2016	0.50–17.25	IS	Pneumonia	310		
Pillarisetti et al., 2019*	0.9–16	Anterior nares, BAL	Bronchiectasis	54	Healthy	26
Ruokolainen et al., 2017	14–17	Anterior nares	Asthma	9	Healthy	118
Sakwinska et al., 2014	0.2–5.0	NP	Pneumonia	14	Healthy	2
van der Gast et al., 2014	0.63–16.85	BAL, sputum	Bronchiectasis	12		
			Cystic fibrosis	18		
			PBB	9		
Wang et al., 2016	0.3–9	BAL	Pneumonia	22	Tracheomalacia	12
Williamson et al., 2017	1.5–1.7	ES, OP	CFTR-related	1		
			Cystic fibrosis	68		
Yi et al., 2014	0–13	OP	Acute infection	25		
Zemanick et al., 2015	8.49–17.89	ES, IS, OP, saliva	Cystic fibrosis	30		
Zemanick et al., 2017	0.166–17.0	BAL	Cystic fibrosis	50	Disease control	11

**Denotes inclusion of multiple samples for some individuals. Diagnoses are as reported in the original papers.*
BAL, bronchoalveolar lavage; CFTR, cystic fibrosis transmembrane conductance regulator; CSLD, chronic suppurative lung disease; ES, expectorated sputum; IS, induced sputum; NP, nasopharyngeal; OP, oropharyngeal; PBB, protracted bacterial bronchitis; RSV, respiratory syncytial virus; URI, upper respiratory infection.

TABLE 2 | Summary of technical factors associated with each of the included studies.

Studys	Sampling site(s)	Sampling method	% eligible samples retained	DNA extraction method	16S rRNA gene region	Sequencing technology
Cardenas et al., 2012	OP	Swab	91.7	QIAamp	V3–V5	454
Cuthbertson et al., 2017	LA	Brushings	66.7	MPBio FastDNA Spin Kit for Soil	V4	MiSeq
de Steenhuijsen Piters et al., 2016	NP	Swab	99.2	NucliSENS	V5–V7	454
Hampton et al., 2014	SP	Induced	100	Gentra PureGene Yeast/Bact. Kit	V4–V6	454
Kelly et al., 2017*	NP	Swab	99.6	In-house protocol	V3	MiSeq
Kim et al., 2017	NP	Swab	69.6	PowerMag RNA/DNA Isolation Kit	V1–V3	454
Langevin et al., 2017**	NP	Unknown	8.3	NucliSENS	V1–V3	MiSeq
Lu et al., 2017	NP	Swab	98.3	PowerSoil	V3–V4	MiSeq
	OP	Swab	97.5	PowerSoil	V3–V4	MiSeq
Luna et al., 2018***	NP	Aspirate	99.9	PowerSoil	V4	MiSeq
Marsh et al., 2016	NP	Swab	7.8	QIAamp	V1–V3	454
	OP	Swab	71.8	QIAamp	V1–V3	454
	LA	BAL	26.3	QIAamp	V1–V3	454
Perez-Losada et al., 2016	NP	Aspirate	96.7	QIAamp	V4	MiSeq
Pettigrew et al., 2016****	SP	Induced	100	NucliSENS	V4	MiSeq
Pillarisetti et al., 2019	AN	Swab	97.3	Qiagen AllPrep	V3–V4	MiSeq
	LA	BAL	61.4	Qiagen AllPrep	V3–V4	MiSeq
Ruokolainen et al., 2017	AN	Swab	70.2	MPBio FastDNA Spin Kit for Soil	V1–V3	454
Sakwinska et al., 2014*****	NP	Swab	32.7	In-house protocol	V4	454
van der Gast et al., 2014	LA	BAL	61.9	In-house protocol	V1–V3	454
	SP	Unknown	74.3	In-house protocol	V1–V3	454
Wang et al., 2016	LA	BAL	100	E.Z.N.A Soil DNA Kit	V3–V4	MiSeq
Williamson et al., 2017	OP	Swab	48.8	Qiagen EZ1	V1–V2	MiSeq
	SP	Expectorated	35.9	Qiagen EZ1	V1–V2	MiSeq
Yi et al., 2014	OP	Swab	37	Qiagen AllPrep	V1–V3	454
	NP	Aspirate	47	Qiagen AllPrep	V1–V3	454
Zemanick et al., 2015	SA	Saliva	63.6	Qiagen EZ1	V1–V2	454
	SP	Induced	58.3	Qiagen EZ1	V1–V2	454
	SP	Expectorated	66.7	Qiagen EZ1	V1–V2	454
	OP	Swab	61.5	Qiagen EZ1	V1–V2	454
Zemanick et al., 2017	LA	BAL	66.3	Qiagen EZ1	V1–V2	MiSeq

AN, anterior nares; LA, lower airways; NP, nasopharynx; OP, oropharynx; SA, saliva; SP, sputum.
**This study provided more data than were contained within the original paper.*
***This study was removed from the analysis due to low sample retention following our processing.*
****This study contained both anterior nare and nasopharyngeal samples from the same individual; to avoid pseudoreplication only nasopharyngeal samples were used in the main analysis.*
*****This study contained both sputum and swab samples, however, only sputum samples were used.*
******This study sequenced two different 16S rRNA gene regions for each sample, however, we selected only the region with the highest average sequencing depth.*

of "Study" to less than 1% (**Table 3**). Clinical and demographic heterogeneity reflected the broad range of diagnoses included, ages spanning infancy to near-adulthood (<18 years), and diverse strategies regarding anatomical site sampled and sample collection technique. For many clinically relevant factors, e.g., antibiotics and other medication usage, data were incomplete or inconsistently reported.

Bacterial Diversity in Health and Disease

Reduced bacterial diversity, reflecting a lower number and/or uneven distribution of bacterial taxa, is sometimes considered a marker of human disease. We therefore calculated bacterial alpha-diversity on aggregated disease vs. controls data, as well as at a more granular level in which disease and control diagnoses were separated into a total of seven groups (**Figure 2**). For the aggregated data, alpha-diversity (described by multiple metrics) was significantly higher in controls than disease for nasal and lower airway sites, with the opposite trend for oral samples (**Figure 2A**). Bacterial richness (observed phylotypes, ACE) differed little between different anatomical sites, though nasal samples did have lower evenness (Shannon, Gini–Simpson), implying dominance by specific taxa. At diagnostic group level (**Figure 2B**), findings varied depending on anatomical site and whether richness or evenness were considered. One notable finding was that of decreased bacterial diversity in the lower airways of CF patients, although as these data were derived from a single study – and reflect varied pulmonary statuses including both clinical stability and exacerbations at the time of sampling (Zemanick et al., 2017) – one must be circumspect if attempting to infer a wider trend.

TABLE 3 | PERMANOVA analysis of technical variables amongst microbiota studies included in this meta-analysis.

Variable combination	Variable	% variation explained	*P*-value
Study alone	Study	12.4	0.001
Extraction method	Extraction method	6.75	0.001
16S rRNA gene region	Gene region	4.76	0.001
Sequencing platform	Sequencing platform	0.438	0.001
Extraction method + study	Extraction method	6.75	0.001
	Study	5.62	0.001
Gene region + study	Gene region	4.76	0.001
	Study	7.61	0.001
Sequencing platform + study	Sequencing platform	0.438	0.001
	Study	11.9	0.001
Extraction method + gene region + study	Extraction method	6.75	0.001
	Gene region	4.74	0.001
	Study	0.878	0.001
Extraction method + sequencing platform + study	Extraction method	6.75	0.001
	Sequencing platform	0.416	0.001
	Study	5.2	0.001
Gene region + extraction method + study	Gene region	4.76	0.001
	Extraction method	6.74	0.001
	Study	0.877	0.001
Gene region + sequencing platform + study	Gene region	4.76	0.001
	Sequencing platform	0.0006	0.072
	Study	7.56	0.001
Sequencing platform + extraction method + study	Sequencing platform	0.438	0.001
	Extraction method	6.73	0.001
	Study	5.2	0.001
Sequencing platform + gene region + study	Sequencing platform	0.438	0.001
	Gene region	4.38	0.001
	Study	7.55	0.001

Percentage of microbiota variation explained was determined using the R^2 score.

Microbiota Taxonomic Differences Between Health and Disease

Having established that bacterial diversity differs between respiratory diseases and controls, we sought to determine which bacterial taxa drive these differences. While for oral and lower airway sites the most abundant genera in samples from diseased individuals largely mirrored those from controls (**Figure 3**), there was far less concordance within the nasal data: disease was associated with clear decreases in relative sequence abundances of *Corynebacterium_1*, *Staphylococcus*, and *Dolosigranulum* but substantial increases in *Streptococcus* and, to a lesser extent, *Haemophilus*. Biomarker analysis of nasal samples *via* LEfSe largely supported these findings, with *Haemophilus* and *Streptococcus* identified as potential markers of disease, while *Corynebacterium_1*, *Staphylococcus*, and *Dolosigranulum* were associated with controls (**Supplementary File B** and **Supplementary Tables E10–16**). Observed minor changes in rank-abundance for oral samples were also supported by LEfSe, with *Veillonella* identified as a marker for disease and *Prevotella_7* a marker for controls. In addition to the abundant taxa, rare taxa – phylotypes present in ≤10% of samples for a given anatomical site which never comprise ≥1% of 16S rRNA gene sequences within a single sample – were more commonly identified by LEfSe as potential markers for controls, though some could represent potential contaminants (Marsh et al., 2018).

Core Microbiota

Clinical samples often contain a wide variety of microbial taxa and identifying which, if any, of these could be relevant to disease pathology is not straightforward. Core microbiota approaches reduce complexity of microbiota analyses by focusing on only the most prevalent (and in some cases abundant) members of a bacterial community (Astudillo-García et al., 2017). Filtering data to retain only genera present in ≥75% of samples with a relative abundance of ≥10% in at least one sample for a given anatomical site revealed that members of the genus *Streptococcus* were present in the core microbiota of almost all diagnostic groups, irrespective of anatomical site (**Figure 4**). The genera *Prevotella*, *Haemophilus*, and *Granulicatella* were also widespread. Notably, there was no 75%-core microbiota for lower airway samples from CF patients, although LEfSe did identify *Pseudomonas* as a marker of this group. Intuitively, cores for specific diagnostic groups were typically larger than those for overall disease or control cores, potentially due to the lower number of samples required to meet the prevalence threshold and/or other factors common to samples within a given diagnostic group.

Microbiota Homogeneity Within and Between Diagnostic Groupings

To determine the extent to which different clinical diagnostic groupings overlap or differ in terms of their microbiota, we analysed bacterial beta-diversity. Bray–Curtis dissimilarity (a common measure of beta-diversity) was similar within and between broad control vs. disease groupings regardless of anatomical site (**Supplementary File A** and **Supplementary Figure E7**). By contrast, in the finer diagnostic groupings Bray–Curtis dissimilarity was highly dependent on both anatomical site and diagnostic grouping. For instance, in nasal samples values within and between groups were similar (indicating equivalent levels of dissimilarity and overall general lack of microbiota distinctiveness for a given diagnosis). In contrast, for some oral (e.g., suppurative, wheezing illness) and lower airway (e.g., acute infections, suppurative) groupings there was greater microbiota homogeneity within compared to between groups, suggesting a more distinct microbiota associated with these diagnostic groupings. According to PERMANOVA analysis, variables contributing most to variability in the microbiota data were individual study (encompassing multiple technical factors; 12.4% of variation explained), anatomical site (2.5%) and diagnostic group (2.4%) (**Supplementary File B** and **Supplementary Table E17**).

Detection of Lower Airway Disease Based on Microbiota Profiles

A key aim was to determine whether lower airway disease could be detected based on composition of upper- and/or

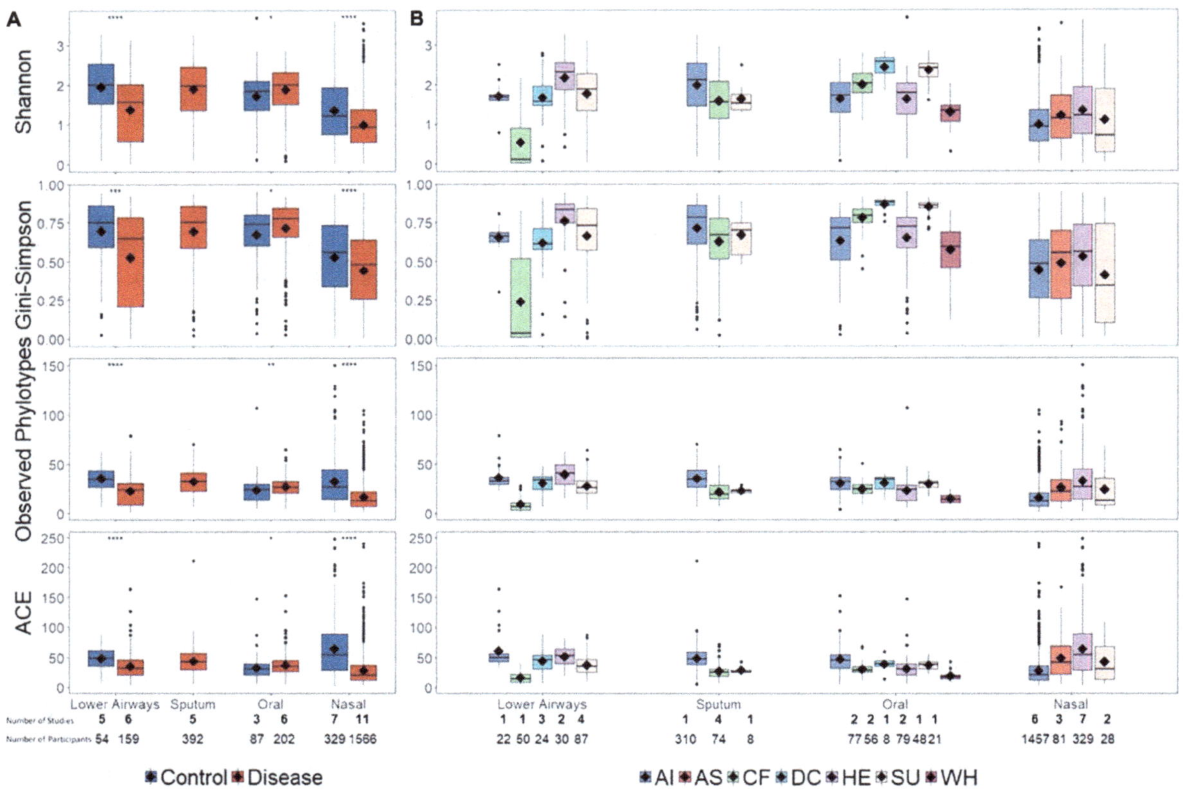

FIGURE 2 | Bacterial alpha-diversity at broad disease **(A)** and specific diagnostic grouping levels **(B)**. Significant differences in **(A)**, as assessed by a Bonferroni corrected *t*-test, are denoted by asterisks ($p < 0.05$). For clarity, statistical significance for **(B)** is presented in **Supplementary Tables E6–9**. Diamonds on each box represent the mean value. Alpha-diversity across different anatomical sites (lower airways, sputum, oral, and nasal) was not explicitly compared. Below the plot the number of studies (bold) and number of contributing samples is reported. AI, acute infections; AS, asthma; CF, cystic fibrosis; DC, disease control; HE, healthy; SU, suppurative; WH, wheezing illness.

lower-airway microbiota. We thus developed a machine learning (random forest) model to predict disease state based upon bacterial distinctiveness of different clinical diagnoses, i.e., is there a distinct microbiota "signature" that allows us to detect different diseases? Machine learning predictions were assessed according to positive predictive value (fraction of calls of a diagnostic grouping which are correct) and sensitivity (fraction of samples within a diagnostic grouping which are correctly identified) for all specific diagnostic groupings. When attempting to use microbiota data alone to predict from which diagnostic group a sample came, success varied with both diagnostic group and anatomical site (**Figure 5**). For example, sputum samples were particularly effective at distinguishing among diagnostic groupings (with both positive predictive value and sensitivity scoring close to 1), while oral samples also performed well. Lower airway samples were poorest overall at identifying lower airway disease, while detection success of nasal samples varied considerably.

Sensitivity Analyses

Sensitivity analyses investigating effects of participant age, sequence data normalisation approach (rarefaction vs. GMPR), and the Wang et al. (2016) and Luna et al. (2018) studies, yielded results largely consistent with those presented above (for details see **Supplementary File A**).

DISCUSSION

Our compilation and re-analysis of 16S rRNA gene data using a uniform bioinformatic pipeline of specimens from >2500 individuals obtained from 20 distinct studies enabled testing of three important hypotheses in childhood respiratory diseases. Inclusion of multiple diseases in the same IPD meta-analysis facilitated the search for overarching microbiota patterns of health and disease. The importance of such an approach was highlighted recently for the gut, where half of all genera linked to specific diseases in a single study were in fact associated with more than one disease (Duvallet et al., 2017). Application of this approach to the respiratory microbiota yielded several novel findings with potential clinical implications.

Airway Microbiota Diversity Differs Between Health and Disease

Observed relationships between bacterial diversity and respiratory disease are complex and vary among different

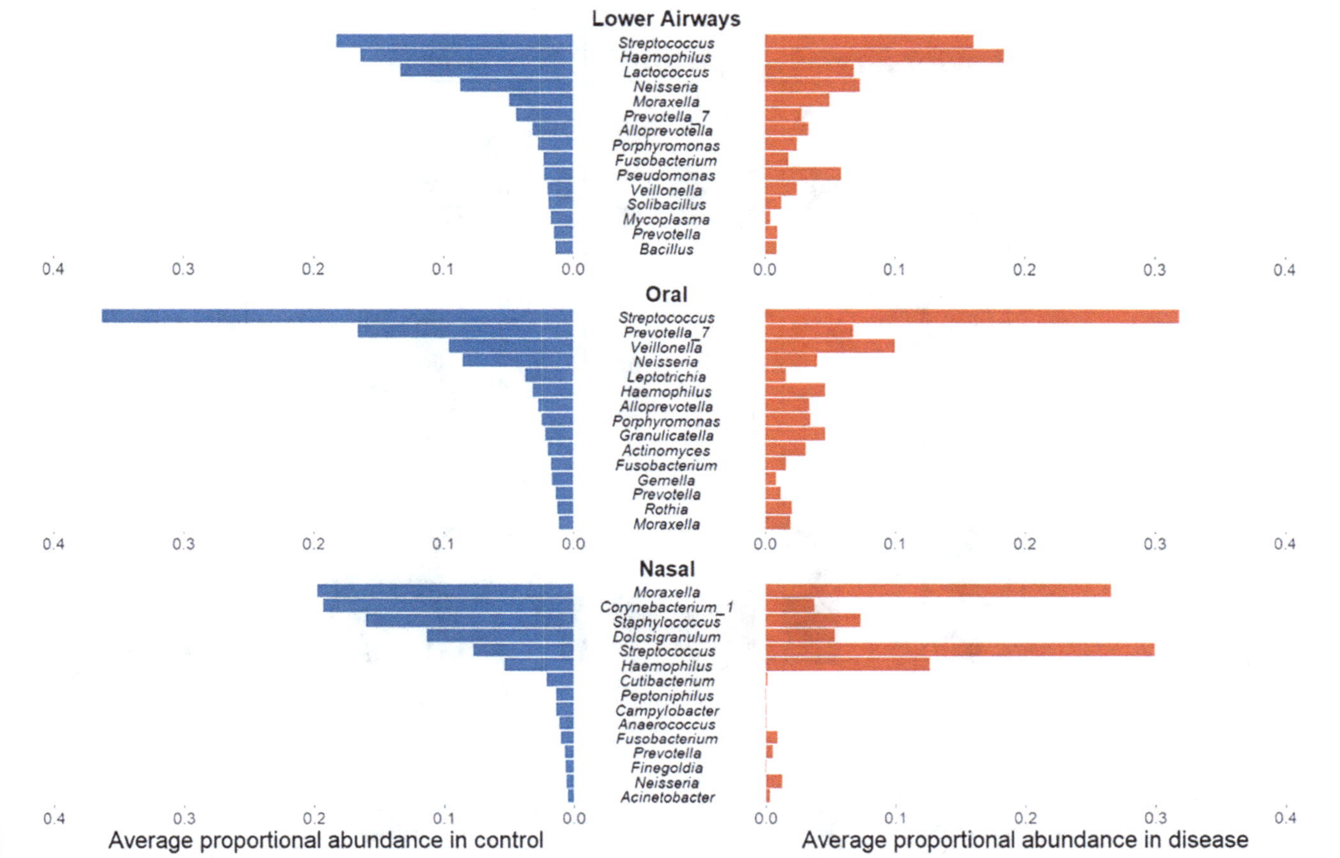

FIGURE 3 | Rank-abundance plots showing the 15 most abundant bacterial phylotypes in control samples (blue) and their respective proportional relative abundance in disease samples (red), for lower airway, oral, and nasal samples. Taxa are ranked based on their relative sequence abundance in controls.

conditions, clinical states and sample types (Man et al., 2017). The primary literature is inconsistent, with reports of both higher (Sakwinska et al., 2014; Cuthbertson et al., 2017) and lower (Marsh et al., 2016; Kim et al., 2017) bacterial diversity in controls compared to disease states. Our IPD meta-analysis revealed significantly lower bacterial diversity with disease in samples of nasal and lower airway origin, but the opposite trend for the oral microbiota. In contrast to diversity, overall microbiota profiles were similar for a given anatomical site, with major bacterial taxa such as *Moraxella*, *Streptococcus*, *Haemophilus*, and *Neisseria* prominent in both health and disease. What *did* sometimes differ was relative abundances of specific genera, with the ubiquitous *Streptococcus* notable for its greatly increased abundance in nasal samples from individuals with disease. Rather than a wholesale shift in microbiota composition, disease may instead manifest more as a decrease in bacterial community evenness, with one or more "bloom" taxa increasing their abundance relative to others. Antibiotic usage, while not explicitly tested here due to a lack of comparable data, may contribute to observed reductions in diversity. The most dramatic example of reduced diversity was in the lower airways of children with CF. Although the exacerbation status of these patients may contribute to this low alpha-diversity, the dataset included a mixture of clinically stable and exacerbating individuals with the original study noting no differences in diversity with exacerbation (Zemanick et al., 2017). Whilst speculative, arresting disease progression *via* microbiota preservation and/or restoration, particularly in long-term or permanent conditions such as CF in which diversity loss may be most marked, may be feasible with wider use of complementary, antibiotic-free approaches such as physiotherapy, anti-inflammatory drugs, probiotics, and vaccines as the first line of defence against disease.

Specific and Non-specific (Overarching) Microbiota Signatures Across Diagnostic Groups

Our analyses revealed that some findings, such as *Pseudomonas* as a potential biomarker of CF in lower airway samples, were specific to an individual diagnostic group and consistent with previous literature (Emerson et al., 2002). We also saw evidence for non-specific signatures of respiratory disease. LEfSe biomarker analysis identified more putative markers for disease overall than for any single diagnostic grouping. This highlights the need for caution when comparing disease to controls for a single condition, in that one may identify apparent markers of that disease which are in fact more general markers of *multiple*

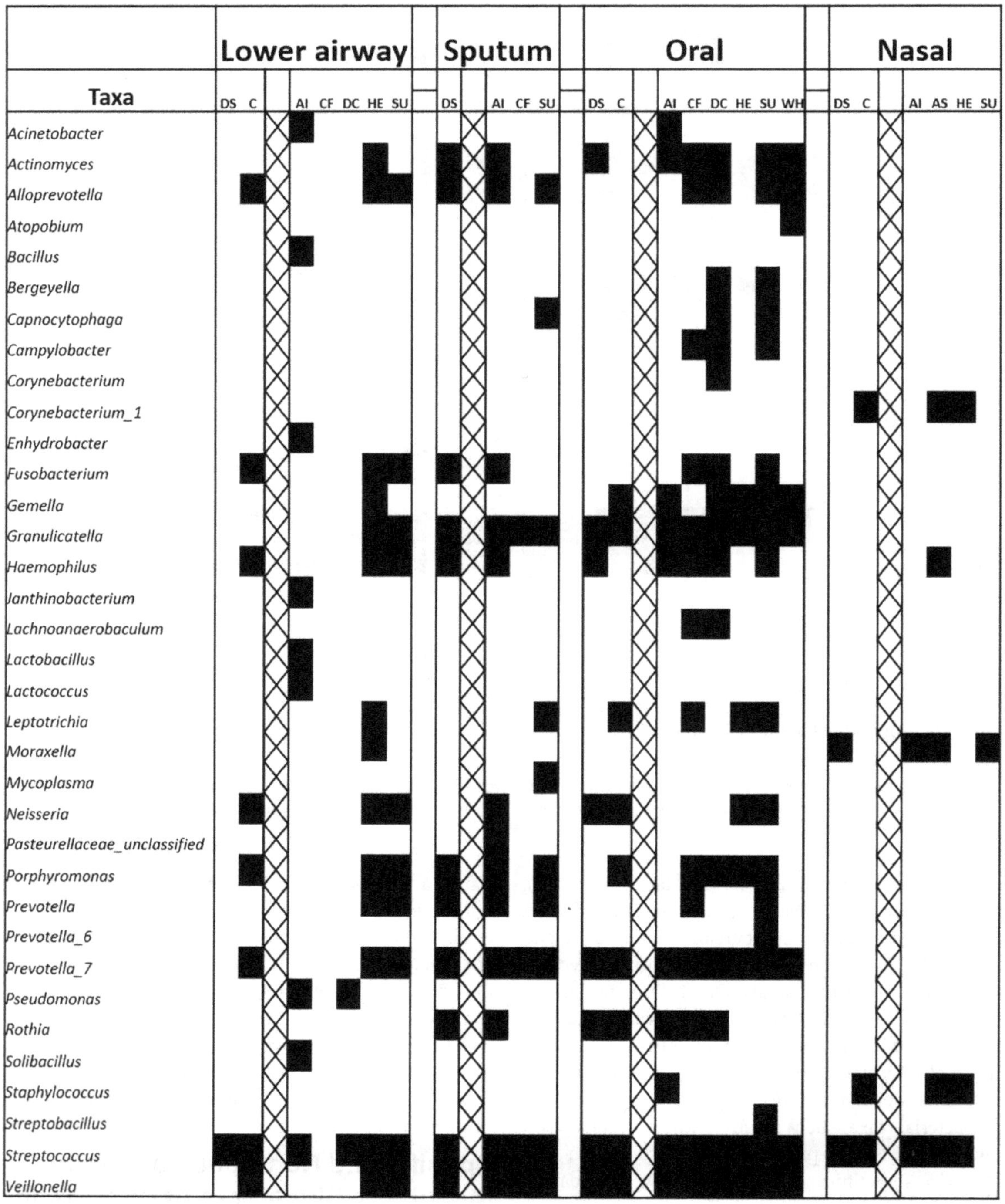

FIGURE 4 | Representation of bacterial genus-level phylotypes in the core microbiota from nasal, oral, sputum, and lower airway samples. A core was defined as presence in at least 75% of samples, based on the rarefied data. An abundance filter was also applied, whereby a genus must represent ≥10% in at least one sample. Cross-hatching separates broad-level comparisons from those involving specific diagnostic groupings, within a given anatomical site. AI, acute infections; AS, asthma; C, control; CF, cystic fibrosis; DC, disease control; DS, disease (any respiratory diagnosis); HE, healthy; SU, suppurative; WH, wheezing illness.

respiratory diseases. Moreover, shared phylotypes in the cores of multiple diagnostic groupings, but not in control cores, provided further evidence for a non-specific disease signature. *Moraxella* within nasal samples is a standout example, being present in all disease group cores but not corresponding control cores. These findings are supported by previous research suggesting a shared core microbiota among different diseases (van der Gast et al., 2014). Caution should therefore be exercised when considering specific bacterial taxa identified *via* microbiota analyses as potentially diagnostic of particular diseases.

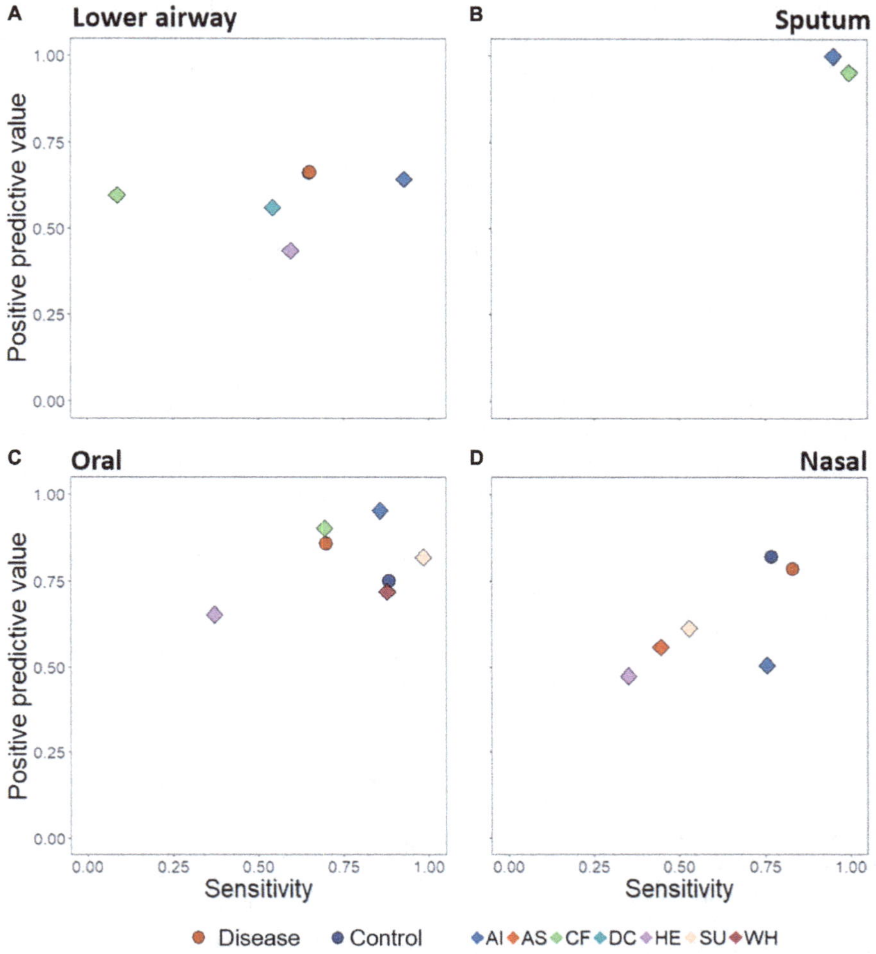

FIGURE 5 | Average positive predictive value (fraction of calls of a diagnostic grouping which are correct) and sensitivity (fraction of samples within a diagnostic grouping which are correctly identified) rates of sample assignments to both broad disease level (circles) and specific diagnostic groupings (diamonds), through use of random forest machine learning. Data are displayed according to anatomical category: lower airways **(A)**, sputum **(B)**, oral **(C)**, and nasal **(D)**. Predictions were made based on rarefied data in which the numbers of samples for each diagnostic grouping were made equal. The Control symbol (blue circles) in **(D)** is hidden behind the red (Disease) circle. AI, acute infections; AS, asthma; CF, cystic fibrosis; DC, disease control; HE, healthy; SU, suppurative; WH, wheezing illness.

Microbiota-Based Detection of Clinical Diagnoses

We used machine learning to evaluate the ability of microbiota profiles to determine clinical diagnostic categories. Sputum and to a lesser extent oral samples yielded the most promising results. Whether this reflects true biological signal or technical biases influencing the random forest model remains unclear. For example, sputum was derived from only two distinct diseases with underlying cohort differences, likely enhancing assignment capabilities beyond that attributable to the microbiota. Indeed, the fact that diagnostic groupings in this meta-analysis were largely reflective of research groups, all of which had distinct methodological characteristics, creates a largely unavoidable bias within the data and presents a challenge for the machine learning model. Such biases could explain the counter-intuitive finding that the microbiota of lower airway specimens appeared to be *least* effective for detecting lower airway disease, implying the lack of a strong disease signal in the lower airway. However, this result should be interpreted with caution and there is a need for further studies using standardised analytic methods to support or refute these preliminary findings. The previously mentioned technical differences among studies may also explain some of our findings, including that related to the lower airways, yet there was still a detectable signal of diagnostic grouping. Parallel PERMANOVA analyses identified a significant albeit minor contribution of diagnostic grouping to underlying variability within the data, even after accounting for technical factors. Ongoing validation of machine learning (using larger datasets and greater standardisation of approaches) may ultimately lead to a complementary diagnostic strategy for diagnosing paediatric lower airway disease *via* relatively non-invasive sampling and analysis of the upper airway microbiota.

Methodological Considerations

While the meta-analysis approach is a powerful one, it does have constraints. Some combinations of diagnostic grouping and anatomical site were represented by a single study, limiting more general conclusions. Moreover, even with such a large dataset (~2800 samples from >2600 individuals) power is quickly lost when attempting to split the data into specific categories. Applying a uniform bioinformatics pipeline removes a potentially substantial source of variation, but clinical (e.g., exacerbation vs. clinical stability) and technical factors (e.g., sampling, DNA extraction) will still contribute to variability within the microbiota data where there is methodological heterogeneity between studies. Indeed, the high explanatory power assigned to individual study by PERMANOVA corroborates the pervasive influence of laboratory-specific approaches and highlights the benefits of a more standardised, cross-laboratory approach. The application of batch correlation tools, particularly where both case and control data are available (Gibbons et al., 2018), also warrants further investigation in an attempt to account for some of these factors. Another useful aspect would be the routine inclusion of both negative technical controls (to detect contaminants) and quantitative approaches such as real-time PCR or droplet digital PCR (to estimate bacterial load). The limited taxonomic resolution of genus-level phylotypes is also noteworthy. The phylotype approach was necessary due to the different 16S rRNA gene regions sequenced, preventing application of operational taxonomic unit or amplicon sequence variant approaches (Callahan et al., 2017). Species- or strain-level differences are likely to be important clinically, and a future focus on deciphering such interactions is warranted. *Streptococcus* provides a salient example: this genus was prevalent and abundant throughout the assembled dataset, but our analyses based on short-read 16S rRNA gene sequences cannot determine whether this was a single species (e.g., pneumococcus) or, more likely, many different species. This is an inherent limitation of 16S rRNA approaches more generally, due to the conserved nature of this gene and the short-read sequences generated by amplicon sequencing techniques. Additionally, while we relied on LEfSe for detecting differential abundance between controls, disease and different diagnostic groups, this is but one of many techniques for identifying differential taxa. Recent comparative studies of various differential abundance approaches have highlighted both considerable variation in outcomes when different techniques are applied and the lack of a clear-cut candidate for the best available tool at present (Nearing et al., 2021; Wallen, 2021). Finally, in our analysis we only considered bacterial members of the respiratory microbiota, whereas viruses and fungi also likely play key roles within the respiratory tract (Wylie, 2017; Cox et al., 2019; Cuthbertson et al., 2020).

CONCLUSION

Despite some limitations, our IPD meta-analysis offered key advantages not available through other approaches. Ethical and logistical considerations associated with sampling the airway microbiota contribute to a paucity of case-control studies (only 60% of included studies contained both cases and controls), constraining the ability of individual studies to explicitly compare health and disease. While this complicates interpretation of broader patterns within the airway microbiota, especially compared with the more accessible microbial communities sampled from human faeces (Duvallet et al., 2017), this meta-analysis enabled disease samples from studies lacking controls to be compared to controls from other studies. Additionally, using sensitivity analyses and the twofold (rarefaction and GMPR) normalisation approach, we were able to evaluate the association of various factors presumed to affect microbiota profiles. Re-analysis of multiple studies also enabled comparison of many more diseases than would be feasible in a single study. While airway bacterial diversity differed between health and disease, other differences were more subtle with a combination of non-specific and anatomical site-dependent contributions to microbiota signatures of any specific diagnostic grouping. Identifying such factors *via* meta-analyses is a further step toward development of novel treatments aimed at rebalancing the airway microbiota, in a manner analogous to faecal transplants and other interventions focused on the gut (Ali and Sweeney, 2020). Moreover, our analysis provides a platform to build future prospective studies where diagnostic categories are uniform.

AUTHOR CONTRIBUTIONS

DB: research design, data collation, bioinformatic analysis, and co-wrote manuscript. DW: bioinformatic pipeline development, data interpretation, and contributed to manuscript writing and editing. MT: conceived study, research design, data interpretation, and co-wrote manuscript. RM, CC, AC, and NP: research design, facilitated access to original data, data interpretation, and contributed to manuscript writing and editing. JH, KH, JM, GO'T, and CvdG: facilitated access to original data, data interpretation, and contributed to manuscript writing and editing. PC, WC, LC, WD, ME, AG, LH, S-JH, LJ, MK, B-SK, YK, SL, AM, LP, MP-L, MPe, MPi, OR, LR, OS, PS, BW, HY, EZ, and YZ: facilitated access to original data, data interpretation, and contributed to manuscript editing. All authors contributed to the article and approved the submitted version.

ACKNOWLEDGMENTS

We gratefully acknowledge the many funders, supporters, and participants of the original studies on which this meta-analysis is based. We also thank the researchers who conducted those studies for their invaluable contributions. Specific funders for each original study are listed in **Supplementary Material**.

REFERENCES

Ali, F., and Sweeney, D. A. (2020). In pursuit of microbiome-based therapies for acute respiratory failure. *Am. J. Respir. Crit. Care Med.* 12, 1616–1618. doi: 10.1164/rccm.202008-3146ed

Astudillo-García, C., Bell, J. J., Webster, N. S., Glasl, B., Jompa, J., Montoya, J. M., et al. (2017). Evaluating the core microbiota in complex communities: a systematic investigation. *Environ. Microbiol.* 19, 1450–1462. doi: 10.1111/1462-2920.13647

Biesbroek, G., Tsivtsivadze, E., Sanders, E. A., Montijn, R., Veenhoven, R. H., Keijser, B. J., et al. (2014). Early respiratory microbiota composition determines bacterial succession patterns and respiratory health in children. *Am. J. Respir. Crit. Care Med.* 190, 1283–1292. doi: 10.1164/rccm.201407-1240oc

Biswas, K., Hoggard, M., Jain, R., Taylor, M. W., and Douglas, R. G. (2015). The nasal microbiota in health and disease: variation within and between subjects. *Front. Microbiol.* 6:134. doi: 10.3389/fmicb.2015.00134

Bui, D. S., Lodge, C. J., Burgess, J. A., Lowe, A. J., Perret, J., Bui, M. Q., et al. (2018). Childhood predictors of lung function trajectories and future COPD risk: a prospective cohort study from the first to the sixth decade of life. *Lancet Respir. Med.* 6, 535–544. doi: 10.1016/S2213-2600(18)30100-0

Callahan, B. J., McMurdie, P. J., and Holmes, S. P. (2017). Exact sequence variants should replace operational taxonomic units in marker-gene data analysis. *ISME J.* 11:2639. doi: 10.1038/ismej.2017.119

Cardenas, P. A., Cooper, P. J., Cox, M. J., Chico, M., Arias, C., Moffatt, M. F., et al. (2012). Upper airways microbiota in antibiotic-naive wheezing and healthy infants from the tropics of rural Ecuador. *PLoS One* 7:e46803. doi: 10.1371/journal.pone.0046803

Charlson, E. S., Bittinger, K., Haas, A. R., Fitzgerald, A. S., Frank, I., Yadav, A., et al. (2011). Topographical continuity of bacterial populations in the healthy human respiratory tract. *Am. J. Respir. Crit. Care Med.* 184, 957–963. doi: 10.1164/rccm.201104-0655OC

Chen, L., Reeve, J., Zhang, L., Huang, S., Wang, X., and Chen, J. G. M. P. R. (2018). A robust normalization method for zero-inflated count data with application to microbiome sequencing data. *PeerJ* 6:e4600. doi: 10.7717/peerj.4600

Cox, M. J., Ege, M. J., and von Mutius, E. (2019). "The lung microbiome," in *European Respiratory Society* eds M. J. Cox, M. J. Ege, and E. von Mutius (Lausanne: European Respiratory Society).

Cuthbertson, L., Craven, V., Bingle, L., Cookson, W. O. C. M., Everard, M. L., and Moffatt, M. F. (2017). The impact of persistent bacterial bronchitis on the pulmonary microbiome of children. *PLoS One* 12:e0190075. doi: 10.1371/journal.pone.0190075

Cuthbertson, L., Felton, I., James, P., Cox, M. J., Bilton, D., Schelenz, S., et al. (2020). The fungal airway microbiome in cystic fibrosis and non-cystic fibrosis bronchiectasis. *J. Cystic Fibros* 20, 295–302. doi: 10.1016/j.jcf.2020.05.013

de Steenhuijsen Piters, W. A., Heinonen, S., Hasrat, R., Bunsow, E., Smith, B., Suarez-Arrabal, M., et al. (2016). Nasopharyngeal microbiota, host transcriptome, and disease severity in children with respiratory syncytial virus infection. *Am. J. Respir. Crit. Care Med.* 194, 1104–1115. doi: 10.1164/rccm.201602-0220OC

Duvallet, C., Gibbons, S. M., Gurry, T., Irizarry, R. A., and Alm, E. J. (2017). Meta-analysis of gut microbiome studies identifies disease-specific and shared responses. *Nat. Commun.* 8:1784. doi: 10.1038/s41467-017-01973-8

Edgar, R. C. (2010). Search and clustering orders of magnitude faster than BLAST. *Bioinformtaics* 26, 2460–2461.

Edgar, R. C., Haas, B. J., Clemente, J. C., Qunice, C., and Knight, R. (2011). UCHIME improves sensitivity and speed of chimera detection. *Bioinformatics* 27, 2194–2200.

Emerson, J., Rosenfeld, M., McNamara, S., Ramsey, B., and Gibson, R. L. (2002). *Pseudomonas aeruginosa* and other predictors of mortality and morbidity in young children with cystic fibrosis. *Pediatr. Pulmonol.* 34, 91–100. doi: 10.1002/ppul.10127

Gibbons, S. M., Duvallet, C., and Alm, E. J. (2018). Correcting for batch effects in case-control microbiome studies. *PLoS Comput. Biol.* 14:e1006102. doi: 10.1371/journal.pcbi.1006102

Grimwood, K., and Chang, A. B. (2015). Long-term effects of pneumonia in young children. *Pneumonia* 6, 101–114. doi: 10.15172/pneu.2015.6/671

Hampton, T. H., Green, D. M., Cutting, G. R., Morrison, H. G., Sogin, M. L., Gifford, A. H., et al. (2014). The microbiome in pediatric cystic fibrosis patients: the role of shared environment suggests a window of intervention. *Microbiome* 2:14. doi: 10.1186/2049-2618-2-14

Huang, Y. J., and Lynch, S. V. (2011). The emerging relationship between the airway microbiota and chronic respiratory disease: clinical implications. *Expert. Rev. Respir. Med.* 5, 809–821. doi: 10.1586/ers.11.76

Jari, O., Blanchet, F. G., Friendly, M., Kindt, R., Legendre, P., McGlinn, D., et al. (2015). *Vegan: Community Ecology Package.* R package version 2.2-1.

Kelly, M. S., Surette, M. G., Smieja, M., Pernica, J. M., Rossi, L., Luinstra, K., et al. (2017). The nasopharyngeal microbiota of children with respiratory infections in Botswana. *Pediatr. Infect. Dis. J.* 36, e211–e218. doi: 10.1097/INF.0000000000001607

Kim, B., Lee, E., Lee, M., Kang, M., Yoon, J., Cho, H., et al. (2017). Different functional genes of upper airway microbiome associated with natural course of childhood asthma. *Allergy* 73, 644–652. doi: 10.1111/all.13331

Langevin, S., Pichon, M., Smith, E., Morrison, J., Bent, Z., Green, R., et al. (2017). Early nasopharyngeal microbial signature associated with severe influenza in children: a retrospective pilot study. *J. Gen. Virol.* 98, 2425–2437. doi: 10.1099/jgv.0.000920

Li, J., Hao, C., Ren, L., Xiao, Y., Wang, J., and Qin, X. (2016). Data mining of lung microbiota in cystic fibrosis patients. *PLoS One*:11:e0164510 doi: 10.1371/journal.pone.0164510

Lu, Z., Dai, W., Liu, Y., Zhou, Q., Wang, H., Li, D., et al. (2017). The alteration of nasopharyngeal and oropharyngeal microbiota in children with MPP and non-MPP. *Genes* 8:380. doi: 10.3390/genes8120380

Luna, P. N., Hasegawa, K., Ajami, N. J., Espinola, J. A., Henke, D. M., Petrosino, J. F., et al. (2018). The association between anterior nares and nasopharyngeal microbiota in infants hospitalized for bronchiolitis. *Microbiome* 6:2. doi: 10.1186/s40168-017-0385-0

Man, W. H., de Steenhuijsen Piters, W. A., Wouter, A. A., and Bogaert, D. (2017). The microbiota of the respiratory tract: gatekeeper to respiratory health. *Nat. Rev. Microbiol.* 15:259. doi: 10.1038/nrmicro.2017.14

Marsh, R. L., Kaestli, M., Chang, A. B., Binks, M. J., Pope, C. E., Hoffman, L. R., et al. (2016). The microbiota in bronchoalveolar lavage from young children with chronic lung disease includes taxa present in both the oropharynx and nasopharynx. *Microbiome* 4:37. doi: 10.1186/s40168-016-0182-1

Marsh, R., Nelson, M. T., Pope, C. E., Leach, A. J., Hoffman, L. R., Chang, A. B., et al. (2018). How low can we go? The implications of low bacterial load in respiratory microbiota studies. *Pneumonia* 10:7. doi: 10.1186/s41479-018-0051-8

Nearing, J. T., Douglas, G. M., Hayes, M., MacDonald, J., Desai, D. K., Allward, N. E., et al. (2021). Microbiome differential abundance methods produce disturbingly different results across 38 datasets. *bioRxiv* [Preprint]. doi: 10.1101/2021.05.10.443486

Pedregosa, F., Varoquaux, G., Gramfort, A., Michel, V., Thirion, B., Grisel, O., et al. (2011). Scikit-learn: machine learning in Python. *J. Mach. Learn. Res.* 12, 2825–2830.

Perez-Losada, M., Crandall, K. A., and Freishtat, R. J. (2016). Two sampling methods yield distinct microbial signatures in the nasopharynges of asthmatic children. *Microbiome* 4:25. doi: 10.1186/s40168-016-0170-5

Pettigrew, M. M., Gent, J. F., Kong, Y., Wade, M., Gansebom, S., Bramley, A. M., et al. (2016). Association of sputum microbiota profiles with severity of community-acquired pneumonia in children. *BMC Infect. Dis.* 16:317. doi: 10.1186/s12879-016-1670-4

Pillarisetti, N., Broderick, D., Ainsworth, A., Mulholland, A., Wagner Mackenzie, B., Middleton, D., et al. (2019). The airway microbiota in children newly diagnosed with bronchiectasis largely retains its diversity. *Eur. Respir. J.* 54:1900704. doi: 10.1183/13993003.00704-2019

Quast, C., Pruesse, E., Yilmaz, P., Gerken, J., Schweer, T., Yarza, P., et al. (2012). The SILVA ribosomal RNA gene database project: improved data processing and web-based tools. *Nucleic Acids Res.* 41, D590–D596. doi: 10.1093/nar/gks1219

R Core Team (2019). *R: A Language and Environment for Statistical Computing*, Vienna, Austria.

Ritchie, A. I., and Singanayagam, A. (2020). Metagenomic characterization of the respiratory microbiome: a pièce de résistance. *Am. J. Respir. Crit. Care Med.* 3, 321–322. doi: 10.1164/rccm.202005-1686ed

Ronchetti, K., Tame, J., Paisey, C., Thia, L. P., Doull, I., Howe, R., et al. (2018). The CF-Sputum Induction Trial (CF-SpIT) to assess lower airway bacterial sampling in young children with cystic fibrosis: a prospective internally controlled interventional trial. *Lancet Respir. Med.* 6, 461–471. doi: 10.1016/S2213-2600(18)30171-1

Ruokolainen, L., Paalanen, L., Karkman, A., Laatikainen, T., Hertzen, L., Vlasoff, T., et al. (2017). Significant disparities in allergy prevalence and microbiota between the young people in Finnish and Russian Karelia. *Clin. Exp. Allergy* 47, 665–674. doi: 10.1111/cea.12895

Sakwinska, O., Bastic Schmid, V., Berger, B., Bruttin, A., Keitel, K., Lepage, M., et al. (2014). Nasopharyngeal microbiota in healthy children and pneumonia patients. *J. Clin. Microbiol.* 52, 1590–1594. doi: 10.1128/JCM.03280-13

Schloss, P. D., Westcott, S. L., Ryabin, T., Hall, J. R., Hartmann, M., Hollister, E. B., et al. (2009). Introducing mothur: open-source, platform-independent, community-supported software for describing and comparing microbial communities. *Appl. Environ. Microbiol.* 75, 7537–7541. doi: 10.1128/AEM.01541-09

Segata, N., Izard, J., Waldron, L., Gevers, D., Miropolsky, L., Garrett, W. S., et al. (2011). Metagenomic biomarker discovery and explanation. *Genome Biol.* 12:R60. doi: 10.1186/gb-2011-12-6-r60

Sokolova, M., Japkowicz, N., and Szpakowicz, S. (2006). "*Beyond accuracy, F-score and ROC: a family of discriminant measures for performance evaluation*", in *Proceedings of the Australasian Joint Conference On Artificial Intelligence*. Vol 4304 (Berlin: Springer).

Teo, S. M., Mok, D., Pham, K., Kusel, M., Serralha, M., Troy, N., et al. (2015). The infant nasopharyngeal microbiome impacts severity of lower respiratory infection and risk of asthma development. *Cell Host Microbe* 17, 704–715. doi: 10.1016/j.chom.2015.03.008

van der Gast, C., Cuthbertson, L., Rogers, G. B., Pope, C., Marsh, R. L., Redding, G. J., et al. (2014). Three clinically distinct chronic pediatric airway infections share a common core microbiota. *Ann. Am. Thorac. Soc.* 11, 1039–1048. doi: 10.1513/AnnalsATS.201312-456OC

Wagner Mackenzie, B., Waite, D. W., Hoggard, M., Douglas, R. G., Taylor, M. W., and Biswas, K. (2017). Bacterial community collapse: a meta-analysis of the sinonasal microbiota in chronic rhinosinusitis. *Environ. Microbiol.* 19, 381–392. doi: 10.1111/1462-2920.13632

Waite, D. W., and Taylor, M. W. (2014). Characterizing the avian gut microbiota: membership, driving influences, and potential function. *Front. Microbiol.* 5:223. doi: 10.3389/fmicb.2014.00223

Wallen, Z. D. (2021). Comparison study of differential abundance testing methods using two large Parkinson disease gut microbiome datasets derived from 16S amplicon sequencing. *BMC Bioinform.* 22:265. doi: 0.1186/s12859-021-04193-6

Wang, H., Dai, W., Qiu, C., Li, S., Wang, W., Xu, J., et al. (2016). *Mycoplasma pneumoniae* and *Streptococcus pneumoniae* caused different microbial structure and correlation network in lung microbiota. *J. Thorac. Dis.* 8, 1316–1322. doi: 10.21037/jtd.2016.04.63

Wickham, H. (2016). *ggplot2: Elegant Graphics For Data Analysis*. Berlin: Springer.

Williamson, K. M., Wagner, B. D., Robertson, C. E., Johnson, E. J., Zemanick, E. T., and Harris, J. K. (2017). Impact of enzymatic digestion on bacterial community composition in CF airway samples. *PeerJ* 5:e3362. doi: 10.7717/peerj.3362

Wylie, K. M. (2017). The virome of the human respiratory tract. *Clin. Chest Med.* 38, 11–19. doi: 10.1016/j.ccm.2016.11.001

Yi, H., Yong, D., Lee, K., Cho, Y., and Chun, J. (2014). Profiling bacterial community in upper respiratory tracts. *BMC Infect. Dis.* 14:583. doi: 10.1186/s12879-014-0583-3

Zemanick, E. T., Wagner, B. D., Robertson, C. E., Ahrens, R., Chmiel, J. F., Clancy, J. P., et al. (2017). Airway microbiota across age and disease spectrum in cystic fibrosis. *Eur. Respir. J.* 50:1700832. doi: 10.1183/13993003.00832-2017

Zemanick, E. T., Wagner, B. D., Robertson, C. E., Stevens, M. J., Szefler, S. J., Accurso, F. J., et al. (2015). Assessment of airway microbiota and inflammation in cystic fibrosis using multiple sampling methods. *Ann. Am. Thorac. Soc.* 12, 221–229. doi: 10.1513/AnnalsATS.201407-310OC

Zhang, W. Z. (2020). The origins of COPD: sometimes the journey matters more than the destination. *Am. J. Respir. Crit. Care Med.* 202, 159–161. doi: 10.1164/rccm.202004-0959ed

21

Revamping of Chronic Respiratory Diseases in Low and Middle-Income Countries

Ling-Hui Zeng[1], Musaddique Hussain[2], Shahzada Khurram Syed[3], Malik Saadullah[4], Qurratulain Jamil[5], Ali M. Alqahtani[6], Taha Alqahtani[6], Nadia Akram[2], Imran Ahmad Khan[2], Sajida Parveen[2], Tehreem Fayyaz[2], Mobeen Fatima[2], Saira Shaukat[2], Najia Shabbir[2], Mehwish Fatima[2], Aisha Kanwal[2], Muhammad Qasim Barkat[1] and Ximei Wu[1*]*

[1] Department of Pharmacology, Zhejiang University City College, Hangzhou, China, [2] Department of Pharmacology, Faculty of Pharmacy, The Islamia University of Bahawalpur, Bahawalpur, Pakistan, [3] Department of Basic Medical Sciences, School of Health Sciences, University of Management and Technology Lahore, Lahore, Pakistan, [4] Department of Pharmaceutical Chemistry, Government College University, Faisalabad, Pakistan, [5] Department of Pharmacy Practice, Faculty of Pharmacy, The Islamia University of Bahawalpur, Bahawalpur, Pakistan, [6] Department of Pharmacology, College of Pharmacy, King Khalid University, Abha, Saudi Arabia

***Correspondence:**
Musaddique Hussain
musaddique.hussain@iub.edu.pk
Ximei Wu
xiwu@zju.edu.cn

Low- and middle-income countries (LMICs) endure an asymmetrically high burden of worldwide disease and death caused by chronic respiratory diseases (CRDs), i.e., asthma, emphysema, bronchiectasis, and post-tuberculosis lung disease (PTLD). CRDs are firmly related with indigence, infectious diseases, and other non-communicable diseases (NCDs) and add to complex multi-disease with great impact on the lives and livelihood of those affected. The pertinence of CRDs to health and demographic wellbeing is relied upon to increment in the long time ahead, as expectations of life rise and the contending dangers of right on time youth mortality and irresistible infections level. The WHO has distinguished the counteraction and control of NCDs as an earnest improvement issue and crucial for the sustainable development goals (SDSs) by 2030. In this review, we center on CRDs in LMICs. We examine the early life roots of CRDs, challenges in their avoidance, identification and administration in LMICs, and the pathways to resolve for accomplish valid widespread wellbeing inclusion.

Keywords: asthma, COPD, tuberculosis, bronchiectasis, emphysema–pneumonia–bronchiolitis–smoking–fibrosis–histiocytosis

INTRODUCTION

Non-communicable diseases (NCDs) are a vital root of morbidity and mortality. In low- and middle-income countries (LMICs) (1), round about 70% of worldwide deaths are reported from NCDs with an elevated threat of dying (2). The purpose of the Sustainable Development Goals (SDGs) of the United Nations is to overcome the threat of precocious fatalities from NCDs by a third by 2030 (3). The ordinary and relatively ignored NCDs that twain the life cycle are chronic respiratory diseases (CRDs), such as asthma, chronic obstructive pulmonary disease (COPD), bronchiectasis, and post-tuberculosis lung disease (PTLD). They are often related with the high level of patient and healthcare prices, morbidity, and threat of mortality by reason of constant manifestation; activity, limitations, and Irregular aggravation need intense care. They inadequately influence poor people in all countries, but mainly in LMICs where assets for research, prevention, and management are rare (4). The recent Lancet Commission on injuries has helped to raise the issues of justice and probity for the poor people of the whole world (5). This evaluation fixates on continual breathing ailment in LMICs. Even though, dearth and social destitution are worldwide matters, we accept that. People who lived in LMICs encountered a specifically hard coalition of destroying early life and environmental exhibition, tasking social and political interpretation, and poor access to prime trait health facilities. We talk about the formative years of CRDs in LMICs and possible strategies to the obstruction of the disease. We propose tactics for research and clinical capacity reinforcement, for both the prevention and management of CRDs. We propose tactics for research and clinical capacity reinforcement, for both the obstruction and regulation of CRDs, and suggest pathways to a solution that would impart to attain international tasks for health including to overcome morbidity and inopportune mortality and attaining worldwide health coverage.

EARLY LIFE ORIGINS OF CRD

Evidence that has mainly been received in high-income countries (HICs) shows that the *in-utero*, infant, child, adults, and surrounding conditions are extremely important for lung development, with preschool lung function, and early adult lung functions, into at least the seventh decade of life (6, 7). Even though, related data from LMICs are rare, the same association probably holds true in these countries (8). Common to both settings are detrimental *in-utero* and early childhood exposures. These can disturb lung development such that individuals fail to reach an optimal peak in early adulthood, with increased CRDs later in life. In LMICs, the increased pervasion and severity of many of these harmful early life exposures might explain the lower lung volumes observed in asymptomatic non-smoking age- and height-matched adults in HICs and in many sub-Saharan African settings (9). Epidemiological evidence is provided to show the association of prenatal or perinatal exposure to air pollutants with various adverse birth outcomes, such as preterm birth, lower birth weight, and lung developmental defects. Interventions to mitigate early life exposures might be crucial for the prevention of CRDs in LMICs (7, 10–12), because of the potential value of *in-utero* and adult lung function and early childhood exposures, the high incidence of these negative effects on one's wellbeing, and the fact that they are so common. In early life exposures and treatments in LMICs, the importance of exposures in the prevention of CRDs may be critical in the least developed countries.

In-utero Exposures

Tobacco smoking changes lung structure and function and affects the immune system of fetus (6). A health study in South Africa—one of first births cohorts in Sub-Saharan Africa-reports, infants of third mothers who smoked during pregnancy had lower tidal volume and higher lung clearance indices at age 6 weeks than infants of non-smoking women (13, 14). Depression, prenatal stress, bad living conditions and intimate partner, and neighborhood violence are issues faced by women around the world. Maternal stress and depression are negatively connected with measures of neonatal health and positively connected with respiratory morbidity in children (15, 16). Maternal alcohol exposure during pregnancy negatively affects lung function at 6 weeks. This effect disappears by 1 year (8, 13). The number of HIV in women of childbearing age is high in many LMICs. The introduction of test and treat approaches to combination antiretroviral treatment (cART) and dedicated programs to prevent mother-based-to-child transmission have decreased rates of perinatal infection (17). Preterm birth is related to increased breathing and lung-related signs of sickness. Premature births occur in 10% of all live births around the world, 80% of these are in LMICs (18, 19).

Childhood Exposures

Maternal smoking and environmental tobacco smoke (ETS) exposure influence infant lung development and are associated with childhood upper and lower respiratory tract infection, wheezing, or asthma (20). Bacterial and viral infections are common in LMICs in early childhood. Some of the most common viral pathogens respiratory syncytial virus, rhinovirus, adenovirus, and influenza A are detected in children with acute lower respiratory tract infections in LMICs (21). A common and serious illness, which affects children of all age groups, is community-acquired pneumonia (22). In LMICs, infectious, maternal, neonatal, and nutritional diseases are still major contributors to disease burden. By contrast, in upper middle income and HICs, NCDs are predominate (23). In LMICs, pneumonia is the major root of mortality in children with an estimated incidence of 0.2–0.3 episodes per-child year (24). In Sub-Saharan Africa, lower respiratory infection in early childhood is an independent risk factor for reduced lung function by 1 year of age; however, pneumococcal vaccine is still only available to ~50% of children around the world, despite its introduction two decades ago (13, 25).

Tuberculosis in the Lungs

Children under the age of 15 account for 11% of new cases of tuberculosis worldwide (26), and pediatricians with LMICs regularly record a high burden of post-tuberculosis squeal, such as bronchiectasis and lung destruction, in children who successfully complete care (27).

HIV Infection That Lasts a Long Time

In LMICs, a large number of children who were initially born with vertically transmitted HIV are now approaching adulthood (28). These long-term survivors have a high prevalence of CRDs, such as bronchiectasis, obliterans bronchiolitis, and reduced lung function (27, 28). Deficits are more serious in people who have been diagnosed late and started antiretroviral treatment late (29).

Dietary Advice

Maternal and childhood malnutrition are becoming more common in LMICs (30), resulting in fetal growth problems. Restriction, stunting, waste, and food isolation are also examples of nutrient isolation. Not only children with deficiencies, but also those who are overweight or obese (31, 32) based on the limited information available. It seems that *in-utero* early childhood, hunger has a negative impact on lung formation that continues into adulthood adolescence. Obesity has also been linked to long-term airway disease in LMICs, it is been linked to asthma and in HICs (33).

Pollution of the Air

Indoor and outdoor air exposures can have an effect on a child's lung health. The connection between the two early childhood biomass fuel exposure and lung development is unknown. Delayed penetration of clean burning stoves into Guatemalan households (child age 18–57 vs. <6 months) was linked to lower lung growth rates (34). Results from a clean stoves intervention sample in rural Malawi revealed a minor but statistically important gap (0.2 Z scores) in the forced vital capacity (FVC) of children from households who had previously received a clean burning stove (35). In HICs, increases in outdoor air emissions over time have been linked with improved lung function (36). There has been a connection between diesel exposure and bad asthma results, and this may be especially true for children. Significant in LMICs, where trucks are often in poor condition maintained, unrestricted petrol, and driving in close quarter's proximity of human settlement (37–39).

Direction of Solutions

In order to prevent CRDs in LMICs, attention must be paid to prenatal and early childhood exposures, which influence the development of the disease. The evolution and health of the lungs over the course of a person's life, many of these exposures can be regulated for public health reasons. Interventions and poverty among mothers are at the root of the problem. Maternal care programs must be reinforced to preserve the physical and mental health of women of childbearing age and mothers, enhance access to high-quality prenatal care, and enhance maternal education on children's nutrition and immunization. Programs that assist HIV-positive mothers in preventing perinatal transmission and providing early HIV testing for their children must be continued. We recommend that early child health programs should be enhanced, with safe access to high-quality nutrition and effective vaccination. Given the anticipated negative consequences of air pollution on lung development, we recommend that endeavor to enhance changes in cooking and ventilation techniques should be continued as a potentially low-cost plan for improving child health (40). Political interventions, such as taxes and successful advertisement regulation legislation, would be necessary to reduce smoking exposure; it will most likely be necessary for cigarettes, nicotine, and indoor and outdoor air pollution (41). Such efforts could be particularly useful due to increased marketing and intervention. LMICs are becoming more vulnerable with public health efforts by tobacco, alcohol, food, inadequate national regulatory mechanisms (4), and soda industries. Many of these healthcare system and policy changes are large in nature and have the potential to help people with diseases other than CRDs. However, without them, the considerable burden of CRDs in LMICs is likely to persist.

CHRONIC OBSTRUCTIVE PULMONARY DISEASE

Chronic obstructive pulmonary disease afflicted 212.33 million adults worldwide in 2019, according to the global burden of disease figures (42). Primary record on the worldwide burden of ailment shows significant variability in the prevalence, reasons, scientific presentation, and mortality among and inside LMICs (43). These discrepancies are mostly due to a lack of spirometry and epidemiological evidence, but they are exacerbated by disagreements about the concept of COPD. For example, it is unknown if fixed percentages, percent expected cutoffs, or lower limit of natural boundaries should be used to distinguish irregular outcomes, what reference ranges should be used for estimation standardization, and whether all patients with fixed airflow obstruction should be considered COPD (9). Despite this problem, community-based evidence shows that airway obstruction is common in Latin America, between 6 and 20% of people are obstructed (44–46). In Sub-Saharan Africa, the rate is 5–24% (47–50). LMICs are thought to be responsible for 71% of global COPD strain, 84% of global COPD deaths, and 84% of global COPD disability-adjusted life year (DALY) around the world (42). Even though, tobacco smoking is still a significant risk factor for airway blockage in LMICs, between a third and a fifth of instances occur in persons who have never smoked, and a significant fraction of these instances are likely connected to biomass usage for cooking and heating, particularly among women (51–55).

The Prognosis

In LMICs, high degrees of under-diagnosis and misdiagnosis of COPD are determined (56, 57). Results from recent national COPD surveys show that more than one-third of the world's population suffers from this disease, 80% of COPD cases detected by spirometry go undiagnosed in normal clinical care (58). Individuals with a minor illness and no prior experience with exacerbations or admissions are less likely to result in a positive outcome. Ethnicity, socioeconomic background, and the lack of interaction with healthcare providers have also been identified as a risk factor for under-diagnosis, suggesting that broader socioeconomic determinants are also important (56–58). As previously mentioned, inadequate worldwide access to spirometry for diagnosis is likely a major stumbling block.

Management

Non-pharmacological therapies are often used in the treatment of smoking-related COPD (supported smoking abstinence, pneumococcal and influenza vaccination, and pulmonary rehabilitation). In addition to pharmacological treatment with inhaled therapies, short-acting beta agonist (SABAs), long-acting beta agonists (LABAs), and short-acting and long-acting muscarinic antagonists, inhaled corticosteroids (ICs) according to the severity of the disease. In LMICs, these measures are underutilized. A population-based survey in Latin America shows that just half of the smokers received medical advice, according to a new study. A quarter were given some kind of respiratory drug, and access to the influenza vaccine was ineffective (59, 60). According to the Public Use Micro data Area (PUMA) survey results, the most commonly used treatment in primary care was SABA-inhaled treatment, with long-acting bronchodilators (LABA) and ICs being used less frequently (61). There have been no clinical trials to determine the best pharmacotherapy for non-smoking-related COPD, such as disease caused by biomass pollutant peril in LMICs, which could vary from those prescribed for smoking-related COPD.

Direction of Solution

Better epidemiological evidence, correct diagnosis, and adequate clinical treatment for COPD in LMICs are all instantly needed (62, 63). Increasing consciousness among patients and clinicians, using licensed standardized protocols for diagnosis and treatment, greater access to spirometry, expanded use of inhaled treatments, improved education for both patients and healthcare providers, and better access to long-term follow-up are some of the interventions that could be needed. COPD, on the other hand, is more common in HICs that has been linked to a variety of systemic consequences, such as cardiovascular disorder, malignancy, osteoporosis, stress, and anxiety (64). As a result, it is important to see if the same results are observed in LMICs, because if they are, programs to overcome this multi-morbidity would almost certainly be required. Increasing access to non-pharmacological treatments that are less expensive, such as smoking abstinence and pulmonary therapy, should be prioritized and tailored to unique cultural environment (65). Smoking is also the leading cause of the COPD worldwide and attempts to transfer lessons learned in HICs about public health and policy approaches to control to LMICs, in order to minimize both direct and passive exposure, would take continued long-term help. In both high- and low-income environments, data on the risks, existence, consequences, and treatment of non-smoking associated airway obstruction are required.

ASTHMA

Asthma is the most ordinary CRD in the world, influencing 262.4 million people in 2019 (42), with LMICs leading 96% of asthma-related worldwide deaths and 84% of DAIY worldwide. Asthma-related diseases and deaths, on the other hand, are entirely avoidable (66).

The Prognosis

In LMICs, the Global Initiative for Asthma (GINA) recommends using a syndromic approach to asthma diagnosis. However, it emphasizes the significance of using peak flow control or spirometry with reversibility checking to measure variations in air flow for validation (67). In LMICs, access to these equipment is limited, substantially limiting diagnostic capabilities (68). In LMICs, asthma is usually under-diagnosed in children and adults, and when it is diagnosed, it is generally more severe (69, 70).

Management

Inhaled corticosteroids are used to treat chronic asthma and improve symptom control and lowering hospital visits and death rates (71). For adolescents and adults in therapy stages 1 and 2, GINA now recommends using inhalers containing ICs and the rapid-onset LABA formoterol as needed (67, 72). Large clinical trials show that this approach is equivalent to or better than using regular ICs with as-needed short-acting 2 agonists (SABAs) for minimizing the threat of acute exacerbations, and that it uses a much lower dose of ICs with no clinically significant difference in symptom control, at least in teenagers and adults over the age of 12 (73–76). Similarly, in moderate-to-extreme asthma, using a mixture of ICs and formoterol for maintenance and reliever treatment decreases severe exacerbations compared to using standard ICs and LABA therapy with a SABA reliever (77). For this reason, if combined ICs and bronchodilator preparations are not available or reasonable for moderate asthma, separate ICs can be used whenever a SABA is taken. Despite these recommendations, ICs are often under-prescribed, inaccessible, or unaffordable to patients and people with asthma in LMICs, who rely on inhaled bronchodilators alone, or take oral bronchodilators Instead, use salbutamol, theophylline, or prednisolone preparations (68, 70, 78, 79). The ability of the healthcare system to provide long-term follow-up and prescription titration for symptom monitoring is limited and patient and clinician awareness of the need for chronic treatment could be inadequate, with 52–76% loss of follow-up seen within 1 year in pilot projects in China, Benin, and Sudan (70, 78, 79).

Direction of Solutions

Global asthma treatment methods for LMICs may be tailored for national use (67). The implementation will necessitate healthcare workers with advice and training a number of cadres to increase clinical identification of asthma, to encourage the use of syndromic identification, and to ensure that adequate preventer treatment are prescribed appropriately. A major need exists for improved access to diagnostic tools (peak flow meters and spirometry) and training in their use. Similarly, access to affordable quality-assured asthma medicines listed on the WHO A list of essential medicines (panel 1) is needed. Education would be necessary to ensure the safety of both patients and caregivers. The proper use of inhalers, with a focus on the value of ICs and inhaler technique preparation and spacer to improve drug delivery in adults and infants will be needed. Healthcare facilities that can accommodate in LMICs, asthma follow-up is uncommon, but it is critical for avoiding over-reliance on emergency care, maintaining long-term symptom management, and reducing morbidity and mortality.

BRONCHIECTASIS

In recent years, the confirmed incidence of non-cystic fibrosis bronchiectasis in HICs has increased to 566 per 100,000 (80), with disease prevalence and severity is linked to rising age and female gender (81). While there are few epidemiological statistics on bronchiectasis in LMICs (82), the few data that are available show that the prevalence, reasons, and risk factors for bronchiectasis vary significantly to those in most HICs, with more post-infectious disease, a correlation with HIV infection, a greater burden of acute disease in younger adults, and distinctions in colonizing or infecting microbiology (80, 83, 84).

The Prognosis

In LMICs, bronchiectasis is difficult to diagnose. The clinical appearance is close to see in people in HIC with persistent cough and sputum production in adults, and children's inability to succeed is often linked with repeated infections and frequent, extreme respiratory symptoms. In several low-resource environments, however, patients with tuberculosis that present with a high tuberculosis rate, these symptoms are mainly managed as tuberculosis suspects who have not been tested for underlying CRDs. The use of CT imaging as the gold standard diagnostic technique for bronchiectasis is highly recommended in international guidelines, but CT imaging is not applicable to the majority of people living in LMICs. There is evidence to justify the use of a simple chest x-ray for the diagnosis of bronchiectasis. Few recommendations advocate the use of a chest x-ray for the investigation in LMICs, with recurrent respiratory problems, in general.

Management

In HIC, management of bronchiectasis is becoming more individualized and based on addressing so-called treatable traits, with the use of airway clearing tools, vaccination against pneumococcal and influenza, treatment of organisms that are infecting or colonizing, and intercurrent fungal and non-tuberculosis mycobacterial disease needs early detection and active management (85). Individualized treatments are not readily available in LMICs, and no recommendations for the diagnosis and treatment of bronchiectasis in resource-poor settings have yet been established to our knowledge.

Direction of Solutions

In LMICs, more effective investigation and treatment methods for persistent cough in children and adults are required. Standardized protocols for decentralized treatment are needed, with an emphasis on programmatic interventions that are both practical and scalable (80). These recommendations must provide adequate inspection for active tuberculosis disease in environments with a high tuberculosis burden, but also recognition of underlying CRD when tuberculosis is ruled out. This will necessitate more seamless incorporation of tuberculosis care with other respiratory or surgical services. Healthcare staff is being educated on persistent productive cough is caused by bronchiectasis, to make this possible, usable and inexpensive diagnostic approaches in the absence of CT imaging are needed. In children in South Africa, patient-centered, low-cost tools, such as airway clearing, have been seen to be appropriate and efficient and should be optimized for use in LMICs (86). To advise population-level antibiotic guidelines, a better understanding of the microbiology of bronchiectasis in both children and adults is needed.

POST-TUBERCULOSIS LUNG DISEASE

Survivors of pulmonary tuberculosis, estimated to number 58 million worldwide so far (26), have a 2-to-4-fold chance of having persistently irregular spirometry (airway obstruction and poor FVC patterns) after tuberculosis treatment compared to those who have never had tuberculosis, Bronchitis, parenchymal cavitation and destruction, and fibrotic alteration are all common conditions (87–90). As seen on imaging, there is a lot of diversity in the world. Residual pathology's prevalence, variations, and severity, however, bronchiectasis or pathological spirometry is believed to be the cause, more than a third of tuberculosis patients had pulmonary tuberculosis survivors (90–92). Long-term persistent respiratory complications, repeated respiratory exacerbations, and increased lung function loss are all risks for people with PTLD. Survivors of tuberculosis are at a high risk of recurrence, reactivation, or reinfection of tuberculosis disease (93). Chronic respiratory problems, on the other hand, put them in jeopardy of being subjected to irrational and unjustified tuberculosis retreatment (94), subjecting them to additional drug side effects, stigma, and healthcare costs are also factors to consider (95). Adult tuberculosis (TB) survivors have a nearly 3-fold higher death rate than the general population, however, the link between PTLD and mortality is uncertain (96). Moreover, 1 million of the 10 million yearly occurrences of acute pulmonary TB in the world occur in children (26), but little is known regarding the burden and consequences of PTLD in this group.

The Prognosis

Spirometry or chest x-ray imaging abnormalities may indicate PTLD, but these procedures are not regularly performed after tuberculosis treatment has been completed and they may not be available at the point-of-care in decentralized TB treatment programs. As a result, the majority of people with residual PTLD are discharged without a diagnosis or a plan for follow-up treatment in LMICs (91). The identification of recurrent TB in people with PTLD can be difficult: nucleic acid amplification tests' sensitivity is lowered in TB survivors, and the effectiveness of screening methods, such as the WHO symptom screen and chest radiography in individuals with PTLD, is unknown (97, 98).

Management

Existing international and national TB recommendations pay little attention to post-tuberculosis morbidity, and there are no evidence-based guidelines for the diagnosis and therapy of PTLD in LMICs (99, 100). Existing strategies are based on COPD and bronchiectasis treatment models and include cannabis and smoking education, which are prevalent co-exposures in patients with TB. Exercises to clear the airways, vaccines according to national standards, and the use of inhaled bronchodilators for reversible airway blockage are all recommended (101). Because of the elevated risk of chronic mycobacterial disease and other respiratory infections, ICs should not be used (102–104). Rehabilitation of the lungs can aid in the enhancement of one's quality of life (105). Even though sputum culture is the gold standard device for the conclusion of recurrent tuberculosis infection and medicates vulnerability testing in this gather, culture is regularly not accessible in LMICs and is not achievable in young children. More research into the effectiveness of TB screening and diagnostic techniques in pulmonary TB survivors and individuals with PTLD is needed.

Direction of Solutions

Following the conclusion of TB treatment, pulmonary TB survivors can be screened for persistent lung pathology, with the goal of continuing to monitor and intervene. However, given the limited resources available, more information is needed in LMICs to support choices on how this should be done, which patients might benefit from continued follow-up, and before implementing this strategy, and the efficacy and cost-effectiveness of healthcare treatment for this population. In addition, clear evidence-based recommendations are required for the prognosis and management of those who are not detected at the end of therapy but re-appear with persistent respiratory problems years later. Improved methods to the identification of recurrent TB illness will necessitate the integration of TB and CRD services in order to enhance PTLD diagnosis and management (106). We propose that any packages of post-TB treatment should also address the larger cardiovascular, psychological, and socioeconomic morbidities that tuberculosis survivors experience (107).

STRENGTHENING OF HEALTHCARE PROGRAMS

Strong health infrastructure, capable of delivering reliable and responsive care throughout the life cycle would be critical for the prevention and treatment of CRDs and NCDs in LMICs and must include the availability of comprehensive maternity care. The WHO has identified six important building elements that must be addressed in the development of these systems: service delivery, health workforce, health information systems, availability to key drugs and vaccinations, finances, and leadership or governance are all important factors to consider (**Figure 1**) (108). Numerous key flaws have been recognized in those regions with respect to respiration care in LMICs. The availability of healthcare surveillance data for respiratory diseases other than tuberculosis is limited (109), limiting the potential of countries to recognize and plan for the healthcare needs of their inhabitants. There are no reliable metrics for monitoring and evaluating priority CRD programs. National guidelines for the management of CRDs are also scarce, with just 64% of countries having them according to the seventh NCD national capability study 2019 (110).

Spirometry and imaging are important diagnostic tools, which are insufficient, in 2019, just 45% of primary care institutions had peak flow or spirometry, compared to 88% for blood glucose testing (111). Preventive interventions, such as the quality of vaccinations, dietary assistance, and smoking abstinence services is inadequate (112). Most importantly, the healthcare workforce is badly equipped to provide respiratory care, with a scarcity of respiratory specialists (113–116), and the majority of care is provided at the primary care level by untrained nurses (117). In the following paragraphs, solutions to some of these challenges are described.

Integrated Delivery of CRD Care

In LMICs, front-line primary care workers are required to offer preventative and curative treatment to both children and adults for infectious and non-infectious illnesses. As a result, CRD services must be well-integrated into larger services and tailored to local requirements. To this purpose, many integrated care techniques have been developed for use in LMICs (118, 119). The WHO Practical Approach to Lung Disease (PAL), which was designed in part to enhance TB case discovery, was one of the first models to focus only on respiratory disorders. These were followed by tools with a more broader reach, such as the WHO Package of Non-communicable Disease Interventions (PEN) (120). Children, adolescents, and adults can benefit from the WHO's Integrated Management of Adolescent and Adult Illness (IMAI) (121) and Package of Care Kit (PACK) (122). For example, PACK offers a decision-making tool that may be used in a variety of clinical scenarios and is accessible in both print and computer formats (123–126). It incorporates local management principles and evidence, is updated on a regular basis, and is backed up by case-based, interactive training on-site (122, 123). Qualitative results show that this integrated care strategy is successful in enhancing CRD services, such as asthma treatment, TB detection, and appropriate hospital referrals (127–129). We believe that in LMICs, respiratory and TB care should be closely connected. Patients with acute and CRD typically appear with exacerbating respiratory symptoms, and in TB-endemic areas, active TB illness is routinely investigated. However, if these tests come back negative, it is critical to examine other respiratory illnesses. Patients with PTLD after the end of TB therapy would benefit from clear and efficient integrated care pathways, as well. Finally, NCD programs in LMICs should think about incorporating palliative care support in their services. This is especially relevant for CRDs, which are typically incurable, progressive, and can cause painful symptoms like severe dyspnea. This type of incorporation would necessitate cultural understanding, personnel and patient education, the advancement of symptom management strategies, and access to opioid drugs (130).

Improving Medical Interface Accessibility

The funding of diagnostic instruments, such as spirometry and imaging, and training of clinical personnel on how to perform tests, maintain quality control, and appropriately interpret data are two specific difficulties in obtaining diagnostic technologies at the primary care level (131). Decentralization may be facilitated by advances in the creation of dependable and portable spirometry, ultrasonography, and chest x-ray equipment for community-based diagnosis, but services might be more sustainable if they are supported by education and access to equipment maintenance services (132). More advanced diagnostics, such as CT imaging, complex lung function testing, and bronchoscopy, will almost certainly remain the domain of tertiary centers in LMICs, but these tools are useful in the training and retention of specialists and the development of

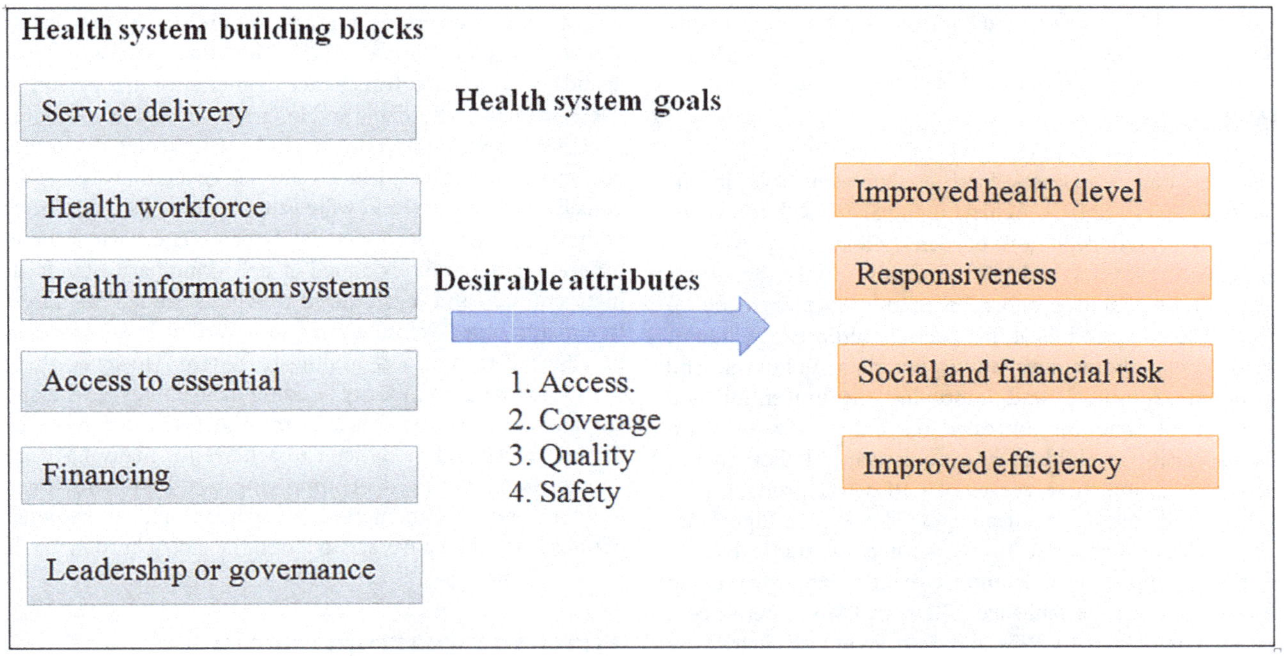

FIGURE 1 | WHO six building blocks of the health system, together with aims and desirable attributes.

research capacity, so some investment in their centralized use may be beneficial.

Enhancing Treatment Accessibility

Inhaled corticosteroids were commonly accessible in 19% of low-income countries in 2019, compared to 96% of HICs, and bronchodilators in 55 and 100%, respectively, despite the fact that numerous important respiratory drugs are on the WHO's list of essential medicines (panel 1). Even when they were accessible, these treatments were typically out of reach for people in LMICs. Despite being among the most cost-effective interventions for CRDs and relevant to the prevention and management of other NCDs, such as cardiovascular disease and cancer, access to non-pharmacological interventions, such as pulmonary rehabilitation and smoking cessation services, is insufficient in LMICs. There are few educational program aimed at improving self-management, promoting health literacy, and combating stigma. Access to these therapies requires immediate advocacy. In LMICs, there are significant data gaps regarding the cost-effectiveness of recently indicated therapies for respiratory disorders, such as ICS–formoterol therapy as needed (and on a frequent basis) in asthma and dual LAMA and LABA treatment in COPD. Rather than presuming unaffordability, the quality pharmacoeconomic analysis should influence plans for broadening the alternatives and tactics offered as necessary medications for respiratory disorders in LMICs. Efforts to adapt and incorporate non-pharmacological therapies into care programs will be necessary and strategies to ease the economical delivery of quality-controlled supplies of these drugs (133). Improving access begins with the establishment of a health staff that is capable of providing CRD services effectively and compassionately.

PRIORITIES FOR RESEARCH AND THE DEVELOPMENT OF RESEARCH CAPABILITIES

This review has uncovered a number of areas of ambiguity, which we have turned into research objectives for CRDs in LMICs (panel 2). These difficulties, however, cannot be solved without a robust critical mass of LMIC researchers. The American Thoracic Society/Pan African Thoracic Society's Methods course and the Structured Operational Research Training Initiative (SORT-IT) course, the Pan African Thoracic Society Methods in Epidemiologic, Clinical and Operations Research (PATS-MECOR) course in epidemiological, clinical, and operational research is an example of a successful respiratory-focused program that provides training and networking opportunities for research-interested individuals, clinicians from LMICs are needed to help enhance this competence. SORT-IT and PATS-MECOR both concentrate on clinical, epidemiological, and operational research, or the "science of doing better" (134, 135). Concept formulation, grant and protocol writing, quality-assured data gathering and analysis, and paper writing are all covered in detail in each session. Participants must meet numerous goals in order to advance, and substantial, hands-on mentoring is provided throughout. Over 1,000 participants from 90 countries contributed to a huge amount of published research that has influenced policy and practice in LMICs (134–139). Graduates have a proven track record of success in the workplace. Graduates have a great track record of staying in research after completing their courses (140–143) or could pursue a career as a course instructor (140–144).

CONCLUSION

Chronic respiratory diseases have a significant role in the burden of illness in LMICs. Achieving the SDGs will necessitate taking steps to reduce illness burdens *via* better prevention and treatment. Poverty reduction initiatives must be at the forefront of preventative efforts, with a particular focus on maternal nutrition and health, lowering airborne pollutants (tobacco smoke, home and atmospheric air pollution, and occupational exposures), and improving the prevention and management of severe or untreated respiratory diseases, such as TB, especially in children and adolescents. Policy actions aimed at addressing these causes of CRDs will produce both short-term and long-term advantages. However, a significant burden of illness is expected to persist, necessitating evidence-based therapy options to minimize continuing disease and death in persons with established CRDs. In LMICs, better data on the epidemiology of CRDs and associated risk factors are required. Many information gaps still exist, and extrapolating data from HICs risks ignoring the particular exposures, health system limits, and social and political factors that define illnesses in LMICs. Understanding the etiology of CRDs and patient outcomes in LMICs and developing diagnostic and treatment techniques that are possible, acceptable, and suitable for local settings, will require renewed efforts. These techniques should take into account heterogeneity both within and across nations. In a world where people are migrating at an increasing rate, the applicability of results from LMICs to groups that have been forced or choose to migrate to other regions of the world should be explored as well (145). The universal health coverage agenda provides a perfect chance to guarantee that persons with CRDs who have affordable and long-term access to adequate and effective diagnostic assessment and pharmacological and non-pharmacological therapy interventions—goals that are applicable globally. CRD services will gain benefit from integration with wider tuberculosis and NCD care. The balance between programmatic methods aimed at delivering basic standardized interventions and customized methods aimed at targeting treatments more accurately requires careful study and should be adjusted to the local healthcare system. However, this will need resources and capacity building in all contexts, with special emphasis directed to the healthcare system's most remote levels. This objective will be difficult to achieve for many LMICs, but it emphasizes the need of improving health systems, capacity building, and implementation research in realizing the potential of universal health coverage to lessen the global burden of CRDs.

AUTHOR CONTRIBUTIONS

MH, MS, NS, and SP: planning. NA, MB, and QJ: data compilation. L-HZ, MoF, AK, MeF, SS, AA, and SKS: writing. L-HZ, TF, AA, IK, TF, and XW: proof reading. All authors contributed to the article and approved the submitted version.

REFERENCES

The World Bank. *Low and Middle Income Countries*. The World Bank. Available online at: https://data.worldbank.org/country/XO

Bennett JE, Stevens GA, Mathers CD, Bonita R, Rehm J, Kruk ME. NCD countdown 2030: worldwide trends in non-communicable disease mortality and progress towards sustainable development goal target 3.4. *Lancet.* (2018) 392:1072–88. doi: 10.1016/S0140-6736(18)31992-5

Global Agenda. *Transforming our World: The 2030 Agenda for Sustainable Development.* New York, NY: Division for Sustainable Development Goals (2015).

Ezzati M, Pearson-Stuttard J, Bennett JE, Mathers CD. Acting on non-communicable diseases in low-and middle-income tropical countries. *Nature.* (2018) 559:507–16. doi: 10.1038/s41586-018-0306-9

Bukhman G, Mocumbi AO, Atun R, Becker AE, Bhutta Z, Binagwaho The lancet NCDI poverty commission: bridging a gap in universal health coverage for the poorest billion. *Lancet.* (2020) 396:991–1044. doi: 10.1016/S0140-6736(20)31907-3

Bush A. Lung development and aging. *Am Thorac Soc.* (2016) 13 (Suppl. 5):S438–46. doi: 10.1513/AnnalsATS.201602-112AW

Agust,í A, Noell G, Brugada J, Faner R. Lung function in early adulthood and health in later life: a transgenerational cohort analysis. *Lancet Respir Med.* (2017) 5:935–45. doi: 10.1016/S2213-2600(17)30434-4

Gray D, Willemse L, Visagie A, Czövek D, Nduru P, Vanker A, et al. Determinants of early-life lung function in African infants. *Thorax.* (2017) 72:445–50. doi: 10.1136/thoraxjnl-2015-207401

Agrawal A, Aggarwal M, Sonnappa S, Bush A. Ethnicity and spirometric indices: hostage to tunnel vision? *Lancet Respir Med.* (2019) 7:743– 4. doi: 10.1016/S2213-2600(19)30204-8

Burney P, Hooper RJT. Forced vital capacity, airway obstruction and survival in a general population sample from the USA. *Thorax.* (2011) 66:49– 54. doi: 10.1136/thx.2010.147041

Burney P, Jithoo A, Kato B, Janson C, Mannino D, Nizankowska-Mogilnicka E. Chronic obstructive pulmonary disease mortality and prevalence: the associations with smoking and poverty—a BOLD analysis. *Thorax.* (2014) 69:465–73. doi: 10.1136/thoraxjnl-2013-204460

Duong M, Islam S, Rangarajan S, Leong D, Kurmi O, Teo K. Mortality and cardiovascular and respiratory morbidity in individuals with impaired FEV1 (PURE): an international, community-based cohort study. *Lancet Glob Health.* (2019) 7:e613–23. doi: 10.1016/S2214-109X(19)30070-1

Gray DM, Turkovic L, Willemse L, Visagie A, Vanker A, Stein DJ, et al. Lung function in African infants in the drakenstein child health study. Impact of lower respiratory tract illness. *Am J Respir Care Med.* (2017) 195:212–20. doi: 10.1164/rccm.201601-0188OC

Lee AG, Kaali S, Quinn A, Delimini R, Burkart K, Opoku-Mensah J. Prenatal household air pollution is associated with impaired infant lung function with sex-specific effects. Evidence from graphs, a cluster randomized Cookstove intervention trial. *Am J Respir Crit Care Med.* (2019) 199:738– 46. doi: 10.1164/rccm.201804-0694OC

MacGinty RP, Kariuki SM, Barnett W, Wedderburn CJ, Hardy A, Hoffman N, et al. Associations of antenatal maternal psychological distress with infant birth and development outcomes: results from a South African birth cohort. *Compr Psychiatry.* (2020) 96:152128. doi: 10.1016/j.comppsych.2019. 152128

Ranabhat CL, Jakovljevic M, Dhimal M, Kim CB. Structural factors responsible for universal health coverage in low-and middle-income countries: results from 118 countries. *Front Public Health.* (2020) 7:414. doi: 10.3389/fpubh.2019.00414

Fowler MG, Qin M, Fiscus SA, Currier JS, Flynn PM, Chipato T. Benefits and risks of antiretroviral therapy for perinatal HIV prevention. *N Engl J Med.* (2016) 375:1726–37. doi: 10.1056/NEJMoa1511691

Bolton CE, Bush A, Hurst JR, Kotecha S, McGarvey L. Lung consequences in adults born prematurely. *Thorax.* (2015) 70:574–80. doi: 10.1136/thoraxjnl-2014-206590

Hurst JR, Beckmann J, Ni Y, Bolton CE, McEniery CM, Cockcroft JR, et al. Respiratory and cardiovascular outcomes in survivors of extremely preterm birth at 19 years. *Am J Respir Crit Care Med.* (2020) 202:422– 32. doi: 10.1164/rccm.202001-0016OC

Vanker A, Gie R, Zar HJ. The association between environmental tobacco smoke exposure and childhood respiratory disease: a review. *Expert Rev Respir Med.* (2017) 11:661–73. doi: 10.1080/17476348.2017.1338949

Famoroti T, Sibanda W, Ndung'u TJB. Prevalence and seasonality of common viral respiratory pathogens, including cytomegalovirus in children, between 0–5 years of age in KwaZulu-Natal, an HIV endemic province in South Africa. *BMC Pediatr.* (2018) 18:240. doi: 10.1186/s12887-018-1222-8

Sinaniotis CJ. Viral pneumoniae in children: incidence and aetiology. *Paediatr Respir Rev.* (2004) 5:S197–200. doi: 10.1016/S1526-0542(04)90037-1

Landrigan PJ, Sly JL, Ruchirawat M, Silva ER, Huo X, Diaz-Barriga F, et al. Health consequences of environmental exposures: changing global patterns of exposure and disease. *Ann Glob Health.* (2016) 82:10– 9. doi: 10.1016/j.aogh.2016.01.005

Zar HJ, Barnett W, Stadler A, Gardner-Lubbe S, Myer L, Nicol MP, et al. Aetiology of childhood pneumonia in a well vaccinated South African birth cohort: a nested case-control study of the drakenstein child health study. *Lancet Respir Med.* (2016) 4:463–72. doi: 10.1016/S2213-2600(16)00096-5

Young S, O'keeffe PT, Arnott J, Landau LI. Lung function, airway responsiveness, and respiratory symptoms before and after bronchiolitis. *Arch Dis Child.* (1995) 72:16–24. doi: 10.1136/adc.72.1.16

Organization WH. *Global Tuberculosis Report 2019.* Geneva: WHO (2018).

Masekela R, Anderson R, Moodley T, Kitchin OP, Risenga SM, Becker PJ. HIV-related bronchiectasis in children: an emerging spectre in high tuberculosis burden areas. *Int J Tuberc Lung Dis.* (2012) 16:114– 9. doi: 10.5588/ijtld.11.0244

Ferrand RA, Desai SR, Hopkins C, Elston CM, Copley SJ, Nathoo K. Chronic lung disease in adolescents with delayed diagnosis of vertically acquired HIV infection. *Clin Infect Dis.* (2012) 55:145–52. doi: 10.1093/cid/cis271

Githinji LN, Gray DM, Hlengwa S, Myer L. Lung function in South African adolescents infected perinatally with HIV and treated long- term with antiretroviral therapy. *Ann Am Thorac Soc.* (2017) 14:722– 9. doi: 10.1513/AnnalsATS.201612-1018OC

Woodruff AW, El Suni A, Kaku M, Adamson EA, Maughan TS, Bundru N. Infants in Juba, southern Sudan: the first twelve months of life. *Lancet.* (1984) 324:506–9. doi: 10.1016/S0140-6736(84)92577-7

Ausloos M, Local Burden of Disease Child Growth Failure Collaborators. Mapping child growth failure across low-and middle-income countries. *J Nat.* (2020) 577:231–4. doi: 10.1038/s41586-019-1878-8

Black RE, Victora CG, Walker SP, Bhutta ZA, Christian P, Onis DM, et al. Maternal and child undernutrition and overweight in low-income and middle-income countries. *Lancet.* (2013) 382:427–51. doi: 10.1016/S0140-6736(13)60937-X

Forno E, Weiner DJ, Mullen J, Sawicki G, Kurland G, Han YY, et al. Obesity and airway dysanapsis in children with and without asthma. *Am J Respir Crit Care Med.* (2017) 195:314–23. doi: 10.1164/rccm.201605- 1039OC

Heinzerling AP, Guarnieri MJ, Mann JK, Diaz JV, Thompson LM, Diaz A, et al. Lung function in woodsmoke-exposed guatemalan children following a chimney stove intervention. *Thorax.* (2016) 71:421–8. doi: 10.1136/thoraxjnl-2015-207783

Rylance S, Nightingale R, Naunje A, Mbalume F, Jewell C, Balmes JR. Lung health and exposure to air pollution in Malawian children (CAPS): a cross-sectional study. *Thorax.* (2019) 74:1070–7. doi: 10.1136/thoraxjnl-2018-212945

Gauderman WJ, Urman R, Avol E, Berhane K, McConnell R, Rappaport E, et al. Association of improved air quality with lung development in children. *N Engl J Med.* (2015) 372:905–13. doi: 10.1056/NEJMoa1414123

Balmes JR. How does diesel exhaust impact asthma? *Thorax.* (2011) 66:4– 6. doi: 10.1136/thx.2010.145391

Brunekreef B, Stewart AW, Anderson HR, Lai CK, Strachan DP. Self- reported truck traffic on the street of residence and symptoms of asthma and allergic disease: a global relationship in ISAAC phase 3. *Environ Health Perspect.* (2009) 117:1791–8. doi: 10.1289/ehp.0800467

Pandya RJ, Solomon G, Kinner A, Balmes JR. Diesel exhaust and asthma: hypotheses and molecular mechanisms of action. *Environ Health Perspect.* (2002) 110:103–12. doi: 10.1289/ehp.02110s1103

Barnes BR. Behavioural change, indoor air pollution and child respiratory health in developing countries: a review. *Int J Environ Res Public Health.* (2014) 11:4607–18. doi: 10.3390/ijerph110504607

Faber T, Kumar A, Mackenbach JP, Millett C, Basu S, Sheikh A. Effect of tobacco control policies on perinatal and child health: a systematic review and meta-analysis. *Lancet Public Health.* (2017) 2:e420– 37. doi: 10.1016/S2468-2667(17)30144-5

IfH M. *Evaluation, Global Burden of Disease Collaborative Network. Global Burden of Disease Study 2016 (GBD 2016) Results.* Institute for Health Metrics and Evaluation Seattle (2017).

Halpin DMG, Celli BR, Criner GJ, Frith P, Varela L, Salvi S, et al. The GOLD summit on chronic obstructive pulmonary disease in low- and middle-income countries. *Int J Tuberc Lung Dis.* (2019) 23:1131– 41. doi: 10.5588/ijtld.19.0397

Caballero A, Torres-Duque CA, Jaramillo C, Bolívar F, Sanabria F, Osorio P, et al. Prevalence of COPD in five Colombian cities situated at low, medium, and high altitude (PREPOCOL study). *Chest.* (2008) 133:343– 9. doi: 10.1378/chest.07-1361

Echazarreta AL, Arias SJ, Del Olmo R, Giugno ER, Colodenco FD, Arce SC, et al. Prevalence of COPD in 6 urban clusters in Argentina: the EPOC. AR study. *Arch Bronconeumol.* (2018) 54:260–9. doi: 10.1016/j.arbr.2017.09.017

Menezes AMB, Perez-Padilla R, Jardim JB, Muiño A, Lopez MV, Valdivia G, et al. Chronic obstructive pulmonary disease in five Latin American cities (the PLATINO study): a prevalence study. *Lancet.* (2005) 366:1875– 81. doi: 10.1016/S0140-6736(05)67632-5

Buist AS, McBurnie MA, Vollmer WM, Gillespie S, Burney P, Mannino DM, et al. International variation in the prevalence of COPD (the BOLD study): a population-based prevalence study. *Lancet.* (2007) 370:741– 750. doi: 10.1016/S0140-6736(07)61377-4

Meghji J, Nadeau G, Davis KJ, Wang D, Nyirenda MJ, Gordon SB. Noncommunicable lung disease in sub-Saharan Africa. A community-based cross-sectional study of adults in urban Malawi. *Am J Respir Crit Care Med.* (2016) 194:67–76. doi: 10.1164/rccm.201509-1807OC

Obaseki DO, Erhabor GE, Gnatiuc L, Adewole OO, Buist SA. Chronic airflow obstruction in a black African population: results of BOLD study, Ile-Ife, Nigeria. *J Chron Obstruct Pulmon Dis.* (2016) 13:42– 9. doi: 10.3109/15412555.2015.1041102

Woldeamanuel GG, Mingude A, Geta B. Prevalence of chronic obstructive pulmonary disease (COPD) and its associated factors among adults in Abeshge District, Ethiopia: a cross sectional study. *BMC Pulm Med.* (2019) 19:181. doi: 10.1186/s12890-019-0946-z

Agust, í A, Faner R. COPD beyond smoking: new paradigm, novel opportunities. *Lancet Respir Med.* (2018) 6:324– 6. doi: 10.1016/S2213-2600(18)30060-2

Salvi SS, Barnes PJ. Chronic obstructive pulmonary disease in non-smokers. *Lancet.* (2009) 374:733–43. doi: 10.1016/S0140-6736(09)61303-9

Perez-Padilla R, Fernandez R, Varela MVL, de Oca MM, Muiño A, Tálamo C, et al. Airflow obstruction in never smokers in five Latin American cities: the PLATINO study. *Arch Med Res.* (2012) 43:159– 65. doi: 10.1016/j.arcmed.2012.03.007

Lamprecht B, McBurnie MA, Vollmer WM, Gudmundsson G, Welte T, Nizankowska-Mogilnicka E, et al. COPD in never smokers: results from the population-based burden of obstructive lung disease study. *Chest.* (2011) 139:752–63. doi: 10.1378/chest.10-1253

Lange P, Celli B, Agust,í A, Boje Jensen G, Divo M, Faner R, et al. Lung-function trajectories leading to chronic obstructive pulmonary disease. *N Engl J Med.* (2015) 373:111–22. doi: 10.1056/NEJMoa14 11532

Tálamo C, de Oca MM, Halbert R, Perez-Padilla R, Jardim JRB, Muino A, et al. Diagnostic labeling of COPD in five Latin American cities. *Chest.* (2007) 131:60–7. doi: 10.1378/chest.06-1149

Casas Herrera A, Montes de Oca M, López Varela MV, Aguirre C, Schiavi E, Jardim JR, et al. COPD underdiagnosis and misdiagnosis in a high-risk primary care population in four Latin American countries. A key to enhance disease diagnosis: the PUMA study. *PLoS ONE.* (2016) 11:e0152266. doi: 10.1371/journal.pone.0152266

Lamprecht B, Soriano JB, Studnicka M, Kaiser B, Vanfleteren LE, Gnatiuc L. Determinants of underdiagnosis of COPD in national and international surveys. *Chest.* (2015) 148:971–85. doi: 10.1378/chest.14-2535

Varela MVL, Muiño A, Padilla RP, Jardim JR, Tálamo C, de Oca MM, et al. Treatment of chronic obstructive pulmonary disease in 5 Latin American cities: the PLATINO study. *Arch Bronconeumol.* (2008) 44:58– 64. doi: 10.1016/S1579-2129(08)60016-6 de Oca MM, Tálamo C, Perez-Padilla R, Lopez MV, Muiño A, Jardim JRB, et al. Use of respiratory medication in five Latin American cities: the PLATINO study. *Pulm Pharmacol Ther.* (2008) 21:788- 93. doi: 10.1016/j.pupt.2008.06.003

Jardim JR, Stirbulov R, Moreno D, Zabert G, Lopez-Varela MV. Respiratory medication use in primary care among COPD subjects in four Latin American countries. *Int J Tuberc Lung Dis.* (2017) 21:458- 465. doi: 10.5588/ijtld.16.0633

Vanjare N, Chhowala S, Madas S, Kodgule R, Gogtay J, Salvi S. Use of spirometry among chest physicians and primary care physicians in India. *NPJ Prim Care Respir Med.* (2016) 26:1-5. doi: 10.1038/npjpcrm.2016.36

Halpin DM, Celli BR, Criner GJ, Frith P, Varela MVL, Salvi S, et al. It is time for the world to take COPD seriously: a statement from the GOLD board of directors. *Eur Respir J.* (2019) 54:1900914. doi: 10.1183/13993003.00914-2019

Divo M, Cote C, de Torres JP, Casanova C, Marin JM, Pinto-Plata V, et al. Comorbidities and risk of mortality in patients with chronic obstructive pulmonary disease. *Am J Respir Crit Care Med.* (2012) 186:155- 61. doi: 10.1164/rccm.201201-0034OC

Singh SJ, Halpin DM, Salvi S, Kirenga BJ. Exercise and pulmonary rehabilitation for people with chronic lung disease in LMICs: challenges and opportunities. *Lancet Respir Med.* (2019) 7:1002–4. doi: 10.1016/S2213-2600(19)30364-9

Asher I, Bissell K, Chiang CY, El Sony A, Ellwood P, García-Marcos L, et al. Calling time on asthma deaths in tropical regions—how much longer must people wait for essential medicines? *Lancet Respir Med.* (2019) 7:13- 5. doi: 10.1016/S2213-2600(18)30513-7

Bateman ED, Hurd SS, Barnes PJ, Bousquet J, Drazen JM, FitzGerald M, et al. Global strategy for asthma management and prevention: GINA executive summary. *Euro Respir J.* (2008) 31:143–78. doi: 10.1183/09031936.00138707

Network GA. *The Global Asthma Report.* Auckland: Global Asthma Network (2018).

Lenney W, Bush A, Fitzgerald DA, Fletcher M, Ostrem A, Pedersen S, et al. Improving the global diagnosis and management of asthma in children. *Thorax.* (2018) 73:662–9. doi: 10.1136/thoraxjnl-2018-211626

Kan XH, Chiang CY, Enarson DA, Rao HL, Chen Q, Aït-Khaled N. Asthma as a hidden disease in rural China: opportunities and challenges of standard case management. *Public Health Action.* (2012) 2:87–91. doi: 10.5588/pha.12.0025

British Thoracic Society Scottish Intercollegiate Guidelines Network. British guideline on the management of asthma. *Thorax.* (2008) 63:iv1- 21. doi: 10.1136/thx.2008.097741

Reddel HK, FitzGerald JM, Bateman ED, Bacharier LB, Becker A, Brusselle G, et al. GINA 2019: a fundamental change in asthma management: treatment of asthma with short-acting bronchodilators alone is no longer recommended for adults and adolescents. *Euro Respir J.* (2019) 53:1901046. doi: 10.1183/13993003.01046-2019

Bateman ED, Reddel HK, O'Byrne PM, Barnes PJ, Zhong N, Keen C. As-needed budesonide–formoterol versus maintenance budesonide in mild asthma. *N Engl J Med.* (2018) 378:1877–87. doi: 10.1056/NEJMoa17 15275

Beasley R, Holliday M, Reddel HK, Braithwaite I, Ebmeier S, Hancox RJ. Controlled trial of budesonide–formoterol as needed for mild asthma. *N Engl J Med.* (2019) 380:2020–30. doi: 10.1056/NEJMoa1901963

Hardy J, Baggott C, Fingleton J, Reddel HK, Hancox RJ, Harwood M, et al. Budesonide-formoterol reliever therapy versus maintenance budesonide plus terbutaline reliever therapy in adults with mild to moderate asthma (PRACTICAL): a 52-week, open-label, multicentre, superiority, randomised controlled trial. *Lancet.* (2019) 394:919–28. doi: 10.1016/S0140-6736(19)31948-8

O'Byrne PM, FitzGerald JM, Bateman ED, Barnes PJ, Zhong N, Keen C, et al. Inhaled combined budesonide–formoterol as needed in mild asthma. *N Engl J Med.* (2018) 378:1865–76. doi: 10.1056/NEJMoa1715274

Sobieraj DM, Weeda ER, Nguyen E, Coleman CI, White CM, Lazarus SC. Association of inhaled corticosteroids and long-acting β-agonists as controller and quick relief therapy with exacerbations and symptom control in persistent asthma: a systematic review and meta-analysis. *JAMA.* (2018) 319:1485–96. doi: 10.1001/jama.2018.2769

Ade G, Gninafon M, Tawo L, Aït-Khaled N, Enarson DA. Management of asthma in Benin: the challenge of loss to follow-up. *Public Health Action.* (2013) 3:76–80. doi: 10.5588/pha.12.0080

El Sony AI, Chiang CY, Malik E, Hassanain SA, Hussien H, Khamis AH. Standard case management of asthma in Sudan: a pilot project. *Public Health Action.* (2013) 3:247–52. doi: 10.5588/pha.13.0019

Dhar R, Singh S, Talwar D, Mohan M, Tripathi SK, Swarnakar R, et al. Bronchiectasis in India: results from the European multicentre bronchiectasis audit and research collaboration (EMBARC) and respiratory research network of India registry. *Lancet Global Health.* (2019) 7:e1269- 79. doi: 10.1016/S2214-109X(19)30327-4

Quint JK, Millett ER, Joshi M, Navaratnam V, Thomas SL, Hurst JR. Changes in the incidence, prevalence and mortality of bronchiectasis in the UK from 2004 to 2013: a population-based cohort study. *Euro Respir J.* (2016) 47:186–93. doi: 10.1183/13993003.01033-2015

Chandrasekaran R, Mac Aogáin M, Chalmers JD, Elborn SJ. Geographic variation in the aetiology, epidemiology and microbiology of bronchiectasis. *BMC Pulm Med.* (2018) 18:83. doi: 10.1186/s12890-018-0638-0

Shoemark A, Ozerovitch L, Wilson RJR. Aetiology in adult patients with bronchiectasis. *Respir Med.* (2007) 101:1163- 70. doi: 10.1016/j.rmed.2006.11.008

Chang AB, Brown N, Toombs M, Marsh RL, Redding GJ. Lung disease in indigenous children. *Paediatr Respir Rev.* (2014) 15:325- 32. doi: 10.1016/j.prrv.2014.04.016

Boaventura R, Sibila O, Agusti A, Chalmers JD. Treatable traits in bronchiectasis. *Eur Respir J.* (2018) 52:1801269. doi: 10.1183/13993003.01269-2018

Morrow BM. Airway clearance therapy in acute paediatric respiratory illness: a state-of-the-art review. *South Afr J Physiother.* (2019) 75:1295. doi: 10.4102/sajp.v75i1.1295

Allwood BW, Myer L, Bateman ED. A systematic review of the association between pulmonary tuberculosis and the development of chronic airflow obstruction in adults. *Respiration.* (2013) 86:76–85. doi: 10.1159/000350917

Byrne AL, Marais BJ, Mitnick CD, Lecca L, Marks GB. Tuberculosis and chronic respiratory disease: a systematic review. *Int J Infect Dis.* (2015) 32:138–46. doi: 10.1016/j.ijid.2014.12.016

Amaral AF, Coton S, Kato B, Tan WC, Studnicka M, Janson C, et al. Tuberculosis associates with both airflow obstruction and low lung function: BOLD results. *Euro Respir J.* (2015) 46:1104–12. doi: 10.1183/13993003.02325-2014

Meghji J, Simpson H, Squire SB, Mortimer K. A systematic review of the prevalence and pattern of imaging defined post-TB lung disease. *PLoS ONE.* (2016) 11:e0161176. doi: 10.1371/journal.pone.0161176

Meghji J, Lesosky M, Joekes E, Banda P, Rylance J, Gordon S, et al. Patient outcomes associated with post-tuberculosis lung damage in Malawi: a prospective cohort study. *Thorax.* (2020) 75:269–78. doi: 10.1136/thoraxjnl-2019-213808

Khosa C, Bhatt N, Massango I, Azam K, Saathoff E, Bakuli A, et al. Development of chronic lung impairment in Mozambican TB patients and associated risks. *BMC Pulm Med.* (2020) 20:127. doi: 10.1186/s12890-020-1167-1

Marx FM, Floyd S, Ayles H, Godfrey-Faussett P, Beyers N. High burden of prevalent tuberculosis among previously treated people in Southern Africa suggests potential for targeted control interventions. *Euro Respir J.* (2016) 48:1227–30. doi: 10.1183/13993003.00716-2016

Balasegaram M, Brigden G. Empiric tuberculosis treatment in retreatment patients in high HIV/tuberculosis-burden settings. *Lancet Infect Dis.* (2014) 14:795–6. doi: 10.1016/S1473-3099(14)70881-3

Houben RM, Lalli M, Kranzer K, Menzies NA, Schumacher SG. What if they don't have tuberculosis? The consequences and trade-offs involved in false-positive diagnoses of tuberculosis. *Clin Infect Dis.* (2019) 68:150- 6. doi: 10.1093/cid/ciy544

Romanowski K, Baumann B, Basham CA, Khan FA, Fox GJ. Long-term all-cause mortality in people treated for tuberculosis: a systematic review and meta-analysis. *Lancet Infect Dis.* (2019) 19:1129–37. doi: 10.1016/S1473-3099(19)30309-3

Dorman SE, Schumacher SG, Alland D, Nabeta P, Armstrong DT, King B. Xpert MTB/RIF Ultra for detection of *Mycobacterium tuberculosis* and rifampicin resistance: a prospective multicentre diagnostic accuracy study. *Lancet Infect Dis.* (2018) 18:76–84. doi: 10.1016/S1473-3099(17)3 0691-6

Kendall EA, Schumacher SG, Denkinger CM, Dowdy DW. Estimated clinical impact of the Xpert MTB/RIF ultra cartridge for diagnosis of pulmonary tuberculosis: a modeling study. *PLoS Med.* (2017) 14:e1002472. doi: 10.1371/journal.pmed.1002472

van Kampen SC, Wanner A, Edwards M, Harries AD, Kirenga BJ, Chakaya J. International research and guidelines on post-tuberculosis chronic lung disorders: a systematic scoping review. *BMJ Glob Health.* (2018) 3:e000745. doi: 10.1136/thorax-2018-212555.379

Allwood BW, Van Der Zalm MM, Amaral AFS, Byrne A, Datta S, Egere U, et al. Post-tuberculosis lung health: perspectives from the first international symposium. *Int J Tuberc Lung Dis.* (2020) 24:820- 828. doi: 10.5588/ijtld.20.0067

Dlodlo RA, Brigden G, Heldal E, Allwood B, Chiang CY, Fujiwara PI, et al. *Management of Tuberculosis: a Guide to Essential Practice.* Paris: International Union Against Tuberculosis and Lung Disease (2020).

Andréjak C, Nielsen R, Thomsen VØ, Duhaut P, Sørensen HT. Chronic respiratory disease, inhaled corticosteroids and risk of non-tuberculous mycobacteriosis. *Thorax.* (2013) 68:256- 62. doi: 10.1136/thoraxjnl-2012-201772

Dong YH, Chang CH, Wu FLL, Shen LJ, Calverley PM, Löfdahl CG, et al. Use of inhaled corticosteroids in patients with COPD and the risk of TB and influenza:

a systematic review and meta-analysis of randomized controlled trials. *Chest.* (2014) 145:1286–97. doi: 10.1378/chest.13-2137

Lee CH, Kim K, Hyun MK, Jang EJ, Lee NR, Yim JJ. Use of inhaled corticosteroids and the risk of tuberculosis. *Thorax.* (2013) 68:1105– 13. doi: 10.1136/thoraxjnl-2012-203175

Jones R, Kirenga BJ, Katagira W, Singh SJ, Pooler J, Okwera A, et al. A pre–post intervention study of pulmonary rehabilitation for adults with post- tuberculosis lung disease in Uganda. *Int J Chron Obstruct Pulmon Dis.* (2017) 12:3533. doi: 10.2147/COPD.S146659

Harries AD, Dlodlo RA, Brigden G, Mortimer K, Jensen P, Fujiwara PI, et al. Should we consider a 'fourth 90'for tuberculosis?. *Int J Tuberc Lung Dis.* (2019) 23:1253–6. doi: 10.5588/ijtld.19.0471

Ranzani OT, Rodrigues LC, Bombarda S, Minto CM, Waldman EA. Long-term survival and cause-specific mortality of patients newly diagnosed with tuberculosis in São Paulo state, Brazil, 2010–15: a population-based, longitudinal study. *Lancet Infect Dis.* (2020) 20:123–32. doi: 10.1016/S1473-3099(19)30518-3

World Health Organization. *Monitoring the Building Blocks of Health Systems: A Handbook of Indicators and Their Measurement Strategies.* Tanzania: World Health Organization (2010). Available online at: https:// www.who.int/healthinfo/systems/WHO_MBHSS_2010_full_web.pdf

Buist AS, Parry V. The American thoracic society methods in epidemiologic, clinical, and operations research program. A research capacity-building program in low-and middle-income countries. *Ann Am Thorac Soc.* (2013) 10:281–9. doi: 10.1513/Anna ls,AT. S.201304-081O. T

WHO. *Assessing, National Capacity for the Prevention and Control of Noncommunicable Diseases.* WHO (2012).

World Health Organization. *Noncommunicable Diseases Country Profiles.* WHO (2018).

Troeger CE, Khalil IA, Blacker BF, Biehl MH, Albertson SB, Zimsen SR, et al. Quantifying risks and interventions that have affected the burden of lower respiratory infections among children younger than 5 years: an analysis for the global burden of disease study 2017. *Lancet Infect Dis.* (2020) 20:60–79. doi: 10.1016/S1473-3099(19)30410-4

Vazquez-Garcia JC, Salas-Hernandez J, Padilla RP, de Oca M. M. Respiratory health in Latin America: number of specialists and human resources training. *Arch Bronconeumol.* (2014) 50:34–9. doi: 10.1016/j.arbr.2013.12.003

Obaseki D, Adeniyi B, Kolawole T, Onyedum C, Erhabor G. Gaps in capacity for respiratory care in developing countries. Nigeria as a case study. *Ann Am Thorac Soc.* (2015) 12:591–8. doi: 10.1513/AnnalsATS.201410-443AR

Zar HJ, Vanker A, Gray D, Zampoli M. The African pediatric fellowship training program in pediatric pulmonology: a model for growing African capacity in child lung health. *Ann Am Thorac Soc.* (2017) 14:500– 4. doi: 10.1513/AnnalsATS.201612-953PS

Wilmshurst JM, Morrow B, du Preez A, Githanga D, Kennedy N. The African pediatric fellowship program: training in Africa for Africans. *Pediatrics.* (2016) 137:1–12. doi: 10.1542/peds.2015-2741

Mash B, Fairall L, Adejayan O, Ikpefan O, Kumari J, Mathee S, et al. A morbidity survey of South African primary care. *PLoS ONE.* (2012) 7:e32358. doi: 10.1371/annotation/3545077e-aded-4eef-a460-be1edbd1845c

Cornick R, Picken S, Wattrus C, Awotiwon A, Carkeek E, Hannington J, et al. The practical approach to care kit (PACK) guide: developing a clinical decision support tool to simplify, standardise and strengthen primary healthcare delivery. *BMJ Glob Health.* (2018) 3:e000962. doi: 10.1136/bmjgh-2018-000962

Fairall L, Cornick R, Bateman E. Empowering frontline providers to deliver universal primary healthcare using the practical approach to care kit. *BMJ.* (2018) 363:k4451. doi: 10.1136/bmj.k4451

World Health Organization. *Implementation Tools: Package of Essential Noncommunicable (PEN) Disease Interventions for Primary Health Care in Low-Resource Settings.* WHO (2013).

World Health Organization. *IMAI District Clinician Manual: Hospital Care Adolescents and Adults: Guidelines for the Management of Illnesess With Limited-Resources.* WHO (2012).

Fairall PL. *The Knowledge Translation Unit, University of Cape Town. Practical Approach to Care Kit (PACK): PACK Overview.* (2020). Available online at: https://knowledgetranslation.co.za/pack/

Picken S, Hannington J, Fairall L, Doherty T, Bateman E, Richards M, et al. PACK child: the development of a practical guide to extend the scope of integrated primary care for children and young adolescents. *BMJ Glob Health.* (2018) 3:e000957. doi: 10.1136/bmjgh-2018-000957

Cornick R, Wattrus C, Eastman T, Ras CJ, Awotiwon A, Anderson L, et al. Crossing borders: the PACK experience of spreading a complex health system intervention across low-income and middle-income countries. *BMJ Glob Health.* (2018) 3(Suppl. 5):e001088. doi: 10.1136/bmjgh-2018-001088

Wattrus C, Zepeda J, Cornick RV, Zonta R, de Andrade MP, Fairall L, et al. Using a mentorship model to localise the practical approach to care kit (PACK): from South Africa to Brazil. *BMJ Glob Health.* (2018) 3(Suppl 5):e001016. doi: 10.1136/bmjgh-2018-001016

Awotiwon A, Sword C, Eastman T, Ras CJ, Ana P, Cornick RV, et al. Using a mentorship model to localise the practical approach to care kit (PACK): from South Africa to Nigeria. *BMJ Glob Health.* (2018) 3:e001079. doi: 10.1136/bmjgh-2018-001079

Zwarenstein M, Fairall LR, Lombard C, Mayers P, Bheekie A, English RG. Outreach education for integration of HIV/AIDS care, antiretroviral treatment, and tuberculosis care in primary care clinics in South Africa: PALSA PLUS pragmatic cluster randomised trial. *BMJ.* (2011) 342:d2022. doi: 10.1136/bmj.d2022

Fairall L, Bachmann MO, Zwarenstein M, Bateman ED, Niessen LW, Lombard C. Cost-effectiveness of educational outreach to primary care nurses to increase tuberculosis case detection and improve respiratory care: economic evaluation alongside a randomised trial. *Trop Med Int Health.* (2010) 15:277–86. doi: 10.1111/j.1365-3156.2009.02455.x

Fairall LR, Folb N, Timmerman V, Lombard C, Steyn K, Bachmann MO, et al. Educational outreach with an integrated clinical tool for nurse-led non-communicable chronic disease management in primary care in South Africa: a pragmatic cluster randomised controlled trial. *PLoS Med.* (2016) 13:e1002178. doi: 10.1371/journal.pmed.1002178

Hannon B, Zimmermann C, Knaul FM, Powell RA, Mwangi-Powell FN. Provision of palliative care in low-and middle-income countries: overcoming obstacles for effective treatment delivery. *J Clin Oncol.* (2016) 34:62– 8. doi: 10.1200/JCO.2015.62.1615

Masekela R, Hall GL, Stanojevic S, Sartorius B. MacGinty R, Saad HB, et al. An urgent need for african spirometry reference equations: the paediatric and adult African Spirometry study. *Int J Tuberc Lung Dis.* (2019) 23:952– 8. doi: 10.5588/ijtld.18.0442

Fonjungo PN, Kebede Y, Messele T, Ayana G, Tibesso G, Abebe A, et al. Laboratory equipment maintenance: a critical bottleneck for strengthening health systems in sub-Saharan Africa?. *J Public Health Policy.* (2012) 33:34– 45. doi: 10.1057/jphp.2011.57

Agodokpessi G, Aït-Khaled N, Gninafon M, Tawo L, Bekou W, Perrin C, et al. Assessment of a revolving drug fund for essential asthma medicines in Benin. *J Pharm Policy Pract.* (2015) 8:1–8. doi: 10.1186/s40545-015-0033-7

Zachariah R, Harries AD, Ishikawa N, Rieder HL, Bissell K, Laserson K. Operational research in low-income countries: what, why, and how?. *Lancet Infect Dis.* (2009) 9:711–7. doi: 10.1016/S1473-3099(09)70229-4

Ramsay A, Harries AD, Zachariah R, Bissell K, Hinderaker SG, Edginton M. The structured operational research and training initiative for public health programmes. *Public Health Action.* (2014) 4:79–84. doi: 10.5588/pha.14.0011

Tripathy JP, Kumar AM, Guillerm N, Berger SD, Bissell K, Reid A, et al. Does the structured operational research and training initiative (SORT IT) continue to influence health policy and/or practice?. *Glob Health Action.* (2018) 11:1500762. doi: 10.1080/16549716.2018.1500762

Kumar AM, Zachariah R, Satyanarayana S, Reid AJ, Van den Bergh R, Tayler-Smith K. Operational research capacity building using 'the union/MSF'model: adapting as we go along. *BMC Res Notes.* (2014) 7:819. doi: 10.1186/1756-0500-7-819

Sagili KD, Satyanarayana S, Chadha SS, Wilson NC, Kumar AM, Moonan PK. Operational research within a global fund supported tuberculosis project in India: why, how and its contribution towards change in policy and practice. *Glob Health Action.* (2018) 11:1445467. doi: 10.1080/16549716.2018.1445467

Zachariah R, Guillerm N, Berger S, Kumar AM, Satyanarayana S, Bissell K. Research to policy and practice change: is capacity building in operational research delivering the goods? *Trop Med Int Health.* (2014) 19:1068– 75. doi: 10.1111/tmi.12343

Guillerm N, Bissell K, Kumar AMV, Ramsay A, Reid AJ, Zachariah R. Sustained research capacity after completing a structured operational research and training (SORT IT) course. *Public Health Action.* (2016) 6:207– 8. doi: 10.5588/pha.16.0057

Guillerm N, Tayler-Smith K, Berger SD, Bissell K, Kumar AMV, Ramsay What happens after participants complete a Union-MSF structured operational research training course? *Public Health Action.* (2014) 4:89– 95. doi: 10.5588/pha.14.0014

Guillerm N, Tayler-Smith K, Dar Berger S, Bissell K, Kumar AMV, Ramsay Research output after participants complete a structured operational research and training (SORT IT) course. *Public Health Action.* (2015) 5:266– 8. doi: 10.5588/pha.15.0045

Bissell K, Harries AD, Reid AJ, Edginton M, Hinderaker SG, Satyanarayana S. Operational research training: the course and beyond. *Public Health Action.* (2012) 2:92–7. doi: 10.5588/pha.12.0022

Fatima R, Yaqoob A, Qadeer E, Hinderaker SG, Heldal E, Zachariah R, et al. Building sustainable operational research capacity in Pakistan: starting with tuberculosis and expanding to other public health problems. *Glob Health Action.* (2019) 12:1555215. doi: 10.1080/16549716.2018.1555215

Garcia-Marcos L, Robertson CF, Ross Anderson H, Ellwood P, Williams HC. Does migration affect asthma, rhinoconjunctivitis and eczema prevalence? Global findings from the international study of asthma and allergies in childhood. *Int J Epidemiol.* (2014) 43:1846–54. doi: 10.1093/ije/dyu145

Permissions

All chapters in this book were first published by Frontiers; hereby published with permission under the Creative Commons Attribution License or equivalent. Every chapter published in this book has been scrutinized by our experts. Their significance has been extensively debated. The topics covered herein carry significant findings which will fuel the growth of the discipline. They may even be implemented as practical applications or may be referred to as a beginning point for another development.

The contributors of this book come from diverse backgrounds, making this book a truly international effort. This book will bring forth new frontiers with its revolutionizing research information and detailed analysis of the nascent developments around the world.

We would like to thank all the contributing authors for lending their expertise to make the book truly unique. They have played a crucial role in the development of this book. Without their invaluable contributions this book wouldn't have been possible. They have made vital efforts to compile up to date information on the varied aspects of this subject to make this book a valuable addition to the collection of many professionals and students.

This book was conceptualized with the vision of imparting up-to-date information and advanced data in this field. To ensure the same, a matchless editorial board was set up. Every individual on the board went through rigorous rounds of assessment to prove their worth. After which they invested a large part of their time researching and compiling the most relevant data for our readers.

The editorial board has been involved in producing this book since its inception. They have spent rigorous hours researching and exploring the diverse topics which have resulted in the successful publishing of this book. They have passed on their knowledge of decades through this book. To expedite this challenging task, the publisher supported the team at every step. A small team of assistant editors was also appointed to further simplify the editing procedure and attain best results for the readers.

Apart from the editorial board, the designing team has also invested a significant amount of their time in understanding the subject and creating the most relevant covers. They scrutinized every image to scout for the most suitable representation of the subject and create an appropriate cover for the book.

The publishing team has been an ardent support to the editorial, designing and production team. Their endless efforts to recruit the best for this project, has resulted in the accomplishment of this book. They are a veteran in the field of academics and their pool of knowledge is as vast as their experience in printing. Their expertise and guidance has proved useful at every step. Their uncompromising quality standards have made this book an exceptional effort. Their encouragement from time to time has been an inspiration for everyone.

The publisher and the editorial board hope that this book will prove to be a valuable piece of knowledge for researchers, students, practitioners and scholars across the globe.

List of Contributors

Andressa Daronco Cereta
Department of Surgery, School of Veterinary Medicine and Animal Sciences, University of São Paulo, São Paulo, Brazil

Vinícius Rosa Oliveira
Department of Physical Therapy, EUSES University School, University of Barcelona/University of Girona (UB-UdG), Barcelona, Spain
Research Group on Methodology, Methods, Models, and Outcomes of Health and Social Sciences (M3O), University of Vic - Central University of Catalonia, Vic, Spain

Ivan Peres Costa
Department of Master's and and Doctoral Programs in Rehabilitation Sciences, Nove de Julho University, São Paulo, Brazil

João Pedro Ribeiro Afonso, Adriano Luís Fonseca, Alan Robson Trigueiro de Souza, Guilherme Augusto Moreira Silva, Diego A. C. P. G. Mello and Luis Vicente Franco de Oliveira
Department of Experimental Cardiorrespiratory Physiology, Postgraduate Program in Human Movement and Rehabilitation, School of Medicine, University Center of Anápolis (UniEVANGELICA), Anápolis, Brazil

Renata Kelly da Palma
Department of Surgery, School of Veterinary Medicine and Animal Sciences, University of São Paulo, São Paulo, Brazil
Department of Physical Therapy, EUSES University School, University of Barcelona/University of Girona (UB-UdG), Barcelona, Spain
Institute for Bioengineering of Catalonia, Barcelona, Spain

Marjolein Ensinck and Marianne S. Carlon
Molecular Virology and Gene Therapy, Department of Pharmaceutical and Pharmacological Sciences, KU Leuven, Leuven, Belgium

Angélique Mottais, Claire Detry and Teresinha Leal
Institut de Recherche Expérimentale et Clinique, Louvain Centre for Toxicology and Applied Pharmacology, Université Catholique de Louvain, Brussels, Belgium

Yanmin Zhao, Jimin Shi, Yi Luo, Yamin Tan, Jian Yu, Huarui Fu, Xiaoyu Lai, Lizhen Liu and He Huang
Bone Marrow Transplantation Center, The First Affiliated Hospital, School of Medicine, Zhejiang University, Hangzhou, China
Institute of Hematology, Zhejiang University, Hangzhou, China

Guifang OuYang
Department of Hematology, Ningbo Hospital of Zhejiang University, Ningbo, China

Xiaofang Yin, Guisong Zhu, Yuan Dong Fu, Juan Wang and Biao Xu
Intensive Care Uint, Nanjing Hospital of Chinese Medicine Affiliated to Nanjing University of Chinese Medicine, Nanjing, China

Qian Wang
Department of Respiration, Jiangsu Province Hospital of Chinese Medicine, Affiliated Hospital of Nanjing University of Chinese Medicine, Nanjing, China

Chengliang Yang
Latner Thoracic Surgery Research Laboratories, Toronto General Hospital Research Institute, University Health Network, Toronto, ON, Canada

Shaf Keshavjee and Mingyao Liu
Latner Thoracic Surgery Research Laboratories, Toronto General Hospital Research Institute, University Health Network, Toronto, ON, Canada
Institute of Medical Science and Department of Surgery, Faculty of Medicine, University of Toronto, Toronto, ON, Canada

Sara Rolandsson Enes
Department of Experimental Medical Science, Faculty of Medicine, Lund University, Lund, Sweden

Anna D. Krasnodembskaya
Wellcome-Wolfson Institute for Experimental Medicine, School of Medicine, Dentistry, and Biomedical Sciences, Queens University, Belfast, United Kingdom

Karen English
Cellular Immunology Laboratory, Biology Department, Kathleen Lonsdale Institute for Human Health Research, Maynooth University, Maynooth, Ireland

Claudia C. Dos Santos
Interdepartmental Division of Critical Care, Department of Medicine and the Keenan Center for Biomedical Research, St. Michael's Hospital, University of Toronto, Toronto, ON, Canada

Daniel J. Weiss
Department of Medicine, 226 Health Science Research Facility, Larner College of Medicine, University of Vermont, Burlington, VT, United States

Shana M. Busch and Zareeb Lorenzana
Hastings Center for Pulmonary Research, Division of Pulmonary, Critical Care and Sleep Medicine, Department of Medicine, University of Southern California, Los Angeles, CA, United States

Amy L. Ryan
Hastings Center for Pulmonary Research, Division of Pulmonary, Critical Care and Sleep Medicine, Department of Medicine, University of Southern California, Los Angeles, CA, United States
Department of Stem Cell Biology and Regenerative Medicine, University of Southern California, Los Angeles, CA, United States

Rui Ye, Cuihong Wang, Pengbo Sun, Shuang Bai and Li Zhao
Department of Pulmonary and Critical Care Medicine, Shengjing Hospital of China Medical University, Shenyang, China

P. Cmielewski, J. Delhove, M. Donnelley and D. Parsons
Respiratory and Sleep Medicine, Women's and Children's Hospital, Adelaide, SA, Australia
Robinson Research Institute, University of Adelaide, Adelaide, SA, Australia
Adelaide Medical School, University of Adelaide, Adelaide, SA, Australia

Katelin M. Allan
School of Women's and Children's Health, Faculty of Medicine, University of New South Wales, Sydney, Australia
Molecular and Integrative Cystic Fibrosis Research Centre (miCF_RC), University of New South Wales and Sydney Children's Hospital, Sydney, Australia

Nigel Farrow and Martin Donnelley
Respiratory and Sleep Medicine, Women's and Children's Health Network, Adelaide, Australia
Robinson Research Institute, The University of Adelaide, Adelaide, Australia
Adelaide Medical School, The University of Adelaide, Adelaide, Australia

Adam Jaffe and Shafagh A. Waters
School of Women's and Children's Health, Faculty of Medicine, University of New South Wales, Sydney, Australia
Molecular and Integrative Cystic Fibrosis Research Centre (miCF_RC), University of New South Wales and Sydney Children's Hospital, Sydney, Australia
Department of Respiratory Medicine, Sydney Children's Hospital, Sydney, Australia

Linda Elowsson Rendin, Anna Löfdahl, Måns Kadefors, Zackarias Söderlund, Emil Tykesson, Sara Rolandsson Enes, Jenny Wigén and Gunilla Westergren-Thorsson
Lung Biology Unit, Department of Experimental Medical Science, Lund University, Lund, Sweden

Nicole Reyne, Patricia Cmielewski, Alexandra McCarron, Juliette Delhove and David Parsons
Adelaide Medical School, University of Adelaide, Adelaide, SA, Australia
Respiratory and Sleep Medicine, Women'sand Children's Hospital, North Adelaide, SA, Australia
Robinson Research Institute, University of Adelaide, Adelaide, SA, Australia

Gwenda F. Vasse
University of Groningen, University Medical Center Groningen, Department of Biomedical Engineering, Groningen, Netherlands
University of Groningen, University Medical Center Groningen, W.J. Kolff Institute for Biomedical Engineering and Materials Science, Groningen, Netherlands
University of Groningen, Department of Molecular Pharmacology, Groningen Research Institute for Pharmacy, Groningen, Netherlands
University of Groningen, University Medical Center Groningen, Groningen Research Institute for Asthma and COPD (GRIAC), Groningen, Netherlands

Lisette Van Os
University of Groningen, University Medical Center Groningen, Groningen Research Institute for Asthma and COPD (GRIAC), Groningen, Netherlands
University of Groningen, University Medical Center Groningen, Department of Pathology and Medical Biology, Groningen, Netherlands

Marina De Jager
University of Groningen, Department of Molecular Pharmacology, Groningen Research Institute for Pharmacy, Groningen, Netherlands

Marnix R. Jonker, Theo Borghuis and L. Tim Van Den Toorn
University of Groningen, University Medical Center Groningen, Groningen Research Institute for Asthma and COPD (GRIAC), Groningen, Netherlands
University of Groningen, University Medical Center Groningen, Department of Pathology and Medical Biology, Groningen, Netherlands

Pytrick Jellema and Martin C. Harmsen
University of Groningen, University Medical Center Groningen, Department of Pathology and Medical Biology, Groningen, Netherlands

Eric S. White
Division of Pulmonary and Critical Care Medicine, University of Michigan Medical School, Ann Arbor, MI, United States

Patrick Van Rijn
University of Groningen, University Medical Center Groningen, Department of Biomedical Engineering, Groningen, Netherlands
University of Groningen, University Medical Center Groningen, W.J. Kolff Institute for Biomedical Engineering and Materials Science, Groningen, Netherlands

Irene H. Heijink
University of Groningen, University Medical Center Groningen, Groningen Research Institute for Asthma and COPD (GRIAC), Groningen, Netherlands
University of Groningen, University Medical Center Groningen, Department of Pathology and Medical Biology, Groningen, Netherlands
University of Groningen, University Medical Center Groningen, Department of Pulmonology, Groningen, Netherlands

Barbro N. Melgert
University of Groningen, Department of Molecular Pharmacology, Groningen Research Institute for Pharmacy, Groningen, Netherlands
University of Groningen, University Medical Center Groningen, Groningen Research Institute for Asthma and COPD (GRIAC), Groningen, Netherlands

Janette K. Burgess
University of Groningen, University Medical Center Groningen, W.J. Kolff Institute for Biomedical Engineering and Materials Science, Groningen, Netherlands
University of Groningen, University Medical Center Groningen, Groningen Research Institute for Asthma and COPD (GRIAC), Groningen, Netherlands
University of Groningen, University Medical Center Groningen, Department of Pathology and Medical Biology, Groningen, Netherlands

Xiaohe Li, Xiaowei Liu, Hao Ruan, Ling Ma, Jingjing Liang, Yunyao Cui, Zeping Li, Honggang Zhou and Cheng Yang
State Key Laboratory of Medicinal Chemical Biology, College of Pharmacy and Tianjin Key Laboratory of Molecular Drug Research, Nankai University, Tianjin, China
Tianjin Key Laboratory of Molecular Drug Research, Tianjin International Joint Academy of Biomedicine, Tianjin, China

Kai Huang, Yanhua Wang, Shuyang Wu, Hailong Li, Yuli Wei and Guang Yang
State Key Laboratory of Medicinal Chemical Biology, College of Pharmacy and Tianjin Key Laboratory of Molecular Drug Research, Nankai University, Tianjin, China

Jingjing Gao
Tianjin Key Laboratory of Molecular Drug Research, Tianjin International Joint Academy of Biomedicine, Tianjin, China

Bo Yang and Xiaoping Li
Department of Thoracic Surgery, Tianjin First Central Hospital, Tianjin, China

Alexandra McCarron and Nigel Farrow
Adelaide Medical School, University of Adelaide, Adelaide, SA, Australia
Robinson Research Institute, University of Adelaide, Adelaide, SA, Australia
Department of Respiratory and Sleep Medicine, Women's and Children's Hospital, Adelaide, SA, Australia

Emma Knight
School of Public Health, University of Adelaide, Adelaide, SA, Australia
South Australian Health and Medical Research Institute, Adelaide, SA, Australia

Anna Valeria Samarelli, Linda Manicardi, Antonio Moretti, Stefania Cerri, Enrico Clini Alessandro Marchioni and Giulia Bruzzi
Laboratory of Cell Therapies and Respiratory Medicine, Department of Medical and Surgical Sciences for Children and Adults University Hospital of Modena and Reggio Emilia, Modena, Italy
University Hospital of Modena, Respiratory Diseases Unit, Department of Medical and Surgical Sciences, University of Modena Reggio Emilia, Modena, Italy

Roberto Tonelli, Ivana Castaniere, Dario Andrisani and Filippo Gozzi
Laboratory of Cell Therapies and Respiratory Medicine, Department of Medical and Surgical Sciences for Children and Adults University Hospital of Modena and Reggio Emilia, Modena, Italy
University Hospital of Modena, Respiratory Diseases Unit, Department of Medical and Surgical Sciences, University of Modena Reggio Emilia, Modena, Italy
Clinical and Experimental Medicine PhD Program, University of Modena Reggio Emilia, Modena, Italy

Irene Heijink
University of Groningen, Departments of Pathology & Medical Biology and Pulmonology, GRIAC Research Institute, University Medical Center Groningen, Groningen, Netherlands

Aina Martin Medina
IdISBa (Institut d'Investigacio Sanitaria Illes Balears), Palma de Mallorca, Spain

Riccardo Fantini, Luca Tabbì and Chiara Nani
University Hospital of Modena, Respiratory Diseases Unit, Department of Medical and Surgical Sciences, University of Modena Reggio Emilia, Modena, Italy

Ilenia Mastrolia
Laboratory of Cellular Therapy, Program of Cell Therapy and Immuno-Oncology, Division of Oncology, Department of Medical and Surgical Sciences for Children & Adults, University Hospital of Modena and Reggio Emilia, Modena, Italy

Massimo Dominici
Oncology Unit, University Hospital of Modena, University of Modena and Reggio Emilia, Modena, Italy

You-Hui Tu, Yan Guo, Shuang Ji and Guang-He Fei
Department of Respiratory and Critical Care Medicine, The First Affiliated Hospital of Anhui Medical University, Hefei, China
Key Laboratory of Respiratory Disease Research and Medical Transformation of Anhui Province, The First Affiliated Hospital of Anhui Medical University, Hefei, China

Ji-Long Shen
Department of Pathogen Biology and Provincial Laboratories of Pathogen Biology and Zoonoses, Anhui Medical University, Hefei, China

J. Mercier, M. Ruffin and L. Guillot
Sorbonne Université, Inserm, Centre de Recherche, Saint Antoine, F-75012, Paris, France

H. Corvol
Pneumologie Pédiatrique, APHP, Hôpital Trousseau, Paris, France

Alexandre Todorovic Fabro
Department of Pathology, Laboratory of Histomorphometry and Lung Genomics, Faculty of Medicine, University of São Paulo, São Paulo, Brazil
Department of Pathology and Legal Medicine, Respiratory Medicine Laboratory, Ribeirão Preto Medical School, University of São Paulo (USP), São Paulo, Brazil

Juliana Machado-Rugolo
Department of Pathology, Laboratory of Histomorphometry and Lung Genomics, Faculty of Medicine, University of São Paulo, São Paulo, Brazil
Health Technology Assessment Center (NATS), Clinical Hospital (HCFMB), Medical School of São Paulo State University (UNESP), Botucatu, Brazil

Camila Machado Baldavira, Tabatha Gutierrez Prieto, Cecília Farhat and Vera Luiza Capelozzi
Department of Pathology, Laboratory of Histomorphometry and Lung Genomics, Faculty of Medicine, University of São Paulo, São Paulo, Brazil

Flavia Regina Rotea ManGone
Laboratory of Molecular Genetics, Center for Translational Research in Oncology, Cancer Institute of São Paulo (ICESP), São Paulo, Brazil

Sabrina Setembre Batah, Heloísa Resende Cruvinel, Maiara Almeida Aldá and Sirlei Siani Morais
Department of Pathology and Legal Medicine, Respiratory Medicine Laboratory, Ribeirão Preto Medical School, University of São Paulo (USP), São Paulo, Brazil

Jhonatas Sirino Monteiro and João Carlos Setubal
Bioinformatic Laboratory, Institute of Chemistry, University of São Paulo (USP), São Paulo, Brazil

Adriana Inacio Pádua, Marcel Koenigkam Santos and José Antônio Baddini-Martinez
Pulmonary Hypertension Care Center, Department of Internal Medicine, Ribeirão Preto Medical School, University of São Paulo (USP), São Paulo, Brazil

Rogério Antônio de Oliveira
Department of Biostatistics, Plant Biology, Parasitology and Zoology, Institute of Biosciences, São Paulo State University (UNESP), Botucatu, Brazil

Claudia Aparecida Rainho
Department of Chemical and Biological Sciences, Institute of Biosciences, São Paulo State University (UNESP), Botucatu, Brazil

Hugo Hyung Bok Yoo
Pulmonary Hypertension Care Center, Department of Internal Medicine, Botucatu Medical School, São Paulo State University (UNESP), São Paulo, Brazil

Pedro Leme Silva
Laboratory of Pulmonary Investigation, Carlos Chagas Filho Biophysics Institute, Federal University of Rio de Janeiro, Centro de Ciências da Saúde, Rio de Janeiro, Brazil
National Institute of Science and Technology for Regenerative Medicine, Rio de Janeiro, Brazil

Maria Aparecida Nagai
Laboratory of Molecular Genetics, Center for Translational Research in Oncology, Cancer Institute of São Paulo (ICESP), São Paulo, Brazil
Department of Radiology and Oncology, Medical School of São Paulo State University (UNESP), São Paulo, Brazil

David T. J. Broderick, David W. Waite and Michael W. Taylor
School of Biological Sciences, University of Auckland, Auckland, New Zealand

Robyn L. Marsh
Child Health Division, Menzies School of Health Research, Charles Darwin University, Darwin, NT, Australia

Carlos A. Camargo Jr. and Kohei Hasegawa
Department of Emergency Medicine, Massachusetts General Hospital, Boston, MA, United States
Department of Epidemiology, Harvard T.H. Chan School of Public Health, Boston, MA, United States
Harvard Medical School, Boston, MA, United States

Paul Cardenas
Colegio de Ciencias Biológicas y Ambientales, Instituto de Microbiología, Universidad San Francisco de Quito, Quito, Ecuador

Anne B. Chang
Child Health Division, Menzies School of Health Research, Charles Darwin University, Darwin, NT, Australia
Department of Respiratory and Sleep Medicine, Queensland Children's Hospital, Brisbane, QLD, Australia
Australian Centre for Health Services Innovation, Queensland University of Technology, Brisbane, QLD, Australia

William O. C. Cookson
National Heart and Lung Institute, Imperial College London, London, United Kingdom
Royal Brompton and Harefield NHS Foundation Trust, London, United Kingdom

Leah Cuthbertson
Royal Brompton and Harefield NHS Foundation Trust, London, United Kingdom

Wenkui Dai
Department of Obstetrics and Gynecology, Peking University Shenzhen Hospital, Shenzhen, China

Mark L. Everard
School of Medicine, University of Western Australia, Perth, WA, Australia

Alain Gervaix
Department of Pediatrics, Gynecology and Obstetrics, Faculty of Medicine, University Hospitals of Geneva, Geneva, Switzerland

J. Kirk Harris and Edith T. Zemanick
Department of Pediatrics, University of Colorado School of Medicine, Aurora, CO, United States

Lucas R. Hoffman
Seattle Children's Hospital, Seattle, WA, United States
Department of Pediatrics and Microbiology, University of Washington, Seattle, WA, United States

Soo-Jong Hong
Department of Pediatrics, Childhood Asthma Atopy Center, Humidifier Disinfectant Health Center, Asan Medical Center, University of Ulsan College of Medicine, Seoul, South Korea

Laurence Josset
Hospices Civils de Lyon, Lyon, France

Matthew S. Kelly
Division of Pediatric Infectious Diseases, Duke University, Durham, NC, United States

Bong-Soo Kim
Department of Life Science, Multidisciplinary Genome Institute, Hallym University, Chuncheon, South Korea

Yong Kong
Department of Biostatistics, Yale School of Public Health, Yale University, New Haven, CT, United States

Shuai C. Li
Department of Computer Science, City University of Hong Kong, Kowloon, Hong Kong SAR, China
Department of Biomedical Engineering, City University of Hong Kong, Kowloon, Hong Kong SAR, China

Jonathan M. Mansbach
Harvard Medical School, Boston, MA, United States
Department of Pediatrics, Boston Children's Hospital, Boston, MA, United States

Asuncion Mejias and Octavio Ramilo
Division of Pediatric Infectious Diseases, Department of Pediatrics, Center for Vaccines and Immunity, Abigail Wexner Research Institute at Nationwide Children's Hospital, The Ohio State University College of Medicine, Columbus, OH, United States

George A. O'Toole
Department of Microbiology and Immunology, Geisel School of Medicine at Dartmouth, Hanover, NH, United States

Laura Paalanen
Finnish Institute for Health and Welfare (THL), Helsinki, Finland

Marcos Pérez-Losada
Department of Biostatistics and Bioinformatics, Computational Biology Institute, Milken Institute School of Public Health, George Washington University, Washington, DC, United States
CIBIO-InBIO, Centro de Investigação em Biodiversidade e Recursos Genéticos, Universidade do Porto, Campus Agrário de Vairão, Vairão, Portugal

Melinda M. Pettigrew
Department of Epidemiology of Microbial Diseases, Yale School of Public Health, New Haven, CT, United States

Maxime Pichon
CHU Poitiers, Infectious Agents Department, Poitiers, France
University of Poitiers, INSERM U1070, Poitiers, France

Lasse Ruokolainen
Department of Biosciences, University of Helsinki, Helsinki, Finland

Olga Sakwinska
Nestlé Research, Lausanne, Switzerland

Patrick C. Seed
Department of Pediatrics, Feinberg School of Medicine, Northwestern University, Chicago, IL, United States

Christopher J. van der Gast
Department of Life Sciences, Manchester Metropolitan University, Manchester, United Kingdom

Brandie D. Wagner
Department of Biostatistics and Informatics, Colorado School of Public Health, University of Colorado, Aurora, Aurora, CO, United States

Hana Yi
School of Biosystem and Biomedical Science, Korea University, Seoul, South Korea

Yuejie Zheng
Shenzhen Children's Hospital, Shenzhen, China

Naveen Pillarisetti
Starship Children's Hospital, Auckland, New Zealand

Ling-Hui Zeng, Muhammad Qasim Barkat and Ximei Wu
Department of Pharmacology, Zhejiang University City College, Hangzhou, China

Musaddique Hussain, Nadia Akram, Imran Ahmad Khan, Sajida Parveen, Tehreem Fayyaz, Mobeen Fatima, Saira Shaukat, Najia Shabbir, Mehwish Fatima and Aisha Kanwal
Department of Pharmacology, Faculty of Pharmacy, The Islamia University of Bahawalpur, Bahawalpur, Pakistan

Shahzada Khurram Syed
Department of Basic Medical Sciences, School of Health Sciences, University of Management and Technology Lahore, Lahore, Pakistan

Malik Saadullah
Department of Pharmaceutical Chemistry, Government College University, Faisalabad, Pakistan

Qurratulain Jamil
Department of Pharmacy Practice, Faculty of Pharmacy, The Islamia University of Bahawalpur, Bahawalpur, Pakistan

Ali M. Alqahtani and Taha Alqahtani
Department of Pharmacology, College of Pharmacy, King Khalid University, Abha, Saudi Arabia

Index

www.ingramcontent.com/pod-product-compliance
Lightning Source LLC
LaVergne TN
LVHW082125200926
848484LV00008B/2006